Morris Sh...

The secondary glaucomas

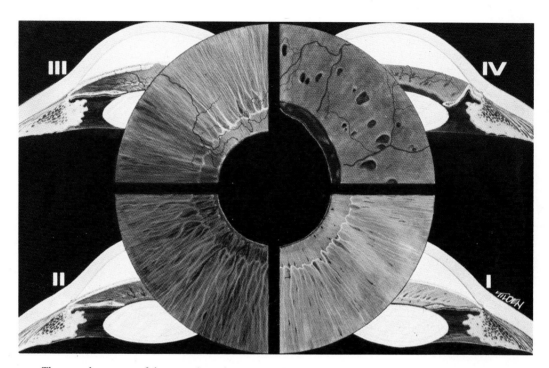

The complex nature of the secondary glaucomas is illustrated by the many phases and mechanisms of neovascular glaucoma.

I, Early rubeosis iridis. Dilated capillary tufts are present only at pupillary margin; angle is not involved. **II,** Moderate rubeosis iridis. New vessels extend radially toward angle, sometimes joining a dilated vessel at collarette; angle is still not involved. **III,** Advanced rubeosis iridis with angle neovascularization. New vessels reach angle and join circumferential ciliary body artery; new vessels come off this artery and cross over scleral spur onto trabecular meshwork, where arborization occurs. One area of synechial closure is shown. Pressure can increase at this stage. **IV,** More advanced neovascular glaucoma. Angle is completely closed; iris is pulled up over whole trabecular meshwork and hides all angle structures posterior to Schwalbe's line; pupil shows ectropion and distortion. A "burned-out" stage can occur later; then there may appear to be little rubeosis iridis, and only an occasional vessel may be seen approaching a completely closed angle. (From Wand, M., Dueker, D.K., Aiello, L.M., and Grant, W.M. Published with permission from the American Journal of Ophthalmology **86:**332-339, 1978. Copyright by the Ophthalmic Publishing Co.)

The secondary glaucomas

Edited by

ROBERT RITCH, M.D.

Associate Professor of Ophthalmology, Department of Ophthalmology,
Mount Sinai School of Medicine, New York, New York; Director,
Department of Ophthalmology, City Hospital Center at Elmhurst,
Queens, New York

M. BRUCE SHIELDS, M.D.

Associate Professor of Ophthalmology, Department of Ophthalmology,
Duke University Medical Center, Durham, North Carolina

*with **298** illustrations*

The C. V. Mosby Company

ST. LOUIS • TORONTO • LONDON   1982

MOSBY

A TRADITION OF PUBLISHING EXCELLENCE

Editor: Eugenia A. Klein
Assistant editor: Kathryn H. Falk
Manuscript editor: Judith Bange
Book design: Susan Trail
Production: Carol O'Leary, Mary Stueck, Carolyn Biby

Printed in the United States of America

The C.V. Mosby Company
11830 Westline Industrial Drive, St. Louis, Missouri 63141

Library of Congress Cataloging in Publication Data

Main entry under title:

The secondary glaucomas.

    Bibliography: p.
    Includes index.
    1. Glaucoma. 2. Glaucoma—Etiology. I. Ritch,
Robert. II. Shields, M. Bruce. [DNLM: 1. Glaucoma.
WW 290 S445]
RE871.S4   617.7'41   81-18686
ISBN 0-8016-4195-0   AACR2

GW/CB/B 9 8 7 6 5 4 3 2 1   02/A/268

CONTRIBUTORS

WILLIAM E. BRUNER, M.D.

Assistant Professor of Ophthalmology, Division of Ophthalmology, Case Western Reserve University; Chief, Ophthalmology Section, Cleveland Veterans Administration Medical Center, Cleveland, Ohio

DAVID G. CAMPBELL, M.D.

Associate Professor of Ophthalmology and Director of Glaucoma Service, Department of Ophthalmology, Emory University School of Medicine, Atlanta, Georgia

MICHAEL COBO, M.D.

Assistant Professor of Ophthalmology, Department of Ophthalmology, Duke University Medical Center, Durham, North Carolina

DAVID L. EPSTEIN, M.D.

Associate Professor of Ophthalmology, Department of Ophthalmology, Massachusetts Eye and Ear Infirmary, Harvard Medical School, Boston, Massachusetts

ALAN H. FRIEDMAN, M.D.

Clinical professor of Ophthalmology and Attending Ophthalmologist, Department of Ophthalmology, and Attending Ophthalmic Pathologist, Department of Pathology, Mount Sinai School of Medicine, New York, New York

JONATHAN HERSCHLER, M.D.

Associate Professor of Surgery (Ophthalmology) and Chief, Section of Ophthalmology, University of Arizona Health Sciences Center, Tucson, Arizona

ELIZABETH A. HODAPP, M.D.

Assistant Professor of Ophthalmology, Department of Ophthalmology, University of Miami School of Medicine, Miami, Florida

MICHAEL A. KASS, M.D.

Associate Professor of Ophthalmology, Department of Ophthalmology, Washington University School of Medicine, St. Louis, Missouri

THEODORE KRUPIN, M.D.

Associate Professor of Ophthalmology, Department of Ophthalmology, Washington University School of Medicine, St. Louis, Missouri

MARVIN L. KWITKO, M.D.

Senior Attending Ophthalmologist, Department of Ophthalmology, St. Mary's Hospital, Montreal, Quebec, Canada

WILLIAM E. LAYDEN, M.D.

Professor of Ophthalmology and Chairman, Department of Ophthalmology, University of South Florida, Tampa, Florida

ROBERT M. MANDELKORN, M.D.

Clinical Instructor in Ophthalmology, Eye and Ear Hospital, University of Pittsburgh; Consultant, St. Francis General Hospital, Pittsburgh, Pennsylvania

CHARLES D. PHELPS, M.D.

Professor of Ophthalmology, Department of Ophthalmology, University of Iowa Hospitals and Clinics, Iowa City, Iowa

MORRIS M. PODOLSKY, M.D.

Clinical Instructor and Attending Ophthalmologist, Department of Ophthalmology, Mount Sinai School of Medicine; Adjunct Surgeon in Ophthalmology, New York Eye and Ear Infirmary, New York, New York

STEVEN M. PODOS, M.D.

Professor of Ophthalmology and Chairman, Department of Ophthalmology, Mount Sinai School of Medicine, New York, New York

THOMAS M. RICHARDSON, M.D.

Clinical Instructor in Ophthalmology, Department of Ophthalmology, Harvard University Medical School, Boston, Massachusetts

ROBERT RITCH, M.D.

Associate Professor of Ophthalmology, Department of Ophthalmology, Mount Sinai School of Medicine, New York, New York; Director, Department of Ophthalmology, City Hospital Center at Elmhurst, Queens, New York

M. BRUCE SHIELDS, M.D.

Associate Professor of Ophthalmology, Department of Ophthalmology, Duke University Medical Center, Durham, North Carolina

RICHARD J. SIMMONS, M.D.

Associate Clinical Professor of Ophthalmology, Department of Ophthalmology, and Surgeon, Massachusetts Eye and Ear Infirmary, Harvard University Medical School, Boston, Massachusetts

WALTER J. STARK, M.D.

Associate Professor of Ophthalmology, The Wilmer Institute, The Johns Hopkins University School of Medicine, Baltimore, Maryland

RICHARD A. STONE, M.D.

Assistant Professor of Ophthalmology, Department of Ophthalmology, University of Pennsylvania School of Medicine; Co-director, Glaucoma Service, Scheie Eye Institute, Philadelphia, Pennsylvania

ALAN SUGAR, M.D.

Associate Professor of Ophthalmology, Department of Ophthalmology, University of Michigan, Ann Arbor, Michigan

JOHN V. THOMAS, M.D.

Clinical Assistant in Ophthalmology, Massachusetts Eye and Ear Infirmary, Harvard University Medical School, Boston, Massachusetts

DAVID S. WALTON, M.D.

Assistant Professor of Ophthalmology, Department of Ophthalmology, Harvard University Medical School, Boston, Massachusetts

MARTIN WAND, M.D.

Research Associate, Joslin Clinic, Boston, Massachusetts; Assistant Clinical Professor of Ophthalmology, Department of Ophthalmology, University of Connecticut Medical School, Farmingham, Connecticut

PETER G. WATSON, M.A., M.B., B.Chir., F.R.C.S., D.O.

Consultant Ophthalmic Surgeon, Addenbrooke's Hospital; Associate Lecturer, University of Cambridge, Cambridge, England; Hon. Consultant Ophthalmic Surgeon, Moorfield's Eye Hospital, London, England

JAYNE S. WEISS, M.D.

Resident, Department of Ophthalmology, Bascom Palmer Eye Institute, University of Miami School of Medicine, Miami, Florida

MICHAEL E. YABLONSKI, M.D., Ph.D.

Associate Professor of Ophthalmology, Department of Ophthalmology, Mount Sinai School of Medicine, New York, New York

THOM J. ZIMMERMAN, M.D., Ph.D.

Chairman, Department of Ophthalmology, Ochsner Clinic; Professor of Ophthalmology, Pharmacology, and Experimental Therapeutics, Louisiana State University Medical Center, New Orleans, Louisiana

To
our parents

PREFACE

The secondary glaucomas are a multiplicity of disorders related by the common denominator of elevated intraocular pressure with a recognizable origin. Some of these conditions, such as the exfoliation syndrome or neovascular glaucoma, are relatively common and account for a significant proportion of the total glaucoma population. Other forms of secondary glaucoma are uncommon but need to be recognized in order to be treated properly. Therapeutic modalities may differ, and what is indicated in one disorder may be contraindicated in another. A missed diagnosis or the wrong treatment may lead to further complications to the patient and irreparable loss of vision.

In this volume we have tried to bring together much diverse information and to provide an approach to the pathogenesis, diagnosis, and management of the secondary glaucomas. We have attempted to organize each chapter within conceptual frameworks that would aid both in establishing the differential diagnosis and in determining choices of therapy. Many interpretations of pathophysiologic processes and their preferred methods of treatment are, and perhaps always will be, more or less controversial. The contributors have been actively involved in advancing our understanding of these forms of glaucoma and have tried to achieve a thorough coverage of each subject. Where differences of opinion exist, we have tried to create a balanced presentation without confining the contributors to our own viewpoints.

We wish to express our appreciation to the contributors and to thank them for making this book possible. We are greatly indebted to colleagues too numerous to mention for their generous and constructive criticism and would like to thank, on behalf of the individual contributors, all those who have assisted with manuscripts or participated in reading them critically. In particular, we would like to thank the two people who served as our mentors—Drs. Steven M. Podos and W. Morton Grant.

Robert Ritch
M. Bruce Shields

CONTENTS

Section I

INTRODUCTION

Chapter 1

CLASSIFICATIONS AND MECHANISMS

M. Bruce Shields and Robert Ritch

For the purpose of discussion in this book, *glaucoma* is defined as any condition leading to a rise in intraocular pressure with or without associated damage to the optic nerve head or visual field. The distinction that is often made between ocular hypertension and glaucoma when one is dealing with primary open-angle glaucoma is not always applicable to the secondary glaucomas. We have no doubt that some patients with a secondary elevation of intraocular pressure are more resistant to glaucomatous optic atrophy than other individuals. However, it is difficult to apply general concepts to all of the secondary glaucomas because of the wide variation in etiologic factors, treatments, and prognoses. In some cases, such as the pigment dispersion syndrome, the criteria for deciding whether to institute treatment may be quite similar to those in primary open-angle glaucoma. On the other hand, with different conditions, such as neovascular glaucoma, the decision to treat or not treat rests less with the state of the optic nerve head and more with the progression of the underlying condition. Therefore all cases of elevated intraocular pressure are referred to in this text as glaucoma, and any distinctions or exceptions are discussed in the respective chapters.

CLASSIFICATIONS

It is convenient to first consider all the glaucomas in two arbitrary divisions: primary and secondary. The primary glaucomas are those that appear to be genetically influenced and are not consistently associated with other ocular or systemic diseases. These include primary open-angle glaucoma, primary angle-closure glaucoma, and primary congenital glaucoma. The secondary glaucomas include all other forms of glaucoma and are the subject of this text. These are glaucomas that can be traced a step back on the etiologic ladder and that would not occur as distinct entities were it not for an underlying predisposing disorder.

The list of secondary glaucomas is long and complex, and no attempt to classify these disorders is completely satisfactory. There is a certain value in considering more than one system of classification, since each offers different disadvantages. In this text the secondary glaucomas have been grouped according to cause. However, it is also helpful to consider these conditions on the basis of anatomic mechanisms, a discussion of which is included in this chapter.

Etiologic classification

The etiologic classification of secondary glaucomas is based on the underlying etiologic factor that ultimately leads to the elevated intraocular pressure. This approach is limited by the fact that the primary etiologic factor is not completely understood in many forms of secondary glaucoma. However, it has the advantage of allowing discussion of a secondary glaucoma under a single heading, unlike systems based on clinical presentations or mechanisms. For example, neovascular glaucoma might be discussed with conditions that give a clinical presentation of rubeosis iridis, hemorrhage, peripheral anterior synechiae, or signs of inflammation, or with those in which the mechanism of aqueous outflow obstruction is either open angle or angle closure, depending on the stage of the disease.

The etiologic classification enables the clinician to think in terms of the underlying disorder and to institute treatment on that basis. Entities that are quite disparate in their manifestations may be grouped together under broader categories, which allows one to think of the underlying disorders as having a common denominator. Such a category is the lens-induced glaucomas, which include such varied entities as phacolytic glaucoma and anterior dislocation of the lens. Although the mechanisms of glaucoma within this group of conditions include both open- and closed-angle forms, treatment may be directed at the lens rather than the secondary manifestation of the glaucoma itself.

Mechanistic classification

The mechanism of intraocular pressure elevation in virtually every form of secondary glaucoma is the obstruction of aqueous outflow. Understanding the precise mechanism that leads to this obstruction provides a helpful framework on which to develop an understanding of the pathophysiology and rationale for therapy for the secondary glaucomas.

Classifying the secondary glaucomas according to the anatomic location of the aqueous outflow obstruction is helpful not only in considering the differential diagnosis, but also in determining the mechanism underlying the intraocular pressure elevation. The tabulation suggested in this chapter represents a systematic arrangement of the various mechanisms of secondary glaucoma. Particularly in the diseases that can cause glaucoma by a number of different mechanisms, it enables one to consider systematically each of the areas of blockage of outflow, to avoid missing a mechanism in cases where more than one may be present and to assist in determining the best treatment.

MECHANISMS

The following outline presents one approach to the mechanistic classification of the secondary glaucomas. In this system all of the secondary glaucomas are arbitrarily divided into two categories on the basis of gonioscopic appearance: open angle and angle closure.

Mechanistic classification*

I. Secondary open-angle glaucomas
  A. Pretrabecular (membrane overgrowth)

---

*Clinical examples cited do not represent an inclusive list of the secondary glaucomas.

    1. Fibrovascular membrane (neovascular glaucoma)
    2. Descemet-like membrane with endothelial layer
      a. Iridocorneal endothelial syndrome
      b. Posterior polymorphous dystrophy
      c. Penetrating and nonpenetrating trauma
    3. Epithelial downgrowth
    4. Fibrous ingrowth
    5. Inflammatory membrane
      a. Fuchs' heterochromic iridocyclitis
      b. Luetic interstitial keratitis
  B. Trabecular
    1. "Clogging" of the meshwork
      a. Red blood cells
        (1) Hemorrhagic glaucoma
        (2) Ghost cell glaucoma
      b. Macrophages
        (1) Hemolytic glaucoma
        (2) Phacolytic glaucoma
        (3) Melanomalytic glaucoma
      c. Neoplastic cells
        (1) Malignant tumors
        (2) Neurofibromatosis
        (3) Nevus of Ota
        (4) Juvenile xanthogranuloma
      d. Pigment particles
        (1) Pigmentary glaucoma
        (2) Glaucoma capsulare
        (3) Uveitis
        (4) Malignant melanoma
      e. Protein
        (1) Uveitis
        (2) Lens-induced glaucoma
      f. Alpha-chymotrypsin–induced glaucoma
      g. Vitreous in anterior chamber
    2. Alterations of the trabecular meshwork
      a. Edema
        (1) Uveitis
        (2) Scleritis and episcleritis
        (3) Alkali burns
      b. Trauma (angle recession)
      c. Intraocular foreign bodies (hemosiderosis, chalcosis)
      d. Steroid-induced glaucoma
  C. Posttrabecular (elevated episcleral venous pressure)
    1. Carotid-cavernous fistula
    2. Cavernous sinus thrombosis
    3. Retrobulbar tumors
    4. Thyrotropic exophthalmos
    5. Superior vena cava obstruction
    6. Mediastinal tumors
    7. Sturge-Weber syndrome
    8. Familial episcleral venous pressure elevation
II. Secondary angle-closure glaucomas
  A. Anterior ("pulling" mechanism)

1. Contracture of membranes
    a. Neovascular glaucoma
    b. Iridocorneal endothelial syndrome
    c. Posterior polymorphous dystrophy
    d. Penetrating and nonpenetrating trauma
2. Contracture of inflammatory precipitates
3. Aniridia
B. Posterior ("pushing" mechanism)
    1. With pupillary block
        a. Intumescent lens
        b. Subluxation of lens
            (1) Traumatic
            (2) Spontaneous
        c. Following lens extraction
            (1) Iris-vitreous block
            (2) Pseudophakia
        d. Iris bombé associated with intraocular inflammation
    2. Without pupillary block
        a. Ciliary block (malignant) glaucoma
        b. Following lens extraction (forward vitreous shift)
        c. Following scleral buckling
        d. Following panretinal photocoagulation
        e. Central retinal vein occlusion
        f. Intraocular tumors
            (1) Malignant melanoma
            (2) Retinoblastoma
        g. Cysts of the iris and ciliary body
        h. Retrolenticular tissue contracture
            (1) Retrolental fibroplasia
            (2) Persistent hyperplastic primary vitreous
C. Congenital
    1. Rieger's syndrome
    2. Axenfeld's anomaly

Secondary open-angle glaucomas

The secondary open-angle glaucomas are those in which the anterior chamber angle structures (i.e., trabecular meshwork, scleral spur, and ciliary band) are visible by gonioscopy. However, this does not necessarily imply that the angle is free of obstructive elements. In the pretrabecular form, a translucent membrane extends across the open angle, leading to the obstruction of aqueous outflow (Fig. 1-1, *A*). In various cases this may be a fibrovascular membrane, an endothelial layer with a Descemet-like membrane, an epithelial membrane, a connective tissue membrane, or a membrane secondary to inflammation.

In the trabecular form of secondary open-angle glaucomas, the obstruction to aqueous outflow is located within the trabecular meshwork (Fig. 1-1, *B*). This may be due to a "clogging" of the meshwork with red blood cells, macrophages, neoplastic cells, pigment particles, protein, lens zonules, or vitreous. In other cases the trabecular obstruction may result from alterations of the trabecular meshwork tissue, such as edema associated with inflammatory conditions, trauma with subsequent scarring, and toxic reactions associated with intraocular foreign bodies. A few conditions, such as steroid-induced glaucoma and certain glaucomas associated with systemic disease, are not well understood but are believed to have obstruction to aqueous outflow in the trabecular meshwork or Schlemm's canal.

A third group of secondary open-angle glaucomas have a mechanism referred to as the posttrabecular form, in which obstruction to aqueous outflow results from increased resistance distal to the meshwork and Schlemm's canal due to elevated episcleral venous pressure (Fig. 1-1, *C*). Conditions in this category include carotid-cavernous fistula, cavernous sinus thrombosis, retrobulbar tumors, thyrotropic exophthalmos, superior vena cava obstruction, mediastinal tumors, Sturge-Weber syndrome, and familial forms of elevated episcleral venous pressure.

Secondary angle-closure glaucomas

The secondary angle-closure glaucomas include those conditions in which the peripheral iris is in apposition to the trabecular meshwork or peripheral cornea. The peripheral iris may be either "pulled" (anterior form) or "pushed" (posterior form) into this position, or, in a few rare cases, the apposition may be the result of a congenital anomaly.

In the anterior form of the secondary angle-closure glaucomas, an abnormal tissue bridges the anterior chamber angle and subsequently undergoes contraction, pulling the peripheral iris into the angle (Fig. 1-1, *D*). The contracting tissue may be a fibrovascular membrane, an endothelial layer with a Descemet-like membrane, inflammatory precipitates, or congenital fibrous bands.

In the posterior form, pressure behind the iris or lens causes the peripheral iris to be pushed into the anterior chamber angle. This may occur with or without pupillary block. In the pupillary block form, there is an apposition between the pupillary portion of the iris and the lens or vitreous (Fig. 1-1, *E*). This apposition obstructs the flow of aqueous into the anterior chamber, resulting in increased pressure in the posterior chamber and caus-

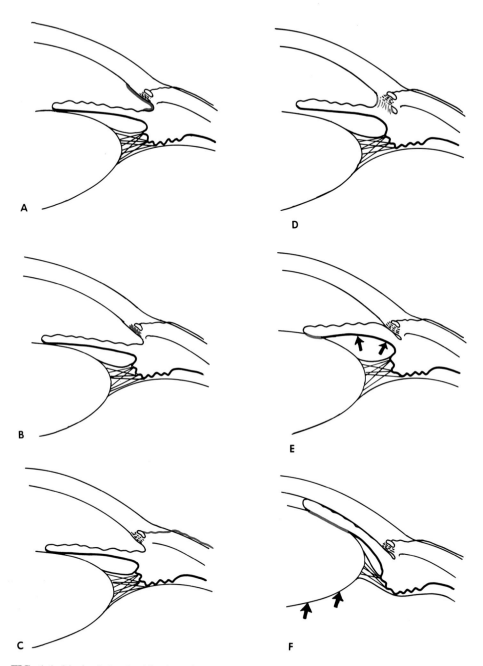

FIG. 1-1. Mechanistic classification of secondary glaucomas. **A,** Pretrabecular form of secondary open-angle glaucoma. **B,** Trabecular form of secondary open-angle glaucoma. **C,** Posttrabecular form of secondary open-angle glaucoma. **D,** Anterior form of secondary angle-closure glaucoma. **E,** Posterior form of secondary angle-closure glaucoma with pupillary block. **F,** Posterior form of secondary angle-closure glaucoma without pupillary block.

ing the peripheral iris to be forced into the anterior chamber angle. The apposition may be functional secondary to a forward shift of the lens or vitreous or following intraocular lens implantation, or it may be synechial apposition, associated with intraocular inflammation.

In the posterior forms of secondary angle-closure glaucoma without pupillary block, increased pressure in the posterior portion of the eye pushes the lens-iris diaphragm or vitreous-iris diaphragm forward (Fig. 1-1, *F*). This may result from alterations in the intraocular tissues following surgery, central retinal vein occlusion, intraocular tumors, cysts of the iris and ciliary body, or contracture of retrolenticular tissue.

In a third form of secondary angle-closure glaucoma, the apposition of the peripheral iris to the trabecular meshwork and peripheral cornea results from a congenital anomaly of the tissue in the anterior chamber angle. These conditions have been grouped under the term mesodermal dysgeneses, and the most significant forms include Rieger's syndrome and Axenfeld's anomaly.

GLAUCOMAS ASSOCIATED WITH DEVELOPMENTAL DISORDERS

Chapter 2

MESODERMAL DYSGENESES OF THE ANTERIOR OCULAR SEGMENT

M. Bruce Shields

HISTORICAL BACKGROUND

Near the turn of the century, reports of congenital abnormalities involving the anterior ocular segment began to appear in the ophthalmic literature. The earliest of these papers dealt primarily with central defects of the cornea and iris. In 1897 von Hippel[40] reported a case with bilateral central opacities of the posterior cornea, adhesions between the corneal defect and the iris, and buphthalmos. He believed that this resulted from intrauterine inflammation and called it an internal corneal ulcer. Peters[27] (1906) described similar cases but suggested a developmental cause, and this central defect of the anterior ocular segment became generally known as Peters' anomaly.

In 1920 Axenfeld[3] reported an abnormality of the peripheral cornea and iris in which a white line, parallel to the limbus at the level of Descemet's membrane, was attached to the iris by delicate fibers. He called this abnormality posterior corneal embryotoxon. Rieger[30] (1935) described similar cases in a family that had the additional features of stromal hypoplasia of the iris, pupillary abnormalities, and dental anomalies. These two conditions, which became known as Axenfeld's anomaly and Rieger's syndrome, respectively, may both be associated with glaucoma and are now recognized as variations within a spectrum of mesodermal abnormalities of the peripheral anterior ocular segment.[1] In addition, rare cases have been reported in which the central features of Peters' anomaly and the peripheral findings of Rieger's syndrome coexist in the same eye.[1,29]

EMBRYOLOGY

The central, peripheral, and combined anomalies discussed in this chapter are believed to result from a primary or secondary mesodermal dysgenesis of the anterior ocular segment. The following is a brief review of the normal development of the related structures.

The lens vesicle begins to develop as an invagination of surface ectoderm during the third week of gestation and separates from the latter structure by the sixth week. By this time the margin of the optic cup (neural ectoderm) has reached the lens equator, and a mass of undifferentiated tissue lies just anterior to it. This tissue has traditionally been considered to be mesoderm, although more recent evidence suggests that it is of neural crest origin.[23] Neural crest cells also contribute to the development of bones, including those of the face, as well as dental papillae, cartilage, and meninges, which may explain the association of developmental glaucomas with malformation of these structures.[23] For this reason, a term other than mesodermal might be more appropriate for developmental defects involving these tissues. Nevertheless, the conventional terms are retained for the purpose of discussion in this chapter.

From the undifferentiated cell mass, three waves of tissue come forward between the surface ectoderm and the lens during the seventh and eighth weeks (listed in order of appearance): (1) corneal endothelium, which later secretes Descemet's membrane; (2) corneal stroma; and (3) stroma of the iris, which is vascularized by the anterior tunica vasculosa lentis (called pupillary membrane after the anterior chamber develops). It is important to note that the corneal endothelium and the stroma of the iris, although practically in contact initially, develop from separate waves of tissue, rather than by the splitting of a common layer.

The same mass of cells that gives rise to the aforementioned layers is also involved in the formation of the anterior chamber angle. Although differentiation of this portion of the tissue begins in the seventh or eighth week, the angle is not completely formed until just before birth. It is not certain whether the changes leading to this development represent atrophy,[25] cleavage,[2] or rarefaction[34] of the cellular mass, but it is significant that development of the central anterior ocular segment is separated by several months from that of the peripheral anterior segment.

CLASSIFICATION

Reese and Ellsworth[29] suggested lumping all the central and peripheral mesodermal anomalies of the anterior ocular segment under the term anterior chamber cleavage syndrome. Other investigators have objected to this classification,[1,10,37] primarily because the central and peripheral defects rarely occur in the same eye, as might be anticipated from the different times at which the related embryologic structures develop. Furthermore, the

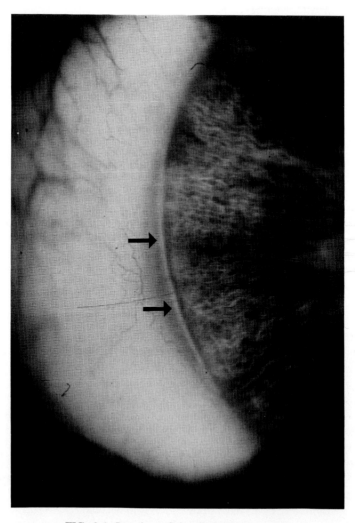

FIG. 2-1. Prominent Schwalbe's ring *(arrows)*.

term cleavage does not accurately describe all the developmental processes that are involved. Alkemade[1] suggested the terms primary dysgenesis mesodermalis of the iris and dysgenesis mesodermalis of the cornea for the pure peripheral and central defects, respectively, and secondary dysgenesis mesodermalis of the iris for combined cases of Rieger's syndrome and Peters' anomaly. Waring et al.[42] used the term anterior chamber cleavage syndrome in their stepladder classification of mesodermal defects of the anterior ocular segment but also pointed out that the anomalies should be subdivided into peripheral, central, and combined forms. A similar three-part classification is used in this chapter: (1) peripheral (prominent Schwalbe's ring, Axenfeld's anomaly, Rieger's syndrome, and other peripheral mesodermal defects of the anterior ocular segment); (2) central (posterior keratoconus, Peters' anomaly, and congenital corneal leukomas and staphylomas); and (3) combined Rieger's syndrome and Peters' anomaly. It should be noted, however, that even within these arbitrary subgroups there may be more than one basic pathogenic mechanism to explain the various clinical entities.

Peripheral mesodermal dysgeneses of the anterior ocular segment
Prominent Schwalbe's ring

During the course of a routine slit-lamp examination, it is not uncommon to observe a thin white line parallel to the limbus at the level of Descemet's membrane in the peripheral cornea (Fig. 2-1). This clinical finding is often referred to by Axenfeld's term, posterior embryotoxon,[3] and its frequency has been variably estimated at 8%[1] and 15%.[5] Burian et al.[5] reported that the white line represents a prominent anterior border ring of Schwalbe (Fig. 2-2). In the vast majority of cases this is an isolated finding in healthy eyes and is considered to be a variant of the normal anatomy.[1] In these cases there is no association with glaucoma, and the only additional gonioscopic finding is occasional hypoplasia of the root of the iris.[1]

The prominent Schwalbe's ring, however, is also associated with many, but not all, cases of mesodermal dysgenesis of the peripheral anterior ocular segment. The finding of a prominent Schwalbe's ring during slit-lamp examination, therefore, should be followed by a gonioscopic

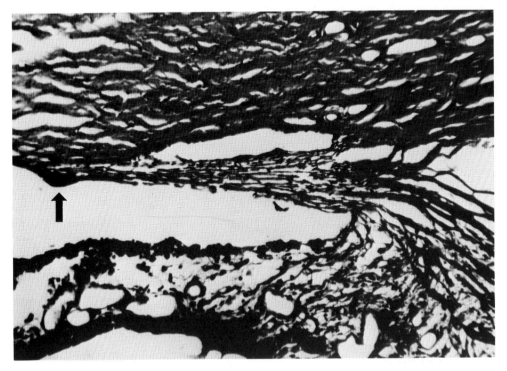

FIG. 2-2. Light microscopic view of prominent Schwalbe's ring *(arrow).* (Masson's trichrome; ×100.)

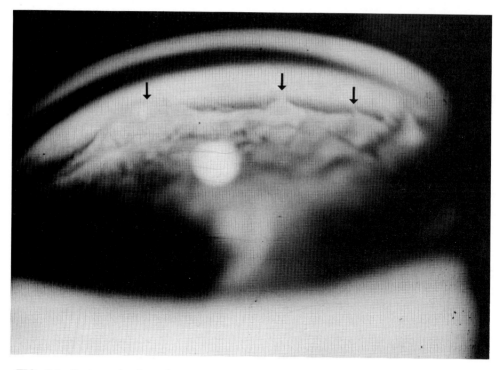

FIG. 2-3. Gonioscopic view of eye with Axenfeld's anomaly showing both delicate and broad strands of iris *(arrows)* traversing anterior chamber angle to prominent Schwalbe's ring.

examination to rule out the possibility of a developmental abnormality of the anterior chamber angle.

Axenfeld's anomaly

The hallmark of Axenfeld's anomaly is strands of iris traversing the anterior chamber angle from the peripheral iris to the prominent Schwalbe's ring (Fig. 2-3). Although the iris is usually otherwise normal in this condition, Axenfeld[3] noted a subtle defect in the iris in his original case study, which makes it difficult to draw a clear distinction between the disorders described by Axenfeld[3] and Rieger.[30] The two conditions most likely represent variations in a spectrum of disease, of which the former anomaly is the milder variant. For this reason, the two disorders are discussed together under the arbitrary heading of Rieger's syndrome.

Rieger's syndrome

As noted above, the term Axenfeld's anomaly is traditionally employed in cases where strands of iris traverse the anterior chamber angle from the peripheral iris to a prominent Schwalbe's ring with minimal or no additional iris defects. The term

Rieger's anomaly is generally reserved for cases in which the aforementioned anterior chamber angle abnormality is associated with hypoplasia of the iris and abnormalities of the pupil. When the latter ocular abnormalities are associated with characteristic facial and dental anomalies, the condition is usually referred to as Rieger's syndrome.

CLINICAL FEATURES. This spectrum of disease is typically bilateral and afflicts both blacks and whites, with an even distribution among males and females.[1] The majority of cases are familial with autosomal dominant transmission and 95% penetrance, but there is considerable variation in expressivity.[1,42]

The characteristic gonioscopic finding throughout this spectrum of disease is the previously described strands that extend from the peripheral iris, across the anterior chamber angle, to a prominent Schwalbe's ring. These strands of iris may be few and delicate or numerous and broad. In rare cases they may extend from the collarette or pupillary margin to the prominent Schwalbe's ring.[42]

In more involved cases the anterior chamber angle anomaly is associated with variable degrees of hypoplasia of the iris. This is limited to the

Post embry. → At Anom → Riegers anomly → At synd
(iris → (At + Pup + iris stroml d's)
strela)
Mesodermal dysgeneses of the anterior ocular segment   **15**

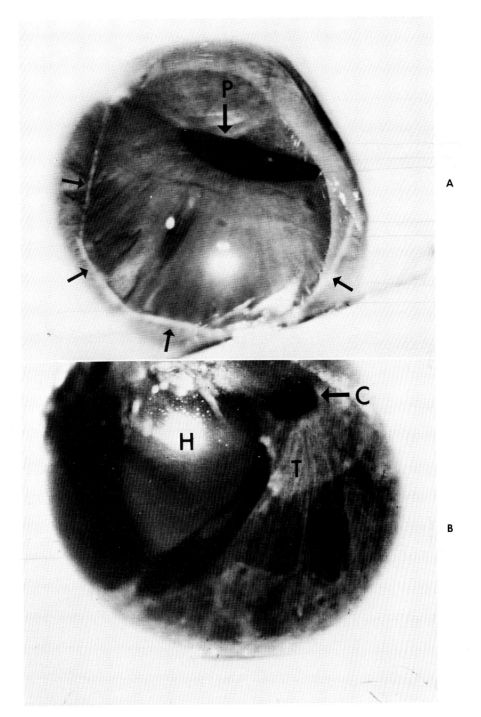

FIG. 2-4. Rieger's anomaly. **A,** Prominent, anteriorly displaced Schwalbe's ring *(arrows)* with ectopic, distorted pupil *(P)*. **B,** Different patient with more advanced changes of iris: corectopia *(C)*, thinning of stroma *(T)*, and large hole *(H)*.

anterior layers of the stroma in most cases, but some eyes may have extensive stromal hypoplasia with associated epithelial defects and holes in the iris. The defects of the iris are frequently associated with abnormalities of the pupil, including dyscoria, corectopia, and ectropion uveae (Fig. 2-4).

The cornea is characteristically clear although frequently enlarged. In his extensive study and review, Alkemade[1] reported that 26% of the eyes

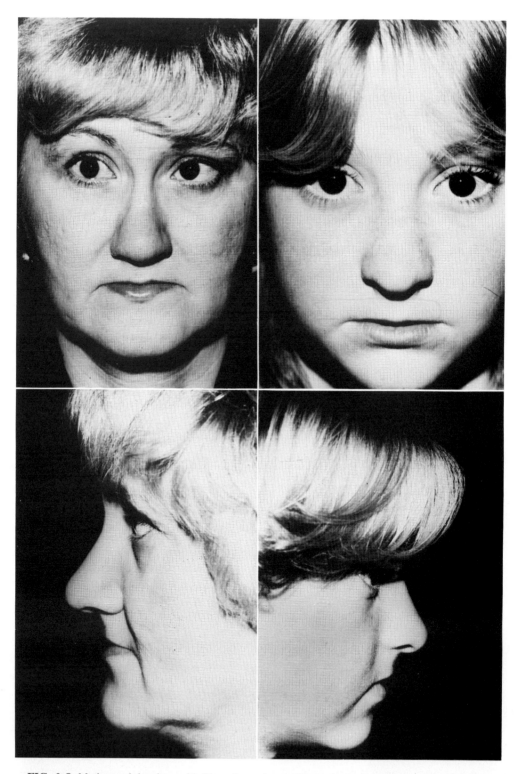

FIG. 2-5. Mother and daughter with Rieger's syndrome demonstrating variable degrees of characteristic facial configuration: broad flat nasal bridge, hypertelorism, flattening of midface, and protruding lower lip.

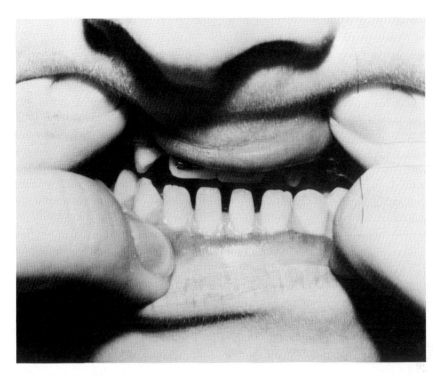

FIG. 2-6. Patient with Rieger's syndrome demonstrating typical dental anomalies of hypodontia (decreased number of teeth) and microdontia (reduction in crown size of teeth).

with Rieger's syndrome had macrocornea, which was usually not associated with congenital glaucoma. In the same study, microcornea was observed in 9% of the eyes, the cornea had an abnormal shape (usually a vertical oval) in 8%, and there was a poorly defined limbus in 75%. The corneal endothelium appeared normal by specular microscopy in a mother and daughter with Rieger's syndrome.[18] Central corneal opacities are rarely observed in Rieger's syndrome (see "Combined Rieger's Syndrome and Peters' Anomaly").

The typical facial configuration in Rieger's syndrome includes a broad flat nasal bridge, frequent telecanthus (wide interorbital distance), occasional hypertelorism (wide intercanthal distance), flattening of the midface due to maxillary hypoplasia, and occasional protruding of the lower lip[1] (Fig. 2-5). Dental anomalies are common in this syndrome and usually consist of hypodontia (decreased number of teeth) and microdontia (reduction in crown size of teeth)[1,10,11] (Fig. 2-6). Other reported abnormalities include hypospadias and redundant periumbilical skin.[10,22]

Glaucoma occurs in approximately half of the patients.[1,17,42] It usually develops during infancy or childhood, although cases occasionally appear in early adulthood, and congenital cases with buphthalmos have also been reported.[42] The presence of glaucoma does not consistently correlate with the extent of the iris strands in the anterior chamber angle.[1]

Alkemade[1] reported that Rieger's syndrome is characteristically a stationary affection unless the intraocular pressure is elevated. Cross and Maumenee,[11] on the other hand, cited six affected individuals with progressive iris dissolution. Two patients,[14,22] including one of Rieger's original patients,[14] have been followed for many years and have shown continuing dissolution of the iris.

HISTOPATHOLOGIC FEATURES. Histopathologic reports of eyes with Rieger's syndrome are scant and do not fully explain all the clinical findings. The most consistent observation is a prominent, anteriorly displaced Schwalbe's ring, connected to the peripheral iris by varying amounts of adhesions. The prominent Schwalbe's ring consists of a core of densely arranged collagen covered by a basement membrane and a single layer of endothelium.[42] In one study, the trabecular meshwork was described as patent but deeply recessed and shallow[36]; others have reported extensive dysplasia of the meshwork[44] and an abnormal[12] or absent[1,44] Schlemm's canal. The stroma of the iris is characteristically hypoplastic,[1,44] especially in the peripheral region, and ectropion uveae may be present.[12,44] Inflammatory cells have been noted in the iris,[1,36] and posterior synechiae have been described.[12]

In several cases a thin layer of tissue has been observed on the anterior surface of the iris, which has been variably described as a delicate membrane, extending from the prominent Schwalbe's ring to the pupillary region[12]; a thin layer of connective tissue[21]; or a proliferation of endothelium with a glass membrane.[39]

MECHANISM OF GLAUCOMA. Alkemade[21] noted that the presence of glaucoma does not always correlate with the extent of gonioscopically visible adhesions in the anterior chamber angle. This led him to suggest that the mechanism of obstruction to aqueous outflow might be defective development of the trabecular meshwork and Schlemm's canal, rather than the adhesions. This theory is supported by the previously noted observations that Schlemm's canal may be abnormal[12] or absent[1,44] and the trabecular meshwork may be defective[44] in some cases. Sugar,[36] on the other hand, noted that the extent of adhesions between the prominent Schwalbe's ring and the peripheral iris correlated with the relative severity of the glaucoma between the two eyes of a child with Axenfeld's anomaly. It may be that more than one mechanism accounts for the glaucoma in this spectrum of disease.

DIFFERENTIAL DIAGNOSIS. The condition that most closely resembles the clinical features of Rieger's syndrome is the iridocorneal endothelial syndrome, which is discussed in Chapter 6. Not only are these two spectra of disease similar in clinical appearance, but they also share the common histopathologic feature of a membrane on the surface of the iris.[6] The latter observation has led some investigators to suggest that Rieger's syndrome and the iridocorneal endothelial syndrome belong to the same broad spectrum of disease.[26,39] However, since many ocular disorders of varied cause are associated with endothelialization of the anterior segment, this finding does not prove that there is a common fundamental defect. Further-

more, clinical and histopathologic features clearly differentiate Rieger's syndrome and the iridocorneal endothelial syndrome. The latter spectrum of disease usually appears in early to middle adulthood, is most often unilateral, and rarely has a positive family history.[33] In addition, the iridocorneal endothelial syndrome appears to have a primary abnormality of the corneal endothelium that may lead to corneal edema,[6] whereas the cornea, as previously noted, is usually normal in Rieger's syndrome except for variation in size and shape.

Posterior polymorphous dystrophy may occasionally have anterior chamber angle and iris changes similar to those seen in Rieger's syndrome.[7] However, this is usually first noted in later childhood or early adulthood and is characterized by the clinical appearance of blisters and vesicles on the posterior cornea with occasional corneal edema.

Congenital iris hypoplasia has been reported in patients with no other characteristics suggestive of Rieger's syndrome.[31] Oculodentodigital dysplasia may occasionally be confused with Rieger's syndrome because of the similar dental abnormalities and the occasional presence of mild iris stromal hypoplasia.[1] Abnormalities of the anterior chamber angle are not characteristic of this syndrome but may occur, along with secondary glaucoma.[21] Aniridia might be confused with Rieger's syndrome because of the abnormal iris and occasional strands in the anterior chamber angle, although it is usually easily distinguished by the rudimentary iris and occasional corneal and lenticular abnormalities. The corectopia in ectopia lentis et pupillae, an autosomal recessive disorder limited to bilateral displacement of the lens and iris,[9] may also resemble changes of the iris in Rieger's syndrome. Iridoschisis is characterized by separation and dissolution of the stromal layers of the iris and is most often seen in elderly individuals. Other peripheral mesodermal dysgeneses of the anterior ocular segment, as discussed later in this chapter, should also be considered in the differential diagnosis.

MANAGEMENT. The primary concern in managing patients with Rieger's syndrome and other mesodermal dysgeneses of the peripheral anterior segment is the potential for glaucoma. As previously noted, the glaucoma may develop at any age, requiring close observation of these patients throughout life.

Management of the glaucoma depends to a degree on the age of the patient. The patient with congenital glaucoma may require surgical treatment (goniotomy, trabeculotomy, or filtering surgery), whereas the individual with a later onset of glaucoma may respond, at least initially, to standard antiglaucoma medications. Since many cases appear to have gross abnormalities of the aqueous outflow system, medications that reduce aqueous production, such as timolol maleate and carbonic anhydrase inhibitors, may be more effective in controlling the intraocular pressure. When the intraocular pressure can no longer be controlled on maximum tolerable medication, filtering surgery is usually required.

Other peripheral mesodermal defects of the anterior ocular segment

Mesodermal dysgenesis of the anterior chamber angle has been described in association with numerous other ocular anomalies. Cases have been cited associating it with Peters' anomaly, congenital miosis, megalocornea, congenital glaucoma, unilateral retinal dysplasia, neuroectodermal developmental defects, cornea plana, congenital nonattachment of the retina, fetal uveitis, and Wagner's syndrome.[1] Goniodysgenesis, hypoplasia of the iris, and juvenile glaucoma in a large pedigree with autosomal dominant inheritance[20] and a similar entity in two brothers with iridogoniodysgenesis and cataracts[16] have been described. Dysembryogenesis of the cornea, iris, and anterior chamber in patients with trisomy 13-15 has also been reported,[19] as well as two cases of unilateral uveal ectropion associated with congenital and late infantile glaucoma, which appeared to result from dysgenesis of the anterior chamber angle.[13] In the broadest sense, congenital glaucoma might be included among the mesodermal anomalies of the anterior chamber angle, but it is omitted from this text because it is considered a primary glaucoma due to the absence of other ocular or systemic defects.

Central mesodermal dysgeneses of the anterior ocular segment

Mesodermal abnormalities involving the central portion of the anterior ocular segment also comprise a spectrum of clinicopathologic entities. The common feature in this group of disorders is a congenital defect involving the central posterior cornea, usually associated with corneal opacification. Alkemade[1] lists these variations, in order of increasing severity, as posterior ketatoconus, Peters' anomaly, and congenital corneal leukomas and staphylomas. However, these conditions not only differ in their clinical manifestations, but also appear to have more than one basic pathogenic mechanism.

Posterior keratoconus

In posterior keratoconus, the central cornea is thinned because of an excessive curvature in the posterior surface of the cornea.[8] Wolter and Haney[43] described the histopathology of a case, noting that Descemet's membrane was thin but present and had many minute ruptures. Adhesions between the cornea and the iris were not observed in this case and are not considered a part of posterior keratoconus. The presence of endothelium and Descemet's membrane distinguishes posterior keratoconus from the other forms of central mesodermal dysgenesis of the anterior segment, but Alkemade[1] believed that this could represent secondary endothelialization and suggested that this might be the mildest form in the spectrum of disorders. The association of glaucoma and systemic abnormalities with posterior keratoconus is rare.

Peters' anomaly

CLINICOPATHOLOGIC FEATURES. The hallmark of Peters' anomaly is a central corneal opacity (Fig. 2-7) associated with a defect in the corresponding portion of the posterior cornea and adhesions from the borders of the corneal defect to the central iris. The condition is most often hereditary, usually with autosomal recessive transmission, although isolated cases have been reported. The defect is present at birth and is bilateral in 80% of cases. Associated ocular findings include frequent microphthalmos and occasional blue sclerae. Cases have also been reported in which anterior segment dysgenesis and keratolenticular adhesion were associated with aniridia.[4] Glaucoma occurs in over 50% of cases and is often present at birth.[1] The lens is frequently cataractous and occasionally adherent to the posterior cornea. Gonioscopically visible abnormalities of the anterior chamber angle are rare.

Townsend et al.[38] subdivided Peters' anomaly into three groups: (1) those not associated with keratolenticular contact or cataract, (2) those associated with keratolenticular contact or cataract, and (3) those associated with Rieger's syndrome.

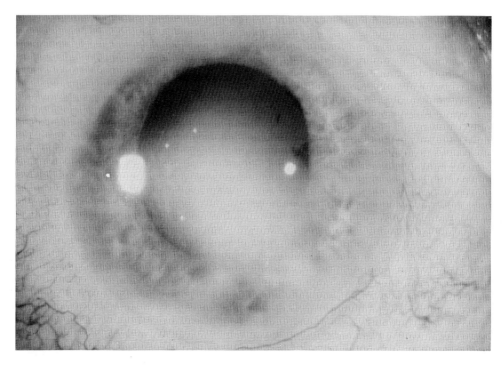

FIG. 2-7. Central corneal opacity with keratolenticular adhesion and cataract in patient with Peters' anomaly and associated glaucoma. (Courtesy George O. Waring, M.D.)

The pathogenesis of these conditions is not fully understood, but the variation in histopathologic findings suggests more than one mechanism. In those cases without lenticular abnormalities, the defect in Descemet's membrane may represent a primary failure of development. However, the adhesions between the cornea and the central iris cannot be explained by failure of separation, since the corneal endothelium and the stroma of the iris, as previously described, develop by individual waves of tissue at different times during gestation and not by cleavage of a common cellular layer. Rather, it appears that the adhesions may be a secondary developmental abnormality, possibly associated with a forward displacement and subsequent adherence of the pupillary membrane to the posterior cornea.[38]

In cases with lenticular abnormalities, Peters[27] postulated that the problem was one of incomplete separation of the lens vesicle from the surface ectoderm, suggesting a primary ectodermal abnormality. However, histopathologic studies of cases with keratolenticular contact suggest that a well-developed lens was secondarily displaced forward

against the cornea, resulting in a secondary loss of Descemet's membrane.[35,38] The cases studied by Townsend et al.[38] indicated that a variety of mechanisms might be responsible for the forward displacement of the lens, including a persistent hyperplastic primary vitreous, a detached and dysplastic retina, iris bombé, and a dislocated, swollen lens. In one case report, unilateral corneal perforation and bilateral central corneal defects at birth appeared to result from a persistent hyperplastic primary vitreous with a forward displacement of the lens-iris diaphragm.[15] However, the possibility remains that incomplete separation of the lens vesicle from the surface ectoderm may be the pathogenic mechanism in some cases of Peters' anomaly. Furthermore, intrauterine inflammation, as postulated by von Hippel,[40] and which gave rise to the term von Hippel's internal ulcer, may be responsible for some cases in this spectrum of disease. Polack and Grave[28] described an infant with a history of rubella syndrome and clinicopathologic features consistent with Peters' anomaly, in which intrauterine inflammation was believed to have caused the condition.

MECHANISM OF GLAUCOMA. In most cases of Peters' anomaly the anterior chamber angle appears to be grossly normal, and the mechanism of aqueous outflow obstruction has not been fully explained. Kupfer et al.[24] reported the ultrastructure of a trabeculectomy specimen from the eye of a 2-year-old child with Peters' anomaly and glaucoma and noted that the trabecular meshwork demonstrated changes characteristic of old age, including fibrous long-spacing collagen and the presence of phagocytosed pigment granules in the endothelium. They suggested that this might represent a failure in the normal differentiation of the mesoderm at the rim of the optic cup into typical endothelial cells or failure of differentiation of neural crest cells destined for corneal or trabecular endothelium.

In other cases the mechanism of aqueous outflow obstruction may be on the basis of less subtle changes in the anterior chamber angle. Scheie and Yanoff[32] described the histopathology of the eye of an infant with Peters' anomaly and total posterior coloboma of the retinal pigment epithelium and choroid. In this case there were total peripheral anterior synechiae, with atrophy of the iris stroma, and no identifiable trabecular meshwork or Schlemm's canal. Other cases have been reported in which Peters' anomaly was associated with mesodermal dysgenesis of the anterior chamber angle, more typical of Rieger's syndrome.

DIFFERENTIAL DIAGNOSIS. The main differential problem in Peters' anomaly is distinguishing the central corneal opacification from other causes of corneal opacification in newborns and infants. In this regard, the differential diagnosis should include congenital glaucoma, birth trauma, mucopolysaccharidosis, and congenital hereditary corneal dystrophy.

MANAGEMENT. An examination with the patient under anesthesia should be performed within the first few weeks of life on all children with congenital corneal opacities. Because the anterior corneal surface may be abnormal, a MacKay-Marg tonometer or pneumotonometer is preferred for intraocular pressure measurement, although a handheld applanation tonometer may be adequate. Elevated intraocular pressure should usually be treated before penetrating keratoplasty is done, and since the mechanism of obstruction to aqueous outflow is not fully understood and Schlemm's canal may be absent, a trabeculectomy probably offers the best surgical approach. Penetrating keratoplasty may subsequently be required, especially if the central corneal opacifications are dense and bilateral. Waring and Parks[41] reported the case of a 6-month-old infant in whom keratolenticular adhesions were separated with a knife-needle and aspirated along with a secondary capsulotomy. When the child was 6 years old, the vision was 20/60 in both eyes.

Congenital corneal leukomas and staphylomas

Congenital leukomas of the cornea may occur with or without sclerocornea and other congenital anomalies, and Alkemade[1] has suggested that these may be closely related, if not identical, to the more severe forms of Peters' anomaly. The most severe form of this spectrum of disease is corneal staphyloma, in which the cornea is markedly thin, scarred, and vascularized and is lined on the posterior surface by an atrophic iris. This condition is frequently associated with glaucoma.

Combined Rieger's syndrome and Peters' anomaly

As noted earlier in this chapter, rare cases have been reported in which the peripheral anomalies of Rieger's syndrome coexisted in the same eye with the central features of Peters' anomaly or other central abnormalities of the anterior ocular segment. Reese and Ellsworth[29] noted that Zimmerman described a 53-year-old woman with reduced vision in her left eye since infancy. Histopathology of that eye revealed the absence of Descemet's membrane in the central cornea, a prominent Schwalbe's ring, iris adhesions to both the central and peripheral corneal defects, and a malformation of the filtration angle. Alkemade[1] described the histopathology of an eye with adhesions from the peripheral iris to a prominent Schwalbe's ring associated with a central corneal defect that was attached by a strand of connective tissue to the anterior surface of a luxated lens. Similar reports have included a case of unilateral Peters' anomaly with mesodermal dysgenesis of the iris, angle, and zonules in the fellow eye[35] and a patient with unilateral Peters' anomaly associated with a prominent Schwalbe's ring.[28]

REFERENCES

1. Alkemade, P.P.H.: Dysgenesis mesodermalis of the iris and the cornea, Springfield, Ill., 1969, Charles C Thomas, Publisher.
2. Allen, L., Burian, H.M., and Braley, A.E.: A new concept of the development of the anterior chamber angle, Arch. Ophthalmol. **53**:783, 1955.
3. Axenfeld, T.: Embryotoxon cornea posterius, Ber. Dtsch. Ophthalmol. Ges. **42**:301, 1920.
4. Beauchamp, G.R.: Anterior segment dysgenesis, keratolenticular adhesion and aniridia, J. Pediatr. Ophthalmol. Strabismus **17**:55, 1980.
5. Burian, H.M., Braley, A.E., and Allen, L.: External and gonioscopic visibility of the ring of Schwalbe and the trabecular zone: an interpretation of the posterior corneal embryotoxon and the so-called congenital hyaline membranes on the posterior corneal surface, Trans. Am. Ophthalmol. Soc. **51**:389, 1955.
6. Campbell, D.G., Shields, M.B., and Smith, T.R.: The corneal endothelium and the spectrum of essential iris atrophy, Am. J. Ophthalmol. **86**:317, 1978.
7. Cibis, G.W., Krachmer, J.H., Phelps, C.D., and Weingeist, T.A.: Iridocorneal adhesions in posterior polymorphous dystrophy, Trans. Am. Acad. Ophthalmol. Otol. **81**:770, 1976.
8. Collier, J.: Le keratocone posterieur, Arch. Ophthalmol. (Paris) **23**:376, 1962.
9. Cross, H.E.: Ectopia lentis et pupillae, Am. J. Ophthalmol. **88**:381, 1979.
10. Cross, H.E., Jorgenson, R.J., Levin, L.S., and Kelly, T.E.: The Rieger syndrome: an autosomal dominant disorder with ocular, dental and systemic abnormalities, Perspect. Ophthalmol. **3**:3, 1979.
11. Cross, H.E., and Maumenee, A.E.: Progressive spontaneous dissolution of the iris, Surv. Ophthalmol. **18**:186, 1973.
12. Delmarcelle, Y., Clerck, P. De., and Pivont, A.: Glaucome congenital associé à des malformations oculaires et somatiques dans deux generations successives, Bull. Soc. Belge Ophthalmol. **120**:638, 1958.
13. Gramer, E., and Krieglstein, G.K.: Infantile glaucoma in unilateral uveal ectropion, Albrecht Von Graefes Arch. Klin. Exp. Ophthalmol. **211**:215, 1979.
14. Gregor, Z., and Hitchings, R.A.: Rieger's anomaly: a 42-year follow-up, Br. J. Ophthalmol. **64**:56, 1980.
15. Heckenlively, J., and Kielar, R.: Congenital perforated cornea in Peters' anomaly, Am. J. Ophthalmol. **88**:63, 1979.
16. Henkind, P., and Friedman, A.H.: Iridogoniodysgenesis with cataract, Am. J. Ophthalmol. **72**:949, 1971.
17. Henkind, P., Siegel, I.M., and Carr, R.E.: Mesodermal dysgenesis of the anterior segment: Rieger's anomaly, Arch. Ophthalmol. **73**:810, 1965.
18. Hirst, L.W., Quigley, H.A., Stark, W.J., and Shields, M.B.: Specular microscopy in iridocorneal endothelial syndrome, Am. J. Ophthalmol. **89**:11, 1980.
19. Hoepner, J., and Yanoff, M.: Ocular anomalies in trisomy 13-15: an analysis of 13 eyes with two new findings, Am. J. Ophthalmol. **74**:729, 1972.
20. Jerndal, T.: Goniodysgenesis and hereditary juvenile glaucoma: a clinical study of a Swedish pedigree, Acta. Ophthalmol. **107**:1, 1970.

21. Judisch, G.F., Martin-Casals, A., Hanson, J.W., and Olin, W.H.: Oculodentodigital dysplasia: four new reports and a literature review, Arch. Ophthalmol. **97**:878, 1979.
22. Judisch, G.F., Phelps, C.D., and Hanson, J.: Rieger's syndrome: a case report with a 15-year follow-up, Arch. Ophthalmol. **97**:2120, 1979.
23. Kupfer, C., and Kaiser-Kupfer, M.I.: Observations on the development of the anterior chamber angle with reference to the pathogenesis of congenital glaucomas, Am. J. Ophthalmol. **88**:424, 1979.
24. Kupfer, C., Kuwabara, T.W., and Stark, W.J.: The histopathology of Peters' anomaly, Am. J. Ophthalmol. **80**:653, 1975.
25. Mann, I.: The development of the human eye, ed. 3, New York, 1964, Grune & Stratton, Inc.
26. Pau, H., Graeber, W., and Holterman, W.: Die "Fortschreitende Atropie des Irisstromas mit Luchbildung und Proliferation des Hornhautendothels," Klin. Monatsbl. Augenheilkd. **141**:568, 1962.
27. Peters, A.: Ueber angeborene defektbildung der Descemetschen Membran, Klin. Montasbl. Augenheilkd. **44**:27, 1906.
28. Polack, F.M., and Grave, E.L.: Scanning electron microscopy of congenital corneal leukomas (Peters' anomaly), Am. J. Ophthalmol. **88**:169, 1979.
29. Reese, A.B., and Ellsworth, R.M.: The anterior chamber cleavage syndrome, Arch. Ophthalmol. **75**:307, 1966.
30. Rieger, H.: Beitrage zur Kenntnis seltener Missbildungen der Iris. II. Uber hypoplasie des Irisvorterblattes mit Verlagerung und Entrundung der Pupille, Albrecht Von Graefe's Arch. Ophthalmol. **133**:602, 1935.
31. Rubell, E.: Angeborene Hypoplasie bzw. Aplasie des Irisvorderblattes, Klin. Monatsbl. Augenheilkd. **51**:174, 1913.
32. Scheie, H.G., and Yanoff, M.: Peters' anomaly and total posterior coloboma of retinal pigment epithelium and choroid, Arch. Ophthalmol. **87**:525, 1972.
33. Shields, M.B., Campbell, D.G., and Simmons, R.J.: The essential iris atrophies, Am. J. Ophthalmol. **85**:749, 1978.
34. Smelser, G.K., and Ozanics, V.: The development of the trabecular meshwork in primate eyes, Am. J. Ophthalmol. **71**:366, 1971.
35. Stone, D.L., Kenyon, K.R., Green, W.R., and Ryan, S.J.: Congenital central corneal leukoma (Peters' anomaly), Am. J. Ophthalmol. **81**:173, 1976.
36. Sugar, H.S.: Juvenile glaucoma with Axenfeld's syndrome, Am. J. Ophthalmol. **59**:1012, 1965.
37. Townsend, W.M.: Congenital corneal leukomas. I. Central defect in Descemet's membrane, Am. J. Ophthalmol. **77**:80, 1974.
38. Townsend, W.M., Font, R.L., and Zimmerman, L.E.: Congenital corneal leukomas. II. Histopathologic findings in 19 eyes with central defect in Descemet's membrane, Am. J. Ophthalmol. **77**:192, 1974.
39. Troeber, R., and Rochels, R.: Histologic findings in Rieger's mesodermal dysgenesis of the iris, Albrecht Von Graefes Arch. Klin. Exp. Ophthalmol. **213**:169, 1980.
40. von Hippel, E.: Uber Hydrophthalmus congenitus nebst Bemerkungen uber die Verfarbung der cornea durch blutfarbstoff: Pathololischeanatomische Untersuchungen, Albrecht Von Graefes Arch. Ophthalmol **44**:539, 1897.

41. Waring, G.O. III, and Parks, M.M.: Successful lens removal in congenital corneolenticular adhesion (Peters' anomaly), Am. J. Ophthalmol. **83:**526, 1977.

42. Waring, G.O. III, Rodrigues, M.M., and Laibson, P.R.: Anterior chamber cleavage syndrome: a stepladder classification, Surv. Ophthalmol. **20:**3, 1975.

43. Wolter, J.R., and Haney, W.P.: Histopathology of keratoconus posticus circumscriptus, Arch. Ophthalmol. **69:**357, 1963.

44. Wolter, J.R., Sandall, G.S., and Fralick, F.B.: Mesodermal dysgenesis of the anterior eye: with a partially separated posterior embryotoxon, J. Pediatr. Ophthalmol. **4:**41, 1967.

Chapter 3

GLAUCOMA IN ANIRIDIA

David S. Walton

Aniridia is an important eye disease characterized by significant congenital and acquired ocular abnormalities. It is a rare entity with an estimated incidence of 1/56,000.[5]

When aniridia is present in multiple family members, evidence of autosomal dominant inheritance is usually seen.[5] Aniridia may rarely be seen in multiple siblings of both sexes born to unaffected parents secondary to a germinal mutation but more commonly occurs sporadically secondary to a spontaneous mutation. In either situation there is a 50% risk to the offspring of the affected person. Autosomal recessive inheritance is rare but has been demonstrated in a syndrome of aniridia, cerebellar ataxia, and mental retardation.[1] Of further importance is the association of aniridia with genitourinary anomalies and mental retardation, a syndrome that is caused by a partial deletion of the short arm of chromosome 11.[4] These patients are also at high risk of developing Wilms' tumor.[4] This association of abnormalities may be familial when the chromosomal defect is derived from defective parental chromosomes.[6]

OCULAR INVOLVEMENT

The congenital ocular defects found in aniridia patients are both functionally and anatomically significant (Fig. 3-1). These defects vary independently of each other in severity. The iris leaf shows a striking absence of tissue with often only a narrow stump of tissue present at the iris root, detectable on gonioscopic examination. Less commonly, sizable portions of iris may be present and even allow the existence of a pupil. The cornea is often slightly small in diameter, a finding that appears exaggerated by the presence of a peripheral zone of vascularized and opacified epithelium. This defect stains well with fluorescein, which facilitates the estimation of its size. Small localized congenital lens opacities are frequently present but rarely are visually significant. However, visually significant congenital lens opacities seem to occur frequently in patients with the aniridia–Wilms' tumor syndrome. Examination of the fundi usually reveals absence of foveal landmarks, and the optic nerve heads may appear small but are usually well vascularized. Typical choroidal colobomas occur with increased frequency in aniridia. External examination may reveal mild bilateral ptosis, and sensory nystagmus is frequently present.

The term traumatic aniridia is sometimes used to describe the occurrence of iris loss secondary to injury. The sequelae of this event are not considered in this chapter, and I have not seen it complicated by changes similar to those that occur with genetically determined aniridia.

MECHANISM OF GLAUCOMA

Secondary glaucoma is suspected to occur in greater than 50% of eyes with aniridia and is always a difficult management problem. The mechanism of this glaucoma has interested investigators for many years. Lembeck[3] (1890) reported the histopathology of aniridia and suggested that the glaucoma was caused by the stump of iris blocking the filtration angle.

Glaucoma in aniridia is usually not caused by a primary defect of filtration tissue alone; it occurs more frequently in eyes that have demonstrated progressive filtration angle abnormalities.[2]

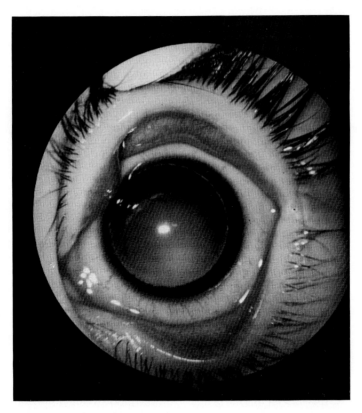

FIG. 3-1. Typical appearance of anterior segment in young patient with aniridia. No iris is visible, and equator of lens is easily seen. Lens is still without opacities in this 4-year-old patient.

The filtration angle in the infant with aniridia usually possesses an unobstructed trabecular meshwork, but this is not always true. Alternatively, slender bridges of tissue extending as strands or sawtooth extensions from the iris root may insert onto the posterior trabecular meshwork or even more anteriorly. Some such extensions may possess fine blood vessels that attach onto the meshwork, course circumferentially, and return to the iris root. Arborization of vessels on the meshwork as found in neovascularization of the angle are not seen. More extensive early obstruction of the trabecular meshwork by the iris and iris extensions seems to occur more frequently in those patients with the aniridia–Wilms' tumor syndrome and may be associated with significant early glaucoma. Alternatively, glaucoma may occur early in life without obstruction of the trabecular meshwork by the iris, but this is unusual.

The presence or absence of glaucoma in aniridia seems to correlate with the extent of gonioscopically visible obstruction of the trabecular meshwork (Fig. 3-2). In aniridic eyes without glaucoma, very little covering of the filtration meshwork by iris tissue is present. With mild elevation of the intraocular pressure, it is common to see partial obstruction of the trabecular meshwork in the form of many individual anterior extensions from the peripheral iris stroma extending across the scleral spur onto the meshwork. In addition, actual blockage of the meshwork by anterior extension of the iris stump is usually present. This abnormality is usually more extensive superiorly, where associated upward sliding by the iris stroma to cover the ciliary body band is frequently seen in this stage. In eyes with moderate to severe glaucoma, adhesion of iris stromal tissue has progressed to cover most meridians of the filtration meshwork. Gonioscopic inspection of the angle frequently reveals a minimal iris stump associated with anterior stromal tissue that appears to have spread onto the face of the angle to cover much of the posterior meshwork. Blood vessels are less visible on the trabecular meshwork at this stage.

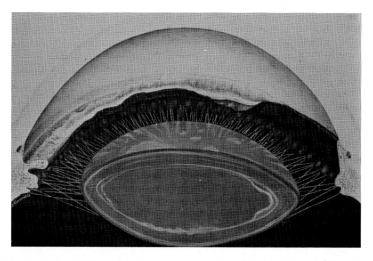

FIG. 3-2. Drawing of aniridic angle showing progression of obstruction of trabecular meshwork as one views angle from left to right. At extreme left, angle is open. Centrally, iris processes are visible over posterior trabecular meshwork. At right, complete obstruction is present secondary to anterior movement of stroma over trabecular meshwork. At extreme right, iris is seen turned anteriorly in apposition with angle face.

This progression of the angle abnormality occurs most frequently in patients from 5 to 15 years of age. I have not seen a spontaneous reversal of any of these angle changes. I have seen this change of iris position in a few patients without glaucoma who appeared to be spared the effects of trabecular meshwork obstruction by virtue of possessing a very wide ciliary body band.

MANAGEMENT

Treatment of glaucoma in aniridia has often proved to be difficult. Medical therapy includes topical miotics, beta-adrenergic blocking agents, adrenergic agonists, and systemic carbonic anhydrase inhibitors, all of which can be helpful. Usually miotics are selected as initial therapy and are well tolerated. However, miotics may also cause the iris leaf to hinge forward to cover the angle structures. An elevation of intraocular pressure can occur secondary to obstruction of the trabecular meshwork as a result of miotic treatment. This effect is reversible by cycloplegics and the discontinuation of miotics. It is not known whether irreversible obstruction may occur secondary to the use of miotics. Therefore aniridia patients treated with miotics require periodic gonioscopy to rule out this occurrence.

Goniotomy for glaucoma in aniridia with advanced angle changes has not been helpful for my patients. In a few patients, when goniotomy was performed at an early stage when only early exten-

sions of iris processes onto the angle were present, it has provided a lasting pressure-lowering effect. When glaucoma is not controlled by medical treatment or when progression of the angle defect occurs even in the presence of adequate medical therapy, this surgery should be considered.

Conventional adult glaucoma procedures, including trabeculectomy, trephination, cyclodialysis, and cyclodiathermy have not proved to be helpful.

Cyclocryotherapy can produce a lasting beneficial effect on the intraocular pressure. I recommend that the freezing probe be placed over the ciliary processes and that not more than one half of the total circumference be treated at one procedure. Lenticular and corneal abnormalities may progress despite improved glaucoma control after cyclocryotherapy.

Based on the observation of progressive angle defects in aniridia associated with the development and worsening of glaucoma, I have attempted prophylactic angle surgery in 15 eyes of 9 patients. This surgery has been done in an attempt to create a permanent separation between the iris and the trabecular meshwork before the iris has a chance to obstruct the meshwork. It has been performed under direct observation with a standard Barkan goniotomy knife. The anterior edge of the curtain of iris tissue extending upward from the iris root is engaged with the tip of the knife and pulled posteriorly with repetitive movements as the knife is moved circumferentially. The anatomic result of this procedure is dramatic, with the creation of an apparent permanent separation between the iris and the angle face. Generally, two operations are done on each eye to achieve a surgical effect of greater than 180 degrees of angle circumference. The postoperative follow-up now ranges from 1 to 9 years. The absence of glaucoma in all eyes treated in this way is encouraging. No complications have been encountered. Familiarity with the gonioscopic appearance of the angle in aniridia and regular experience with goniotomy surgery would seem to be important personal preparation for considering this surgical procedure.

REFERENCES

1. Gillespie, F.D.: Aniridia, cerebellar ataxia and oligophrenia in siblings, Arch. Ophthalmol. **73:**338, 1965.
2. Grant, W.M., and Walton, D.S.: Progressive changes in the angle in congenital aniridia with development of glaucoma, Am. J. Ophthalmol. **78:**842, 1974; Trans. Am. Ophthalmol. Soc. **74:**207, 1974.
3. Lembeck, H.: Ueber die Pathologische Anatomie der Irideremia totalis congenita, 19 July 1890 (inaugural dissertation).
4. Riccardi, V.M., Sujansky, E., Smith, A.C., and Francke, U.: Chromosomal imbalance in the Aniridia-Wilms' tumor association: 11p interstitial deletion, Pediatrics **61:**604, 1978.
5. Shaw, M.W., Falls, H.G., and Neel, J.V.: Congenital aniridia, Am. J. Hum. Genetics **12:**389, 1960.
6. Yunis, J.J., and Ramsay, N.K.C.: Familial occurrence of the aniridia-Wilms' tumor syndrome with deletion 11p13-14.1, J. Pediatr. **96:**1027, 1980.

Chapter 4

GLAUCOMA IN THE PHAKOMATOSES

Jayne S. Weiss and Robert Ritch

The phakomatoses (*phakos,* birthmark), or disseminated hamartomatoses, are a group of ophthalmologically important hereditary disorders exhibiting variable penetrance and expressivity (see outline below). These disorders are characterized by the formation of hamartias and hamartomas in viscera, skin, the central nervous system, and ocular structures. The classic features of the phakomatoses are:

1. Nontumorous growths on the skin or mucous membranes that arise from cells normally found in the tissue at the involved site (hamartias)
2. Localized hyperplastic tumor formations arising from cells normally found in the tissue at the site of growth (hamartomas)
3. True neoplasms originating from undifferentiated embryonic cells or dedifferentiated mature cells
4. Other associated congenital abnormalities

Phakomatoses

A. Glaucoma common
   1. Encephalotrigeminal angiomatosis (Sturge-Webber)
B. Glaucoma occurs
   1. Neurofibromatosis (von Recklinghausen)
   2. Angiomatosis retinae (von Hippel-Lindau)
   3. Oculodermal melanocytosis (Nevus of Ota)
C. Rarely associated with glaucoma
   1. Basal cell nevus syndrome
   2. Tuberous sclerosis (Bourneville)
   3. Klippel-Trenaunay-Weber (in pure form)
   4. Diffuse congenital hemangiomatosis
D. Unassociated with glaucoma
   1. Ataxia-telangiectasia (Louis-Bar)

   2. Racemose angioma of the retina (Wyburn-Mason)

Derivatives of all three germ layers may be affected. Francois[39] has listed three important factors in their pathogenesis:

1. The developmental stage in which the abnormal gene intervenes. Estimates have ranged from between the thirtieth day[58] to the third month[65] to sometime between the third and seventh months.[22]
2. The phakomatoses may be differentiated embryologically based on the particular germinal layer affected. In neuroectodermal dysplasias, such as neurofibromatosis and tuberous sclerosis, interference with the migration and differentiation of neuroblasts and spongioblasts results in proliferation of spongiocytes. In the mesodermal disorders, such as encephalotrigeminal angiomatosis, angiomatosis retinae, and Klippel-Trenaunay-Weber syndrome, irregularity in the distribution and structure of small vessels results in abnormal proliferation of perivascular cells. Rarely, more than one phakomatosis may occur in a single patient.
3. Multiple malformations may arise from interference with the process of induction.

Glaucoma in the phakomatoses can develop by a number of different mechanisms, even within a single disease entity. Many mechanisms have been suggested, few of which have been proved. Diagnosis is frequently straightforward, based on the presence of buphthalmos and/or other signs of congenital glaucoma in infancy or early childhood,

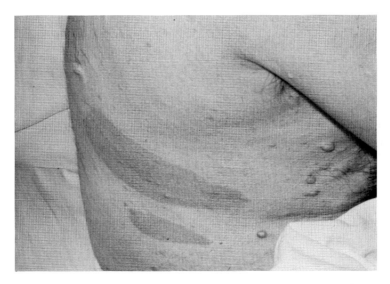

FIG. 4-1. Large café au lait spots on trunk of patient with neurofibromatosis. Cutaneous neurofibromas and slight axillary freckling are also present.

and on an elevated intraocular pressure in children and adults. Treatment, however, often depends on the underlying mechanism of the glaucoma, when a mechanism can be defined. One should make every effort to define one, both for patient benefit through institution of proper treatment and to further elucidate our understanding of these relatively uncommon entities.

Although no universal mechanism explaining the pathogenesis of glaucoma in the phakomatoses exists, there are obvious similarities among the syndromes. Hypertrophy and developmental anomalies have been postulated to cause ocular hypertension in both neurofibromatosis and encephalotrigeminal angiomatosis. The anterior chamber angle may be occluded by a neurofibroma in neurofibromatosis, neovascularization in encephalotrigeminal angiomatosis, or melanocytes in oculodermal melanocytosis. A ciliary body or choroidal neurofibroma, or an iris hemangioma may cause the root of the iris to obstruct the anterior chamber angle. Neovascular glaucoma has been reported in neurofibromatosis, encephalotrigeminal angiomatosis, angiomatosis retinae, and tuberous sclerosis.

NEUROFIBROMATOSIS

Neurofibromatosis is primarily a neuroectodermal dysplasia characterized by tumorlike formations derived by the proliferation of peripheral nerve elements. Von Recklinghausen[108] (1882) was the first to identify the clinical and pathologic complex of neurofibromatosis as a distinct entity. Schiess-Gemuseus[92] (1884) first reported the association of neurofibromatosis with congenital glaucoma. The disease is inherited by means of an autosomal dominant gene with irregular penetrance and a mutation rate of 1×10^{-4}. It is reported to occur in 1 of 2500 to 3300 births.[17] Though congenital, tumors may first present in late childhood or adult life. Mental retardation and seizure disorders may occur, but intelligence is usually normal.

Systemic involvement

The usual clinical appearance is one of multiple circumscribed areas of hyperpigmentation of the skin accompanied by multiple dermal nodules and neurofibromas. Tumors of the central and peripheral nervous system include neurofibromas, optic and chiasmal gliomas, neurinomas, astrocytomas, and meningiomas. The brain, meninges, spinal cord, and peripheral, cranial, or sympathetic nerves may be involved. Acoustic neuroma is the most frequent intracranial lesion.

Cutaneous manifestations are common and form the hallmark of diagnosis. Café au lait spots are regularly circumscribed, brown macules typically found on the trunk (Fig. 4-1). The presence of five or more of these greater than 1.5 cm in diameter is considered diagnostic. Plexiform neuromas are large, ramifying cords of neurofibromas caused by enlarged nerves and thickened perineural sheaths. Fibroma mollusca are pedunculated, pigmented nodules caused by an increased number of Schwann's cells, connective tissue elements, and enlarged cutaneous nerves (Fig. 4-2). Regional giantism, or hemihypertrophy of the face or extremities, may be caused by diffuse proliferation of mesodermal tissue near a plexiform neuroma. Frecklelike or diffuse pigmentation of the axillae is characteristic and almost pathognomonic.

Occasionally a neurofibroma may undergo sarcomatous change and develop into a malignant schwannoma. Skeletal defects occur in 29% of patients, whereas endocrine, vascular, and visceral disturbances are less common.[44]

Recently evidence has accumulated that elevated nerve growth factor levels exist in patients with neurofibromatosis.[32,96] Decreased binding of epidermal growth factor by fibroblasts of patients with neurofibromatosis suggests that a receptor deficiency or membrane abnormality may play a role in the cause of the disease.[128]

Ocular involvement

In decreasing order of frequency, neurofibromatosis involves the eyelids, orbit, uvea, optic nerve, retina, cornea, tarsal conjunctiva, and bulbar conjunctiva. Only the lens and vitreous are unaffected.

The lids may be involved by plexiform neuromas with characteristic palpable stringlike swellings (Figs. 4-3 to 4-5). These usually affect the upper lid unilaterally but rarely may be bilateral[78] or affect primarily the lower lid.[39] In addition to the upper lid, the skin above the orbit and on the adjacent temple may be involved. This lesion is identical histologically to the neurofibroma. The combination of plexiform neuroma of the lid, facial hemihypertrophy, and buphthalmos has been termed François' syndrome.[40] Café au lait spots, pigmented nevi, elephantiasis neuromatosa, fibroma molluscum, and diffuse palpebral neuro-

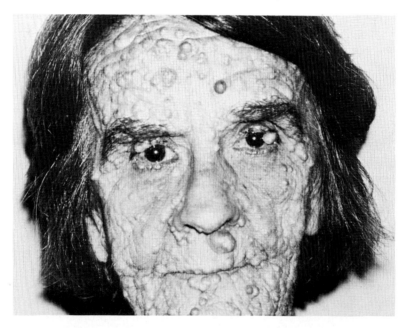

FIG. 4-2. Diffuse cutaneous neurofibromas, or fibroma mollusca, are hallmark of this disease. (From Gass, J.D.M.: The phakotomatoses. In Smith, J.L., editor: Neuro-ophthalmology, vol. 2, St. Louis, 1965, The C.V. Mosby Co.)

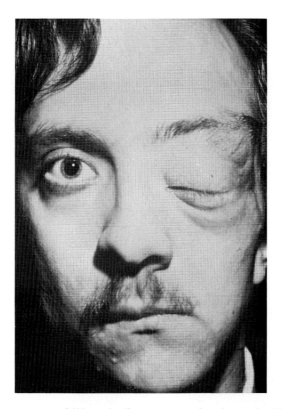

FIG. 4-3. Plexiform neuroma of lids and adjacent temporal region and mild facial hemihypertrophy. When buphthalmos is present, triad is referred to as François' syndrome.

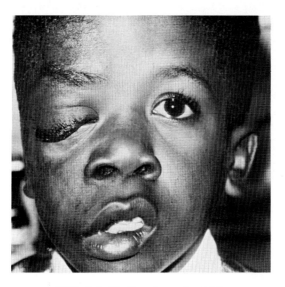

FIG. 4-4. Similar picture in child.

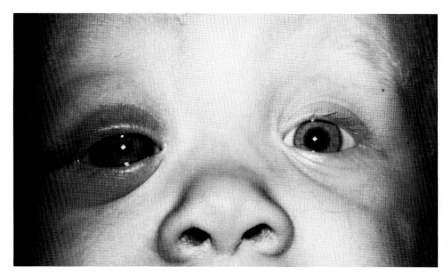

FIG. 4-5. Plexiform neuroma of upper and lower lids in association with congenital glaucoma in infant. (From Satran, L., et al.: Am. J. Dis. Child. **134:**182, 1980. Copyright 1980, American Medical Association.)

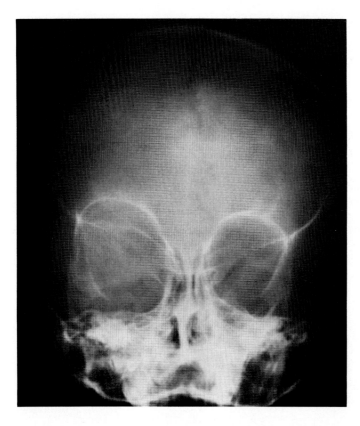

FIG. 4-6. Significant orbital asymmetry due to extensive orbital plexiform neuroma in same patient as in Fig. 4-5. (From Satran, L., et al.: Am. J. Dis. Child. **134:**182, 1980. Copyright 1980, American Medical Association.)

fibromatosis with absence of cordlike structures may also occur in the lid.

Glial neoplasms or meningoblastomas of the optic nerve may cause loss of vision, proptosis, and optic atrophy. Rarely, neurofibroma of the disc occurs, and glial hamartomas or nerve fiber medullation may involve the retina.[68]

Orbital neurofibroma (Fig. 4-6) or plexiform neurofibromatosis causes displacement of the globe with proptosis. Pulsating exophthalmos

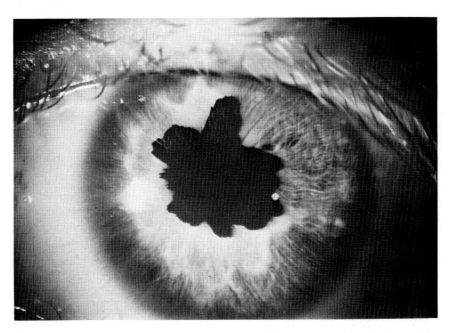

FIG. 4-7. Congenital ectropion uveae in 10-year-old boy with juvenile glaucoma and neurofibromatosis. Plexiform neuroma of lids is not present in this patient.

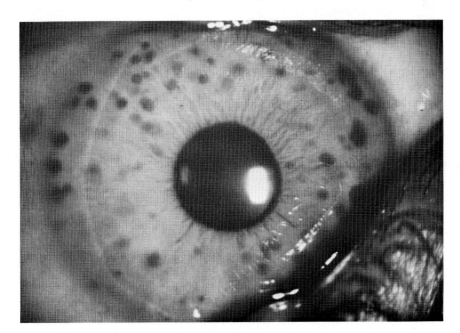

FIG. 4-8. Numerous iris hamartomas (Lische nodules) are characteristically found in neurofibromatosis.

unassociated with bruits results from orbital wall defects or meningoceles. Pulsating muscle palsies may be secondary to orbital expansion caused by congenital defects or tumor erosion.

Conjunctival nodules, or diffuse infiltration of the episclera by nerve fibers or small tumors, and scleral melanosis occur rarely. Hyperplasia of nerve fibers or tumor formation may involve the cornea.

Ectropion uveae (Fig. 4-7), Lische nodules (variably pigmented nodules comprising focal collections of spindle cells) (Fig. 4-8), or heterochromia may involve the iris. Hyperplastic neurons, Schwann's cells, fibroblasts, and/or melanocytes may cause thickening of the choroid and ciliary body. Circumscribed tumors that ophthalmoscopically resemble malignant melanomas may occur in the region of the ciliary nerves.

Glaucoma associated with neurofibromatosis

There are no reports of the incidence of glaucoma in neurofibromatosis, but despite the frequent mention of the subject in the literature, it appears to be rather rare in proportion to the number of patients with the disease. Of 300 cases of congenital glaucoma in a large series, only one (0.3%) was related to neurofibromatosis.[48] In almost all reported cases, the association of glaucoma with neurofibromatosis occurred at birth or shortly thereafter. Late-onset glaucoma occasionally occurs, however, and patients should be followed routinely if there is any question of orbital or ocular involvement. Open-angle glaucoma appearing in late adulthood should be considered to be primary unless proved otherwise.

Glaucoma associated with neurofibromatosis is almost always unilateral.[63] Neurofibromatous involvement of the upper lid is classically present, especially with buphthalmos (Fig. 4-5), although exceptions have been reported.[41,48] Lid involvement is not necessarily accompanied by glaucoma. Glaucoma is present in only 50% of all eyes with plexiform neuroma.[63] Nevertheless, a high index of suspicion should be maintained in these cases and patients watched for the development of glaucoma.

Buphthalmos occurring in the absence of elevated intraocular pressure has been reported in neurofibromatosis.[4,52,121] This is an important point to consider in diagnosis to prevent unnecessary surgery. Hoyt and Billson[52] reported an infant with buphthalmos in which enlargement of the globe continued after control of the intraocular pressure. They concluded that the buphthalmos resulted from a factor other than increased intraocular pressure secondary to anterior chamber angle obstruction and that it represented an effect of regional giantism similar to the hypertrophy of adjacent structures.

Many mechanisms have been postulated as causes of glaucoma in neurofibromatosis. Sachsalber[89] (1897) hypothesized that an abnormality of choroidal innervation led to connective tissue overgrowth and lymphatic (aqueous) blockage along the vortex veins, which impeded aqueous outflow, resulting in buphthalmos. Verhoeff[105] de-

scribed three patients with plexiform neuroma, intraocular nerve involvement, and unilateral buphthalmos. He concluded that a disturbance of the ciliary nerves resulted in buphthalmos but later rescinded this theory. Most tenable hypotheses for glaucoma in neurofibromatosis relate to developmental or mechanical abnormalities.

Persistence of embryonal tissue in the filtration angle has been reported.[52,63,120,121] This may result in blockage of aqueous outflow and increased intraocular pressure, but pressure may also be normal.[52] Incomplete cleavage of the iridocorneal angle may give a picture similar to that of primary congenital glaucoma[45] (Fig. 4-9).

Malformation[71] or absence of Schlemm's canal* may accompany the cleavage anomaly as part of the developmental disorder or, in some cases, may have been a secondary change due to long-standing glaucoma and sclerosis or distortion of the angle structures.

The presence of compact iris processes[16,63,73,92] and marked anterior insertion of the iris[63] have been described in children with neurofibromatosis and buphthalmos. However, patients may have increased numbers of iris processes and normal intraocular pressure.[48] In addition to an anterior iris insertion (actually a defect in angle cleavage), the ciliary processes may be abnormal and anterior, even extending onto the posterior iris surface.

Collins and Batten[16] found adhesions between the iris and the posterior cornea suggestive of incomplete cleavage of these structures during embryogenesis. Other authors have postulated that neurofibromatous thickening of the ciliary body and choroid might cause anterior displacement of the iris diaphragm, narrowing of the angle, peripheral anterior synechiae, and resultant glaucoma[20,44,69] (Fig. 4-10). The choroid may be thickened to as much as six to eight times normal (Fig. 4-11). It is difficult to determine what is primary and what is secondary in these instances, particularly because most eyes coming to enucleation have had previous surgery, which may be responsible for many of the pathologic changes. However, neurofibromatous involvement of the choroid is characteristically present when glaucoma is also present.

In most cases patients with the preceding intraocular pathologic findings have had buphthal-

---

*References 16, 60, 74, 89, 97, 120-122.

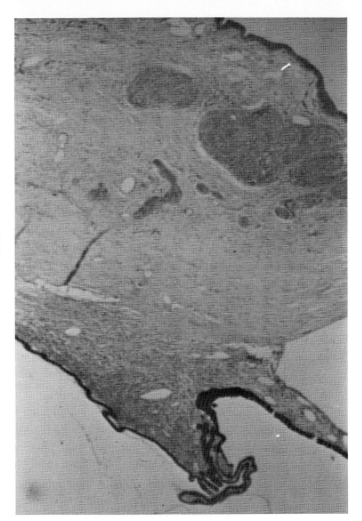

FIG. 4-9. Anterior chamber angle cleavage anomaly in eye exenterated because of diffuse orbital neurofibromatosis and long-standing blindness secondary to congenital glaucoma.

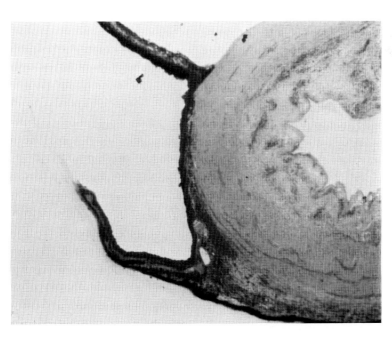

FIG. 4-10. Extensive vascular enlargement and massive thickening of limbus in neurofibromatosis. Angle is sealed by broad peripheral anterior synechiae. Nodular areas of neurofibromatous tissue are present. Angle closure in this case appears to have been secondary to posterior synechiae between iris sphincter and lens, with resultant peripheral iris bombé, after anterior chamber hemorrhage. (From Friedman, M.W., and Ritchey, C.L.: Arch. Ophthalmol. **70:**294, 1963. Copyright 1963, American Medical Association.)

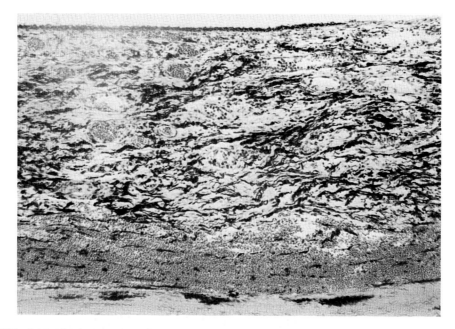

FIG. 4-11. Massive choroidal thickening due to diffuse neurofibroma in same patient as in Fig. 4-10. Although termed choroidal neurofibroma in the literature, this is really a hyperplasia of schwannian elements and melanocytes. (From Friedman, M.W., and Ritchey, C.L.: Arch. Ophthalmol. **70**:294, 1963. Copyright 1963, American Medical Association.)

mos.* There have been case reports of adults with choroidal involvement, peripheral anterior synechiae, and glaucoma, without buphthalmos.[13,69] Choroidal involvement may also be present without glaucoma.[13,41]

Infiltration of the angle[48] or root of the iris[20] with neurofibromatous tissue may lead to peripheral anterior synechiae (PAS) formation. Neovascular glaucoma may result from invasion of the chamber angle by new fibrovascular tissue with resultant synechial closure of the angle. Wolter and Butler[123] reported a patient with neurofibromatosis, ectropion uveae, neovascularization of the iris, and angle-closure glaucoma.

A single eye may be affected by more than one mechanism over a period of time. Friedman and Ritchey[44] described a patient with congenital buphthalmos and abnormal tissue in the angle on gonioscopy that was similar to the appearance of the angle in primary congenital glaucoma, and the intraocular pressure was controlled after goniotomy. Six years later the patient had sudden onset of severe pain with increased pressure. Examination of the enucleated globe revealed total peripheral anterior synechiae, a rudimentary ciliary body, and a markedly thickened choroid. Apparently, thickening of the choroid and ciliary body produced an anterior displacement of the uveal tract and subsequent PAS formation with angle closure.

Management

The choice of treatment depends on the severity of the glaucoma, its age of onset, and the mechanism. Mild elevations of intraocular pressure may be treated medically, particularly if buphthalmos is not present. A patient with buphthalmos and a clear cornea should not be assumed to have glaucoma without definite evidence of elevated intraocular pressure.

Surgery for glaucoma in neurofibromatosis has reflected the development of glaucoma surgery in general, and goniotomy, goniopuncture, trabeculotomy, trabeculectomy, cyclodiathermy, and cyclocryotherapy have all been reported. The overall rate of success, however, is much lower than that for primary congenital glaucoma. Because of the rarity, it is difficult to generalize as to the reason, but it may be that, in addition to anomalies of cleavage, abnormal tissue in the angle or an abnormal meshwork prevent aqueous outflow even after goniotomy in some cases. In others the

_____

*References 12, 43, 48, 60, 71, 74, 84, 89, 97, 102, 116, 120-122, 124.

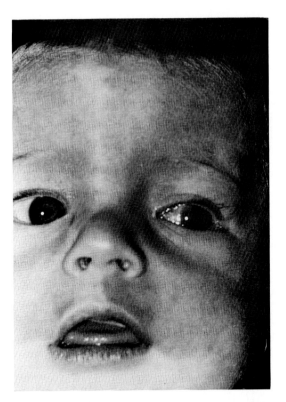

FIG. 4-12. Encephalotrigeminal angiomatosis involving first and second divisions of trigeminal nerve. Congenital glaucoma is present.

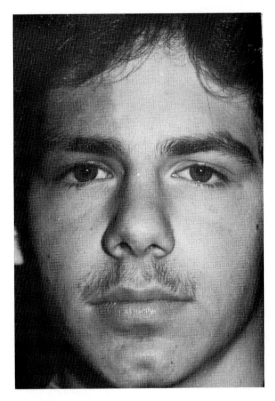

FIG. 4-13. Encephalotrigeminal angiomatosis involving first division of trigeminal nerve. Juvenile-onset glaucoma is present.

hypertrophic effect of the disease itself may contribute to progressive buphthalmos in the absence of marked elevation of intraocular pressure.

It is important to remember that angle closure due to choroidal enlargement may supervene even after successful goniotomy. Therefore these patients should be followed with repeated gonioscopy even if goniotomy is successful. A reasonable approach, therefore, would be to perform goniotomy initially if the angle is open but has the appearance of incomplete cleavage. If the angle is closed at diagnosis or cannot be seen because of corneal edema, trabeculectomy is probably a better choice. If goniotomy is successful, the patient should be followed with routine gonioscopy and trabeculectomy performed when there is obvious progressive closure of the angle.

ENCEPHALOTRIGEMINAL ANGIOMATOSIS

The first case of encephalotrigeminal angiomatosis was probably reported when Schirmer[93] (1860) described a patient with a facial angioma and glaucoma. Sturge[100] (1879) described a hemi-

paretic epileptic girl with a facial angioma and ipsilateral congenital glaucoma and hypothesized that a cerebral angioma resulted in the neurologic defect. Kalischer[56] (1897) confirmed the association between facial and intracranial angiomas at autopsy. Weber[114] and Dimitri[24] independently demonstrated radiologic evidence of intracranial calcification. Elschnig[31] and Nakamura[76] were the first to realize an etiologic relationship between the angioma and the glaucoma. The disease has little familial tendency and no sexual or racial predisposition. Chromosomal abnormalities have been reported in some patients, and the disorder may be a dominant trait with incomplete penetrance. Ocular manifestations occur between birth and early childhood.

Systemic involvement

The hallmark of the disorder is a facial cutaneous angioma (nevus flammeus, port wine stain), which is present at birth, is usually unilateral, and involves the region of distribution of the first and second divisions of the trigeminal nerve[30] (Figs. 4-12 and 4-13). The angioma is a variably sized, burgundy-colored, macular vascular malformation resulting from a loose arrangement of dilated thin-walled capillaries in the dermis and subcutaneous tissue. Bilaterality occurs in 10%[28] to 30%[95] of cases. The supraorbital region is almost always affected, although exceptions have been reported.[25,104] Occasionally hemangiomas of the oral and nasal cavities occur concomitantly. Facial hypertrophy in the region associated with the angioma is common.

A meningeal racemose hemangioma usually occurs ipsilateral to the facial hemangioma. It is ordinarily confined to the pia mater and develops close to the cerebrum, usually over the occipital lobe. Progressive calcification frequently occurs in the subintimal layer of the meningeal arteries and may obliterate the vascular lumen. Calcification and atrophy of the external layers of the cerebral cortex may result in mental retardation. Seizure disorders are common. Focal motor seizures contralateral to the facial nevus may begin at age 1 to 2. The course is characterized by partial or complete remission followed by increased severity of attack. Postepileptic lesions such as hemiparesis, hemiplegia, and homonymous hemianopsia are common.

Various combinations of involved structures may occur. The trisymptomatic form, classically known as Sturge-Weber syndrome, affects the leptomeninges, eyes, and face. Bisymptomatic forms affect the face and eyes or face and leptomeninges. There are no descriptions of a form involving the leptomeninges and eyes and sparing the face. Monosymptomatic forms also occur.

Skeletal malformations such as hemihypertrophy of the face and body have also been reported. Localized or diffuse visceral angiomas may occur in the kidneys, spleen, intestine, pancreas, lungs, and thyroid.

Ocular involvement

Hemangiomas may affect the lid, episclera, conjunctiva, iris, and ciliary body. Anderson's rule states that when the nevus flammeus involves the upper lid, there is ipsilateral intraocular involvement.[3] If the upper lid is spared, the ipsilateral eye is spared. Exceptions may occur.[110] Rarely, orbital involvement results in exophthalmos. Iris hyperchromia occurs in 7% to 8% of cases.[1] Tortuous retinal vessels and scleral melanosis may occur.

Choroidal hemangiomas, which occur in 40% of cases,[28] are the most common ocular abnormality, except perhaps for conjunctival involvement. They are usually diffuse, flat, and involve the posterior pole. The hemangioma is easily overlooked in younger patients and grows slowly. It may appear as an orange-yellow, slightly elevated mass. Pathologically these are cavernous hemangiomas, consisting of thin-walled, blood-filled sinuses, lined by a single layer of endothelium (Fig. 4-14).

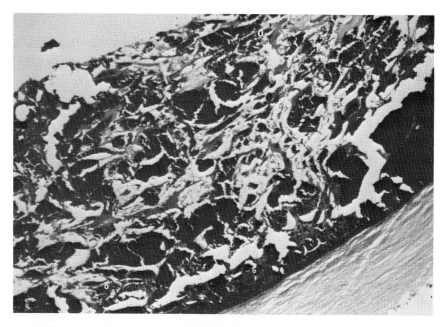

FIG. 4-14. Choroidal hemangioma. (Courtesy R. Cordero Moreno, M.D.)

Exudative retinal detachments may occur after a long period of growth. In some cases a diffuse uveal involvement occurs, which has been termed "tomato catsup" fundus.[101] The hemangioma may be so large as to involve nearly the entire choroid, a situation that sets the stage for surgical disaster by predisposing the patient to expulsive choroidal hemorrhage. Exact calculation of the prevalence of hemangiomas at autopsy is difficult, because the lesion may contract artifactitiously during fixation and not be recognized. Of all cases of choroidal hemangiomas noted on examination of enucleation specimens, 50% occur in encephalotrigeminal angiomatosis.[27]

Glaucoma associated with encephalotrigeminal angiomatosis

One third of patients with the Sturge-Weber syndrome have increased intraocular pressure.[2] Usually this occurs only when the hemangioma involves the eyelid, tarsus, and conjunctiva.

When the cutaneous angioma is unilateral, the buphthalmos or glaucoma is nearly always unilateral and ipsilateral to it. Exceptions have been reported where the glaucoma was contralateral to the hemangioma.[26,98] Bilateral glaucoma rarely occurs with unilateral cutaneous angioma.[31] Bilateral angiomas may be accompanied by either unilateral or bilateral glaucoma.

Of 174 patients with increased intraocular pressure in a large series, 84 had buphthalmos.[19] Alexander and Norman[2] reported that two thirds of their 73 patients had buphthalmos ipsilateral to the nevus and the remaining one third had glaucoma without buphthalmos. Sixty percent of the glaucomas were congenital and 40% adult onset. Buphthalmos without increased intraocular pressure has been reported.[34,57]

Eighty-eight percent of patients with choroidal hemangiomas develop glaucoma,[36] which may be congenital with buphthalmos, adult onset, or secondary to inflammation and uveal reaction, usually following retinal detachment. Some authors have concluded that the presence of choroidal hemangioma in encephalotrigeminal angiomatosis results in glaucoma. However, patients with choroidal hemangiomas who do not have the Sturge-Weber syndrome rarely develop glaucoma. Furthermore, choroidal hemangiomas are frequently associated with anterior segment structural anomalies, which themselves may result in glaucoma.

Numerous mechanisms have been postulated to explain the pathogenesis of glaucoma in encephalotrigeminal angiomatosis. Hudelo[53] theorized that clinically silent meningeal angiomas obstructed ocular drainage into the cavernous sinus, thereby raising intraocular pressure. The neural theory[18,42,88,106] hypothesized that a congenital abnormality of the sympathetic innervation of the eye resulted in uveal capillary dilation, stasis, and glaucoma. Cabannes postulated that the choroidal hemangioma provided an increased blood supply, leading to congenital hypertrophy of ocular structures and glaucoma.[12]

These theories are historically interesting, but vascular or mechanical explanations offer more plausible mechanisms. The mechanical theories are based on occlusion of the anterior chamber angle, leading to blockage of aqueous outflow, increased intraocular pressure, and glaucoma.

Numerous authors have believed that glaucoma is secondary to developmental anomalies that result in chamber angle malformations. Histologic specimens reveal a poorly developed scleral spur, thickened uveal meshwork, and iris root inserted "anteriorly" on the base of the trabecular meshwork (Figs. 4-15 and 4-16).* In some cases a superficial iris stroma appears to cover the meshwork and extend to an insertion on or near Schwalbe's line (Fig. 4-15). This is similar to the description sometimes reported in neurofibromatosis.[48] Posterior displacement and incomplete development of Schlemm's canal has been described.[14,29,90] Persistent embryonic mesodermal tissue may also be found in the angle.[94,115] Patients who develop glaucoma during adolescence or later may have a milder expression of the angle cleavage anomaly, a forme fruste of the disorder, or unrelated primary open-angle glaucoma. In these patients gonioscopy usually reveals a normal-looking angle and the glaucoma is generally more easily controlled, although angle cleavage abnormalities have been found on pathologic examination. Other authors have reported no abnormalities in the angle even in the presence of buphthalmos.[15,114,115]

Hemorrhage from the choroidal hemangioma may result in subretinal hemorrhage and retinal detachment with forward displacement of the iris and angle closure secondary to PAS formation either on a mechanical basis or secondary to neo-

---

*References 3, 7, 10, 14, 36, 45, 61, 90, 91, 117.

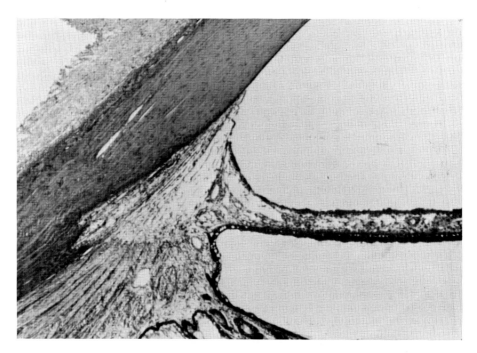

FIG. 4-15. Congenital angle deformity with incomplete cleavage and apparent "anterior insertion of iris" in encephalotrigeminal angiomatosis. (From Weiss, D.I.: Trans. Ophthalmol. Soc. U.K. **93:**477, 1973.)

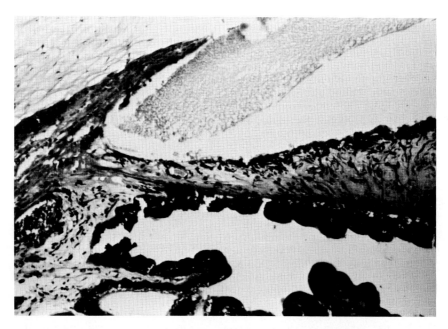

FIG. 4-16. This patient with glaucoma and encephalotrigeminal angiomatosis underwent enucleated at age 16 after hemorrhage from choroidal hemangioma had resulted in a blind, painful eye with elevated intraocular pressure. Angle was partially sealed with peripheral anterior synechiae. In this photograph it is open, but meshwork is compressed and sclerosed. Serosanguinous exudate is present in anterior chamber. (Courtesy R. Cordero Moreno, M.D.)

vascularization.* Most eyes coming under pathological examination have had this severe outcome.

The vascular theories relate the elevation of intraocular pressure to the presence of vascular malformations that might increase production, decrease outflow, or actually change the components of aqueous fluid, or interfere with extrascleral drainage.

Tyson[103] administered fluorescein to a patient with encephalotrigeminal angiomatosis and noted that it appeared in the aqueous in the glaucomatous eye more quickly than in the normal eye. He concluded that increased vascular permeability in the affected eye had caused increased ocular fluid density, which resulted in blockage of the iris angle by "plasmoid aqueous." Intravenous injection of 50% dextrose was found not to lower intraocular pressure in the glaucomatous eye but did in the opposite eye.[29,54] Dunphy[29] postulated a rapid equalization of osmotic pressure due to increased vascular permeability. Others found the protein content of the aqueous to be increased in the glaucomatous eye.[54,70] Subsequently this theory has been experimentally refuted.

Many authors have invoked vascular hypertrophy as the cause for glaucoma.† Increased number and/or size of choroidal vessels has been postulated to cause choroidal congestion with increased transudation and/or decreased outflow of aqueous.[9,29,46,99] There is no experimental proof for these theories.

Mansheim[66] and Miller[72] found glaucomatous eyes in the Sturge-Weber syndrome to have a normal coefficient of outflow and concluded that elevated intraocular pressure was due to increased aqueous production. Fluorophotometric analysis of aqueous production has not been reported.

More recently Weiss[117] found vascular hamartias of the anterior episclera and conjunctiva in all patients examined (Figs. 4-17 and 4-18). Although in the earlier literature patients without episcleral angiomas were reported, these angiomas may be very subtle and occasionally evident only at surgery. Weiss hypothesized that the increased pulse pressure present on tonography was indicative of an arteriovenous fistula and that a combination of elevated episcleral venous pressure, indirectly deduced by the presence of engorged vessels, and a congenital angle malformation contributed in variable proportions to the elevated intraocular pressure.

Phelps[82] examined 19 patients with encephalotrigeminal angiomatosis and glaucoma. All of these patients had episcleral hemangiomas, the extent of which correlated roughly with the severity of the glaucoma. Elevated episcleral venous pressure was present in 11 of 12 eyes in which this was measured. Two patients without glaucoma had small episcleral hemangiomas. Angle deformities of a congenital nature were seen in only two patients. Phelps concluded that an elevation in episcleral venous pressure due to arteriovenous shunts was etiologically responsible for the glaucoma. However, no predictable correlation between the episcleral and intraocular pressures in individual eyes was found.

The most likely cause for elevated intraocular pressure seems to be a combination of angle cleavage anomalies and elevated episcleral venous pressure. The contribution of each to the glaucoma is dependent on the individual case. Careful gonioscopy, tonography, and measurement of episcleral venous pressure are useful in the determination of the cause (Fig. 4-19).

Management

Because the glaucoma in encephalotrigeminal angiomatosis is variable in its severity, medical treatment is warranted if buphthalmos is not present and if the pressure can be adequately controlled. If intraocular pressure is high but outflow is normal or nearly so, drugs that decrease aqueous production, such as timolol or carbonic anhydrase inhibitors, will be most helpful, whereas if outflow is also reduced, miotics and epinephrine compounds may contribute to lowering pressure.

If medical treatment fails, as frequently happens, or if the glaucoma is congenital, surgical intervention is necessary. Goniotomy is the treatment of choice in congenital glaucoma when gonioscopy suggests cleavage abnormalities, and it may be tried if gonioscopy is inconclusive. Nevertheless, this procedure, even repeated, is frequently unsuccessful.[111] Numerous surgical procedures have been reported in the literature, but trabeculectomy appears to be the best choice at the present time. Trabeculectomy bypasses any component of the glaucoma due to elevated episcleral venous pressure, whereas goniotomy does not.

Two serious complications may result from filtering procedures in this disease. Expulsive cho-

---

*References 19, 21, 29, 36, 50, 51, 62, 81.
†References 6, 15, 31, 46, 127.

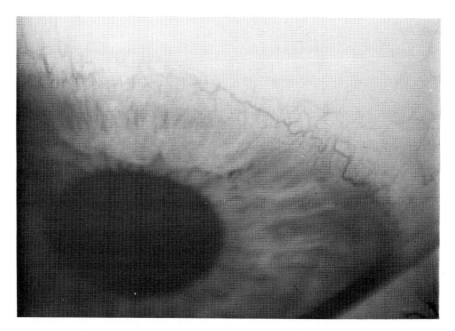

FIG. 4-17. Arteriovenous anastomoses at limbus in same patient as in Fig. 4-13.

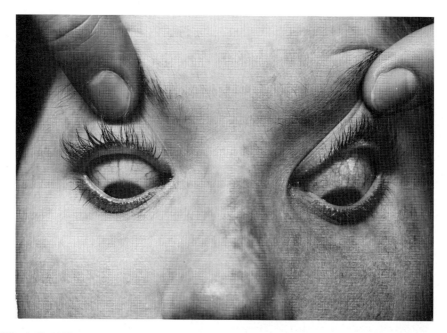

FIG. 4-18. Diffuse involvement of conjunctiva and episclera in patient with glaucoma and encephalotrigeminal angiomatosis. (From Schaffer, R.N., and Weiss, D.I.: Congenital and pediatric glaucomas, St. Louis, 1970, The C.V. Mosby Co.)

roidal hemorrhage may result as soon as the globe is entered or immediately thereafter, because of the presence of a choroidal hemangioma.[14] Precautionary measures should be taken before surgery to reduce intraocular pressure as much as possible, and hyperosmotic agents are strongly recommended. Vitreous loss and bleeding from episcleral vessels are also more common.

The second serious complication is that of sudden onset of choroidal effusion after opening the

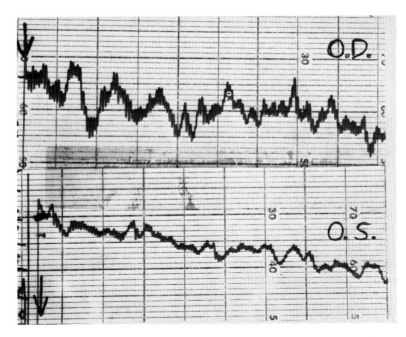

FIG. 4-19. Prominent arterial pulse pressure is present in involved eye *(OD)*, whereas outflow coefficient is not significantly reduced. (From Weiss, D.I.: Trans. Ophthalmol. Soc. U.K. **93:**477, 1973.)

globe due to rapid transudation of fluid from the intravascular to the extravascular space in the face of elevated episcleral (and choroidal) venous pressure when the intraocular pressure is suddenly lowered.[8] Adverse consequences of this may be minimized by performing a posterior sclerotomy before opening the eye.[8,111]

Phelps[82] has suggested that electrocautery or laser photocoagulation might partially obliterate the anterior episcleral vascular anomaly and result in decreased intraocular pressure.

If external filtration fails, cyclocryotherapy can be attempted as a last resort.

Results of therapy for glaucoma in encephalotrigeminal angiomatosis are often disappointing. Hopefully, with further delineation of the mechanisms responsible for the glaucoma, we may develop more successful modalities of treatment.

KLIPPEL-TRENAUNAY-WEBER SYNDROME

Klippel and Trenaunay[59] (1900) described a syndrome characterized by a triad of cutaneous hemangioma extending over one limb, varicosities in the affected limb, and hypertrophy of bone and soft tissue. Parkes Weber[113] (1907) described a similar triad of findings.

Arteriovenous fistulas, vascular hyperplasia, and osseous hypertrophy occur in both syndromes. In the Klippel-Trenaunay syndrome, the fistulas are small, numerous, and of little consequence; in the Parkes Weber syndrome, they are large, few, and may lead to circulatory disturbances.[33] Frequently the two diseases are not differentiated and are included under the heading Klippel-Trenaunay-Weber syndrome.

The disease may be inherited in an irregular dominant pattern.[109] Formes frustes occur, in which one of the three major findings is absent. The congenital hemangioma varies in size, location, and color. Frequently it follows a radicular distribution and may increase in size. Osteohypertrophy is usually present at birth but may develop afterward. The limbs are most commonly involved and may further increase in size with age.

Although the varices in the Klippel-Trenaunay syndrome are congenital in origin, they may first become evident years after birth. They are unilateral and ipsilateral to the skin lesion. The Parkes Weber syndrome is characterized by the occurrence of large arteriovenous fistulas, cirsoid aneurysms, and angiectasias.

Neurologic involvement[79] is demonstrated by electroencephalographic (EEG) abnormalities, seizures, mental retardation, and cerebral hemangiomas.

Ocular findings include enophthalmos, conjunctival telangiectasis, heterochromia iridis, iris coloboma, oculosympathetic palsy, retinal varicosities, choroidal angiomas, Marcus Gunn pupil, strabismus, orbital varices, disc anomalies, glaucoma, and buphthalmos.[79] Ocular findings may occur in the absence of a facial hemangioma.

Glaucoma, with or without buphthalmos, has been described in patients with the Klippel-Trenaunay-Weber syndrome.[49,76,83] Unilateral congenital glaucoma has been reported.[109] In most of these cases patients have also had a facial nevus. In the one patient with a pure form of the Klippel-Trenaunay-Weber syndrome (i.e., not combined with the Sturge-Weber syndrome), elevated intraocular pressures, and unilateral vein occlusion,[49] the association may have been circumstantial.

ANGIOMATOSIS RETINAE

A retinal hemangioma was illustrated for the first time in 1879 by Panas and Remy.[80] Von Hippel[107] described the progression of retinal involvement (1904) and later identified the lesion as a hemangioblastoma. Lindau[64] (1926) discovered angiomatous cysts of the cerebellum in many cases of von Hippel's disease. Subsequently, the combination of angiomas of the retina and central nervous system was referred to as von Hippel–Lindau disease (retinocerebellar angiomatosis). Ballantyne[5] (1930) first reported the occurrence of secondary glaucoma. Nicholson et al.[77] (1976) classified the lesion as a capillary hemangioma on the basis of ultrastructural findings.

The inheritance pattern is autosomal dominant with incomplete penetrance, and the disease usually presents in the second and third decades of life. In addition to the retinal and cerebellar hemangiomas, other viscera may be involved. Symptoms are usually related to the retinal and cerebellar lesions and include headache, vertigo, and cerebellar dysfunction.

The retinal hemangioma is a reddish, globular tumor approximately 1 to 2 disc diameters in size. It is usually located in the midperiphery and contains arteriovenous capillary shunts (Fig. 4-20). The artery and vein leading to and from the hemangioma are characteristically dilated and tortuous. Some 50% of cases occur bilaterally, and

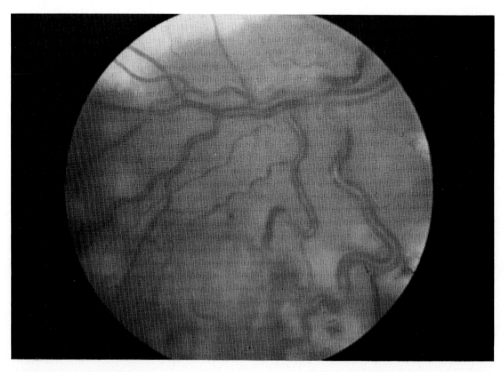

FIG. 4-20. Retinal angioma in von Hippel–Lindau syndrome. Artery and vein feeding and draining angioma are markedly enlarged.

approximately one third of patients have more than one angioma per eye. Occasionally the angioma may occur adjacent to or involve the disc. The presence of a retinal angioma should alert the examiner to search carefully for others that might be at a much earlier stage of development. Fluorescein angiography is often helpful.

The retinal involvement, when untreated, progresses from vascular dilation to transudation into the retina and subretinal space, and to exudation and hemorrhage. Exudation may occur at sites distant from the angioma, and macular exudates with star figures may be the presenting symptom. At this stage the patient may appear to have Coats' disease. Eventually, massive exudation, retinal detachment, and neovascular glaucoma may develop.

The usual course in untreated eyes consists of relentless progression. The hemangiomas should be treated as soon as they are discovered by either cryotherapy or photocoagulation or a combination of the two.[112]

TUBEROUS SCLEROSIS

Tuberous sclerosis was described by Bourneville[11] in 1880. It is inherited through an autosomal dominant gene with low penetrance and variable expressivity. Signs of the disease may be manifest at birth, but the clinical diagnosis is usually made in the first or second decade of life.

The most frequent clinical manifestations consist of a triad of epilepsy, adenoma sebaceum, and mental deficiency. The "ash leaf" sign, seen under ultraviolet light, is believed to be pathognomonic. Intracranial calcified harmartomas ("brainstones") seen radiologically are diagnostic. A wide range of other lesions occurs, including subungual fibromas, cardiac rhabdomyomas, and hamartomas of the kidney, liver, thyroid, and gastrointestinal tract.

The classic ocular lesion is the peripapillary astrocytic hamartoma, or "mulberry lesion," which may be single or multiple. These may undergo cystic degeneration but rarely lead to loss of vision. Sebaceous adenomas of the upper lid and glands of Zeis are less common.

One case of primary glaucoma has been reported.[86] Secondary glaucoma is also extremely rare and results from vitreous hemorrhage,[87] rubeosis iridis, and retinal detachment.[125]

OCULODERMAL MELANOCYTOSIS

Oculodermal melanocytosis, or nevus of Ota, is a hereditary disease usually found in Orientals, most commonly women, characterized by unilateral pigmented nevi in the distribution of the first and second divisions of the trigeminal nerve (Fig. 4-21). Most patients concomitantly have hyperpigmentation of the globe, which may involve the

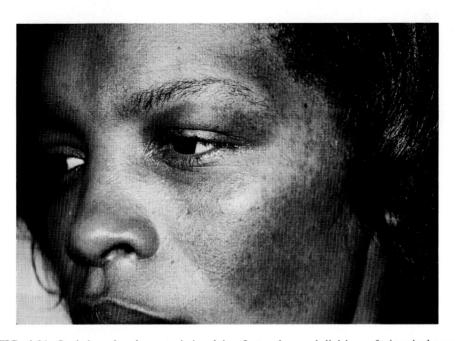

FIG. 4-21. Oculodermal melanocytosis involving first and second divisions of trigeminal nerve.

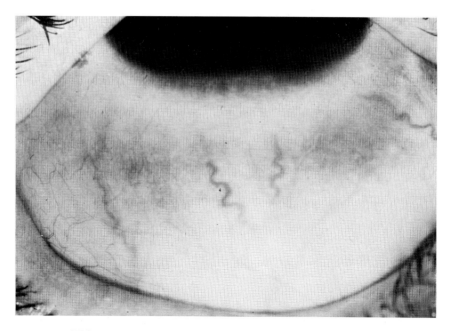

FIG. 4-22. Involvement of sclera in oculodermal melanocytosis.

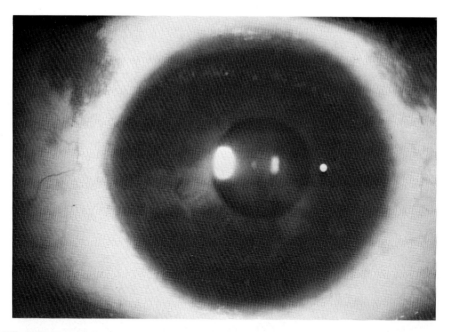

FIG. 4-23. Extensively involved iris in patient with oculodermal melanocytosis. Sclera is involved superiorly.

sclera (Fig. 4-22), conjunctiva, cornea, iris (Fig. 4-23), and fundus. The iridocorneal angle may be extremely hyperpigmented without elevation of intraocular pressure.

What appear to be primary angle-closure[35] and open-angle[35,38] glaucomas have been reported.

Shaffer and Weiss[95] reported elevated intraocular pressure in a patient with nevus of Ota and melanocytic infiltration of the anterior chamber angle. Weiss and Krohn[118] postulated that the melanocytes increased outflow resistance, resulting in "benign melanocytic glaucoma." Secondary glaucomas have been associated with increased numbers of iris processes,[23] malignant melanoma of the iris,[37] and nevus flammeus with retinal angiomatosis.[85]

BASAL CELL NEVUS SYNDROME

The basal cell nevus syndrome is a rare disease transmitted by a highly penetrant autosomal dominant gene. It is characterized by multiple skin tumors, histologically indistinguishable from basal cell carcinomas. Dental cysts, frontal bossing, and skeletal, neurologic, genital, and skin anomalies are seen. Defective renal tubular phosphate reabsorption is common. Hermans et al.[50] classified the disease as a phakomatosis on the basis of the characteristic ocular findings.

The skin tumors may be present at birth but usually become noticeable in adolescence. They are found on the eyelids, nose, cheeks, and trunk and less often on the face, scalp, and neck.[67] Clinically they may resemble nevi, neurofibromas, or skin tags, and their true nature may not be appreciated until pathologic diagnosis. Most lesions are benign but may become invasive. Unlike basal cell carcinoma, the nevus appears in younger individuals and in areas not exposed to sunlight.

Reported ocular findings have included orbital involvement by tumor, hypertelorism, congenital cataract, strabismus, coloboma of the choroid and optic nerve, corneal leukoma, and glaucoma.[47,55] The mechanisms involved and incidence of glaucoma have not been described.

DIFFUSE CONGENITAL HEMANGIOMATOSIS

Diffuse congenital hemangiomatosis is a rare disease in which multiple small cutaneous hemangiomas are associated with visceral hemangiomas. Death usually occurs within the first few months of life, usually as a result of cardiac failure associated with a large hepatic hemangioma.

One case has been associated with infantile glaucoma.[119] Neovascularization of the iris was present and extended into the angles, which were open. The pressures were normalized with a combination of cyclocryotherapy in both eyes and goniotomy in the left eye after the abnormal vessels had cleared. In a second case, a cavernous hemangioma of the iris compressed the ciliary body and occluded the angle adjacent to it, but glaucoma was not present.[75]

REFERENCES

1. Alexander, G.L.: The Sturge-Weber syndrome. In Vinken, P.J., and Bruyn, G.W., editors: Handbook of clinical neurology, the phakomatoses, vol. 14, Amsterdam, 1972, North Holland Publishing Co.
2. Alexander, G.L., and Norman, R.M.: The Sturge-Weber syndrome, Bristol, England, 1960, John Wright & Sons, Ltd.
3. Anderson, J.R.: Hydrophthalmia or congenital glaucoma, London, 1939, Cambridge University Press.
4. Babel, J., and Younessian, S.: Buphthalmie ohne Hypertension: ein Fall von familiärer Neurofibromatose, Ber. Dtsch. Ophthalmol. Ges. **69**:221, 1968.
5. Ballantyne, A.: Buphthalmos with facial nevus and allied conditions, Br. J. Ophthalmol. **14**:481, 1930.
6. Bär, C.: Ein bemerkenswerter Fall von Feuermal und Glaukom, Z. Augenheilkd. **57**:628, 1925.
7. Barkan, O.: Goniotomy for glaucoma associated with nevus flammeus, Am. J. Ophthalmol. **43**:545, 1957.
8. Bellows, A.R., Chylack, L.T., Jr., Epstein, D.L., and Hutchinson, B.T.: Choroidal effusion during glaucoma surgery in patients with prominent episcleral vessels, Arch. Ophthalmol. **97**:493, 1979.
9. Beltman, J.: Ueber angeborene Telangiektasien des Auges als Ursache von Glaucoma simplex, Albrecht Von Graefes Arch. Ophthalmol. **59**:502, 1904.
10. Berkow, T.W.: Retinitis pigmentosa associated with Sturge-Weber syndrome, Arch. Ophthalmol. **75**:72, 1966.
11. Bourneville, D.M.: Sclérose tubéreuse des circonvolutions cérébrales: idiotie et épilepsie hémiplégigue, Arch. Neurol. (Paris) **1**:390, 1881.
12. Cabannes, C.: La buphthalmie congénitale dans ses rapports avec l'hémihypertrophie de la face, Arch. d'Ophthalmol. **29**:368, 1909.
13. Callender, G.R., and Thigpen, C.A.: Two neurofibromas in one eye, Am. J. Ophthalmol. **13**:121, 1930.
14. Christensen, G.R., and Records, R.E.: Glaucoma and expulsive hemorrhage mechanisms in the Sturge-Weber syndrome, Ophthalmology **86**:1360, 1979.
15. Clausen, W.: Discussion on Voegel's paper, Klin. Monatsbl. Augenheilkd. **81**:393, 1928.
16. Collins, T., and Batten, R.D.: Neurofibroma of the eyeball and its appendages, Trans. Ophthalmol. Soc. U.K. **25**:248, 1905.
17. Crowe, F.W., Schull, W.J., and Neil, J.W.: A clinical, pathological and genetic study of multiple neurofibromatosis, Springfield, Ill., 1956, Charles C Thomas Publisher.
18. Cushing, H.: Cases of spontaneous intracranial hemorrhage associated with trigeminal naevi, J.A.M.A. **47**:178, 1906.
19. Danis, P.: Aspects ophthalmologiques des angiomatoses du système nerveux, Acta Neurol. Psychiatr. Belg. **50**:615, 1950.
20. Davis, F.A.: Plexiform neurofibromatosis of orbit and globe with associated glioma of the optic nerve and brain: report of a case, Arch. Ophthalmol. **22**:761, 1939.
21. de Haas, H.L.: Glaukom bei naevus flameus, Ned. Tijdschr. Geneeskd. **2**:4326, 1928.
22. Dejean, C., Hervouet, F., and Leplat, G.: L'embryologie de l'oeil et sa tératologie, Paris, 1958, Masson, Editeur.

23. Dev, S., Jain, I.S., and Nayo, K.: Naevus of Ota associated with glaucoma, Orient. Arch. Ophthalmol. **7**:251, 1969.

24. Dimitri, V.: Tumeur cérébrale congénitale (angiome caverneux), Rev. Assoc. Med. Argent. **6**:63, 1923.

25. Djacos, C., and Joannidès, T.: La Maladie de Sturge-Weber-Krabbe, Ann. Ocul. **184**:994, 1951.

26. Duhamel, E., and Goetz, G.: A propos de l'angiomatose encéphalo-trigéminée, Bull. Soc. Ophthalmol. Fr. **6**: 541, 1954.

27. Duke-Elder, S.: System of ophthalmology, vol. 9, Diseases of the uveal tract, St. Louis, 1966, The C.V. Mosby Co., p. 808.

28. Duke-Elder, S.: System of ophthalmology, vol. 11, Diseases of the lens and vitreous; glaucoma, and hypotony, St. Louis, 1969, The C.V. Mosby Co., p. 639.

29. Dunphy, E.B.: Glaucoma accompanying nevus flammeus, Am. J. Ophthalmol. **18**:709, 1935.

30. Ehrlich, L.M.: Bilateral glaucoma associated with unilateral nevus flammeus, Arch. Ophthalmol. **25**:1002, 1941.

31. Elschnig, A.: Naevus vasculosus mit gleichseitigem Hydrophthalmus, Z. Augenheilkd. **39**:189, 1918.

32. Fabricant, R.N., Todaro, G.J., and Eldridge, R.: Increased levels of a nerve-growth-factor cross-reacting protein in "central" neurofibromatosis, Lancet **1**:4, 1979.

33. Faivre, G., Pernot, C., Gilgenkrantz, J.M., and Cherrier, F.: Les shunts arterioveneux des emembres: à propos d'une observation, Soc. Med. Nancy, May 11, 1960.

34. Falk, W.: Beitrag zur Aetiologie und Klinik der Sturge Weberschen Krankheit, Osten. Z. Kinderheilkd. **5**:175, 1950.

35. Fishman, F.R.A., and Anderson, R.: Nevus of Ota, Am. J. Ophthalmol. **54**:453, 1962.

36. Font, R.L., and Ferry, A.P.: The phakomatoses, Int. Ophthalmol. Clin. **12**:1, 1972.

37. Font, R.L., Reynolds, A.N., and Zimmerman, L.E.: Diffuse malignant melanoma of the iris in the nevus of Ota, Arch. Ophthalmol. **77**:513, 1967.

38. Foulks, G.N., and Shields, M.B.: Glaucoma in oculodermal melanocytosis, Ann. Ophthalmol. **9**:1299, 1977.

39. François, J.: Ocular aspects of the phakomatoses. In Vinken, P.J., and Bruyn, G.W., editors: Handbook of clinical neurology, the phakomatoses, vol. 14, Amsterdam, 1972, North Holland Publishing Co.

40. François, J., and Katz, C.: Association homolatérale d'hydrophalmie de névrome plexiforme de la paupière supérieure et d'hémihypertrophie faciale dans la maladie de Recklinghausen, Ophthalmologica **142**:549, 1961.

41. Freeman, D.: Neurofibromata of the choroid, Arch. Ophthalmol. **11**:641, 1934.

42. Freese, L.: Hydrophthalmus beim Erwachsenen, Verchardl. Berl. Augenarztl. Ges., Nov. 25, 1910.

43. Freidenwald, J.S.: Ophthalmic pathology atlas and textbook, Philadelphia, 1952, W.B. Saunders Co., p. 431.

44. Friedman, M.W., and Ritchey, C.L.: Unilateral congenital glaucoma, neurofibromatosis and pseudoarthrosis, Arch. Ophthalmol. **70**:294, 1963.

45. Gass, J.D.M.: The phakomatoses. In Smith, J.L., editor: Neuro-ophthalmology, vol. 2, St. Louis, 1965, The C.V. Mosby Co.

46. Ginzburg, J.: Glaukom und Feuermal mit Akromegalie, Klin. Monatsbl. Augenheilkd. **76**:393, 1926.

47. Gorlin, R.J., Vickers, R.A., Kellen, E., and Williamson, J.J.: The multiple basal-cell nevi syndrome, Cancer **18**:89, 1965.

48. Grant, W.M., and Walton, D.S.: Distinctive gonioscopic findings in glaucoma due to neurofibromatosis, Arch. Ophthalmol. **79**:127, 1968.

49. Heinhold, P., and Nover, A.: Augenveränderungen beim Klippel-Trenaunay-Weber Syndrom, Fortschr. Med. **89**: 91, 1971.

50. Hermans, E.H., Grosfeld, J.C.M., and Valk, L.E.M.: Naevus epitheliomatides multiplex, een vijfde Facomatose, Ned. Tijdschr. Geneeskd. **103**:1795, 1959.

51. Hogan, M., and Zimmerman, L.: Ophthalmic pathology, an atlas and textbook, Philadelphia, 1962, W.B. Saunders Co., p. 433.

52. Hoyt, C.M., and Billson, F.: Buphthalmos in neurofibromatosis: Is it an expression of regional giantism? J. Pediatr. Ophthalmol. **14**:228, 1977.

53. Hudelo, A.: Glaucome et naevus facial, Ann. Ocul. **166**: 889, 1929.

54. Joy, H.H.: Nevus flammeus associated with glaucoma, Trans. Am. Ophthalmol. Soc. **47**:93, 1949.

55. Kahn, L.B., and Gordon, W.: Basal cell naevus syndrome, S. Afr. Med. J. **41**:832, 1967.

56. Kalischer, S.: Demonstration des Gehirns eines Kindes mit Telangiectasie der linksseitigen Gesichtskopfhaut und Hirnoberflache, Berl. Klin. Wochenschr. **34**:1059, 1897.

57. King, G., and Schwartz, G.A.: Sturge-Weber syndrome, Arch. Int. Med. **94**:743, 1954.

58. Kissel, P., and Dureux, J.B.: Limites nosologiques et conception générale des phakomatoses. In Michaux, L., and Feld, M., editors: Les phakomatoses cérébrales, Paris, 1963, S.P.E.I.

59. Klippel, M., and Trenaunay, P.: Du naevus variqueux ostéo-hypertrophique, Arch. Gén. Méd. **77**:641, 1900.

60. Knight, M.S.: A critical survey of neoplasms of the choroid, Am. J. Ophthalmol. **8**:791, 1925.

61. Kwitko, M.L.: Glaucoma in infants and children, New York, 1973, Appleton-Century-Crofts, pp. 344-347.

62. Lawford, J.B.: Naevus of left side of face: naevus of choroid, subretinal hemorrhage and detached retina in left eye, Trans. Ophthalmol. Soc. U.K. **5**:136, 1885.

63. Lieb, W.A., Wirth, W.A., and Geeraets, W.J.: Hydrophthalmos and neurofibromatosis, Confin. Neurol. **19**:230, 1958.

64. Lindau, A.: Studien uber Kleinhirncysten, Acta Pathol. Microbiol. Scand. **1**(suppl):1, 1926.

65. Mann, I.: Developmental abnormalities of the eye, London, 1957, British Medical Association.

66. Mansheim, B.J.: Aqueous outflow measurements by continuous tonometry in some unusual forms of glaucoma, Arch. Ophthalmol. **50**:580, 1953.

67. Markovits, A.S., and Quickert, M.H.: Basal cell nevus, Arch. Ophthalmol. **88**:397, 1972.

68. Martyn, I., and Knox, D.L.: Glial hamartoma of the retina in generalized neurofibromatosis, Br. J. Ophthalmol. **56**:487, 1972.

69. Meeker, L.H.: Two tumors of the eye, Arch. Ophthalmol. **16**:152, 1936.

70. Mehney, G.H.: Naevus flammeus associated with glaucoma, Arch. Ophthalmol. **17**:1018, 1937.

71. Michelson-Rabinowitsch, C.: Beitrag zur Kenntnis des Hydrophthalmus congenitus, Arch. Augenheilkd. **55:** 245, 1906.

72. Miller, S.J.H.: Symposium: the Sturge-Weber syndrome, Proc. R. Soc. Med. **56:**419, 1963.

73. Moore, R.F.: Diffuse neurofibromatosis with propotosis, Br. J. Ophthalmol. **15:**272, 1931.

74. Murakami, S.: Zur pathologischen Anatomie und Pathogenese des Buphthalmus bei Neurofibromatosis, Klin. Monatsbl. Augenheilkd. **51:**514, 1913.

75. Naidoff, M.A., Kenyon, K., and Green, W.: Iris hemangioma and abnormal retinal vasculature in a case of diffuse congenital hemangiomatosis, Am. J. Ophthalmol. **72:**633, 1971.

76. Nakamura, B.: Angeborener halbseitiger Naevus flammeus mit Hydrophthalmus und Knochenverdickung derselben Seite, Klin. Monatsbl. Augenheilkd. **69:**312, 1922.

77. Nicholson, D.H., Green, W.R., and Kenyon, R.K.: Light and electron microscopic study of early lesions in angiomatosis retinae, Am. J. Ophthalmol. **82:**193, 1976.

78. Nicolai, C.: Un névrome plexiforme, Arch. Ophthalmol. (Paris) **29:**59, 1909.

79. O'Connor, P.S., and Smith, J.D.: Optic nerve variant in the Klippel-Trenaunay-Weber syndrome, Ann. Ophthalmol. **10:**131, 1978.

80. Panas, F., and Remy, D.A.: Anatomie Pathologique de l'Oeil, Paris, 1879, Delahaye & Cie, p. 88.

81. Paton, L., and Collins, E.T.: Angioma of the choroid, Trans. Ophthalmol. Soc. U.K. **39:**157, 1919.

82. Phelps, C.D.: The pathogenesis of glaucoma in Sturge-Weber syndrome, Ophthalmology **85:**276, 1978.

83. Pietruschka, G.: Zur Symptomatic der Syndrome nach Sturge-Weber und Klippel-Trenaunay, Klin. Monatsbl. Augenheilkd. **137:**545, 1960.

84. Politi, F., Sachs, R., and Barishak, R.: Neurofibromatosis and congenital glaucoma, Ophthalmologica **176:**155, 1978.

85. Reinke, R.T., Haber, K., and Josselson, A.: Ota nevus, multiple hemangioma and Takayasu arteritis, Arch. Dermatol. **110:**447, 1974.

86. Renard, G.: Aspects Pathologiques du Fond d'Oeil dans les Affections de la Retine, Paris, 1946, Masson, Editeur.

87. Robertson, D.M.: Ophthalmic findings. In Gomez, M., editor: Tuberous sclerosis, New York, 1979, Raven Press.

88. Rotth, A.: Muttermal und Glaukom (abstract), Zentralbl. Gesamte. Ophthalmol. **20:**588, 1929.

89. Sachsalber, A.: Uber das Rankenneurom der Orbita mit sekundaren Buphthalmus, Beitr. Z. Prakt. Augenheilkd. **27:**1, 1897.

90. Safar, K.: Histologischer Beitrag zur Frage des ursächlichen Zusammenhanges zwischen Hydrophthalmus congenitus und Naevus flammeus, Z. Augenheilkd. **51:**301, 1923.

91. Salus, R.: Glaukom und Feuermal, Klin. Monatsbl. Augenheilkd. **71:**305, 1923.

92. Schiess-Gemuseus: Vier Fälle angeborener Anomalie des Auges, Albrecht Von Graefes Arch. Ophthalmol. **30:** 191, 1884.

93. Schirmer, R.: Ein Fall von Teleangiektasie, Albrecht Von Graefes Arch. Ophthalmol. **7:**119, 1860.

94. Sedlacek, J., and Vrabec, F.: Angioma of the choroid and Sturge-Weber-Krabbe's syndrome, Cesk. Oftal. **17:** 232, 1961.

95. Shaffer, R.N., and Weiss, D.I.: Congenital and pediatric glaucomas, St. Louis, 1970, The C.V. Mosby Co., pp. 60-75.

96. Siggers, D.C., Boyer, S.H., and Eldridge, R.: Nerve growth factor in disseminated neurofibromatosis, N. Engl. J. Med. **292:**1134, 1978.

97. Snell, S., and Collins, E.T.: Plexiform neuroma of temporal region, orbit, eyelid and eyeball, Trans. Ophthalmol. Soc. U.K. **23:**157, 1903.

98. Stoermer, J.: Krankheitsbild und Ätiologie der Sturge-Weberschen Erkrankung, Medizinische **6:**221, 1956.

99. Stoll, K.L.: Nevus flammeus and glaucoma, Trans. Am. Acad. Ophthalmol. Otolaryngol. **41:**534, 1936.

100. Sturge, W.A.: A case of partial epilepsy due to a lesion of one of the vasomotor centers of the brain, Trans. Clin. Soc. London **12:**162, 1879.

101. Susac, J.O., Smith, J.L., and Scelfo, R.J.: The "tomato-catsup" fundus in Sturge-Weber syndrome, Arch. Ophthalmol. **92:**69, 1974.

102. Sutherland, G.A., and Mayou, M.S.: Neurofibromatosis of the fifth nerve with buphthalmus, Trans. Ophthalmol. Soc. U.K. **27:**79, 1907.

103. Tyson, H.H.: Nevus flammeus of the face and the globe, Arch. Ophthalmol. **8:**365, 1932.

104. Vannas, M.: Naevus flammeus pa hogra armen och handen och glaucoma pa hogra ogat, Finska Lak.-Sallsk. Handl. **76:**399, 1934.

105. Verhoeff, F.H.: Discussion of paper by Snell and Collins, Trans. Ophthalmol. Soc. U.K. **23:**176, 1903.

106. Von Baerensprung: Naevus unius lateris, Ann. Charite-Krankenh. Berlin **11:**91, 1863.

107. von Hippel, E.: Über eine sehr seltene Erkrankung der Netzhaut, Albrecht Von Graefes Arch. Ophthalmol. **59:** 83, 1904.

108. von Recklinghausen, F.: Über die multiplen Fibrome der Haut und ihre Beziehung zu den multiplen Neuromen, Berlin, 1882, Hirschwald.

109. Waardenburg, P.J., Franceschetti, A., and Klein, D.: Genetics and ophthalmology, vol. 2, Springfield, Ill., 1973, Charles C Thomas, Publisher, p. 1381.

110. Walsh, F.B., and Hoyt, W.F.: Clinical neuroophthalmology, vol. 3, ed. 3, Baltimore, 1969, The Williams & Wilkins Co.

111. Walton, D.S.: Hemangioma of the lid with glaucoma. In Chandler, P.A., and Grant, W.M., editors: Glaucoma, Philadelphia, 1979, Lea & Febiger.

112. Watzke, R.C., Weingeist, T.A., and Constantine, J.B.: Diagnosis and management of von Hippel-Lindau disease. In Peyman, G.A., Apple, D.J., and Sanders, D.R., editors: Intraocular tumors, New York, 1977, Appleton-Century-Crofts.

113. Weber, F.P.: Angioma-formation in connection with hypertrophy of limbs and hemihypertrophy, Br. J. Dermatol. **19:**231, 1907.

114. Weber, F.P.: On the association of extensive hemangiomatosis nevus of the skin with cerebral (meningeal) hemangioma, Proc. R. Soc. Med. **22:**431, 1928.

115. Weekers, R., Prijot, E., Delmarcelle, Y., et al.: Le diagnostic précoce du glaucome débutant, Bull. Soc. Belge Ophthalmol. **121:**1, 1959.

116. Weinstein, A.: Ein Fall von Buphthalmus mit kongenitaler Hypertrophie des Oberlides, Klin. Monatsbl. Augenheilkd. **47:**577, 1909.

117. Weiss, D.I.: Dual origin of glaucoma in encephalotrigeminal angiomatosis, Trans. Ophthalmol. Soc. U.K. **93:**477, 1973.

118. Weiss, D.I., and Krohn, D.L.: Benign melanocytic glaucoma complicating oculodermal melanocytosis, Ann. Ophthalmol. **3:**958, 1971.

119. Weiss, M.J., and Ernest, J.T.: Diffuse congenital hemangiomatosis with infantile glaucoma, Am. J. Ophthalmol. **81:**216, 1976.

120. Wheeler, J.M.: Plexiform neurofibromatosis involving the choroid, ciliary body and other structures, Am. J. Ophthalmol. **20:**368, 1937.

121. Wiener, A.: A case of neurofibromatosis with buphthalmus, Arch. Ophthalmol. **54:**481, 1925.

122. Wolter, J.R.: Nerve fibrils in ovoid bodies, Arch. Ophthalmol. **73:**696, 1965.

123. Wolter, J.R., and Butler, R.: Pigment spots of the iris and ectropion uveae with glaucoma in neurofibromatosis, Am. J. Ophthalmol. **56:**964, 1963.

124. Wolter, J.R., Gonzales-Sirit, R., and Mankin, W.J.: Neurofibromatosis of the choroid, Am. J. Ophthalmol. **54:**217, 1962.

125. Wolter, J.R., and Mertus, J.M.: Exophytic retinal astrocytoma in tuberous sclerosis, J. Pediatr. Ophthalmol. **6:**186, 1969.

126. Yamanaka, R.: Naevus Flammeus mit gleichseitigem Glaukom, Klin. Monatsbl. Augenheilkd. **78:**372, 1927.

127. Zaun, W.: Ueber die Beziehungen zwischen Naevus flammeus und angeborenem Glaukom, Klin. Monatsbl. Augenheilkd. **72:**57, 1924.

128. Zelkowitz, M., and Stambouly, J.: Diminished epidermal growth factor binding by neurofibromatosis fibroblasts, Ann. Neurol. **8:**296, 1980.

Chapter 5

GLAUCOMA ASSOCIATED WITH CONGENITAL DISORDERS

Alan H. Friedman, Marvin L. Kwitko, and Robert Ritch

Glaucoma may occur as a feature of many congenital disorders. In many cases the congenital glaucoma is primary congenital glaucoma, whereas in others it may be secondary. In some cases the line between primary and secondary begins to blur. Disorders that affect numerous tissues and organs within the body often affect the eye as well, and developmental anomalies of the iridocorneal angle are one manifestation of what may be a protean list of abnormalities.

In this chapter we have not attempted an exhaustive listing of all syndromes associated with developmental glaucomas, primary or secondary, but instead give an overview of the more important disorders not covered elsewhere in this book.

GLAUCOMA ASSOCIATED WITH CHROMOSOMAL ABNORMALITIES
Trisomy 13 (Trisomy D; Patau's syndrome)

The systemic[34] and ocular[2,17] findings in trisomy 13 are summarized as follows:
A. Systemic findings
 1. Mental retardation
 2. Low-set, malformed ears
 3. Cleft lip and palate
 4. Sloping forehead
 5. Facial angiomas
 6. Cryptorchidism
 7. Narrow, hyperconvex nails
 8. Flexed or overlapping fingers
 9. Posterior prominence of heels
 10. Transverse palmar creases
 11. Cardiac and renal anomalies
 12. Arrhinencephaly
 13. Bicornuate uterus
 14. Apneic spells
 15. Deafness
 16. Seizures
 17. Hypotonia
B. Ocular findings
 1. Microphthalmos
 2. Cyclopia (rare)
 3. Epicanthal folds
 4. Iridogoniodysgenesis
 5. Coloboma of iris, ciliary body, and choroid
 6. Retinal dysplasia
 7. Persistent hyperplastic primary vitreous (PHPV)
 8. Cataract
 9. Glaucoma; immature anterior chamber angle

The most common findings are microphthalmos, colobomas, retinal dysplasia, and cataracts. The condition is usually severe and incompatible with life, although milder forms have been reported.[25] Congenital glaucoma associated with anterior chamber angle dysgenesis may occur.[12] If the general condition of the patient warrants it, surgical treatment (goniotomy, trabeculotomy, or trabeculectomy) should be performed.

Chromosome 18 deletion syndrome

The systemic[32] and ocular[46] findings in the chromosome 18 deletion syndrome are summarized as follows:
A. Systemic findings

1. Low-set ears
2. Nasal abnormalities
3. External genital abnormalities
4. Hepatosplenomegaly
5. Cardiovascular abnormalities
6. Holoprosencephaly
B. Ocular findings
   1. Hypertelorism
   2. Epicanthus
   3. Ptosis
   4. Strabismus
   5. Nystagmus
   6. Myopia
   7. Microphthalmos
   8. Microcornea
   9. Corneal opacities
   10. Posterior keratoconus
   11. Uveal colobomas
   12. Retinal abnormalities
   13. Optic atrophy
   14. Glaucoma; immature anterior chamber angle

Although three separate types of deletion defects have been reported (deletion of a short arm, or 18p⁻; deletion of a long arm, or 18q⁻; and deletion of parts of the long and short arms, producing a ring 18 chromosome), no specific ocular abnormalities relate to the different forms of deletion. Congenital glaucoma may occur in association with developmental abnormalities of the anterior chamber angle.

Trisomy 18 (Edward's syndrome)

Trisomy 18 consists of a multitude of inconsistent malformations affecting every organ system. Ocular findings[31,42] include corneal and lens opacities, amaurosis, optic atrophy, blue sclerae, disc colobomas, and congenital glaucoma.

Trisomy 21 (Down's syndrome)

Down's syndrome is usually due to nondysjunction of chromosome 21 or, more rarely, a translocation of chromosome 21 with centric fusion between chromosomes 21 and 15 or between 21 and 22. In the case of translocation, the karyotype contains 46 chromosomes. The systemic and ocular findings are summarized as follows:
A. Systemic findings
   1. Mental retardation
   2. Short stature
   3. Flat occiput
   4. Low-set, malformed ears

5. Small nose
6. Large fissured tongue
7. Simian crease across palms
8. Congenital heart defects
9. Dry, scaly skin
B. Ocular findings
   1. Hypertelorism
   2. Mongoloid slant
   3. Epicanthal folds
   4. Blepharitis
   5. Ectropion
   6. Hyperopia
   7. High myopia
   8. Keratoconus
   9. Brushfield's spots
   10. Esotropia
   11. Congenital glaucoma

Congenital glaucoma may occur rarely, and one patient with Down's syndrome and Rieger's anomaly has been described[7] (Fig. 5-1).

Turner's syndrome

Approximately 1 of 5000 phenotypic females has an XO karyotype (45 chromosomes), presumably because of nondysjunction during maternal

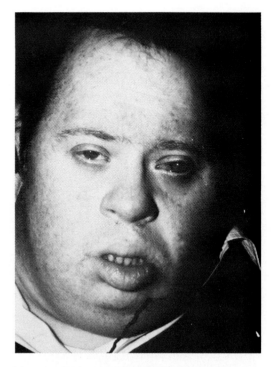

FIG. 5-1. Clinical photograph of patient with trisomy 21 and keratoconus with corneal hydrops OS.

or paternal gametogenesis. Other sex chromosome abnormalities, such as mosaicism (XO/XX), have also been demonstrated. The female has either an absent X chromosome, a mosaic sex chromosome pattern, or a so-called isochromosome for the long arm of the X or ring X chromosome.

Females with Turner's syndrome are characterized clinically by a short stature, webbed neck, undeveloped breasts, ovarian dysgenesis, and primary amenorrhea. Coarctation of the aorta, diabetes, and hypothyroidism may occur.

Male patients with the classic nonurogenital female clinical characteristics of Turner's syndrome have occasionally been reported. The male has small testes with unilateral or bilateral cryptorchidism and a small prostate. The 17-ketosteroid excretion is low to normal, and the urinary gonadotropins are elevated. The buccal smear and karyotype are usually normal and may cause some confusion as to the precise definition of male Turner's syndrome.

Ocular anomalies[23] in females include bilateral epicanthal folds, ptosis, hypertelorism, nystagmus, strabismus, refractive errors, color blindness, blue sclerae, corneal nebulae, and iris colobomas. Concomitant Coats' disease has been described.[4] Congenital glaucoma may occur,[22] whereas associated primary open-angle glaucoma is probably coincidental.[23] Angle-closure glaucoma may occur and is usually primary. A male patient was reported to have angle-closure glaucoma secondary to a long-standing retinal detachment and intumescent lens.[18]

GLAUCOMA ASSOCIATED WITH "GENERALIZED" SYNDROMES
Oculocerebrorenal syndrome (Lowe's syndrome)

Over 150 cases of the oculocerebrorenal syndrome have been reported since it was first described by Lowe et al.[26] in 1952. It is characterized by mental retardation, hypotonia, hyperaminoaciduria, ketonuria, glycosuria, slight albuminuria, and rickets. There is a decrease in serum CO_2 and phosphorus.

The condition occurs in males and is probably sex linked. A few cases have been reported in females. Both proximal and distal renal tubular disease are present, causing the systemic metabolic acidosis, alkaline urinary pH, and low urine specific gravity with proteinuria and glycosuria. Lack of renal reabsorption of phosphorus causes phosphaturia and hypophosphatemia. Bone reabsorption occurs partially under the influence of secondary hyperparathyroidism, which leads to osteomalacia in the infant. Phosphorus is lost from bone to plasma and then into the urine. Further, the alkaline urine creates an increase in calcium loss, since calcium accompanies the excretion of bicarbonate. Diminished serum calcium adds to the parathyroid stimulus and bone reabsorption.

The basic enzymatic abnormality remains unknown. Recently urinary excretion of a large amount of bound sialic acid and of undersulfated chondroitin sulfate A was reported.[1] The primary defect may reside in an abnormality of sulfation of glycosaminoglycans.

The two principal ocular abnormalities are cataracts, which are usually bilateral and occur in nearly all cases, and glaucoma, which occurs in approximately 70% of cases. Other ocular findings include microphthalmos, strabismus, nystagmus, miosis, and iris atrophy.

The lens is probably involved before the fifth week of development, whereas other ocular abnormalities occur later in embryogenesis. The lens capsule is irregularly thickened anteriorly and in the equatorial region, where wartlike excrescences are observed. In the region of the posterior pole, the capsule becomes thin and defective, giving rise to a prominent convexity (posterior lenticonus). Here the lens and vitreous appear to be fused. Proliferated and metaplastic cells from the migrated lens epithelium may be observed among fibrils of the anterior hyaloid membrane.

Female carriers frequently show scattered punctate lens opacities detectable by slit-lamp examination.[45] These are not associated with visual impairment but are a valuable clue in detection of the carrier state (Fig. 5-2).

There is little precise information on the character of the glaucoma. The mechanism appears to be related to faulty development of the filtration angle. Gonioscopy often reveals nothing specific, although the extension of the hypoplastic iris stroma onto the trabecular meshwork and covering the anterior ciliary face and scleral spur has been described.[43] Histopathologic examination has generally revealed incomplete angle differentiation, with partial failure of separation of the iris root from the trabecular meshwork, anterior displacement of ciliary processes onto the posterior iris, and insertion of fibers of the ciliary muscle into

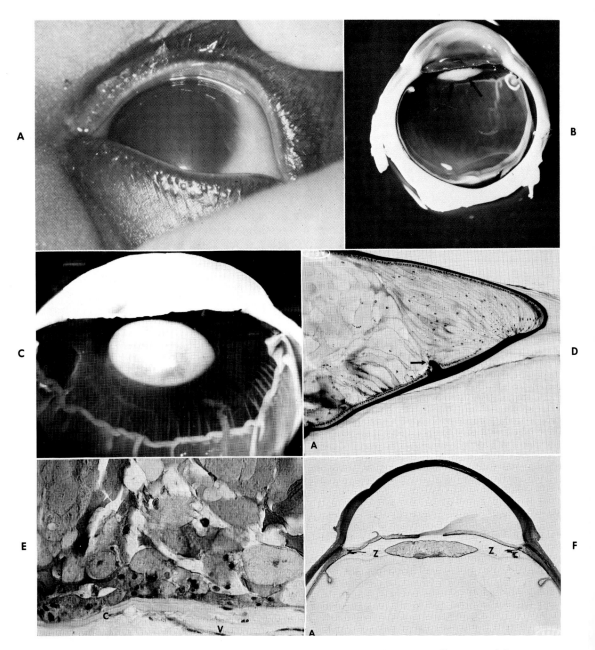

FIG. 5-2. A, Clinical photograph of patient with Lowe's syndrome revealing corneal haze. **B,** Gross photograph of autopsy specimen taken from 8-month-old boy with Lowe's syndrome. Cataractous lens is quite small and disc shaped. There is a densely opaque subcapsular lesion with prominent convexity projecting from posterior pole *(arrows)*. Cornea and anterior chamber are larger than normal because of congenital glaucoma. **C,** Oblique view of posterior surface of same lens. **D,** Photomicrograph showing irregular thickening of lens capsule. Wartlike excrescences *(arrow),* posterior migration of lens epithelium, and disorganization of cortical architecture are evident. **E,** In region of posterior polar opacity, lens capsule *(c)* is deficient, and proliferated lenticular cells are observed among fibrils of anterior vitreous *(V)*. **F,** Anterior chamber angle is incompletely formed. Iris is incompletely separated from trabecular meshwork. Ciliary processes appear to be drawn in toward small lens by taut zonular ligaments *(Z)* and are farther forward than normal. Ora serrata is also farther forward than normal. (**B** to **F** from Zimmerman, L.E., and Font, R.L.: J.A.M.A. **196:**684, 1966. Copyright 1966, American Medical Association.)

both the trabecular meshwork and the scleral spur.[6,14,27]

The glaucoma is particularly unresponsive to treatment, and goniotomy is only rarely successful. Filtration surgery also has a low rate of success but should be attempted.

Oculodentodigital dysplasia

Oculodentodigital dysplasia is characterized systemically by diffuse skeletal dysplasia, syndactyly, hypoplastic dental enamel, microdontia, and a characteristic thin nose.[30] Multiple ocular anomalies may be found, most of which are inconsistent, except for microcornea.[15]

Glaucoma is an inconsistent feature of the disorder but appears to occur more frequently than randomly. Many patients develop glaucoma in early adulthood, but congenital glaucoma has been described.[21] Iris stromal hypoplasia and fine iris processes extending to Schwalbe's line may be present.[15] One case of chronic angle-closure glaucoma associated with bilateral microcornea has been reported.[41]

Patients previously recorded as having normal intraocular pressures have gone on to develop glaucoma,[8,15] and these patients should be watched regularly.

Hallermann-Streiff syndrome

Micrognathia and dwarfism in the Hallermann-Streiff syndrome may be associated with ocular abnormalities, including cataracts and microphthalmos. Glaucoma may also be present in association with absorption of lens material.

Rubinstein-Taybi syndrome

Patients with the Rubinstein-Taybi syndrome have unusually large thumbs and toes. Other features include hypertelorism, myopia, mental retardation, and congenital glaucoma.[3,24,28]

Familial histiocytic dermatoarthritis

Patients with familial histiocytic dermatoarthritis have multiple histiocytic cutaneous and subcutaneous nodules; thickened, lichenified skin; and an arthropathy with symmetric destructive arthritis, primarily of the hands and wrists. Ocular findings include uveitis, cataracts, and glaucoma.[48] The mechanism of the glaucoma is uncertain.

Pierre Robin syndrome

The Pierre Robin syndrome is characterized by micrognathia, a cleft palate, and glossoptosis. Pa-

tients are often described as having an "Andy Gump" or "birdlike" face. Other abnormalities include flattening of the base of the nose, finger and toe anomalies, hearing loss, and hydrocephalus. Once the diagnosis is made postnatally, these children must be observed carefully, since they may have difficulty swallowing, choking spells, and bouts of cyanosis due to glossoptosis. Respiratory tract infections and failure to thrive occur at a later age. Five of the 39 cases reported by Smith and Stowe[40] in four generations of a pedigree died from congenital heart disease, and nine had cardiac murmurs. The heart defects included patent ductus arteriosus and foramen ovale, auricular septal defect, and cor triloculare with coarctation of the aorta. Since these children frequently require surgery, these defects must be remembered.

Opitz et al.[33] have suggested that all patients with the Pierre Robin syndrome, dominantly inherited myopia with or without retinal detachment and deafness, dominantly inherited cleft palate, and dominantly inherited mild spondyloepiphyseal dysplasia should be suspected of having Stickler's syndrome (see Chapter 11).

Congenital glaucoma may occur.[30] Schreiner et al.[38] described a patient with glaucoma secondary to retinal detachment and a dislocated lens in one eye and glaucoma (mechanism not mentioned) in the other. Neovascular glaucoma has also been reported in association with Stickler's syndrome.[47] No doubt, more will be learned about the nature and frequency of glaucoma in these syndromes as Stickler's syndrome becomes more widely recognized.

GLAUCOMA RELATED TO OTHER OCULAR DISORDERS
Microphthalmos

Three general types of microphthalmos have been described. They are "pure" microphthalmos, or nanophthalmos; microphthalmos with a cyst; and microphthalmos associated with other systemic anomalies.

Nanophthalmos is a rare clinical syndrome with a suggested familial predisposition and is characterized by a globe 13 to 17 mm in diameter. The features of the condition include hypermetropia of +13 to +18 D, small corneal diameters (about 10 mm), extremely thickened sclera, narrow anterior chamber angles, and glaucoma occurring at age 30 to 55. The glaucoma is usually of the angle-closure type. Glaucoma surgery is fraught with

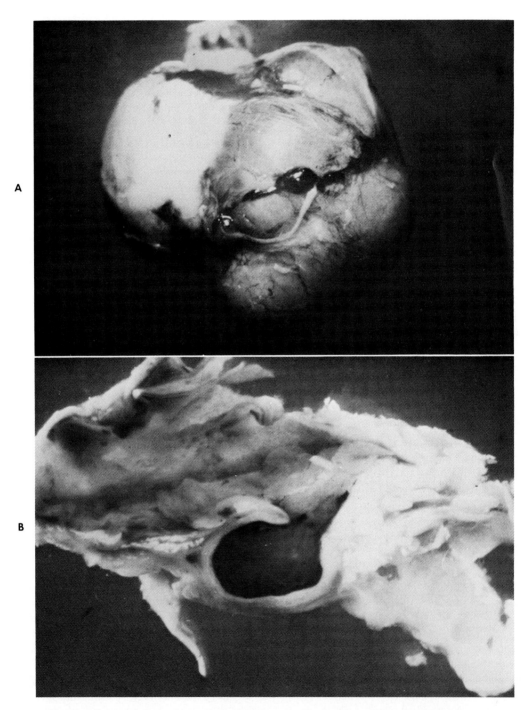

FIG. 5-3. Microphthalmos with orbital cyst. **A,** Gross photograph of globe at left with large orbital cyst attached to globe. **B,** Cut section reveals globe at right with communication to cyst above and at left.

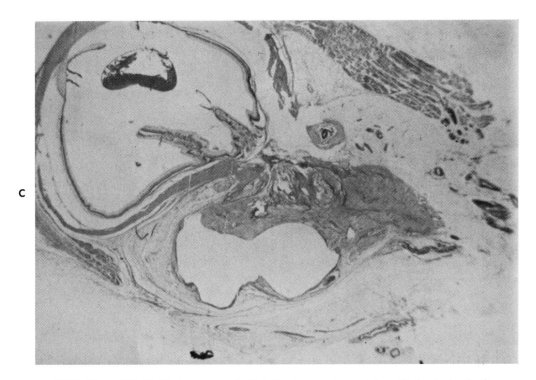

C

FIG. 5-3 cont'd. C, Photomicrograph of globe above and cyst below. Retina is dysplastic.

disaster and is usually followed by choroidal effusion and secondary retinal detachment. This is discussed more fully in Chapter 11.

Microphthalmos with an orbital cyst is due to the failure of the choroidal fissure to close during embryologic development. Proliferating retinal tissue extends into the orbital space and is eventually covered by connective tissue, thus producing a cyst. The globe is small and usually malformed, whereas the cyst may be quite large and cause proptosis. Treatment consists of surgical excision of the orbital cyst plus the globe (Fig. 5-3).

Microphthalmos may also be seen with a wide variety of congenital systemic disorders, including:

  1. Trisomy 13 (Patau's syndrome)
  2. Chromosome 18 deletion syndrome
  3. Congenital rubella
  4. Hallermann-Streiff syndrome
  5. LSD embryopathy
  6. Goldenhar's syndrome
  7. Oculodentodigital dysplasia
  8. Pierre Robin syndrome
  9. Oculocerebrorenal syndrome
10. Focal dermal hypoplasia
11. François' syndrome
12. Ullrich's syndrome

Megalocornea

Megalocornea is a bilateral, nonprogressive condition in which the corneal diameter is usually greater than 13 mm (range 14 to 17 mm). It is usually inherited as an x-linked recessive but may be autosomal dominant or recessive. Vision is unaffected, although high astigmatism is common. There appear to be two clinical types.[37] In the first, the cornea and anterior segment are normal, whereas in the second, megalocornea is associated with posterior embryotoxon, a cataract or dislocated lens, iridodonesis, and lax zonules.

Megalocornea may occur with congenital glaucoma in the same pedigree.[9,37] Gonioscopy reveals iris processes inserting higher than usual on the trabecular meshwork or intense pigmentation of the meshwork. Cataracts and lens subluxation can occur in adulthood, producing a secondary glaucoma. For treatment of the secondarily dislocated lens, see Chapter 10.

Sclerocornea

Sclerocornea is an unusual congenital abnormality that may affect the periphery or the entire cornea and is due to vascularized scleral tissue extending onto the cornea.[13] It may occur as an iso-

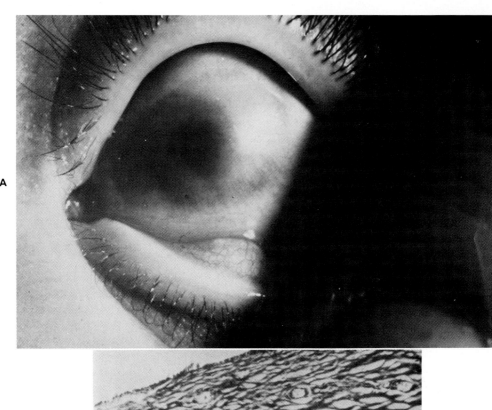

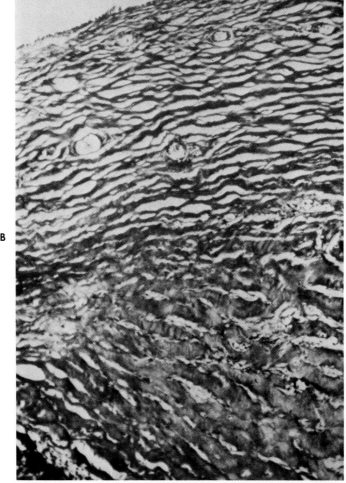

FIG. 5-4. Sclerocornea. **A,** Clinical photograph of left eye of 8-month-old child with sclerocornea. Condition was present bilaterally. Central cornea is translucent. Peripheral cornea is very hazy and quite vascularized. There is no corneoscleral sulcus. Scleral curvature is continuous with corneal curvature. **B,** Photomicrograph of cornea revealing marked vascularization at all levels. Note markedly thickened corneal lamellae inferiorly.

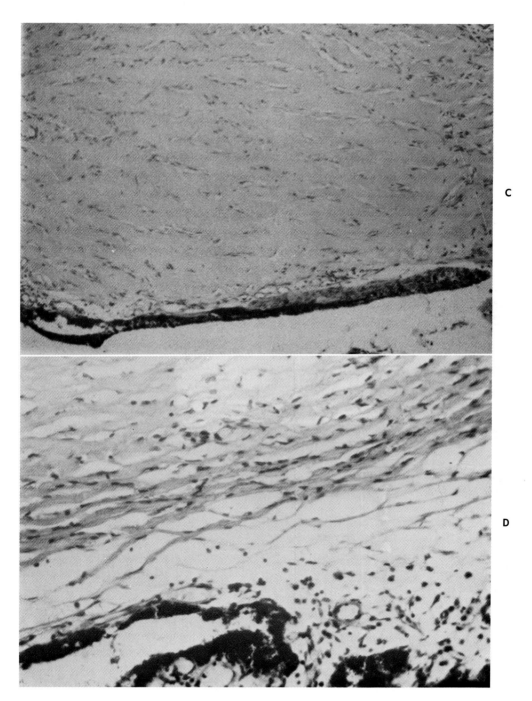

FIG. 5-4 cont'd. C, Photograph showing obliteration of anterior chamber with total iridocorneal adhesion. Corneal lamellae are markedly thickened. Iris possesses no stroma. There is no Descemet's membrane or endothelium of cornea. **D,** There are no angle structures. There is total iridocorneal adhesion but no ciliary musculature, scleral spur, or trabecular meshwork.

lated condition or in association with the following ocular or systemic abnormalities:

A. Systemic findings
   1. Trisomy 18
   2. (17p, 10q) translocation
   3. Dandy-Walker cyst
   4. Mental retardation
   5. Cerebellar dysfunction
   6. Deafness
   7. Craniofacial anomalies
   8. Digital anomalies
   9. Cryptorchidism
B. Ocular findings
   1. Micropthalmos
   2. Iridocorneal synechiae
   3. Iridogoniodysgenesis
   4. Defective mesodermal migration
   5. Congenital glaucoma
   6. Nystagmus
   7. Strabismus

Sclerocornea is almost always bilateral. Visual acuity is severely decreased in most patients. Cornea plana is concurrent in about 80% of severe cases (Fig. 5-4).

Sclerocornea has been associated with an unbalanced translocation (17p, 10q)[36] and a presumed trisomy 18,[19] as well as with the Smith-Lemli-Opitz syndrome.[11]

A possible relationship between sclerocornea, Peters' anomaly, and Rieger's anomaly has been hypothesized,[13] and congenital glaucoma may occur.[10,13] Mechanisms for the development of glaucoma include (1) total iridocorneal adhesion obliterating the anterior chamber, (2) iridogoniodysgenesis, and (3) defective mesodermal migration with total absence of angle structures (e.g., trabecular meshwork and Schlemm's canal). In those cases of sclerocornea unassociated with glaucoma, corneal transplantation has been successful. The presence of congenital glaucoma is nearly always a hopeless sign.

Retinopathy of prematurity (retrolental fibroplasia)

Retrolental fibroplasia is invariably bilateral and is not present at birth.[16] It usually occurs in premature infants who have a history of oxygen exposure to immature retinal vessels but has been reported in the full-term infant.[20]

In the peripheral retina, endothelial cells proliferate and neovascular tufts eventually break through the inner limiting membrane into the sub-vitreal space. Fibrovascular tissue forms, retracts, and produces retinal detachment and hemorrhage or displacement of the macular region and posterior retinal vessels. As the condition develops, the eyes become microphthalmic and may develop shallow anterior chambers. Ciliary processes become elongated and are incorporated into the fibrovascular retrolental mass (Fig. 5-5).

The active phase of retrolental fibroplasia lasts 3 to 6 months and is followed by a cicatricial stage. This is characterized by dragging of the optic nerve head, retinal folds, retinal pigment epithelial proliferation, chorioretinal scarring, and vitreous membranes.

When retrolental fibroplasia is complicated by glaucoma, it is usually angle-closure glaucoma, which most commonly appears after the age of 1[44] or 2[35] years but may occur as late as the third decade of life.[44]

The anterior chamber is usually shallow in severely affected eyes. Cohen et al.[5] found a "smaller than normal" cornea in 19 of 54 eyes (35%) in 27 school-age children. The anterior chamber was shallow in 21 eyes (39%) and flat in 14 (26%), and finger tension was elevated in 17% of the patients tested.

When angle closure occurs in these patients, they frequently have flat rather than shallow anterior chambers. The mechanism of the glaucoma appears to be a forward movement of the lens-iris diaphragm, probably secondary to the retrolental mass. Patients with severe posterior segment disease, perilenticular membrane formation, shallow anterior chambers, and narrow angles should be followed for progression of these findings, and parents should be warned regarding the signs and symptoms of angle closure. Prophylactic iridectomy has been recommended when these signs indicate a present and increasing risk of acute angle closure.[44] There have as yet been no reports of the use of laser iridectomy in therapy for this disorder.

A complication unique to retrolental fibroplasia is the closure of a peripheral iridectomy due to a gradual drawing of the coloboma into the angle, where it becomes obliterated with contact with the peripheral cornea and angle wall, necessitating reoperation, and Walton[44] has recommended performance of a sector iridectomy.

Lens removal, either by needling and aspiration[29] or by pars plana lensectomy with vitrectomy,[35] has been reported to be successful in relieving the glaucoma.

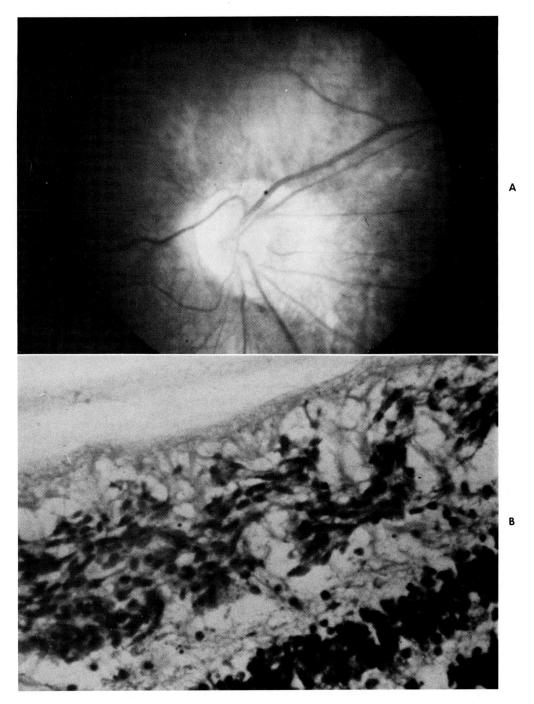

FIG. 5-5. Retinopathy of prematurity. **A,** Fundus photograph of young child with arrested retinopathy of prematurity with traction of retinal vessels. Note how vessels are all pulled to right side, which is temporally in left eye. **B,** Photomicrograph revealing glomeruloid tufts of proliferated endothelial cells in peripheral temporal retina of child.   *Continued.*

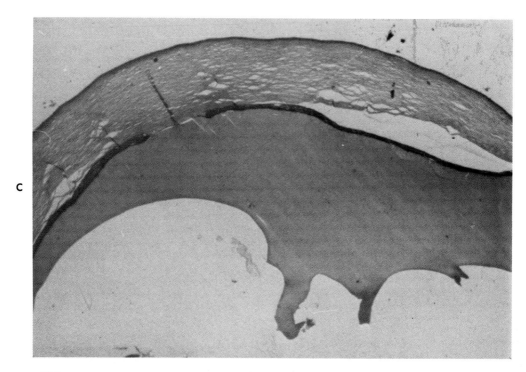

FIG-5-5 cont'd. C, End-stage retinopathy of prematurity with totally obliterated anterior chamber. Lens has fallen out in processing.

Neovascular glaucoma may also occur with retrolental fibroplasia, particularly when there is a long-standing retinal detachment.

Persistent hyperplastic primary vitreous

Persistent hyperplastic primary vitreous (PHPV) is a unilateral congenital anomaly that is recognizable at birth. Complications intrinsic to PHPV include intraocular hemorrhage, secondary glaucoma, and corneal opacification. PHPV presents at birth as a partial or complete leukocoria, usually in a microphthalmic eye.

The fundamental abnormality is a persistence and overgrowth of the primary vitreous and its associated blood vessels: the hyaloid artery, vasa hyaloidea propria, and branches contributed by the ciliary vessels. The ciliary processes are incorporated into the periphery of the membrane and are drawn centrally as the eye grows. The result is a dense fibrovascular retrolental mass. Almost invariably there is rupture of the posterior lens capsule, which results when the lens and the remainder of the eye grow at a rate that exceeds that of the vascular retrolental membrane. A secondary cataract, which may be slow or rapid in onset, is a common sequela finally leading to intumescence. Spontaneous hemorrhage may occur into the membrane, vitreous, and lens. Fibrous tissue and blood vessels may extend to the defect in the posterior lens capsule (Fig. 5-6).

Elements of the peripheral retina are continuous with the mass. Other findings include rupture of the anterior lens capsule, unusual vascularity of the iris, ectopia lentis, and coloboma of the iris, choroid, and optic nerve. The anterior chamber is shallow, and the iridocorneal angle may show retarded development.

PHPV may be complicated by angle-closure glaucoma. When indications are present for the treatment of PHPV, the lens and retrolental membrane should be removed with vitrectomy instruments. The mechanism for the occurrence of secondary glaucoma may be swelling of the lens resulting from rupture of the posterior lens capsule, which leads to pupillary block or angle-closure glaucoma, or a forward movement of the iris-lens diaphragm associated with contracture of the retrolental membrane.

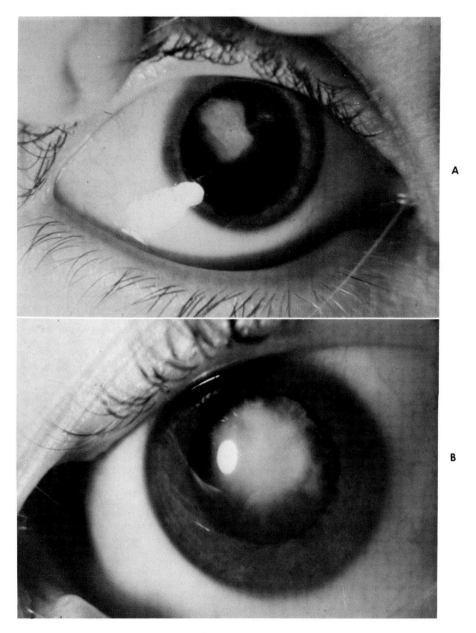

FIG. 5-6. Persistent hyperplastic primary vitreous. **A,** Clinical photograph revealing localized white retrolental opacity. **B,** More advanced example. Eye is microphthalmic as well. *Continued.*

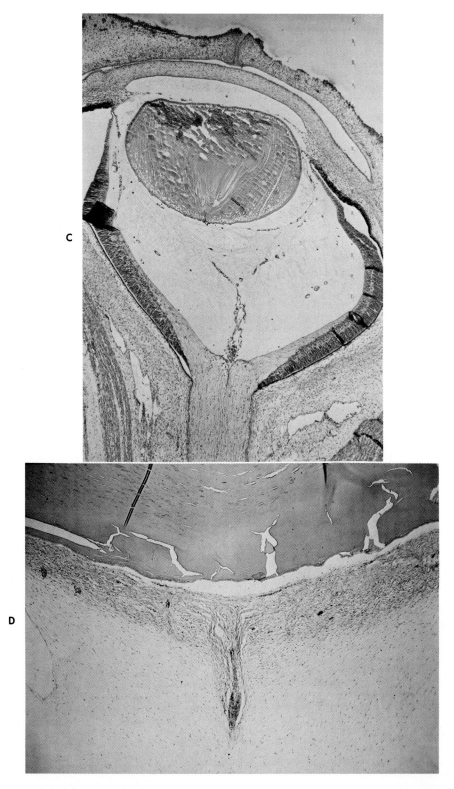

FIG. 5-6, cont'd. C, Fully developed hyaloid system in 16-mm embryonic eye. Note that lids have not separated. **D,** PHPV with retrolental fibrovascular mass.

REFERENCES

1. Akasaki, M., Fukui, S., Sakano, T., et al.: Urinary excretion of a large amount of bound sialic acid and of undersulfated chondroitin sulfate A by patients with the Lowe syndrome, Clin. Chim. Acta **89:**119, 1978.
2. Apple, D.J., Holden, J.D., and Stallworth, B.: Ocular pathology of Patau's syndrome, Am. J. Ophthalmol. **74:** 729, 1972.
3. Blanck, F., Braun-Vallon, S., and Guillaumat, L.: Deux cas de nanisme constitutionnel (syndrome de Rubenstein et Taybi) avec glaucome, Bull. Soc. Ophthalmol. Fr. **68:**588, 1968.
4. Cameron, J.D., Yanoff, M., and Frayer, W.C.: Coats' disease and Turner's syndrome, Am. J. Ophthalmol. **78:** 852, 1974.
5. Cohen, J., Alfano, J.E., Boshes, A.D., and Palmgren, C.: Clinical evaluation of school-age children with retrolental fibroplasia, Am. J. Ophthalmol. **57:**41, 1964.
6. Curtin, V.T., Joyce, E.E., and Ballin, N.: Ocular pathology in the oculo-cerebro-renal syndrome of Lowe, Am. J. Ophthalmol. **64:**533, 1967.
7. Dark, A.J., and Kirkhan, T.H.: Congenital corneal opacities in a patient with Rieger's anomaly and Down's syndrome, Br. J. Ophthalmol. **52:**631, 1968.
8. Dudgeon, J., and Chisholm, I.A.: Oculo-dento-digital dysplasia, Trans. Ophthalmol. Soc. U.K. **94:**203, 1974.
9. Friedman, A.I., and Etzine, S.: Familial coexistence of congenital glaucoma and megalocornea, Ophthalmologica **142:**629, 1961.
10. Goldstein, J.E., and Cogan, D.G.: Sclerocornea and associated congenital anomalies, Arch. Ophthalmol. **67:** 761, 1962.
11. Harbin, R.L., Katz, J.I., Frias, J.L., et al.: Sclerocornea associated with the Smith-Lemli-Opitz syndrome, Am. J. Ophthalmol. **84:**72, 1977.
12. Hoepner, J., and Yanoff, M.: Ocular anomalies in trisomy 13-15, Am. J. Ophthalmol. **74:**721, 1972.
13. Howard, R.O., and Abrahams, I.W.: Sclerocornea, Am. J. Ophthalmol. **71:**1254, 1971.
14. Johnson, B.L., and Hiles, D.A.: Ocular pathology of Lowe's syndrome in a female infant, J. Pediatr. Ophthalmol. **13:**204, 1976.
15. Judisch, F.G., Martin-Casals, A., Hanson, J.W., and Olin, W.H.: Oculodentodigital dysplasia, Arch. Ophthalmol. **97:**878, 1979.
16. Karlsberg, R.C., Green, W.R., and Patz, A.: Congenital retrolental fibroplasia, Arch. Ophthalmol. **89:**122, 1973.
17. Keith, C.G.: The ocular manifestations of trisomy 13-15, Trans. Ophthalmol. Soc. U.K. **86:**435, 1966.
18. Khodadoust, A., and Paton, D.: Turner's syndrome in a male, Arch. Ophthalmol. **77:**630, 1967.
19. Kolbert, G.S., and Seelenfreund, M.: Sclerocornea, anterior cleavage syndrome, and trisomy 18, Ann. Ophthalmol. **2:**26, 1970.
20. Kraushar, M.F., Harper, R.G., and Sia, C.G.: Retrolental fibroplasia in a full-term infant, Am. J. Ophthalmol. **80:** 106, 1975.
21. Lalive d'Epinay, S., and Reme, C.: Clinical and morphological studies in a case of congenital glaucoma combined with an ocular-dental-digital dysplasia, Klin. Monatsbl. Augenheilkd. **168:**113, 1976.
22. Laurent, C., Royer, J., and Noel, G.: Syndrome de Turner et glaucome congenitale, Bull. Soc. Ophthalmol. Fr. **5:** 367, 1961.
23. Lessell, S., and Forbes, A.P.: Eye signs in Turner's syndrome, Arch. Ophthalmol. **76:**211, 1966.
24. Levy, N.S.: Juvenile glaucoma in the Rubenstein-Taybi syndrome, J. Pediatr. Ophthalmol. **13:**141, 1976.
25. Lichter, P.R., and Schmickel, R.D.: Posterior vortex vein and congenital glaucoma in a patient with trisomy 13 syndrome, Am. J. Ophthalmol. **80:**939, 1975.
26. Lowe, C.U., Terrey, M., and MacLachlan, E.A.: Organic-aciduria, decreased renal ammonia production, hydrophthalmos, and mental retardation: a clinical entity, Am. J. Dis. Child. **83:**164, 1952.
27. Lythgoe, C., and Ramsey, M.S.: A possible case of oculo-cerebro-renal (Lowe's) syndrome in a female infant, Can. J. Ophthalmol. **8:**591, 1973.
28. Manzitti, E., and Lavin, J.R.: Le glaucome congenitale dans le syndrome de Rubenstein-Taybi, Ann. Ocul. **205:** 1005, 1972.
29. McCormick, A.Q., and Pratt-Johnson, J.A.: Angle closure glaucoma in infancy, Ophthalmic Surg. **2:**91, 1971.
30. Meyer-Schwickerath, G., Gruterich, E., and Weyers, H.: Microphthalmos-syndrom, Klin. Monatsbl. Augenheilkd. **131:**18, 1957.
31. Mullaney, J.: Ocular pathology in trisomy 18 (Edward's syndrome), Am. J. Ophthalmol. **76:**246, 1976.
32. Nev, R.L., and Takashi, K.: Partial deletion of long arm chromosome 18 and deletion of short arms of chromosome 18. In Gardner, L.I., editor: Endocrine and genetic diseases of childhood, Philadelphia, 1969, W.B. Saunders Co., p. 655.
33. Opitz, J.M., France, T., Herrmann, J., and Spranger, J.W.: The Stickler syndrome, N. Engl. J. Med. **286:**546, 1972.
34. Patau, K., Smith, D.W., and Therman, E.: Multiple congenital anomalies caused by an extra autosome, Lancet **1:**790, 1960.
35. Pollard, Z.F.: Secondary angle-closure glaucoma in cicatricial retrolental fibroplasia, Am. J. Ophthalmol. **89:** 651, 1980.
36. Rodrigues, M.M., and Calhoun, J., and Weinreb, S.: Sclerocornea with an unbalanced translocation (17p, 10q), Am. J. Ophthalmol. **78:**49, 1974.
37. Rogers, G.L., and Polomeno, R.C.: Autosomal-dominant inheritance of megalocornea associated with Down's syndrome, Am. J. Ophthalmol. **78:**526, 1974.
38. Schreiner, R.L., McAlister, W.H., Marshall, R.E., and Shearer, W.T.: Stickler syndrome in a pedigree of Pierre Robin syndrome, Am. J. Dis. Child. **126:**86, 1973.
39. Schweitzer, N.M.J.: Megalocornea, Ophthalmologica **144:**304, 1962.
40. Smith, J.L., and Stowe, F.: The Pierre Robin syndrome (glossoptosis, micrognathia, cleft palate): a review of 39 cases with emphasis on associated ocular lesions, Pediatrics **27:**128, 1961.
41. Sugar, H.S.: Oculodentodigital dysplasia syndrome with angle-closure glaucoma, Am. J. Ophthalmol. **86:**36, 1978.
42. Townes, P.L., Manning, J.A., and DeHart, G.K., Jr.: Trisomy-18 (16-18) associated with congenital glaucoma and optic atrophy, J. Pediatr. **61:**755, 1962.
43. Walton, D.S.: Congenital glaucoma associated with congenital cataract. In Chandler, P.A., and Grant, W.M., edi-

tors: Glaucoma, ed. 2, Philadelphia, 1979, Lea & Febiger.

44. Walton, D.S.: Retrolental fibroplasia with glaucoma. In Chandler, P.A., and Grant, W.M.: Glaucoma, ed. 2, Philadelphia, 1979, Lea & Febiger.

45. Wilson, W.A., Richards, W., and Donnell, G.N.: Oculo-cerebral-renal syndrome of Lowe, Arch. Ophthalmol. **70:**5, 1963.

46. Yanoff, M., Rorke, L.B., and Niederer, B.J.: Ocular and cerebral abnormalities in chromosome 18 deletion defect, Am. J. Ophthalmol. **70:**391, 1970.

47. Young, N.J.A., Hitchings, R.A., Sehmi, K., and Bird, A.C.: Stickler's syndrome and neovascular glaucoma, Br. J. Ophthalmol. **63:**826, 1979.

48. Zayid, I., and Farraj, S.: Familial histiocytic dermato-arthritis: a new syndrome, Am. J. Med. **54:**793, 1973.

Section III

GLAUCOMAS ASSOCIATED WITH OCULAR DISEASE

Chapter 6

GLAUCOMA ASSOCIATED WITH PRIMARY DISORDERS OF THE CORNEAL ENDOTHELIUM

M. Bruce Shields

IRIDOCORNEAL ENDOTHELIAL SYNDROME
Historical background and terminology

In 1903 Harms[15] described a disease with unilateral glaucoma and extensive atrophy of the iris, which became generally known as progressive essential iris atrophy. Approximately one-half century later, Chandler[5] reported a similar condition that differed in that corneal endothelial dystrophy, often associated with corneal edema, was consistently present and the atrophy of the iris was mild and limited to the stroma. Chandler and Grant[6] suggested that this disorder, which became known as Chandler's syndrome, and progressive essential iris atrophy represented basic variations of the same disease process. In 1969 Cogan and Reese[9] described a third entity that differed from the aforementioned by the presence of pigmented nodules on the surface of the iris. Scheie and Yanoff[29] reported similar cases with both nodular and diffuse lesions of the iris and suggested the term iris nevus (Cogan-Reese) syndrome.

Studies have indicated that the three disorders described above represent major clinical variations within a spectrum of disease.[4,10,31-33] The collective term essential iris atrophy has been used for this group of disorders, although clinical and histologic evidence indicates that the basic defect is an abnormality of the corneal endothelium rather than of the iris.[4] Therefore Yanoff[40] proposed the term iridocorneal endothelial (ICE) syndrome for the spectrum of disease, and the term progressive iris atrophy has been suggested for the clinical variation previously called progressive essential iris atrophy. The three major clinical variations of the ICE syndrome are summarized in Table 6-1. It should also be noted that overlapping of progressive iris atrophy and Chandler's syndrome leads to intermediate variations in some patients.

Clinicopathologic features

The ICE syndrome is typically a unilateral disease that occurs predominantly in white women. The medical and family histories are usually non-

TABLE 6-1
Iridocorneal endothelial (ICE) syndrome

Major clinical variations	Characteristic features of iris*
Progressive iris atrophy	Marked corectopia and atrophy of the iris with hole formation
Chandler's syndrome	Mild or absent corectopia and mild atrophy of the iris
Cogan-Reese syndrome (Iris nevus syndrome)	Nodular or diffuse pigmented lesions of the iris with full spectrum of atrophy of the iris

*All variations of the ICE syndrome have similar corneal and anterior chamber angle features, although the clinically apparent changes of the cornea may be more consistent in Chandler's syndrome.

69

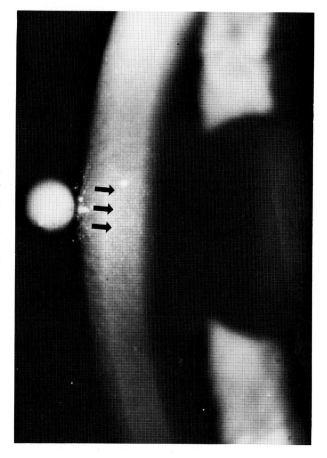

FIG. 6-1. Slit-lamp biomicroscopic view showing fine-hammered silver appearance of posterior cornea *(arrows)* in patient with ICE syndrome. (From Shields, M.B., Campbell, D.G., and Simmons, R.J. Published with permission from the American Journal of Ophthalmology **85:**749-759, 1978. Copyright by the Ophthalmic Publishing Co.)

contributory, although familial cases have been reported. The condition is most often recognized in early to middle adulthood, and the first clinical manifestation is usually a change in the iris or a disturbance of vision.

Alterations in the cornea are characteristic of all variations of the ICE syndrome, although they may be more consistently apparent in Chandler's syndrome. The typical appearance of the posterior cornea by slit-lamp biomicroscopy is that of fine-hammered silver, similar to Fuchs' dystrophy, but less coarse[5] (Fig. 6-1). Specular microscopy reveals diffuse abnormalities of the corneal endothelial cells, characterized by variable degrees of pleomorphism in size and shape, dark areas within the cells, and loss of the clear hexagonal margins (Fig. 6-2).[16,30] The endothelial defect alone is asymptomatic and is the only abnormality of the cornea in some eyes. In other cases there is associated corneal edema, which may be mild, with blurred vision in the first few hours of the morning, or severe, with pain and persistent reduc-

tion in vision. Ultrastructural studies of the cornea from eyes with all variations of the ICE syndrome reveal attenuated, grossly abnormal cells lining a thickened, multilayered Descemet's membrane[10,24,25,34] (Fig. 6-3).

A second characteristic feature found in all variations of the ICE syndrome is peripheral anterior synechiae, which usually extend to or beyond Schwalbe's line (Fig. 6-4). Histologic studies of the anterior chamber angle in all variations of the ICE syndrome have revealed a membrane, composed of a single layer of endothelial cells and a Descemet-like basement membrane, covering an open angle in some areas (Fig. 6-5) and associated with synechial closure elsewhere.* Secondary glaucoma usually develops with progressive synechial closure of the anterior chamber angle, although the correlation between glaucoma and the degree of synechiae is not precise,[32] and glaucoma

---

*References 1, 4, 10, 26, 27, 34.

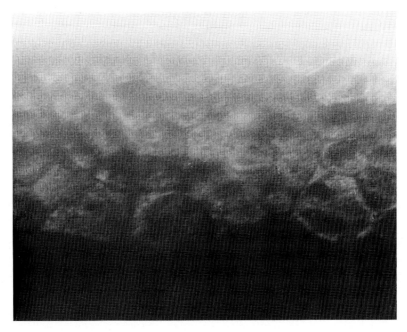

FIG. 6-2. Specular microscopic view of corneal endothelium in ICE syndrome showing pleomorphism in size and shape of cells, dark areas within cells, and loss of clear hexagonal margins. (Courtesy L.W. Hirst, M.D.)

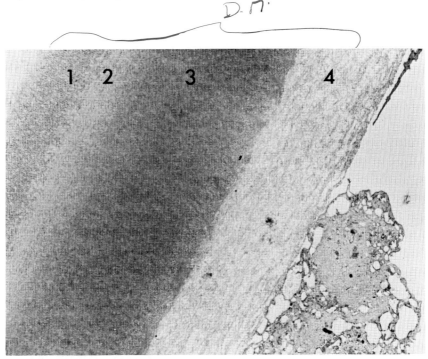

FIG. 6-3. Transmission electron microscopic view of posterior cornea from eye with ICE syndrome and advanced corneal edema showing isolated, abnormal cell on four-layered acellular collagenous membrane: *1,* normal anterior banded portion of Descemet's membrane; *2,* thin posterior nonbanded portion of Descemet's membrane; *3* and *4,* abnormal posterior layers of collagen. (×6875.) (From Shields, M.B., McCracken, J.S., Klintworth, G.K., and Campbell, D.G.: Ophthalmology **86:**1533, 1979.)

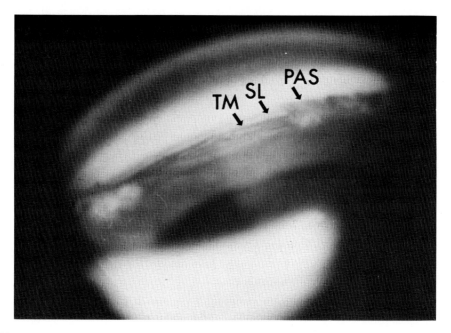

FIG. 6-4. Gonioscopic view of eye with ICE syndrome showing broad-based peripheral anterior synechiae *(PAS)* extending beyond trabecular meshwork *(TM)* to Schwalbe's line *(SL)*. (From Shields, M.B., Campbell, D.G., and Simmons, R.J. Published with permission from the American Journal of Ophthalmology **85:**749-759, 1978, Copyright by the Ophthalmic Publishing Co.)

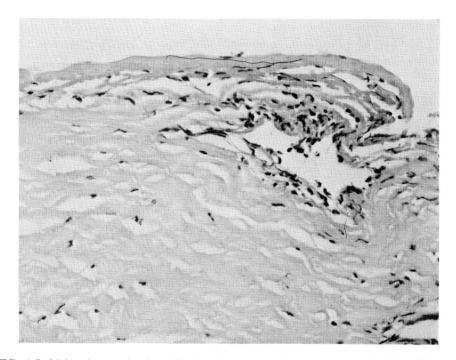

FIG. 6-5. Light microscopic view of trabeculectomy specimen from eye with Chandler's syndrome showing Descemetlike membrane extending across trabecular meshwork. (Hematoxylin and eosin; ×250.) (From Shields, M.B., McCracken, J.S., Klintworth, G.K., and Campbell, D.G.: Ophthalmology **86:**1533, 1979.)

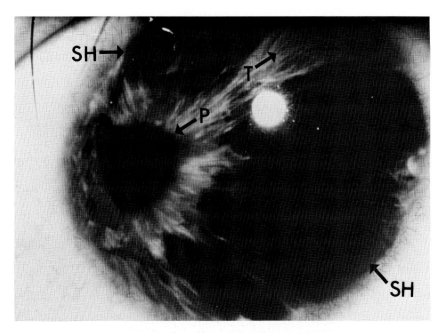

FIG. 6-6. Example of progressive iris atrophy showing distortion of pupil *(P)*, thinning of iris stroma *(T)*, and "stretch holes" *(SH)*. (From Shields, M.B.: Surv. Ophthalmol. **24:**3, 1979; courtesy Richard J. Simmons, M.D.)

has been reported when the entire angle was open but covered by the membrane.[1]

Abnormalities of the iris complete the triad of clinicopathologic features in the ICE syndrome and are the primary basis for classifying the clinical variations within the spectrum of disease. Progressive iris atrophy is characterized by extreme thinning of the iris, ultimately leading to complete hole formation. In some cases there is marked corectopia and ectropion uveae with thinning of the iris and "stretch holes" in quadrants away from the direction of the pupillary displacement[32] (Fig. 6-6). Other cases are characterized by "melting holes" (Fig. 6-7), which are not associated with significant corectopia or thinning of the iris but have been demonstrated by anterior segment fluorescein studies to be surrounded by ischemia and leaking vessels (Fig. 6-8).[32] In Chandler's syndrome, the corectopia is mild or absent, and thinning of the iris is limited to the superficial stroma[5] (Fig. 6-9). Intermediate clinical variations may also be seen, in which atrophy of the iris and corectopia are more than in the typical case of Chandler's syndrome but hole formation in the iris is not present. Eyes with the Cogan-Reese syndrome may have any degree of atrophy of the iris but differ from the aforementioned variations by

the presence of pigmented, pedunculated nodules[29,33] (Fig. 6-10), diffuse, pigmented lesions (Fig. 6-11),[29] or both,[29] on the surface of the iris.

Histologic studies of the iris in all variations of the ICE syndrome reveal the previously described membrane, extending across the anterior chamber angle and onto the surface of the iris.[4,10] The membrane is characteristically found in that portion of the iris toward which the pupil is distorted, and the iris in the opposite quadrant usually has loss of variable amounts of stroma and in some cases pigment epithelium.[4] The characteristic lesions of the iris in the Cogan-Reese syndrome are always in the area of the membrane.[4,10] The electron microscopic appearance of the nodular type of lesion has been described as spindle pigmented cells with fusiform nuclei.[10] They are surrounded by the basement membrane but are continuous with the underlying stroma of the iris through a central aperture in the membrane.[10] Diffuse nevi involving the iridic stroma have also been described.[10,29]

Pathogenesis

Several theories have been proposed for the cause of the ICE syndrome, including inflammation, primary vascular insufficiency, and a fundamental defect of the iris. However, Campbell et

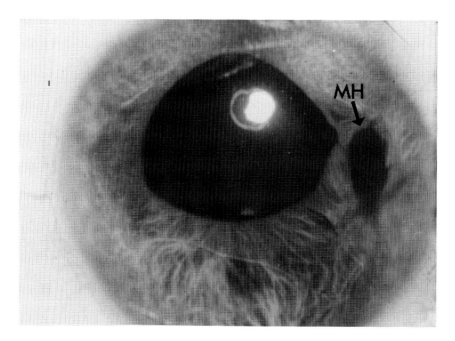

FIG 6-7. Example of progressive iris atrophy showing "melting hole" *(MH)*, pupillary irregularity, and ectropion uveae, but no significant stretching of iris. (From Shields, M.B., Campbell, G.D., and Simmons, R.J. Published with permission from the American Journal of Ophthalmology **85:**749-759, 1978. Copyright by the Ophthalmic Publishing Co.)

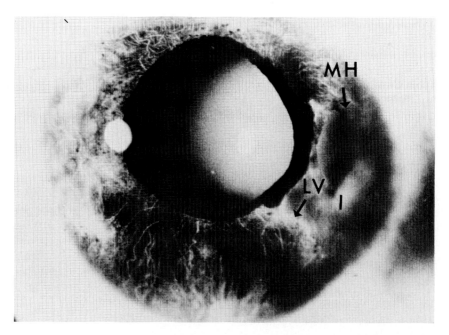

FIG. 6-8. Fluorescein angiographic view of eye in Fig. 6-7 showing area of ischemia *(I)* and leaking vessels *(LV)* around melting hold *(MH)*. (From Shields, M.B., Campbell, D.G., and Simmons, R.J. Published with permission from the American Journal of Ophthalmology **85:**749-759, 1978. Copyright by the Ophthalmic Publishing Co.)

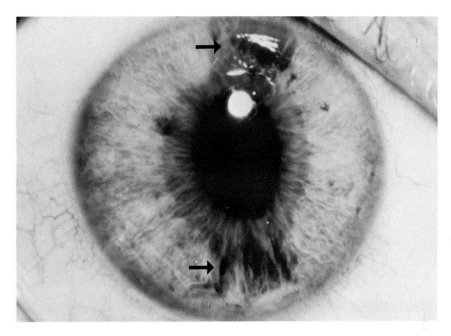

FIG. 6-9. Example of Chandler's syndrome with oval pupil and mild atrophy of iris stroma *(arrows)*. (From Shields, M.B., Campbell, D.G., and Simmons, R.J. Published with permission from the American Journal of Ophthalmology **85:**749-759, 1978. Copyright by the Ophthalmic Publishing Co.)

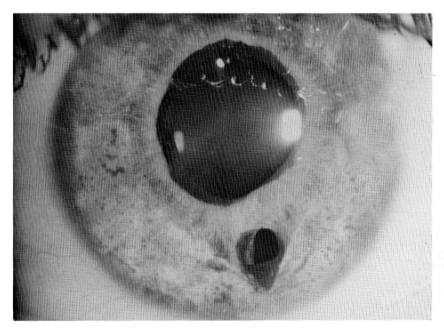

FIG. 6-10. Example of Cogan-Reese syndrome with fine, pigmented nodules on iris and matting of underlying iris stroma. (From Shields, M.B., Campbell, D.G., Simmons, R.J., and Hutchinson, B.T.: Arch. Ophthalmol. **94:**406, 1976. Copyright 1976, American Medical Association.)

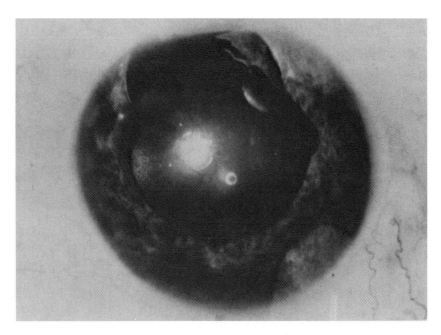

FIG. 6-11. Example of Cogan-Reese syndrome with diffuse, pigmented lesion on surface of iris. (From Scheie, H.G., and Yanoff, M.: Arch. Ophthalmol. **93:**963, 1975. Copyright 1975, American Medical Association.)

al.[4] have provided clinical and histologic evidence that the abnormality of the corneal endothelium is the basic defect in this spectrum of disease, and this concept has been supported by other investigators.[10] The endothelial defect not only causes the corneal edema, but also leads to growth of the membrane across the anterior chamber angle and onto the anterior surface of the iris. According to the membrane theory of Campbell et al.,[4] contraction of the membrane leads to the formation of peripheral anterior synechiae with secondary glaucoma and to the variable changes in the iris. This concept has been supported by a case report of unilateral glaucoma with a corneal endothelial abnormality and an endothelial membrane across the open anterior chamber angle but with no changes in the iris, suggesting an early case of the ICE syndrome.[1] Clinical studies show that the pupil is distorted toward the quadrant with the most prominent peripheral anterior synechiae,[32] which corresponds histologically with the location of the membrane.[4] In the opposite quadrant stretching of the iris is usually associated with thinning and in some cases hole formation (Fig. 6-12). In addition to the mechanical stretching, other factors such as secondary ischemia of the iris are probably involved in the changes. There is also evidence

that the membrane creates the nodules of the iris in the Cogan-Reese syndrome by squeezing clusters of stromal cells into the elevated structures.[3]

Differential diagnosis

The changes in the posterior cornea and associated corneal edema may occasionally be confused with those of posterior polymorphous dystrophy or Fuchs' endothelioepithelial dystrophy, which are discussed later in this chapter. Dissolution of the iris in the ICE syndrome may be confused with the changes of iridoschisis, in which stromal layers of the iris spontaneously separate (Fig. 6-13), occasionally leading to secondary glaucoma.[22] However, this condition characteristically occurs in the elderly and is usually bilateral. Rieger's syndrome and aniridia may also mimic the iris changes in some patients with the ICE syndrome, but both of these conditions are congenital and nearly always bilateral. The nodular and diffuse pigmented lesions of the iris in the Cogan-Reese syndrome may be confused with the changes in neurofibromatosis, malignant melanomas of the iris (eyes have been enucleated because of this suspicion),[29] and anterior uveitis with nodules of the iris, such as in sarcoidosis.

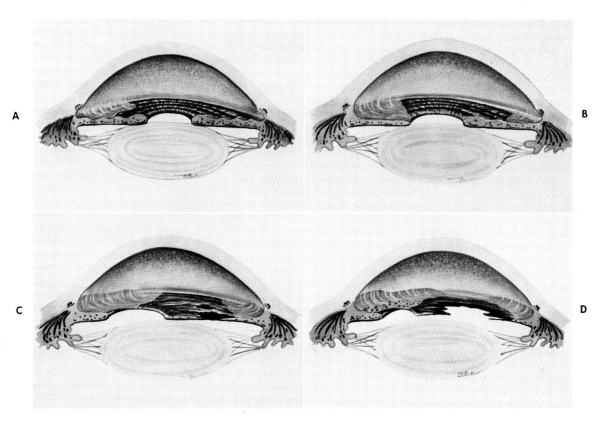

FIG. 6-12. Membrane theory of Campbell suggests that **(A)** membrane grows from abnormal cornea, across anterior chamber angle, onto iris; **(B)** contracture of membrane leads to formation of peripheral anterior synechiae and distortion of pupil; **(C)** corectopia is associated with stretching and thinning of iris stroma (eyes with Chandler's syndrome do not progress beyond this phase); and **(D)** eyes with progressive iris atrophy eventually develop iris holes, whereas those with Cogan-Reese syndrome acquire nodular or diffuse pigmented lesions on iris in area of membrane. (From Shields, M.B.: Surv. Ophthalmol. **24**:3, 1979.)

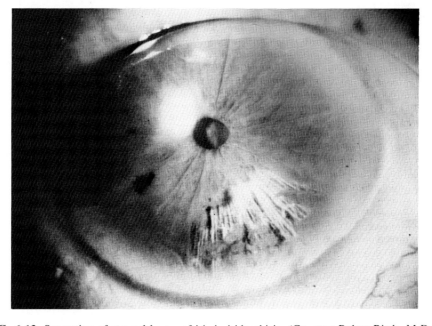

FIG. 6-13. Separation of stromal layers of iris in iridoschisis. (Courtesy Robert Ritch, M.D.)

Management

The management of patients with the ICE syndrome may involve treating the corneal edema, the secondary glaucoma, or both. In some cases these two aspects of the disease may both be controlled by medical or surgical reduction of the intraocular pressure. In the early phases of the disease process, miotics and epinephrine may be effective in controlling the intraocular pressure. However, in patients with advanced synechial closure of the anterior chamber angle, drugs with a greater effect on aqueous production, such as timolol maleate or a carbonic anhydrase inhibitor, may be more effective. Some patients require additional measures for the corneal edema, such as hypertonic saline solutions or soft contact lenses.

When medical therapy is no longer effective in controlling the corneal edema or the secondary glaucoma, surgical intervention is usually indicated. A filtering operation appears to be the procedure of choice when there is progressive glaucomatous optic atrophy and visual field loss despite maximum tolerable medical therapy.[32] Filtering surgery has also been used in an attempt to control the corneal edema in eyes without glaucomatous damage, although this is frequently unsuccessful, since corneal edema may persist despite very low intraocular pressures.[34] Penetrating keratoplasty has been successful in these cases and is probably the initial surgical procedure of choice when the corneal edema is marked and the intraocular pressure is normal or only moderately elevated and not associated with progressive glaucomatous damage.[34]

POSTERIOR POLYMORPHOUS DYSTROPHY
Historical background and classification

In 1916 Koeppe[19] described congenital pits on the posterior surface of the cornea in six patients and called the condition keratitis bullosa interna. One patient had glaucoma, although no description of the anterior chamber angle or iris was provided. Numerous reports have subsequently described similar abnormalities of the posterior cornea, which are now referred to collectively as the posterior polymorphous dystrophies. Soukup[35] (1964) reported peripheral anterior synechiae and iris rarefaction with posterior polymorphous dystrophy, and Cibis et al.,[7] in a large clinical study, emphasized this association as well as the occasional presence of glaucoma.

Considerable confusion has resulted from the many reported variations in the clinical and histologic picture of this disorder. Grayson[12] and Cibis et al.[8] have emphasized that posterior polymorphous dystrophy represents a broad spectrum of abnormalities involving the posterior cornea, the anterior chamber angle, and the iris. One of the less common forms within this group of diseases has the corneal changes in association with broad peripheral anterior synechiae, atrophy of the iris, and glaucoma. It is this clinical variant that is discussed here.

Clinicopathologic features

Posterior polymorphous dystrophy is a familial disorder, usually inherited by an autosomal dominant, although occasionally by an autosomal recessive, mode. It is typically bilateral, occurs in both blacks and whites, and has no significant sex predilection.[39]

The condition is probably congenital, although it is rarely observed in children, other than in family studies, because in most patients it is asymptomatic and stationary and there is good visual acuity.[39] However, the posterior corneal abnormality may occasionally be associated with secondary stromal and epithelial edema, which has required penetrating keratoplasty in several reported cases.*

With slit-lamp biomicroscopy, the cornea has an appearance of blisters or vesicles at the level of Descemet's membrane, which are often linear or in groups and surrounded by an aureole of gray haze (Fig. 6-14). Other findings include a thickening of Descemet's membrane, which may appear as excrescences projecting into the anterior chamber with isolated or diffuse white patches on the posterior corneal surface, a peau d'orange texture with retroillumination, and bandlike lesions at the level of Descemet's membrane.[8] As previously noted, the corneal abnormality is limited to the posterior layers, and in most cases the patients remain symptom free, although secondary stromal and epithelial edema may occur in some cases.

Light microscopic studies of the cornea in cases of posterior polymorphous dystrophy reveal fusiform excrescences of Descemet's membrane, which are occasionally vacuolated[23] or contain calcium crystals.[17] Ultrastructural studies of the cor-

---

*References 2, 13, 14, 17, 18, 23.

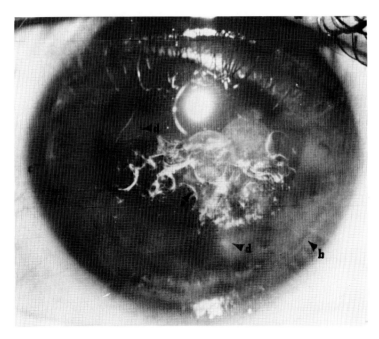

FIG. 6-14. Example of posterior polymorphous dystrophy with iridocorneal adhesions showing *(a)* semicircular, brush stroke–like opacities of cornea; *(b)* prominent Schwalbe's ring; *(c)* atrophic iris extending to posterior surface of cornea; and *(d)* deep opacities of cornea. (From Grayson, M.: Trans. Am. Ophthalmol. Soc. **72:**516, 1974.)

nea reveal an unusually thin Descemet's membrane covered by multiple layers of collagen[2,13,14,18] and lined by cells variably described as having features of abnormal endothelium,[13] fibroblasts,[14,18] or epithelium[2,28] (Fig. 6-15).

A small number of patients with posterior polymorphous dystrophy have broad iridocorneal adhesions that often extend anterior to Schwalbe's line and occasionally onto the peripheral cornea. This may be associated with corectopia, ectropion uveae, and rarefaction of the iris. A translucent sheetlike "glass membrane" has been observed clinically to extend from the posterior corneal surface onto the iris.[7] In some cases the pupil has been noted to be displaced toward this membrane on the iris. The diagnosis of iridocorneal adhesions and posterior polymorphous dystrophy is usually made after the patient reaches adulthood, and these changes are typically bilateral.

A small percentage of patients with posterior polymorphous dystrophy have glaucoma. In some patients this is associated with iridocorneal adhesions, although other patients with glaucoma have open, normal-appearing anterior chamber angles.[7]

Rodrigues et al.[26] studied the ultrastructure of the anterior chamber angle and iris in two trabecu-

lectomy and peripheral iridectomy specimens from eyes with posterior polymorphous dystrophy. They reported that the trabecular beams were covered by Descemet's membrane and transformed endothelial cells that resembled epithelial cells with numerous microvillous projections and desmosomal attachments (Fig. 6-16). The downgrowth of the membrane and endothelium with epithelial-like cells was also present on the surface of the iris.

Pathogenesis

Many early investigators believed that the posterior corneal lesion might be the result of the herpes simplex virus. Subsequent clinical and histologic studies, however, have suggested that the disorder is most likely developmental. In those cases associated with iridocorneal adhesions, a mesodermal dysgenesis of the anterior segment has been postulated, since the corneal endothelium was once believed to be of mesodermal origin.[39] However, Cibis et al.[7] have postulated that the Descemet-like glass membrane, which was observed to extend from the posterior cornea onto the iris, may be a result of the dystrophic endothelium and may lead to the secondary synechiae formation, a mechanism similar to the one in the

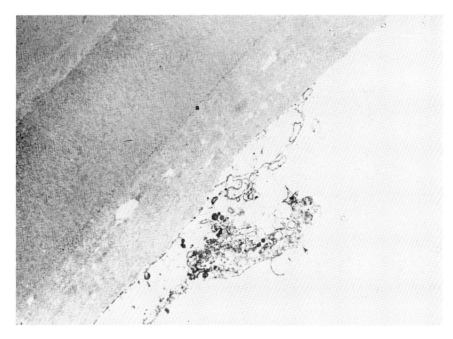

FIG. 6-15. Transmission electron microscopic view of posterior cornea in posterior polymorphous dystrophy showing dying endothelial cells on abnormal basement membrane. (From Grayson, M.: Trans. Am. Ophthalmol. Soc. **72:**516, 1974.)

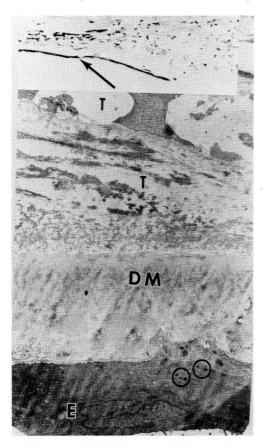

FIG. 6-16. Transmission electron microscopic view of trabeculectomy specimen from eye with posterior polymorphous dystrophy showing trabecular beams *(T)* covered by Descemet's membrane *(DM)* and transformed endothelial cells *(E)*. The latter have numerous microvillous projections and desmosomal attachments *(circles)*. (×8200.) Inset shows light microscopic appearance of membrane on trabecular meshwork *(arrow)*. (Toluidine blue; ×130.) (From Rodrigues, M.M., Phelps, C.D., Krachmer, J.H., et al.: Arch. Ophthalmol. **98:**688, 1980. Copyright 1980, American Medical Association.)

membrane theory of Campbell et al.[4] for the pathogenesis of the ICE syndrome.

In those patients with iridocorneal adhesions and glaucoma, it is likely that the synechial obstruction of the trabecular meshwork is responsible for the elevated intraocular pressure. However, in patients with posterior polymorphous dystrophy and glaucoma with open, normal-appearing anterior chamber angles, the mechanism of glaucoma is less clear. It may be that the trabecular endothelium is affected by the same dystrophic process as the cornea, or that the meshwork is covered by the epithelial-like layer, which has not yet led to synechiae formation. The previously noted study of Rodrigues et al.[26] is consistent with this theory.

Differential diagnosis

Cases of posterior polymorphous dystrophy with abnormalities limited to the cornea must be distinguished from other dystrophies of the corneal endothelium, such as Fuchs' endothelioepithelial dystrophy and congenital hereditary endothelial dystrophy. When the condition is associated with iridocorneal adhesions and glaucoma, the differential diagnosis must include Rieger's syndrome and the ICE syndrome.

Management

Although most patients with posterior polymorphous dystrophy are asymptomatic, some require treatment for corneal edema, secondary glaucoma, or both. The edema of the cornea may be controlled with hypertonic saline solutions or soft contact lenses, although some patients eventually require penetrating keratoplasty. Medical management of the secondary glaucoma is the same as for primary open-angle glaucoma in those patients with open, normal-appearing angles. When the angle is obstructed by broad peripheral anterior synechiae, drugs that reduce aqueous production, such as carbonic anhydrase inhibitors and timolol maleate, may be more efficacious. In cases of secondary glaucoma that cannot be controlled by maximum tolerable medical therapy, glaucoma filtering surgery is usually indicated.

FUCHS' ENDOTHELIOEPITHELIAL DYSTROPHY
Historical background

In 1910 Fuchs[11] described a primary, chronic edema of the cornea that usually appeared in middle-aged patients and had a strong predilection for women. Six years later, Koeppe[19] reported the first slit-lamp study of this entity, in which he described fine defects in the endothelial layer of the cornea. Subsequent studies established the correlation between the primary endothelial dystrophy and the secondary edema of the corneal stroma and epithelium in what became known as Fuchs' endothelioepithelial dystrophy.

The recognition of glaucoma in association with Fuchs' dystrophy has come about in more recent years, with two forms having been described: open-angle[20] and angle-closure glaucoma.[37]

Clinicopathologic features

Fuchs' dystrophy is a bilateral condition with a familial tendency and is usually first detected between the ages of 40 and 70 years (mean in the sixth decade) with a marked preponderance of women. The typical appearance of the posterior cornea by slit-lamp examination is that of beaten silver, which is often difficult to distinguish from the ICE syndrome. This stage of the disease, usually referred to as cornea guttata, is common and rarely leads to the full picture of Fuchs' endothelioepithelial dystrophy with edema of the corneal stroma and epithelium.

Histologically Descemet's membrane is thickened and contains many excrescences, which project posteriorly, and the endothelial cells are attenuated as they cross over the excrescences, or warts. In eyes with corneal edema, the stromal lamellae are loosened by fluid infiltration and the corneal epithelial cells are vacuolized and in some areas separated from Bowman's membrane by fluid and cellular debris. In advanced cases there may also be subepithelial collagenous tissue.[37] Secondary complications of Fuchs' dystrophy include infection of ruptured epithelial bullae and glaucoma. It has been estimated that 10% to 15% of patients with Fuchs' dystrophy have open-angle glaucoma,[20] although a study of 71 patients with Fuchs' endothelioepithelial dystrophy revealed only one case of open-angle glaucoma.[21] A few cases of associated angle-closure glaucoma have also been described.[37]

Mechanism of glaucoma

In cases of open-angle glaucoma, the cause of obstruction to aqueous outflow has not been determined. These cases resemble primary open-angle glaucoma, although Waltman et al.[38] found that only 2 of 16 patients with Fuchs' dystrophy had the in vitro lymphocyte responsiveness to corticosteroids that is commonly found in patients with primary open-angle glaucoma. It has been speculated that the endothelial dystrophy may involve the endothelium of the trabecular meshwork, leading to the obstruction of aqueous outflow.[20]

Stocker[37] reported patients with shallow anterior chamber angles in whom gradual thickening of the corneal stroma eventually led to closure of the anterior chamber angle and an acute attack of angle-closure glaucoma. Prophylactic measures with 1% pilocarpine did not prevent such attacks.

Management

Although most cases of Fuchs' dystrophy are not associated with glaucoma, further reduction of a normal intraocular pressure is occasionally used to minimize the corneal edema by reducing the hydrostatic pressure exerted on the damaged endothelium. Stocker[36] reported that acetazolamide was particularly effective in such cases, which he believed might be related to both the diuretic and the intraocular pressure–reducing action of the drug. Other measures to manage the corneal edema include the use of topical hypertonic saline solutions, soft contact lenses, and penetrating keratoplasty.

When elevated intraocular pressure is present in cases of Fuchs' dystrophy, measures to reduce the pressure are indicated to minimize the corneal edema as well as to protect the optic nerve head. Patients with the open-angle type of glaucoma are managed in the same manner as those with primary open-angle glaucoma: with medical therapy and filtering surgery when indicated. Patients with the angle-closure type of glaucoma are treated with iridectomy or filtering surgery if there are extensive peripheral anterior synechiae. As previously noted, prophylactic miotic therapy has not been effective in patients with impending angle closure.[37]

REFERENCES

1. Benedikt, O., and Roll, P.: Open-angle glaucoma through endothelialization of the anterior chamber angle, Glaucoma **2**:368, 1980.
2. Boruchoff, S.A., and Kuwabara, T.: Electron microscopy of posterior polymorphous degeneration, Am. J. Ophthalmol. **72**:879, 1971.
3. Campbell, D.G.: Formation of iris nodules in primary proliferative endothelial degeneration, paper presented at the meeting of the Association for Research in Vision and Ophthalmology, Sarasota, Fla., April 30 to May 4, 1979.
4. Campbell, D.G., Shields, M.B., and Smith, T.R.: The

corneal endothelium in the spectrum of essential iris atrophy, Am. J. Ophthalmol. **86**:317, 1978.
5. Chandler, P.A.: Atrophy of the stroma of the iris: endothelial dystrophy, corneal edema, and glaucoma, Am. J. Ophthalmol. **41**:607, 1956.
6. Chandler, P.A., and Grant, W.M.: Lectures on glaucoma, Philadelphia, 1965, Lea & Febiger, pp. 276-285.
7. Cibis, G.W., Krachmer, J.H., Phelps, C.D., and Weingeist, T.A.: Iridocorneal adhesions in posterior polymorphous dystrophy, Trans. Am. Acad. Ophthalmol. Otol. **81**:770, 1976.
8. Cibis, G.W., Krachmer, J.A., Phelps, C.D., and Weingeist, T.A.: The clinical spectrum of posterior polymorphous dystrophy, Arch. Ophthalmol. **95**:1529, 1977.
9. Cogan, D.G., and Reese, A.B.: A syndrome of iris nodules, ectopic Descemet's membrane, and unilateral glaucoma, Doc. Ophthalmol. **26**:424, 1969.
10. Eagle, R.C., Jr., Font, R.L., Yanoff, M., and Fine, B.S.: Proliferative endotheliopathy with iris abnormalities: the iridocorneal endothelial syndrome, Arch. Ophthalmol. **97**:2104, 1979.
11. Fuchs, E.: Dystrophia epithelialis cornea, Albrecht Von Graefes Arch. Ophthalmol. **76**:478, 1910.
12. Grayson, M.: The nature of hereditary deep polymorphous dystrophy of the cornea: its association with iris and anterior chamber dysgenesis, Trans. Am. Ophthalmol. Soc. **72**:516, 1974.
13. Hanna, C., Fraunfelder, F.T., and McNair, J.R.: An ultrastructure study of posterior polymorphous dystrophy of the cornea, Ann. Ophthalmol. **9**:1371, 1977.
14. Hanselmayer, H.: Zur Histopathologie der hinteren polymorphen Hornhautdystrophie nach Schlichting. II. Ultrastrukturelle Befunde, pathogenetische und pathophysiologische Bemerkungen, Albrecht. Von Graefes Arch. Klin. Exp. Ophthalmol. **185**:53, 1972.
15. Harms, C.: Einseitige spontane Luckenbildung der Iris durch Atrophie ohne mechanische Zerrung, Klin. Monatsbl. Augenheilkd. **41**:522, 1903.
16. Hirst, L.W., Quigley, H.A., Stark, W.J., and Shields, M.B.: Specular microscopy in iridocorneal endothelial syndrome, Am. J. Ophthalmol. **89**:11, 1980; Aust. J. Ophthalmol. **8**:139, 1980.
17. Hogan, M.J., and Bietti, G.: Hereditary deep dystrophy of the cornea (polymorphous), Am. J. Ophthalmol. **68**:777, 1969.
18. Johnson, B.L., and Brown, S.I.: Posterior polymorphous dystrophy: a light and electron microscopic study, Br. J. Ophthalmol. **62**:89, 1978.
19. Koeppe, L.: Klinische Beobachtungen mit der lampe und dem Hornhaupmikroskop, Albrecht Von Graefes Arch. Ophthalmol. **91**:363, 1916.
20. Kolker, A.E., and Hetherington, J., Jr.: Becker-Shaffer's diagnosis and therapy of the glaucomas, ed. 4, St. Louis, 1976, The C.V. Mosby Co., pp. 265-266.
21. Krachmer, J.H., Purcell, J.J., Jr., Young, C.W., and Bucher, K.D.: Corneal endothelial dystrophy: a study of 64 families, Arch. Ophthalmol. **96**:2036, 1978.
22. Lisch, W.: Iridoschesis, Klin. Monatsbl. Augenheilkd. **168**:228, 1976.
23. Morgan, G., and Patterson, A.: Pathology of posterior polymorphous degeneration of the cornea, Br. J. Ophthalmol. **51**:433, 1967.
24. Quigley, H.A., and Forster, R.F.: Histopathology of cor-

nea and iris in Chandler's syndrome, Arch. Ophthalmol. **96:**1878, 1978.

25. Richardson, T.M.: Corneal decompensation in Chandler's syndrome: a scanning and transmission electron microscopic study, Arch. Ophthalmol. **97:**2112, 1979.

26. Rodrigues, M.M., Phelps, C.D., Krachmer, J.H., and others: Glaucoma due to endothelialization of the anterior chamber angle: a comparison of posterior polymorphous dystrophy of the cornea and Chandler's syndrome, Arch. Ophthalmol. **98:**688, 1980.

27. Rodrigues, M.M., Streeten, B.W., and Spaeth, G.L.: Chandler's syndrome as a variant of essential iris atrophy, Arch. Ophthalmol. **96:**643, 1978.

28. Rodrigues, M.M., Sun, T.T., Krachmer, J., and Newsome, D.: Epithelialization of the corneal endothelium in posterior polymorphous dystrophy, Invest. Ophthalmol. Vis. Sci. **19:**832, 1980.

29. Scheie, H.G., and Yanoff, M.: Iris nevus (Cogan-Reese) syndrome: a cause of unilateral glaucoma, Arch. Ophthalmol. **93:**963, 1975.

30. Setala, K., and Vannas, A.: Corneal endothelial cells in essential iris atrophy: a specular microscopic study, Acta Ophthalmol. **57:**1020, 1979.

31. Shields, M.B.: Progressive essential iris atrophy, Chandler's syndrome, and the iris nevus (Cogan-Reese) syndrome: a spectrum of disease, Surv. Ophthalmol. **24:**3, 1979.

32. Shields, M.B., Campbell, D.G., and Simmons, R.J.: The essential iris atrophies, Am. J. Ophthalmol. **85:**749, 1978.

33. Shields, M.B., Campbell, D.G., Simmons, R.J., and Hutchinson, B.T.: Iris nodules in essential iris atrophy, Arch. Ophthalmol. **94:**406, 1976.

34. Shields, M.B., McCracken, J.S., Klintworth, G.K., and Campbell, D.G.: Corneal edema in essential iris atrophy, Ophthalmology **86:**1533, 1979.

35. Soukup, F.: Polymorfni zadni degenerace rohovky, Cesk. Oftalmol. **20:**181, 1964.

36. Stocker, F.W.: Use of acetazoleamide (Diamox) for endothelial corneal dystrophy and diseased corneal grafts, Am. J. Ophthalmol. **41:**203, 1956.

37. Stocker, F.W.: The endothelium of the cornea and its clinical implications, ed. 2, Springfield, Ill., 1971, Charles C Thomas, Publisher, pp. 79-140.

38. Waltman, S.R., Palmberg, P.F., and Becker, B.: In vitro corticosteroid sensitivity in patients with Fuchs' dystrophy, Doc. Ophthalmol. Proc. Ser. **18:**321, 1979.

39. Waring, G.O. III., Rodrigues, M.M., and Laibson, P.R.: Corneal dystrophies. II. Endothelial dystrophy, Surv. Ophthalmol. **23:**147, 1978.

40. Yanoff, M.: In discussion of Shields, M.B., McCracken, J.S., Klintworth, G.K., and Campbell, D.G.: Corneal edema in essential iris atrophy, Ophthalmology **86:**1549, 1979.

Chapter 7

PIGMENTARY GLAUCOMA

Thomas M. Richardson

CLINICAL PICTURE

Pigmentary glaucoma is a bilateral disorder predominantly affecting young myopic men. It is characterized by loss of pigment from the pigmented epithelium of the iris, particularly in the midperipheral region (Fig. 7-1). This loss of pigment gives rise to radial transillumination defects in the iris and a dispersion of melanin pigment into the aqueous humor. The pigment is deposited on various surfaces in the anterior segment, including the lens, zonules, iris, cornea (Krukenberg's spindle), and trabecular meshwork (Fig. 7-2). It is the general belief that it is the accumulation of pigment in the aqueous outflow system that causes glaucoma. Such a dispersion of pigment may also occur without causing glaucoma.

While pigmentary glaucoma is usually a progressive disease requiring medical or surgical management to prevent damage to the optic disc and glaucomatous visual field loss, it sometimes has a mild course or occasionally becomes less severe, particularly with age. In a series of 102 patients, Lichter and Shaffer[29] observed a definite decrease in the amount of pigment in the trabecular meshwork in 10% of cases, leading them to conclude that the pigment could pass out of the meshwork as the patient aged. On occasion, transilluminating areas of the iris have been observed to disappear,[10,13] suggesting that these areas can be resurfaced by pigment or pigment-containing cells. In a few rare patients the intraocular pressure has even been noted to return toward normal within a few years.[13,18,37] In such patients it has been possible to reduce or discontinue treatment for glaucoma.

HISTORICAL BACKGROUND

The relationship between pigment particles in the anterior segment and elevation of intraocular pressure was suspected more than three quarters of a century ago, when von Hippel[43] suggested that glaucoma was caused by obstruction of the aqueous outflow system by pigment. Levinsohn[27] detected pigment in the angle of the anterior chamber of certain patients with glaucoma, and he believed that these particles originated from the pigmented layer of the iris. The view that there was a cause-and-effect relationship between pigment and glaucoma was supported by some investigators (e.g., Koeppe[24] and Jess[22]) but was opposed by others (e.g., Vogt,[42] Birch-Hirschfeld,[6] and Evans et al.[15]). In recent times more investigators have supported the concept that the pigment particles observed in this condition arise from the pigmented neuroepithelium of the iris and perhaps the ciliary body.[4,35,39] In 1940 Sugar[38] described a 29-year-old man with a form of glaucoma that was accompanied by degeneration of the pigment epithelium of the iris and ciliary body and deposition of pigment on surfaces within the anterior chamber. By 1949 Sugar and Barbour[41] had applied the term pigmentary glaucoma to this disease and delineated the clinical features that are now well recognized as the hallmarks of an unusual type of glaucoma.

In the years that followed, many cases of pigmentary glaucoma were reported in the literature, and in 1966 Sugar[39] reviewed 147 cases in which several additional features of this disease were highlighted. These included bilateral occurrence, frequent association with a moderate degree of

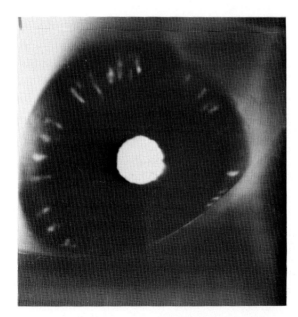

FIG. 7-1. Donaldson photograph of transilluminated iris from patient with pigmentary glaucoma showing radial defects in midperiphery resulting from loss of pigment from pigmented epithelium.

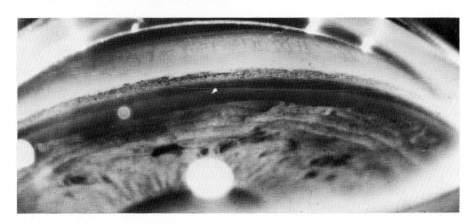

FIG. 7-2. Goniophotograph of angle from patient with pigmentary glaucoma showing dense band of pigment in trabecular meshwork.

myopia, greater incidence in men than in women, and a relatively youthful onset of the disease in comparison with that of primary open-angle glaucoma. Pigmentary glaucoma typically occurs in men at about age 35 and in women at about age 50. These features have been confirmed in a report by Scheie and Cameron[34] describing a series of 104 patients with pigmentary glaucoma.

Although the clinical features of pigmentary glaucoma have been recognized in detail, knowledge of its pathophysiology remains obscure, perhaps because of the limited availability of histopathologic material, but more probably because of the lack of a readily available animal model in

which to test various hypotheses relative to the pathophysiology of the disease.

CLASSIFICATION
Pigment dispersion syndrome

Pigment dispersion in the anterior segment of the eye can occur without elevated intraocular pressure and may be encountered in routine eye examinations as frequently as true pigmentary glaucoma.[13] Some of these patients go on to develop glaucoma, although the time period between the diagnosis of pigment dispersion and the onset of glaucoma varies considerably and may take from 12 to 20 years.[39,40] Some patients with diffuse pigment dispersion have not developed abnormal pressures even after 20 years of follow-up.[13]

Pigment dispersion syndrome with glaucoma

Individuals with pigmentary glaucoma appear clinically exactly like those with the pigment dispersion syndrome except for their elevated pressures and sometimes secondary changes in the optic disc. Pigmentary glaucoma is a relatively rare disease that appears to have an age, sexual, and racial predilection (young white men). The disease can have a rather mild course, but frequently it is not managed adequately by medical therapy and requires surgery to prevent progressive compromise of the optic disc with characteristic glaucomatous visual field loss.

PATHOPHYSIOLOGY AND MECHANISMS
Development of glaucoma

The pathogenetic mechanism that adequately explains the cause-and-effect relationship between pigment in the anterior segment and the elevation of intraocular pressure has been a topic of debate since Sugar and Barbour[41] first clinically distinguished pigmentary glaucoma as a disease directly related to the accumulation of pigment in the aqueous outflow system. Subsequently, a variety of hypotheses have emerged that attempt to explain the pathogenesis of the glaucoma that frequently accompanies the dispersion of pigment. One view suggests that patients who develop pigmentary glaucoma suffer from a mesodermal angle anomaly[9,28,29] and that the presence of pigment in the trabecular meshwork is secondary to a developmental defect in angle structures. However, as pointed out by Epstein,[13] these anomalies (abnormal iris processes) seem to occur with equal frequency in similarly myopic eyes that have wide angles and no excessive pigment in the meshwork. Other iris abnormalities, namely hyperplasia of the iris dilator muscle and degeneration of iris nerve fibers, have been observed in the pigment dispersion syndrome,[16,26] but their relevance to the development of glaucoma is unknown.

Another view of the pathogenesis of pigmentary glaucoma suggests that it is simply a variant of primary open-angle glaucoma. This is supported by a study indicating that patients with the pigment dispersion syndrome who develop elevated intraocular pressure after the administration of topical corticosteroids are inherently susceptible to glaucoma due to a defective gene.[1] It is believed that such patients belong to a class of individuals who have a genetic predisposition for open-angle glaucoma. Results from that study, however, have not been confirmed. Rather, other studies of pressure responses to corticosteroids indicate that pigmentary glaucoma is not simply a variant of primary open-angle glaucoma but is in fact a separate and distinct entity.[2,45]

Yet another view of pigmentary glaucoma, and one that seems to gain support as time passes, is that the elevation of intraocular pressure that accompanies the pigment dispersion syndrome is caused, at least initially, by accumulation of melanin pigment in the trabecular meshwork (Fig. 7-3) and that this blocks the flow of aqueous humor through the outflow channels.[39] This concept gained considerable support when it was shown that pigment particles obtained from the pigmented epithelium of the iris and perfused into enucleated human and primate eyes caused an increase in the resistance to fluid flow through the aqueous outflow system.[3,17] This is confirmed clinically by tonography when patients with the pigment dispersion syndrome who develop a shower of pigment in the aqueous humor, either spontaneously or after vigorous exercise, have an acute rise in intraocular pressure and a concomitant decrease in the facility of outflow.[14]

Transient rises in intraocular pressure have also been observed clinically after a shower of pigment was released into the aqueous humor by mydriasis.[25] It is well known that topically administered mydriatics, especially a sympathomimetic such as phenylephrine, often result in the liberation of pigment into the aqueous humor.[19,30] However, in normal individuals or those with chronic open-angle glaucoma, phenylephrine administered topically either reduces or has no effect on intraocular pressure.[19] In Kristensen's study,[25] patients with either pigmentary glaucoma or exfoliation glaucoma developed an acute rise in intraocular pressure associated with excessive pigment release, suggesting that these individuals are more susceptible to temporary obstruction of the aqueous outflow system by pigment particles. A similar conclusion can be reached from Mapstone's study.[30]

To determine whether pressure responses to phenylephrine could be used as a prognostic indi-

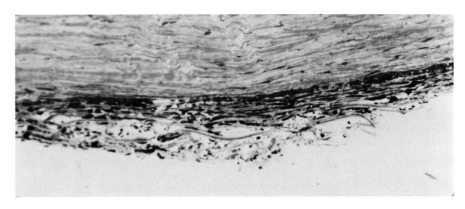

FIG. 7-3. Light microscopic appearance of trabecular meshwork in pigmentary glaucoma. Heavy deposits of melanin pigment extend through entire depth of meshwork.

cator to identify those patients predisposed to pressure elevation as a result of the release of pigment showers, Epstein et al.[14] performed phenylephrine provocative testing on a selected group of patients who had the pigment dispersion syndrome bilaterally, with or without glaucoma. Patients were evaluated for the liberation of pigment and a rise in intraocular pressure in response to phenylephrine 10% administered topically to one eye while the second eye served as the control. Only 2.5% of the patients in the study developed 4+ pigment reaction in the anterior chamber, and less than 15% developed a rise in intraocular pressure greater than 2 mm Hg as a result of the provocative test. As in Kristensen's study,[25] the majority of patients who tended to develop a rise in pressure already had either pigmentary or exfoliation glaucoma. Few, if any, with only the pigment dispersion syndrome developed increased pressure.

It is interesting that in the study by Epstein et al.,[14] pigment liberation tended to be greatest in the older patient with pigment dispersion who already had glaucoma and who also had been treated with topical antiglaucoma medication. It seems paradoxical that pigment liberation should be increased with increasing age, when it is well known that the incidence of pigmentary glaucoma actually decreases with advancing years. Although there seems to be no correlation between the extent of iris transillumination and the grade of phenylephrine-induced pigment liberation, Kristensen[25] showed that repeated mydriasis resulted in smaller and smaller showers of pigment into the anterior chamber. However, mydriasis induced after about

2 weeks' recovery from mydriatics produced pigment liberation approximately the same as in the initial response. This suggests that pigment or pigment-containing cells expand to cover the sites of previously liberated pigment.[10]

While the above studies demonstrate that pigment particles can temporarily obstruct aqueous outflow, at least in some individuals, heavy pigmentation of the trabecular meshwork can occur without pressure elevation.[16] Some individuals with a clinically well defined dispersion of pigment in the anterior segment may not develop an elevated pressure or abnormal facility of outflow even after 20 years of observation.[13] The mere presence of pigment particles in the meshwork is not sufficient, then, to account for the severe, persistent form of pigment-induced glaucoma.

What, then, are the factors that determine the fate of pigment particles in the aqueous outflow system, and how are these factors translated into elevation of intraocular pressure? It is common to find on gonioscopy a dense band of pigment in the trabecular meshwork of persons with the pigment dispersion syndrome (Fig. 7-2). Light and electron microscopy has established that the pigment particles are located both within and outside of the cells that line the trabeculae* (Figs. 7-4 and 7-5). Occasionally a pigment-containing cell, ostensibly derived from the iris stroma, is seen in the intertrabecular spaces. Frequently, from the examination of histopathologic specimens, the amount of pigment within and outside the cells of

---

*References 16, 20, 21, 31, 32.

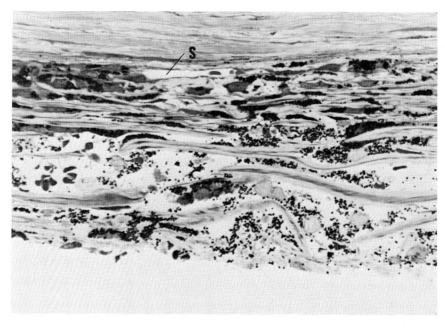

FIG. 7-4. Light micrograph of trabecular meshwork and portion of Schlemm's canal *(S)* from patient with pigmentary glaucoma. Free pigment granules are located mainly in uveal meshwork and beginning of corneoscleral meshwork. Deeper deposits of pigment are mainly intracellular. Free pigment is not found within lumen of Schlemm's canal.

the trabecular meshwork appears to severely restrict the intertrabecular spaces. Such restriction alone is probably sufficient to impede the flow of aqueous and cause elevation of pressure in the eye.

There seems, however, to be another stage in the obstructive process in the patient who is unresponsive to medical therapy. Electron microscopic studies of such patients have revealed degeneration of endothelial cells of the trabecular meshwork, trapping of cell debris or breakdown products of pigment-containing cells (Fig. 7-6), and sclerosis of the trabecular beams[31] (Figs. 7-7 and 7-8). There is evidence that the endothelial cells that line the trabeculae behave as local purveyors of materials passing through the corneoscleral meshwork.[5,10] These cells appear to have a selective capacity to phagocytize various types of particles and cells that can potentially obstruct the outflow channels.[33,36] Excessive phagocytosis often appears to lead to migration of the endothelial cells away from the trabeculae[33,36] (Fig. 7-9) and/or to autolysis of the cells in situ[31] (Fig. 7-6), which contributes to the cell debris. In either case the trabeculae are left denuded and unprotected from the aqueous humor and its contents.[31] A similar process occurs in pigmentary glaucoma, where denud-

ation of the trabeculae leads to breakdown and collapse of the intertrabecular spaces with degeneration and sclerosis of the trabeculae (Figs. 7-7 and 7-8).

These observations have led us to postulate that obstruction of the aqueous outflow system and the development of glaucoma probably occur in two stages, as diagrammed in Fig. 7-10. In the first stage, pigment liberated mainly from the iris neuroepithelium accumulates in the cells and spaces of the otherwise normal-appearing trabecular meshwork. Accumulation of pigment in moderate amounts over a short period may acutely obstruct the intertrabecular space and result in transient elevation of intraocular pressure. Excessive phagocytosis of pigment leads to migration of the trabecular cells away from the beams. These cells may undergo autolysis, resulting in further accumulation of cell debris and pigment in the meshwork. The remaining attached cells spread over the denuded portions of the trabeculae in an apparent attempt to keep them covered (Fig. 7-11).

During the first stage, the pigment dispersion cycle probably remains static, with only an occasional or low-grade elevation of intraocular pressure. This stage is probably clinically reversible,

Text continued on p. 93.

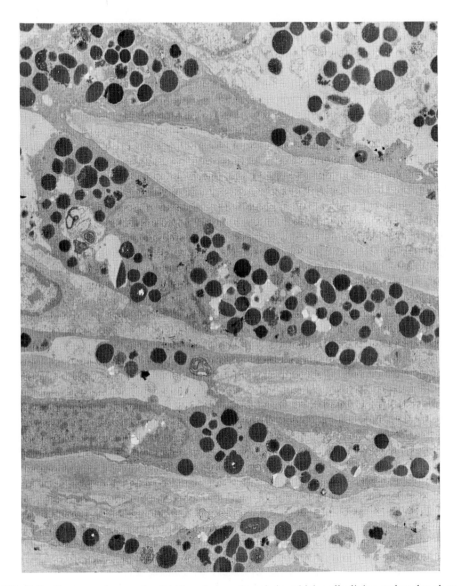

FIG. 7-5. Electron micrograph of trabecular meshwork in which cells lining trabecular sheets are heavily laden with pigment granules. Some granules are fragmented and could be undergoing digestion. Except for heavy pigment deposits, trabecular cells appear relatively healthy. A few free pigment granules are located in intertrabecular spaces.

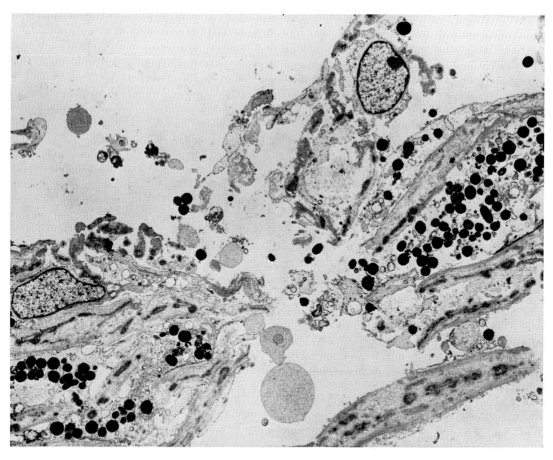

FIG. 7-6. Electron micrograph of trabecular meshwork in which trabecular cells have undergone degeneration and left beams partially denuded of cells. Connective tissue of some beams is disorganized. Pigment particles and cell debris fill intertrabecular spaces.

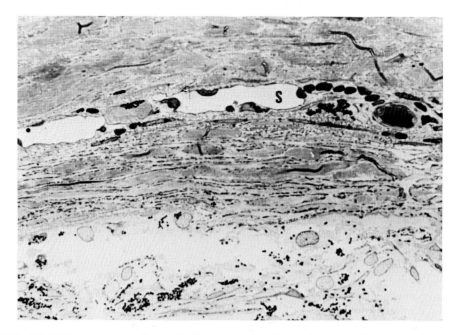

FIG. 7-7. Light micrograph of severely damaged trabecular meshwork in pigmentary glaucoma. Corneoscleral meshwork is collapsed and appears relatively acellular. Schlemm's canal *(S)* is patent and free of pigment particles.

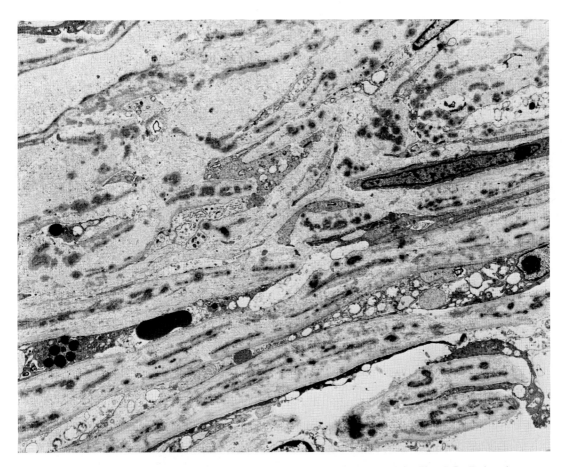

FIG. 7-8. Electron micrograph of trabecular meshwork demonstrated in Fig. 7-7. Trabecular sheets have collapsed and fused, leading to obliteration of aqueous pathway. Cell debris, scattered pigment-containing cells, and an occasional normal-appearing cell are located throughout sclerotic tissue.

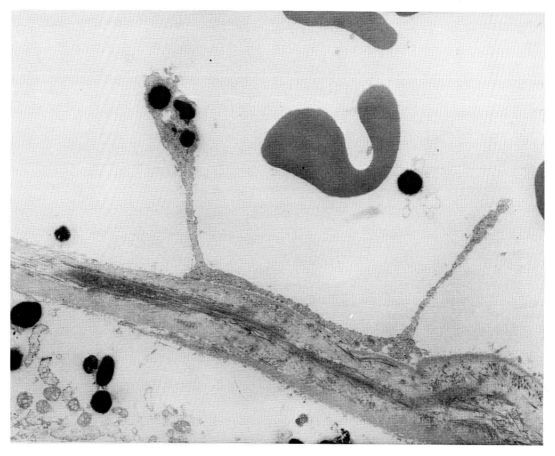

FIG. 7-9. Portion of trabecular cell in contact with trabecular beam. Trabecular cell contains ingested pigment particles. Portions of cell have lost contact with beam, leaving underlying connective tissue exposed.

PATHOPHYSOLOGY of PIGMENTARY GLAUCOMA

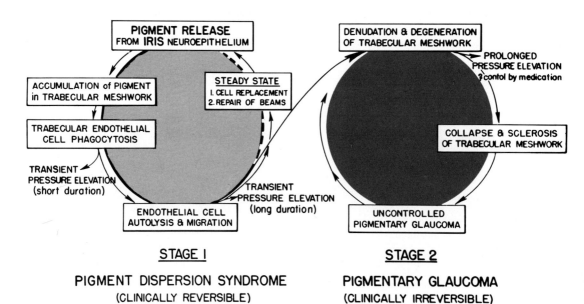

PIGMENT RELEASE
FROM **IRIS** NEUROEPITHELIUM

DENUDATION & DEGENERATION
OF TRABECULAR MESHWORK

PROLONGED
PRESSURE ELEVATION
?contol by medication

ACCUMULATION of PIGMENT
in TRABECULAR MESHWORK

STEADY STATE
1. CELL REPLACEMENT
2. REPAIR OF BEAMS

TRABECULAR ENDOTHELIAL
CELL PHAGOCYTOSIS

COLLAPSE & SCLEROSIS
OF TRABECULAR MESHWORK

TRANSIENT
PRESSURE ELEVATION
(short duration)

TRANSIENT
PRESSURE ELEVATION
(long duration)

ENDOTHELIAL CELL
AUTOLYSIS & MIGRATION

UNCONTROLLED
PIGMENTARY GLAUCOMA

STAGE 1

PIGMENT DISPERSION SYNDROME
(CLINICALLY REVERSIBLE)

STAGE 2

PIGMENTARY GLAUCOMA
(CLINICALLY IRREVERSIBLE)

FIG. 7-10. Hypothetical mechanism that may explain pathophysiology of pigmentary glaucoma. First stage of disease is clinically reversible and gives rise to transient rises in intraocular pressure. Second stage, characterized by irreparable damage to trabecular tissues, is irreversible and is accompanied by uncontrolled glaucoma.

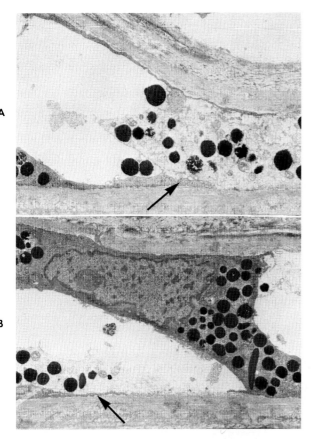

FIG. 7-11. Trabecular meshwork in which single trabecular cells support opposing beams. Thin processes of healthy trabecular cells spread to cover denuded beams or replace damaged or degenerating cells. **A,** Pale, disintegrating trabecular cell has partially lifted from beam and is being undermined by process from healthier trabecular cell *(arrow)*. Bottom surface of upper beam has been covered by thin cell process, whereas upper surface of beam is still denuded of cells. **B,** A small cell process from large trabecular cell has extended to cover portion of denuded lower beam. A second healthy trabecular cell has extended under and is replacing damaged trabecular cell *(arrow)*.

provided that the trabecular meshwork maintains the capacity to undergo self-repair. When it loses this capacity, the trabecular beams degenerate and the second stage is entered. The second stage is probably irreversible and is the result of irreparable damage to the trabeculae (Fig. 7-8).

Such a scheme could explain the great variability in individual behavior in this disease. The transient rises in pressure that have been observed clinically after a pigment shower in the aqueous humor after mydriasis or physical disturbance of the eye and the acute obstruction of outflow that has been reported after iris pigment was injected into the anterior chamber of human or animal eyes fits well with the first stage, which can be transient with only a temporary rise in intraocular pressure.[29] The key to reversibility in this disease appears to reside in the capacity of trabecular endothelial cells to migrate away from the beams and be replaced by new or healthier cells (Fig. 7-11) to repair mildly damaged trabecular sheets before they undergo degeneration and collapse. Inability of the trabecular meshwork to achieve the latter

may represent a primary defect in the endothelial cells. This would explain why certain individuals with the pigment dispersion syndrome go on to develop severe glaucoma whereas others with an identical clinical picture might have no persistent elevation of intraocular pressure. Those individuals who have mild to moderate pressure elevation and who apparently recover from the disease can be thought of as having a less severe endothelial incapacitation.

Loss of pigment from the iris

The spontaneous loss of pigment from the iris neuroepithelium in the comparatively young myopic eye has long been considered to be due to congenital atrophy or degeneration of the iris neuroepithelium.[8,19,32] Campbell[10] has documented a pathogenetic mechanism that appears to account for the release of pigment from the posterior surface of the iris (Fig. 7-12). It appears that friction created by alternate back-and-forth rubbing of the posterior peripheral iris surface against packets of zonules inserted anteriorly on the lens surface

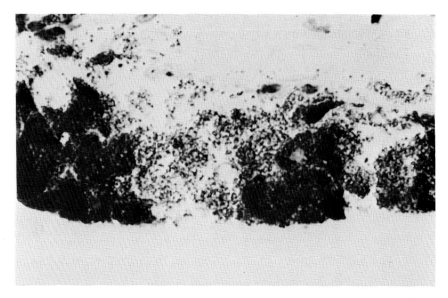

FIG. 7-12. Light micrograph of region of pigmented epithelium of iris where pigment has been liberated. Sharply delineated regions of pigment loss may represent paths of zonular fibers.

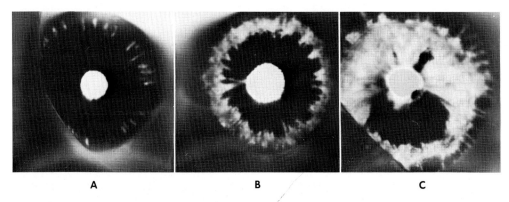

A   B   C

FIG. 7-13. Donaldson photographs of transilluminated irides depicting three stages of pigment loss in pigmentary glaucoma. Characteristic early midperipheral pattern of transillumination defects shown in **A** may become confluent in some patients and extend toward pupillary margin as shown in **B**. Rarely, pigment loss may progress to involve most of iris as shown in **C**.

causes pigment granules to be mechanically dislodged from the pigmented epithelium of the iris. The loss of pigment and cells that overlie the zonules corresponds well with the characteristic midperipheral radial pattern of iris transillumination defects in the irides of patients with the pigment dispersion syndrome (Fig. 7-13). This loss of pigment, however, can progress to involve the entire neuroepithelial layer. Kampik et al.[23] used scanning electron microscopy to study four eyes with pigment dispersion and have confirmed that the iris defects consistently follow the course of the zonular fibers.

This theory also answers two questions of major interest regarding the pathophysiology of pigmentary glaucoma. First, why does it predominantly affect younger white men with mild to moderate myopia; second, why does the severity and incidence of the disease decrease with increasing age? Regarding the first question, Campbell[10] believes that the eyes of patients predisposed to pigmentary glaucoma have an anterior segment structured in such a way that the peripheral iris assumes a concave configuration. This allows the normal physiologic movement of the iris to rub against the zonules and cause the liberation of pigment. Apparently, neither normal eyes nor eyes that are simply enlarged tend to have the necessary configuration for the iridozonular contact. The young myopic eye may continue to enlarge into the patient's 20s or early 30s, and this increase in diameter of the globe may be associated with an enlargement of the ciliary body ring in relation to the lens.[10] Such an enlargement causes the peripheral iris to sag and establish contact with the zonules. Male predominance may occur because men naturally have larger eyes than women, and this greater relative size increases the chance of having sufficient iris convexity to permit iridozonular rubbing. Except for the young myope, the eye generally ceases to enlarge when maturity is reached. The lens, however, continues slow growth until late in life. Since the average size of the pupil decreases with increasing age, this combination of increasing lens diameter and decreasing pupil size creates a relative pupillary block, which causes an anterior shift in the peripheral iris away from the zonules. This may explain the decrease in incidence and severity of pigmentary glaucoma in elderly patients.

Another puzzling feature of pigmentary glaucoma is that blacks tend not to get the disease, even though their uveae are heavily endowed with pigment and pigment in the angle is not an infrequent finding. The incidence of pigmentary glaucoma in the nonwhite population is believed to be rather small, being almost nonexistent in blacks and rare in Orientals. A physiologic basis for the difference in black and white patients was sought by Boles-Carenini et al.,[7] who made a comparative study of aqueous dynamics in normotensive eyes. However, they were unable to demonstrate a difference in the intraocular pressure, facility of outflow, or rate of aqueous production in the two groups. The higher incidence in whites might be related more specifically to the degree of iris pigmentation and stromal compactness.

The iris in darkly pigmented individuals is heavily laden with pigment, and the anterior surface of the iris frequently appears velvety smooth and homogeneously compact. By contrast, in lighter pigmented persons the iris is not only lighter in color, but also appears to have a more lacy texture, deep crypts, and easily visible stromal blood vessels. The lightest colored irides also appear thinner, often to a point where the slit beam can be focused through the entire stroma to the level of the ectodermal pigmented layer. Attempts

to demonstrate histologically that the darker iris is thicker have not been successful. It does appear, however, to be more compact with a larger number of melanocytes in the stroma.[44] The velvety appearance of the iris under slit-lamp observation is borne out histologically by evidence of a semiconfluent anterior surface.

Evidence of a more tightly compact stroma in darkly pigmented individuals is provided in studies demonstrating that the darker iris does not respond initially as well as the lighter colored iris to miotics or mydriatics. The effects of several different mydriatics on the pupils of whites, Orientals, and blacks were studied systematically by Chen and Poth[11] in 1929. They found that whites were most responsive, blacks were least responsive and Orientals had an intermediate response to the drugs.

A possible explanation for the slower response of blacks to miotics and mydriatics was provided by Emiru.[12] Comparing African blacks with European whites, he administered homatropine 4% to one eye and phenylephrine 4% to the other. Both the onset of mydriasis and the attainment of full mydriasis took less time in the European than in the heavily pigmented African. Interestingly, the irides of albino Africans dilated more briskly than those of either group, suggesting that these differences are more related to iris color than to race. Furthermore, homatropine, a cholinergic blocking agent, had a faster onset of action than phenylephrine, an adrenergic stimulator. The site of action of homatropine is the sphincter pupillae, and the site of action of phenylephrine is the dilator pupillae, which lies deeper in the stroma. The difference in accessibility to these muscles by topically applied drugs is argued as being the reason for the different individual responses found in such studies.[12] One may suppose that the more heavily pigmented compact stroma of dark irides not only would impede the penetration of various drugs, but would also limit the extent to which such irides could dilate. Such stromal characteristics as heavy pigmentation and compactness might well prevent peripheral iris sagging, which is believed to be essential in persons who develop the pigment dispersion syndrome.[10]

In many secondary glaucomas, such as pigmentary, exfoliation, corticosteroid-induced, lens-induced, ghost cell, and uveitic glaucoma, the usual cause of elevated intraocular pressure is an acquired abnormality in the trabecular meshwork. As pigmentary glaucoma comes more into focus, the anatomic and physiologic role of the iris appears increasingly important in understanding the pathogenetic mechanism as well as the natural history and racial predilection of this disease.

DIAGNOSIS
Special diagnostic techniques

The central feature of the pigmentary dispersion syndrome, whether or not there is a concomitant elevation of pressure, is the presence of a dense band of pigment in the trabecular meshwork. The details of the filtration angle can be observed by gonioscopy. The Koeppe lens, a separate hand-held light source (Barkan light), and a low-powered biomicroscope provide versatility, a direct view, controlled illumination, and excellent magnification for making out fine details of the angle structures.

Essential to the diagnosis of pigmentary glaucoma is the characteristic iris transillumination pattern. The defects can best be observed when the examiner is dark adapted. For a light source, a fiberoptic transilluminator is preferred. The probe of the illuminator is positioned over the sclera so as to achieve a bright red reflex from the posterior pole through the pupil. Any defects in the iris will transmit light, and the radial pattern common to pigmentary glaucoma should be present if one is to make the diagnosis reliably.

Differential diagnosis

Pigmentary dispersion, with or without elevated intraocular pressure, can usually be easily distinguished from most other abnormalities in which dissemination of pigment is part of the disease process. Several potentially confusing disease entities, such as uveitis, pigment in the angle due to dispersion of melanoma cells (e.g., melanomalytic dispersion), cysts of the iris and ciliary body, postoperative conditions, and aging can be eliminated from consideration rather early, because their occurrence is usually unilateral. In addition, trabecular pigmentation is less dense and is usually unevenly distributed throughout the entire circumference of the trabecular meshwork in these conditions.

The one disease process that clinically comes closest to mimicking pigmentary glaucoma is exfoliation glaucoma. In this condition, there is loss of pigment from the iris neuroepithelium with iris transillumination, pigment dispersion in the anterior segment including Krukenberg's spindle, trabecular pigmentation, and elevation of intraocular pressure. Even here, however, the clinical history combined with careful biomicroscopic examination easily separates the two diseases.

The age of onset for exfoliation glaucoma is generally over 60, and onset is rare under 40; there is no sexual or racial predilection for the exfoliation syndrome, although reports seem to indicate a higher prevalence of the disease in Scandinavians; the size and shape of the eye (myopia) appear to bear no relationship to the incidence of the disease; the accumulation of pigment in the trabecular meshwork is not as intense as in pigmentary glaucoma; the pattern of iris transillumination characteristically begins at the pupillary border and not the midperiphery; unlike pigmentary dispersion, approximately 50% of patients with the exfoliation syndrome are clinically affected in only one eye; and finally, the presence of white, flaky material at the pupillary border and the anterior lens surface unequivocally makes the diagnosis exfoliation syndrome.

MANAGEMENT
Medical therapy

Consideration for the institution of medical therapy in pigmentary glaucoma may be different from the rationale used in other forms of open-angle glaucoma. In pigmentary glaucoma, there is often a rather insidious rise in intraocular pressure, with ocular tensions frequently rising to 60 mm Hg or more. One would do well to remember, however, that this disease is subject to rather wide fluctuations in intraocular pressure, especially in the younger patient. Thus alarmingly elevated pressure may be followed spontaneously by lower pressure.

Since pigmentary glaucoma is basically a secondary open-angle glaucoma with the major site of resistance in the trabecular meshwork, the approach to medical therapy is the same as for primary open-angle glaucoma. The use of miotics in young individuals is rarely tolerated because of the associated spasm of accommodation and blurring of vision. Also, cautious use of miotics should be exercised in young myopic patients with pigmentary glaucoma, since there has been a reported association with retinal detachment in such patients who have peripheral chorioretinal degeneration.

Epinephrine continues to be the first line of topical therapy for pigmentary glaucoma. This drug alone or in combination with miotics has proved very effective in controlling this disease.[13]

Timolol, a beta-adrenergic blocking agent, because of its relatively low incidence of undesirable side effects and its effectiveness in lowering intraocular pressure, is gaining considerable appeal as treatment of pigmentary glaucoma. Carbonic anhydrase inhibitors are used on a short-term basis to lessen the severity of an acute pressure rise or on a long-term basis when indicated and tolerated by the patient.

Pigmentary glaucoma appears rather unique in its expression and behavior. The early age at which it comes on and the wide fluctuations in intraocular pressure require a somewhat different approach to management than that of primary open-angle glaucoma. It appears that if the trabecular meshwork in such patients has the capacity to undergo self-repair and remain in stage one of the disease, only the occasional ''crisis'' of pressure elevation will require therapy and the individual may perhaps eventually go into remission. However, if the patient's trabecular meshwork has limited or no capacity to recover and the disease goes into the second stage, the management will be determined by the effectiveness of the medication and the ability of the trabecular meshwork to undergo repair sufficient to maintain aqueous flow.

If the iridozonular mechanism of pigment release is true, then, theoretically, pigmentary glaucoma could be controlled by any drug that would constrict the pupil and make the peripheral iris taut. This would effectively decrease iridozonular rubbing and eliminate pigment accumulation in the meshwork. An alpha-adrenergic blocking agent such as thymoxamine hydrochloride, which constricts the pupil but does not affect accommodation or aqueous dynamics, could be beneficial to such patients.[10]

At the time of writing, thymoxamine hydrochloride is not an approved drug for this purpose and is unavailable for general use. In addition, in its present formulation, the ocular irritation that the drug causes makes it unlikely that patients would tolerate it. Mechanistically, however, such a drug has interesting possibilities, and its usefulness should be explored.

Surgical therapy

The surgical management of patients with pigmentary glaucoma follows the same principles and considerations used in the management of primary

open-angle glaucoma. The appearance and change in the optic nerve along with visual field defects should be the principal guidelines used in deciding whether surgery is needed. Most patients respond well to standard filtration operations.

REFERENCES

1. Becker, B., and Podos, S.M.: Krukenberg's spindles and primary open-angle glaucoma, Arch. Ophthalmol. **76:** 635, 1966.
2. Becker, B., Shin, D.H., Cooper, D.G., and Kass, M.A.: The pigment dispersion syndrome, Am. J. Ophthalmol. **83:**161, 1977.
3. Bellows, A.R., Jocson, V.L., and Sears, M.L.: Iris pigment granule obstruction of the aqueous outflow channels in enucleated monkey eyes, paper presented at ARVO National Meeting, 1974.
4. Bick, M.W.: Pigmentary glaucoma in females, Arch. Ophthalmol. **58:**483, 1957.
5. Bill, A.: Blood circulation and fluid dynamics in the eye, Physiol. Rev. **55:**383, 1975.
6. Birch-Hirschfeld, A.: Menschlichen Auges durch Röntgenstrahlen, Z. Augenheilkd. **45:**199, 1921.
7. Boles-Carenini, B., Buten, R.E., Spurgeon, W.M., and Ascher, K.W.: Comparative tonographic study of normotensive eyes of white and Negro persons, Am. J. Ophthalmol. **40:**224, 1955.
8. Brini, A., Porte, A., and Roth, A.: Atrophie des couches epitheliales de l'iris: etude d'un cas de glaucome pigmentaire au microscope optique et au microscope electronique, Doc. Ophthalmol. **26:**403, 1969.
9. Calhoun, F.P., Jr.: Pigmentary glaucoma and its relation to Krukenberg's spindles, Am. J. Ophthalmol. **36:**1398, 1953.
10. Campbell, D.G.: Pigmentary dispersion and glaucoma: a new theory, Arch. Ophthalmol. **97:**1667, 1979.
11. Chen, K.K., and Poth, E.J.: Racial difference as illustrated by the mydriatic action of cocaine, euphthalmine, and ephedrine, J. Pharmacol. Exp. Ther. **36:**429, 1929.
12. Emiru, V.P.: Response to mydriatics in the African, Br. J. Ophthalmol. **55:**538, 1971.
13. Epstein, D.L.: Pigment dispersion and pigmentary glaucoma. In Chandler, P.A., and Grant, W.M., editors: Glaucoma, Philadelphia, 1979, Lea & Febiger, p. 122.
14. Epstein, D.L., Boger, W.P. III, and Grant, W.M.: Phenylephrine provocative testing in the pigmentary dispersion syndrome, Am. J. Ophthalmol. **85:**43, 1978.
15. Evans, W.H., Odom, R.E., and Wenass, E.J.: Krukenberg's spindle: a study of 202 collected cases, Arch. Ophthalmol. **26:**1023, 1941.
16. Fine, B.S., Yanoff, M., and Sheie, H.G.: Pigmentary ''glaucoma'': a histologic study, Trans. Am. Acad. Ophthalmol. Otolaryngol. **78:**314, 1974.
17. Grant, W.M.: Experimental aqueous perfusion in enucleated human eyes, Arch. Ophthalmol. **69:**783, 1963.
18. Grant, W.M.: Personal communication, 1981.
19. Havener, V.H.: Ocular pharmacology, ed. 4, St. Louis, 1978, The C.V. Mosby Co., pp. 240-241.
20. Hoffmann, F., Dumitrescu, L., and Hager, H.: Pigmentglaucom, Klin. Monatsbl. Augenheilkd. **166:**609, 1975.

21. Iwamoto, T., Witmer, R., and Landolt, E.: Light and electron microscopy in absolute glaucoma with pigment dispersion phenomena and contusion angle deformity, Am. J. Ophthalmol. **72:**420, 1971.

22. Jess, A.: Zur Frage des Pigmentglaukoms, Klin. Monatsbl. Augenheilkd. **71:**175, 1923.

23. Kampik, A., Green, W.R., Quigley, H.A., and Pierce, L.H.: Scanning and transmission electron microscopic studies of two cases of pigment dispersion syndrome, Am. J. Ophthalmol. **91:**573, 1981.

24. Koeppe, L.: Die Rolle des Irispigment beim Glaukom, Ber. Dtsch. Ophthalmol. Ges. **40:**478, 1916.

25. Kristensen, P.: Mydriasis-induced pigment liberation in the anterior chamber associated with acute rise in intraocular pressure in open-angle glaucoma, Acta. Ophthalmol. **43:**714, 1965.

26. Kupfer, C., Kuwabara, T., and Kaiser-Kupfer, M.: The histopathology of pigmentary dispersion syndrome with glaucoma, Am. J. Ophthalmol. **80:**857, 1975.

27. Levinsohn, G.: Beitrag zur pathologische Anatomie und Pathologie des Glaukoms, Arch. Augenheilkd. **62:**131, 1909.

28. Lichter, P.R.: Pigmentary glaucoma: current concepts, Trans. Am. Acad. Ophthalmol. Otolaryngol. **78:**309, 1974.

29. Lichter, P.R., and Shaffer, R.M.: Diagnostic and prognostic signs in pigmentary glaucoma, Trans. Am. Acad. Ophthalmol. Otolaryngol. **74:**984, 1970.

30. Mapstone, R.: Pigment release, Br. J. Ophthalmol. **65:** 258, 1981.

31. Richardson, T.M., Hutchinson, B.T., and Grant, W.M.: The outflow tract in pigmentary glaucoma: a light and electron microscopic study, Arch. Ophthalmol. **95:**1015, 1977.

32. Rodrigues, M.M., Spaeth, G.L., Weinreb, S., and Sivalingam, E.: Spectrum of trabecular pigmentation in open-angle glaucoma: a clinicopathologic study, Trans. Am.

Acad. Ophthalmol. Otolaryngol. **81:**258, 1976.

33. Rohen, J.W., and van der Zypen, E.: The phagocytic activity of the trabecular meshwork endothelium: an electron microscopic study of the vervet (cercopithecus aethiops), Albrecht Von Graefes Arch. Klin. Exp. Ophthalmol. **175:**143, 1968.

34. Scheie, H.G., and Cameron, J.D.: Pigment dispersion syndrome: a clinical study, Br. J. Ophthalmol. **65:**264, 1981.

35. Scheie, H.G., and Fleischauer, H.W.: Idiopathic atrophy of the epithelial layers of the iris and ciliary body, Arch. Ophthalmol. **59:**216, 1958.

36. Sherwood, M., and Richardson, T.M.: Evidence for in vivo phagocytosis by trabecular endothelial cells, Invest. Ophthalmol. Vis. Sci. **6**(suppl.):66, 1980.

37. Speakman, J.S.: Pigmentary dispersion, Br. J. Ophthalmol. **65:**249, 1981.

38. Sugar, H.S.: Concerning the chamber angle. I. Gonioscopy, Am. J. Ophthalmol. **23:**853, 1940.

39. Sugar, H.S.: Pigmentary glaucoma: a 25-year review, Am. J. Ophthalmol. **62:**499, 1966.

40. Sugar, H.S.: Symposium: glaucoma—discussion of the three preceding papers, Trans. Am. Acad. Ophthalmol. Otolaryngol. **78:**328, 1974.

41. Sugar, H.S., and Barbour, F.A.: Pigmentary glaucoma: rare clinical entity, Am. J. Ophthalmol. **32:**90, 1949.

42. Vogt, A.: Atlas der Spaltlampenmikroskopie, Klin. Monatsbl. Augenheilkd. **81:**711, 1928.

43. von Hippel, E.: Zur pathologischen Anatomie des Glaucoma, Arch. Ophthalmol. **52:**498, 1901.

44. Yanoff, M., and Fine, B.S.: Ocular pathology: a text and atlas, New York, 1975, Harper & Row, Publishers, Inc.

45. Zink, H.A., Palmberg, P.F., Sugar, A., et al.: Comparison of in vitro corticosteroid response in pigmentary glaucoma and primary open-angle glaucoma, Am. J. Ophthalmol. **80:**478, 1975.

Chapter 8

EXFOLIATION SYNDROME

William E. Layden

HISTORICAL BACKGROUND

The terms proposed for the exfoliation syndrome have varied throughout the years. Lindberg[46] (1917) described the presence of grayish or bluish gray flecks on the pupillary border in 50% of his patients with chronic glaucoma. Malling[48,49] (1923) further described this condition. The terms senile exfoliation of the lens capsule and glaucoma capsulare were suggested by Vogt[81] (1925), who considered exfoliation to originate from the lens capsule. Other investigators argued that there was a deposit of material on the capsule.[15,48] The term glaucoma due to senile uveal exfoliation was coined by Weekers et al.[82] (1951). Wilson[83] (1953) suggested the term glaucoma senilis, indicating that exfoliation and glaucoma capsulare were a result of the aging process. The term pseudoexfoliation of the lens capsule was proposed by Dvorak-Theobald[23] (1954) to differentiate this entity from the true exfoliation seen in glassblowers or iron industry workers. Audibert[8] (1957) suggested the term iridociliary exfoliation with capsular pseudoexfoliation. Sunde[72] (1956) proposed the term exfoliation syndrome, which may be the most appropriate.

Jones[41] (1960) proposed the term exfoliation of the pseudocapsule, and Bertelson et al.[14] (1964) suggested the term fibrillopathia epitheliocapsularis. The term complex pigmentary glaucoma, coined by Simon Tor[68] (1961) was used to separate the primary pigmentary glaucoma complex from exfoliation. Electron microscopic investigations by Bertelson et al.,[14] Dark et al.,[18] Ashton et al.,[7] Ghosh and Speakman,[25,27] Ringvold,[58,59,61] and Ringvold and Vegge[65] indicate that not only the lens capsule but other ocular structures such as the ciliary body, iris, and conjunctiva contain depositions of exfoliative material. Eagle et al.[24] (1979) found short–posterior ciliary artery involvement and suggested that the exfoliation syndrome is a basement membrane disease, terming it the basement membrane exfoliation syndrome.

INCIDENCE
Incidence without glaucoma

The incidence of exfoliation without glaucoma may be as low as 0.001% or as high as 53%.[47,74] The original report by Lindberg[46] noted a 20% incidence of exfoliation without glaucoma. Age is an important determinant in the incidence of exfoliation in patients both with and without glaucoma.[1] Sveinsson[73] found an incidence of 1.7% to 2.9% in Iceland, and in the series by Taylor et al.,[77] the range was 1.3% to 16%, depending on the age, again being higher in the elderly. Thus the reported incidence of exfoliation in normal population studies varies widely but is consistently lower when compared with age-matched samples in populations with primary open-angle glaucoma.

Incidence with glaucoma

The incidence of exfoliation in patients with glaucoma varies according to author and population studied, with reported incidences ranging from 0% to 93%.[5,12,34,74] Luntz,[47] in South Africa, found exfoliation in 1.4% of a white population and in 20% of a black population with open-angle glaucoma. Australian aborigines were reported to have an incidence of glaucoma of 8.1% of patients with exfoliation,[77] and in Iceland Sveinsson[73] found an incidence of 46% to 57%. In all the reviews, the incidence of exfoliation and glaucoma increases with age, being much higher after age 60. Odland and Aasved[51] studied the occurrence of glaucoma in eyes with exfoliation followed for 2 to 9 years and found the greatest risk of glaucoma to be in the initial years.

Geographic incidence

Reports from various areas of the world indicate that virtually no area is spared.* Classically, there has been a higher incidence of exfoliation in the general population in Norway, England, and Germany, with reports of 3.3%, 2.7%, and 7.7%, respectively. In the United States the incidence of exfoliation in eyes with open-angle glaucoma has been cited at 4% and 28%.[38,74] It should be noted that many cases go undetected because of failure to dilate the pupil or to examine the lens by the slit lamp after dilation, and because of a low index of suspicion.[45,66] This may explain the wide variation in findings in both geographic and incidence studies among investigators.

Monocular versus binocular involvement

Tarkkanen[74] described unchanged unilateral occurrence in 47 patients followed for 5 years. Hansen and Sellevold[35] found, however, that exfoliation developed in the second eye in 40% of men and in 31% of women over 5 years. Aasved[2] found that 43% of patients with unilateral occurrence developed binocular involvement after 6 or 7 years. Most evidence would point to the fact that unilateral exfoliation is often the precursor of bilateral exfoliation. Tarkkanen[74] and Gifford[28] both noted that patients with monocular involvement were generally younger than those with binocular involvement.

SYSTEMIC ASSOCIATIONS

No clear-cut association of exfoliation with any systemic disease has been shown. Systemic hypertension and diabetes mellitus occur with the same frequency in patients with exfoliation as in the general population.[74] Tsukahara and Matsuo[78] described patients with both primary familial amyloidosis and exfoliation, but age was a predominant factor in both conditions, and a cause-and-effect association could not be established.

---

*References 1, 11, 38, 47, 74, 77.

HEREDITY

The nature and mode of inheritance of exfoliation remain unclear. Gifford[28] reported a father and son with exfoliation. Tarkkanen[74] found no clear familial tendency but did note such an association in open-angle glaucoma. He postulated that a gene was responsible for open-angle glaucoma, exfoliation, and pigment dispersion. However, Tarkkanen,[75] Pohjola,[56] and Gillies[29] found no significant steroid responsiveness in patients with exfoliation but without glaucoma. Pohjanpelto and Hurskainen[55] suggested that the occurrence of exfoliation depends on hereditary factors but that open-angle glaucoma and the exfoliation syndrome are not genetically identical. Jerndal and Svedbergh[40] also postulated an inheritance pattern but believed most cases to be sporadic.

CLINICAL PICTURE OF THE EXFOLIATION SYNDROME
Conjunctiva

Clinically the conjunctiva has no abnormalities except for angiographic evidence of involvement. Loss of the regular limbal vascular pattern and areas of neovascularization in advanced cases, as well as congestion of the anterior ciliary vessels, have been reported (Fig. 8-1).[44]

Cornea

Small areas of flakes or clumps of exfoliation may be found on the endothelial surface of the cornea.[17,42] There is usually also a small amount of pigment on the central endothelium. In contrast to pigmentary glaucoma, however, Krukenberg's spindles are only rarely noticed, and the pigment is often distributed unevenly.[71] Vannas et al.[80] noted that the endothelial cell count by specular microscopy was decreased in affected eyes. This decrease could not be correlated with the duration of treatment or severity of the glaucoma. Spheroidal degeneration of the cornea has also been noted in eyes with exfoliation, but this may be incidental.[13]

Iris and pupil

Small flakes on the pupillary border of the iris are one of the hallmarks of the diagnosis[17,42,45,66] (Fig. 8-2). The diagnosis can be made in the majority of cases by observation of this area before dilation. Defects of the pigmented pupillary ruff have been reported, in contrast to the midstromal slitlike transillumination defects found in pigmen-

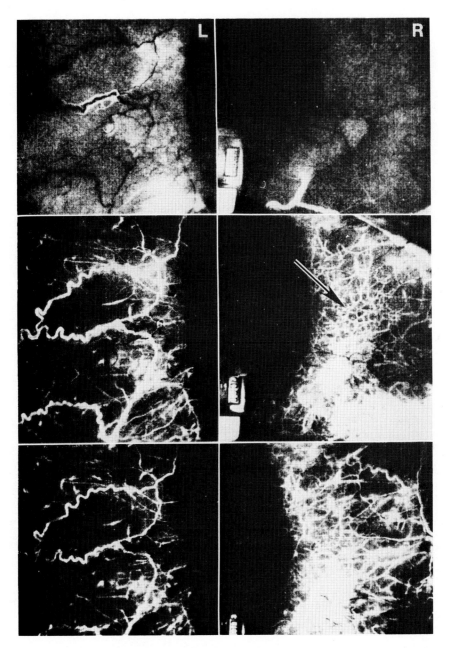

FIG. 8-1. Fluorescein angiography of limbus. *L,* Eye with open-angle glaucoma. *R,* Exfoliation glaucoma. Arrow illustrates loss of regular pattern and neovascularization. (From Laatikainen, L.: Acta Ophthalmol. Suppl. **111:**3, 1971.)

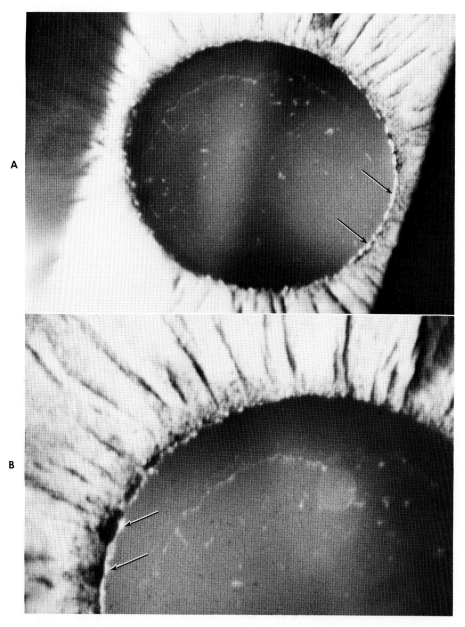

FIG. 8-2. A, Flecks in pupillary border *(arrows).* **B,** Close-up view of material lining pupil edge *(arrows).*

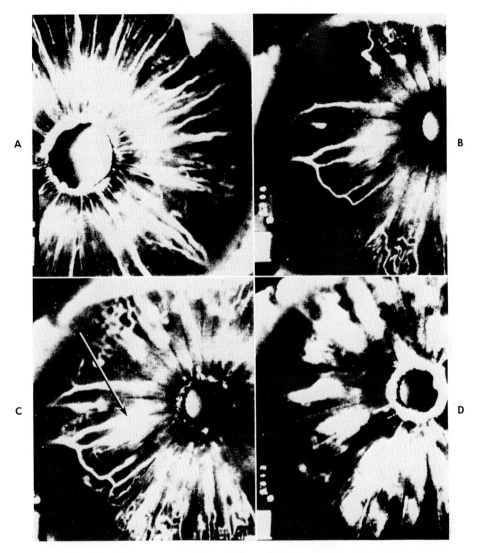

FIG. 8-3. A, Healthy fellow eye. **B** to **D,** Exfoliation with progressive filling showing neovascularization and profound leakage of dye *(arrow).*

tary glaucoma.[6] The iris sometimes has areas of gross pigment deposition on the anterior surface. In contrast to pigmentary glaucoma, iridodonesis is not usually found in exfoliation.[42] Angiographic abnormalities of the iris vessels include diminution in number, lack of normal radial pattern, neovascular clumps, and leakage of fluorescein[79] (Fig. 8-3).

Anterior chamber
Aqueous humor

The aqueous is not prominently involved in the undilated eye. Rarely, small pigment floaters can be found. After mydriasis, pigment floaters are often seen more distinctly in exfoliation cases, somewhat reminiscent of the liberation of pigment into the anterior chamber during mydriasis in the pigment dispersion syndrome.[43]

Angle

A hallmark of the diagnosis is pigmentation of the trabecular meshwork[17,22,42,71] (Fig. 8-4). The pigmented ring on the meshwork is much less distinct than that seen in the pigment dispersion syndrome, and the pigment band is spotty and not as well defined. A pigment line (Sampaolesi's line) can also be detected over Schwalbe's line (Fig. 8-5) in the exfoliation syndrome, similar to the

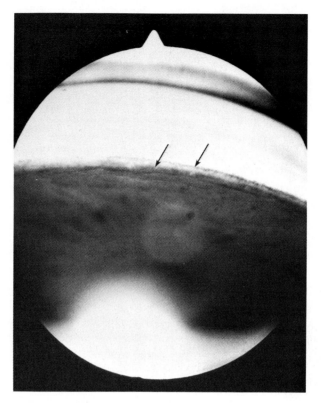

FIG. 8-4. Exfoliation with trabecular pigment. Arrows denote uneven and poorly defined pigment band.

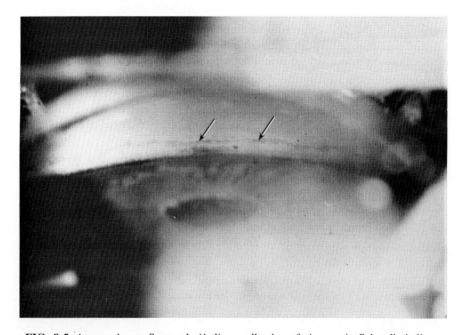

FIG. 8-5. Arrows denote Sampaolesi's line, collection of pigment in Schwalbe's line.

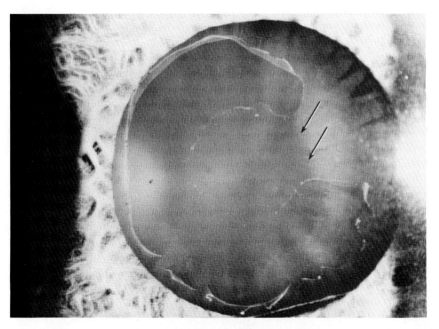

FIG. 8-6. Three zones on anterior lens capsule. Clear area is between central disc and peripheral zone with exception of bridge of material illustrated by double arrows.

one seen in the pigment dispersion syndrome. Less commonly, discrete flecks of exfoliation material can be observed in the angle. Angle-closure glaucoma may be associated with exfoliation, but the majority of patients have open angles.[33,45]

Lens and zonules

The formation of exfoliation material on the surface of the lens is the most consistent and important diagnostic feature.* Three distinct zones may be present: a translucent central disc, a granular girdle around the periphery, and a clear zone separating these two areas (Fig. 8-6). The central disc is absent in approximately 20% of cases, accounting for the occasional lack of pupillary flecks.[45] The peripheral zone is always present, and radial striations are often seen (Fig. 8-7). The clear ring between the central and peripheral zones may be a result of contact with the moving iris.[71] A curled-up edge of the central zone may be seen after dilation (Fig. 8-8).

No observations of exfoliation material on the back of the lens have been noted. In the pigment dispersion syndrome, by contrast, a pigmentary band may be seen on the posterior equatorial side

*References 7, 46, 67, 72, 74.

of the lens. There is apparently no increased incidence of lens opacities with exfoliation.[74] Zonules have been noted to contain deposits of exfoliation material (Fig. 8-9), which may explain the tendency to spontaneous subluxation or dislocation of the lens in the advanced exfoliation syndrome.[9,10,28,71]

Ciliary body

The ciliary processes and zonules were examined clinically by Mizuno and Muroi[50] with a special type of gonioscopy lens. Almost all eyes (77%) with exfoliation showed accumulations of material on the zonules and ciliary processes (Fig. 8-10).

Vitreous and retina

Deposits occur on the anterior vitreous hyaloid face[28,70] (Fig. 8-11). Continued deposition after lens extraction has been observed, suggesting that the lens is not the only source of exfoliation material.[28,70] Other vitreous disease, such as asteroid hyalosis, has no association with exfoliation.[74] No correlation with macular degeneration has been found.[74] No exfoliation material has been found behind the ora serrata, and no association with detachment has been discovered.[72]

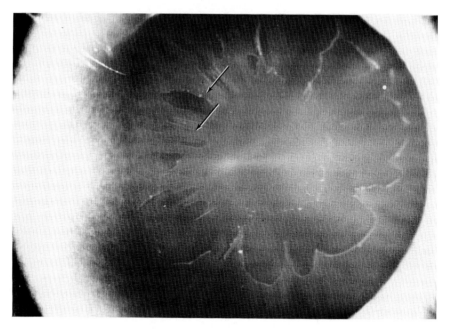

FIG. 8-7. Radial striations of material in lens capsule, perhaps reflection of iris movement *(arrows)*.

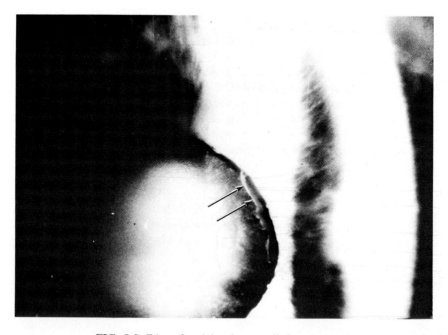

FIG. 8-8. Edge of peripheral zone rolled up *(arrows)*.

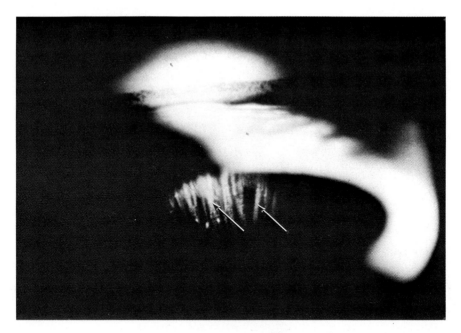

FIG. 8-9. Zonules coated with exfoliation material *(arrows).* (Courtesy R.N. Shaffer, M.D.)

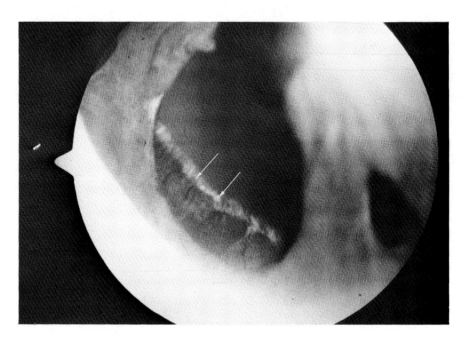

FIG. 8-10. Ciliary processes coated with exfoliation seen in aphakic eye. (Courtesy R.N. Shaffer, M.D.)

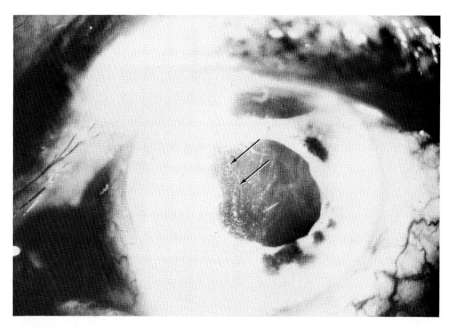

FIG. 8-11. Deposits on hyaloid face after cataract extraction *(arrows).* (Courtesy R.N. Shaffer, M.D.)

CLINICAL PICTURE OF ASSOCIATED GLAUCOMA

Increased intraocular pressure may be found in 55% to 81% of the reported series.[74] Only rarely is low-tension glaucoma associated with the presence of exfoliation.[71] The level of intraocular pressure is usually higher when the disease is first detected than it is in primary open-angle glaucoma. It has been thought that the degree of pigmentation may play a role in the very high pressures encountered in some cases, but the extent of pigmentation and the severity of the glaucoma do not always correlate.[45]

Aasved[4] found the distribution curve for intraocular pressures in eyes with exfoliation to be displaced toward a higher range in comparison with glaucomatous eyes without exfoliation, supporting the work of Hansen and Sellevold,[36] who also found unusually high intraocular pressures in patients with exfoliation. Aasved[3] also found that optic nerve damage in simple glaucoma and capsular glaucoma was the same in a screening group, but in treated patients optic nerve damage was definitely more common in exfoliation glaucoma than in primary open-angle glaucoma (74% versus 45%). Surgical treatment for glaucoma was carried out more often in the eyes with exfoliation (35% versus 21%).

Visual field damage is usually greater in patients with exfoliation glaucoma than in patients with primary open-angle glaucoma, which probably reflects the effects of the higher intraocular pressure on the optic nerve.

PATHOPHYSIOLOGY
Conjunctiva

Routine light microscopy shows no conjunctival alteration. With transmission electron microscopy, characteristic fibrillar granular material occurs near the basement membranes of the endothelial cells of the limbal conjunctival vessels[45,58,67] (Figs. 8-12 and 8-13). Drainage of aqueous material does not account for the presence of the material in the conjunctiva.[59]

Iris

Sunde,[72] by gross anatomic dissection, found flakes on the pupillary border in all cases studied. Only occasional exfoliation deposits occur on the anterior surface of the iris. Aggregates of exfoliation material within the anterior iris surface occur in involved eyes with both normal and elevated pressure.[60] Electron microscopy reveals exfoliation material deposits around the iris vessels[27,45,58] (Figs. 8-14 and 8-15). Iris vessels also contain fibrillar granular material in their walls. Pigment

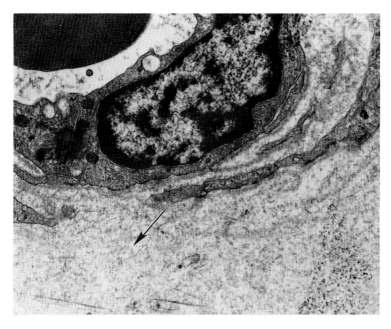

FIG. 8-12. Conjunctival vessel of open-angle glaucoma patient. Arrow denotes absence of fibrillar material. (×16,000.) (From Layden, W.E., and Shaffer, R.N. Published with permission from the American Journal of Ophthalmology **78:**835-841, 1974. Copyright by the Ophthalmic Publishing Co.)

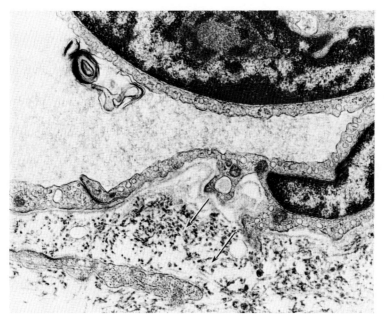

FIG. 8-13. Conjunctival vessel of exfoliation glaucoma. Arrows denote fibrillar material. (×32,00.) (Courtesy R.N. Shaffer, M.D.)

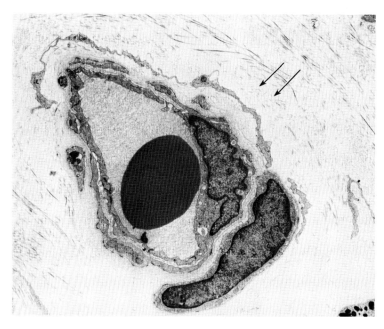

FIG. 8-14. Iris vessel of open-angle glaucoma *(arrows),* no material seen. (×8,000.) (Courtesy R.N. Shaffer, M.D.)

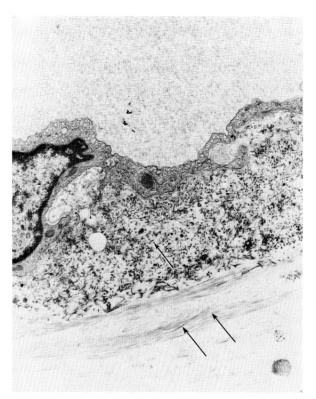

FIG. 8-15. Iris vessel of exfoliation glaucoma. Arrow denotes fibrillar material; double arrows denote normal collagen. (×16,000.) (From Layden, W.E., and Shaffer, R.N. Published with permission from the American Journal of Ophthalmology **78:**835-841, 1974. Copyright by the Ophthalmic Publishing Co.)

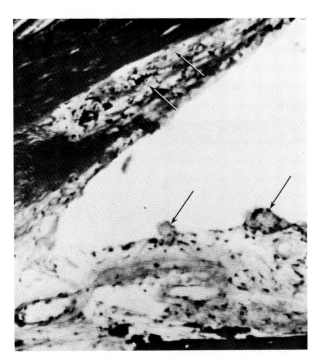

FIG. 8-16. Arrows illustrate deposits on iris surface and in trabecular meshwork. (From Devork-Theobold, G.: Trans. Am. Ophthalmol. Soc. **51,** 1953.)

epithelial cells with extensive atrophy have been noted in those eyes studied. Light microscopy reveals deposits on the posterior surface of the iris,[15,23] and Dickson and Ramsay[21] also found involvement of the posterior surface of the iris by scanning and transmission electron microscopy.

Trabecular meshwork

Deposits occur on the trabecular meshwork and in the intertrabecular spaces[15,23,72] (Fig. 8-16). Ringvold and Vegge[65] found eyes with higher pressures to have greater involvement of the trabecular meshwork by exfoliation material. Ringvold and Davanger[64] reported exfoliation material in the intertrabecular spaces, the trabecular endothelium, and the juxtacanalicular tissue, but none in Schlemm's canal. Material may be brought to the angle by the aqueous humor, as well as produced by the basement membrane of trabecular endothelial cells. Harnisch[37] described both intercellular and intracellular pigment granules in the trabecular cells.

Lens and zonules

In light microscopic studies of the lens by Busacca,[15] minute vacuoles appeared in the deep and superficial layers of the lens capsule, with exfoliation material appearing to flake off the capsular surface. Dvorak-Theobald[23] described the typical

deposits on the lens as well as other structures of the anterior segment (Fig. 8-17). Several other investigators also indicated involvement of the lens capsule[7,14,18,25] (Fig. 8-18).

However, debate continues as to whether there is primary involvement of the capsule and epithelial cells of the lens, or whether it is a secondary deposit. Sugar et al.[71] suggested the lens, iris, and ciliary body epithelia as likely sources of exfoliation fibrils. Scanning electron microscopic studies by Dickson and Ramsay[21] again confirmed the presence of material on the lens capsule (Fig. 8-19), but the fibrillar material may come from the iris pigment epithelium and involve the lens capsule secondarily.

Zonular involvement was discussed by Dvorak-Theobald,[23] who supposed that they may be fragile and lead to lens displacement as described by Bartholomew[9] in 1970. No histologic confirmation of zonular weakness has been forthcoming. Sunde[72] found flakes on the zonules but described elasticity of the zonular fibers as being normal.

Ciliary body

Histologic evidence of exfoliation deposits on ciliary processes[15,23] were confirmed by transmission electron microscopy showing fibrils deposited on the surface and within the basement membrane of the nonpigmented epithelium (Fig. 8-20).[26]

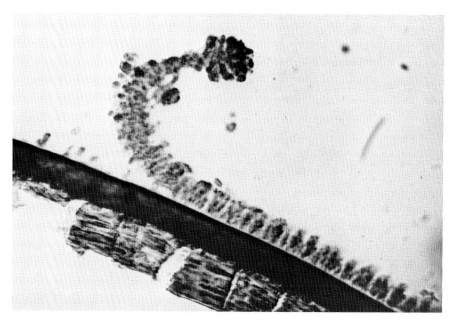

FIG. 8-17. Exfoliation material peeling off anterior capsule of lens. (From Devork-Theobold, G.: Trans. Am. Ophthalmol. Soc., 1953.)

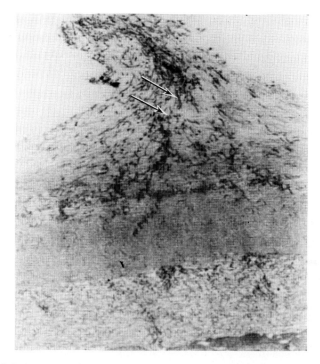

FIG. 8-18. Exfoliation material near zonular insertion. Arrows denote fibrillar material. (Courtesy J.S. Speakman, M.D.)

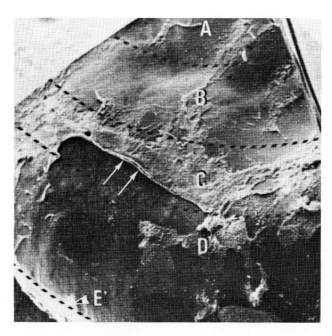

FIG. 8-19. Scanning electron micrographs of anterior lens surface with exfoliation material *(arrows).* (×35.) *A,* Central area; *B,* connection of peripheral-central area; *C,* peripheral zone; *D,* far periphery; *E,* equator. (From Dickson, D.H., and Ramsay, M.S.: Can. J. Ophthalmol. **10:**148, 1975.)

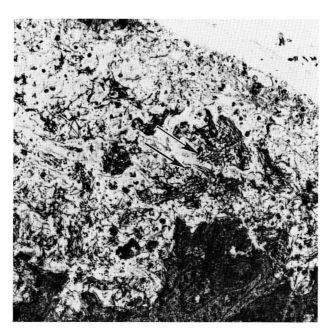

FIG. 8-20. Exfoliation material *(arrows)* within basement membrane of nonpigmented ciliary epithelium. (×16,400.) (From Ghosh, M., and Speakman, J.S.: Can. J. Ophthalmol. **8:**394, 1973.)

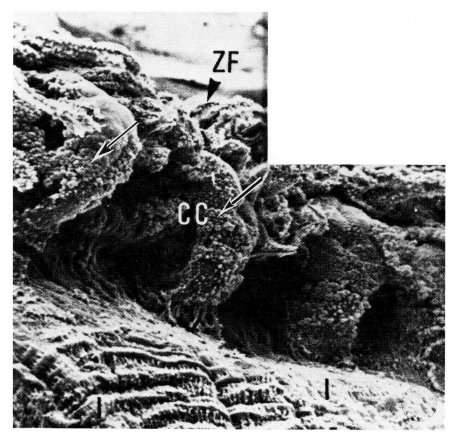

FIG. 8-21. Scanning electron micrograph of ciliary processes showing accumulation of material *(arrows).* (×55.) *ZF,* zonular fibers; *CC,* ciliary concretions (exfoliation material). (From Dickson, D.H., and Ramsay, M.S.: Can. J. Ophthalmol. **10:**154, 1975.)

By scanning electron microscopy, Dickson and Ramsay[21] found involvement of the ciliary processes (Fig. 8-21). Sunde[72] found exfoliation of the ciliary processes and, in about 50% of eyes, on the pars plana. No exfoliation material has been found in the vessels or the stroma of the ciliary body or processes.

Other tissues

Deposition of exfoliation material on the hyaloid face after lens extraction has been noted clinically.[28,57,70] Although the palpebral conjunctiva may be involved, biopsies of the skin or oral mucosa do not reveal any abnormal material, suggesting an absence of systemic involvement.[61] In an important study, Eagle et al.[24] found exfoliation material in the anterior iris stroma adjacent to a newly formed abnormal endothelial basement membrane. Typical exfoliation material was also found in the wall of a short posterior ciliary artery

in the orbit. They suggested that exfoliation material is an abnormal basement membrane synthesized at multiple sites by aging cells.

Nature of the exfoliation material

The biochemical nature of the exfoliation material is as yet unknown, although both histochemical and electron microscopic studies have suggested a close association with amyloid.[62,63] The material consists of an irregular meshwork of randomly oriented cross-banded fibrils measuring about 30 nm in diameter. The core of the fibril appears to be a fibrillar protein with a periodicity of 50 to 55 nm. The core is surrounded by a fuzzy material protruding from the fibers. Davanger[19,20] concluded that the filament is a proteoglycosaminoglycan (mucopolysaccharide) consisting of a protein core surrounded by polysaccharide side chains. The amino acid content of the exfoliation material is different from the amino acid content of collagen.[62] The exfoliation fibers examined by transmission electron microscopy and scanning electron microscopy are identical to each other.[19]

Origin of the exfoliation material

Sunde[72] maintained that exfoliation originated as a degenerative condition of the lens capsule and that the characteristic deposition patterns were caused by the iris rubbing the material away from the anterior capsular surface. Involvement of the iris, ciliary processes, zonules, and pars plana lent confusion as to the origin of the exfoliation debris. The origin of the material is multifocal. Lens epithelium, ciliary body epithelium, iris pigment epithelium, and even trabecular endothelial cells have all been proposed to play a role. The disease process may be a result of abnormal basement membrane synthesis at multiple sites by aging cells. These may lead to replacement of normal basement membranes and subsequent epithelial atrophy.[24]

MECHANISM OF GLAUCOMA

The causative mechanism of glaucoma in exfoliation is not clear. Whether it is primary open-angle glaucoma, a true secondary glaucoma, or a combination of both is still subject to speculation. Eyes with exfoliation and glaucoma do not respond to topical steroid testing as do eyes with open-angle glaucoma; rather, they are more like those of the normal population.[29,56,75] Exfoliation exists in the absence of glaucoma[75] and may arise independently of glaucoma in some patients.[16] In addition, the presence of exfoliation may increase the intraocular pressure without the actual development of glaucoma.[4] In a few patients with an elevated pressure in both eyes, exfoliation may exist in one eye, suggesting an underlying defect in the aqueous dynamics.[53,74] The observation that some patients with unilateral exfoliation have bilateral glaucoma counters the idea of a simple obstruction. Therefore in eyes with normal aqueous dynamics, exfoliation may exist without glaucoma, whereas in eyes with underlying impaired aqueous dynamics, glaucoma may result. Severe pigment dispersion in exfoliation may also cause a secondary glaucoma. Jerndal and Svedbergh[40] have suggested that gonidodysgenesis may play a role. Patients with exfoliation who do have glaucoma tend to be younger than those who do not have glaucoma.[3,32,74] It appears, then, that patients with

exfoliation may have either primary open-angle glaucoma, a secondary glaucoma, or no glaucoma. There is no genetic pattern for those with exfoliation and glaucoma as compared with that for open-angle glaucoma.[29,55,56,76]

DIAGNOSIS
Slit-lamp techniques

Careful examination of the pupillary border is of great help in the diagnosis. If, after dilation, the diagnosis is still in question, placement of the slit beam at 45 degrees to the axis of observation may help to highlight the deposits on the lens surface (Figs. 8-22 and 8-23). Careful attention to the patterns of pigment deposition on the endothelium of the cornea and slit-lamp transillumination of the pupillary edge may also be helpful.

Gonioscopy and cycloscopy

Koeppe gonioscopy appears to be more revealing than gonioscopy with Zeiss or Goldmann lenses. When one sweeps across the iris to the angle, small deposits on the pupillary border can be highlighted (Fig. 8-24).

Cycloscopy may also be helpful in making the diagnosis. However, the identification of small amounts of pigment on the endothelium of the cornea, elevated intraocular pressure, characteristic pigmentation on gonioscopy, and deposits on the anterior surface of the pupil and lens are generally sufficient to diagnose the exfoliation syndrome.

Differential diagnosis

The pigment dispersion syndrome is clinically most similar but differs by usually having a denser pigment band in the angle and Krukenberg's spindle. It occurs in myopic eyes of younger patients, and transillumination defects are peripheral and slitlike in contrast to those found in the exfoliation syndrome.

Iritis with secondary glaucoma can be distinguished by the presence of a flare and cells in the aqueous. The presence of peripheral anterior synechiae or posterior synechiae may also be helpful diagnostic features and may be associated with systemic findings such as one finds in juvenile rheumatoid arthritis. Also, iritis with secondary glaucoma usually occurs in younger patients.

True lens exfoliation is associated with a secondary heat-induced cataract and is usually not associated with glaucoma. The deposit from the

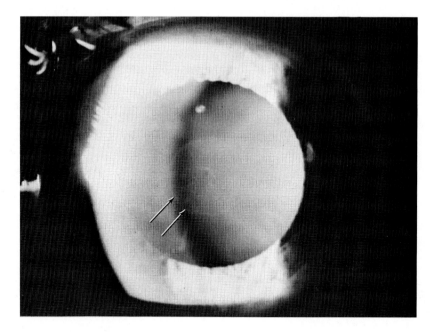

FIG. 8-22. Oblique illumination highlights central disc *(arrows)*.

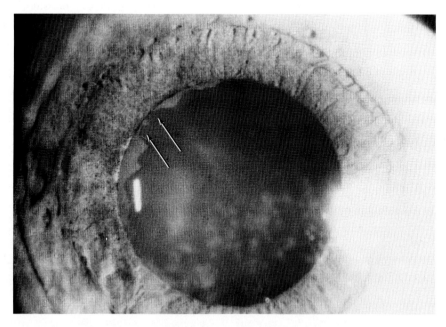

FIG. 8-23. Oblique illumination highlights serrated edges of peripheral zone *(arrows)*.

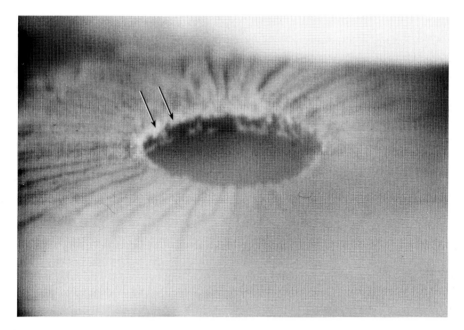

FIG. 8-24. Arrows highlight material on pupil viewed through Koeppe lens. (Courtesy R.N. Shaffer, M.D.)

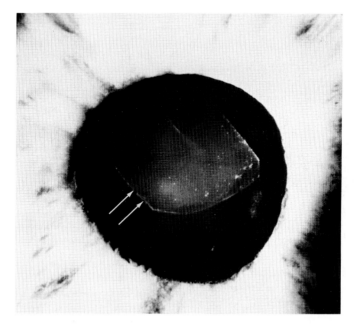

FIG. 8-25. True exfoliation *(arrows)*—splitting of capsule—seen in glassblower's cataract.

heat-induced cataract is rolled up in a characteristic thin sheet in contrast to the frosty appearance of exfoliation (Fig. 8-25).

Other conditions characterized by pigment changes, such as Fuch's heterochromic iridocyclitis, pigmentation of the chamber angle with aging, and pigmentation secondary to intraocular tumors can usually be readily distinguished.

MANAGEMENT
Medical therapy

Cholinergic agents, such as pilocarpine, can sometimes be employed to control the glaucoma associated with the exfoliation syndrome. Because of the older age of the population with exfoliation, anticholinesterase drugs should be avoided. The medical control with any agents usually is not as satisfactory in exfoliation glaucoma as it is in open-angle glaucoma.*

Adrenergic agents are often helpful, because many of these patients have nuclear sclerosis and need to avoid miosis. Topical epinephrine or the newer beta-blocking agents have been successfully employed in many cases.

Carbonic anhydrase inhibitors can be routinely prescribed in order to forestall surgery. However, again because of the older age of the population involved, the systemic drug-induced side effects are often profound.

Surgical therapy

Despite occasional reports that lens extraction in exfoliation might help pressure control, most investigators have noted that deposition of material on the hyaloid membrane continues after lens extraction.[28,30,57,70] Therefore although lens extraction may be temporarily beneficial, the confirmed reports of continued deposits of material and widespread sites of ocular involvement suggest that it is unwise to depend solely on lens extraction to control the glaucoma. Trabeculectomy may be effective in up to 80% of cases.[39] This parallels my experience with those patients with exfoliation who have required surgery.

Trabeculotomy has been advocated as an alternative surgical procedure,[31] although the effectiveness of this procedure in adult patients is subject to question. Argon laser treatment of the anterior chamber angle (laser gonioplasty) may offer some

---

*References 17, 22, 40, 42, 45, 52.

alternative surgical control in exfoliation as recently reported by Pohjanpelto.[54]

SUMMARY

The exfoliation syndrome is characterized clinically by the presence of deposits of fibrillar material on the pupillary border, anterior lens surface, corneal endothelium, and anterior chamber angle in association with pigment deposits. It occurs also on the lens equator, zonules, and ciliary processes and in the stroma and basement membrane area of certain intraocular and even orbital and conjunctival vessels. This syndrome is often accompanied by an elevation of intraocular pressure. In these cases a diagnosis can be made of secondary glaucoma associated with the exfoliation syndrome. Such glaucoma has proved to be more refractory to conventional treatment than a primary open-angle glaucoma without exfoliation.

The frequency of diagnosis can be increased significantly by suitable knowledge of the condition and clinical suspicion on the part of the examiner. The exact origin and pathogenesis of the abnormal exfoliation material has not been elucidated. It remains to be discovered whether it is chiefly ocular or perhaps an ocular and systemic degeneration of some tissue such as the basement membrane of small vessels and epithelial cells.

REFERENCES

1. Aasved, H.: The geographical distribution of fibrillopathia epitheliocapsularis, Acta Ophthalmol. **47**:792, 1969.
2. Aasved, H.: The frequency of fibrillopathia epitheliocapsularis (so-called senile exfoliation or pseudoexfoliation) in patients with open-angle glaucoma, Acta Ophthalmol. **49**:194, 1971.
3. Aasved, H.: The frequency of optic nerve damage and surgical treatment in chronic simple glaucoma and capsular glaucoma, Acta Ophthalmol. **49**:589, 1971.
4. Assved, H.: Intraocular pressure in eyes with and without fibrillopathia epitheliocapsularis, Acta Ophthalmol. **49**:601, 1971.
5. Aasved, H.: Mass screening for fibrillopathia epitheliocapsularis, Acta Ophthalmol. **49**:334, 1971.
6. Aasved, H.: Incidence of defects in the pigmented pupillary ruff in eyes with and without fibrillopathia epitheliocapsularis, Acta Ophthalmol. **51**:710, 1973.
7. Ashton, N., Sharit, M., Coelzer, R., and Black, R.: Electron microscopic study of pseudoexfoliation of the lens capsule. I. Lens capsule and zonular fibers. Invest. Ophthalmol. **4**:141, 1965.
8. Audibert, J. Cited in Tarkkanen, A.: Pseudoexfoliation of the lens capsule, Acta Ophthalmol. Suppl. **71**:1, 1962.
9. Bartholomew, R.S.: Lens displacement associated with pseudocapsular exfoliation, Br. J. Ophthalmol. **54**:744, 1970.

10. Bartholomew, R.S.: Phakodonesis, Br. J. Ophthalmol. **54:**663, 1970.

11. Bartholomew, R.S.: Pseudocapsular exfoliation in the Bantu of South Africa, Br. J. Ophthalmol. **55:**693, 1971.

12. Bartholomew, R.S.: Pseudocapsular exfoliation in the Bantu of South Africa. II. Occurrence and prevalence, Br. J. Ophthalmol. **57:**41, 1973.

13. Bartholomew, R.S.: Spheroidal degeneration of the cornea, Doc. Ophthalmol. **43:**325, 1977.

14. Bertelson, R.I., Drablos, P.A., and Flood, P.R.: The so-called senile exfoliation (pseudoexfoliation) of the anterior lens capsule, a product of the lens epithelium, Acta Ophthalmol. **42:**1096, 1964.

15. Busacca, A.: Struktur und Bedeutung der Hautchennieder-Schlaze in der vorderen und hinteren Augendammer, Albrecht Von Graefes Arch. Ophthalmol. **119:**135, 1927.

16. Ceban, L., and Smith, R.J.H.: Pseudoexfoliation of lens capsule and glaucoma, Br. J. Ophthalmol. **60:**279, 1976.

17. Chandler, P.A., and Grant, W.M.: Glaucoma, ed. 2, Philadelphia, 1979, Lea & Febiger.

18. Dark, A.J., Streeten, B.W., and Conward, C.C.: Pseudoexfoliative diseases of the lens: a study in electron microscopy and histochemistry, Br. J. Ophthalmol. **61:**462, 1977.

19. Davanger, M.: A note on the pseudoexfoliation fibrils, Acta Ophthalmol. **56:**114, 1978.

20. Davanger, M.: Studies on the pseudoexfoliation material, Albrecht Von Graefes Arch. Klin. Exp. Ophthalmol. **208:**65, 1978.

21. Dickson, D.H., and Ramsay, M.S.: Fibrillopathia epitheliocapsularis (pseudoexfoliation): a clinical and electron microscope study, Can. J. Ophthalmol. **10:**148, 1975.

22. Duke-Elder, S.: System of ophthalmology, vol. 11, Diseases of the lens and vitreous; glaucoma and hypotony, St. Louis, 1969, The C.V. Mosby Co.

23. Dvorak-Theobald, G.: Pseudoexfoliation of the lens capsule: relation to ''true'' exfoliation of the lens capsule as reported in the literature and role in the production of glaucoma capsulocuticulare, Trans. Am. Ophthalmol. Soc. **51,** 1953.

24. Eagle, R.C., Jr., Font, R.L., and Fine, B.S.: The basement membrane exfoliation syndrome, Arch. Ophthalmol. **97:**510, 1979.

25. Ghosh, M., and Speakman, J.S.: Anterior central opacities of the capsule in senile lens exfoliation, Can. J. Ophthalmol. **6:**273, 1971.

26. Ghosh, M., and Speakman, J.S.: The ciliary body in senile exfoliation of the lens, Can. J. Ophthalmol. **8:**394, 1973.

27. Ghosh, M., and Speakman, J.S.: The iris in senile exfoliation of the lens, Can. J. Ophthalmol. **9:**289, 1974.

28. Gifford, H., Jr.: A clinical and pathologic study of exfoliation of the lens capsule, Am. J. Ophthalmol. **46:**508, 1958.

29. Gillies, W.E.: Corticosteroid-induced ocular hypertension in pseudoexfoliation of lens capsule, Am. J. Ophthalmol. **70:**90, 1970.

30. Gillies, W.E.: Effect of lens extraction in pseudoexfoliation of the lens capsule, Br. J. Ophthalmol. **57:**46, 1973.

31. Gillies, W.E.: Trabeculotomy in pseudoexfoliation of the lens capsule, Br. J. Ophthalmol. **61:**297, 1977.

32. Gillies, W.E.: Secondary glaucoma associated with pseu-

33. Gnanadoss, A.S., and Parasuraman, A.: Pseudoexfoliation and narrow angle glaucoma, Orient Arch. Ophthalmol. **10:**55, 1972.

34. Hansen, E., and Sellevold, O.J.: Pseudoexfoliation of the lens capsule. I. Clinical evaluation with special regard to the presence of glaucoma, Acta Ophthalmol. **46:**1095, 1968.

35. Hansen, E., and Sellevold, O.J.: Pseudoexfoliation of the lens capsule. II. Development of the exfoliation syndrome, Acta Ophthalmol. **47:**161, 1969.

36. Hansen, E., and Sellevold, O.J.: Pseudoexfoliation of the lens capsule. III. Ocular tension in eyes with pseudoexfoliation, Acta Ophthalmol. **48:**446, 1970.

37. Harnisch, J.P.: Exfoliation material in different sections of the eye, Albrecht Von Graefes Arch. Klin. Exp. Ophthalmol. **203:**181, 1977.

38. Horven, I.: Exfoliation syndrome, Arch. Ophthalmol. **76:**505, 1966.

39. Jerndal, T., and Kriisa, U.: Results of trabeculectomy for pseudoexfoliative glaucoma, Br. J. Ophthalmol. **58:**927, 1974.

40. Jerndal, T., and Svedbergh, B.: Goniodysgenesis in exfoliation glaucoma, Adv. Ophthalmol. **35:**45, 1978.

41. Jones, B. Cited in Tarkkanen, A.: Pseudoexfoliation of the lens capsule, Acta Ophthalmol. Suppl. **71:**1, 1962.

42. Kolker, A.E., and Hetherington, J., Jr.: Becker and Shaffer's diagnosis and therapy of the glaucomas, ed. 4, St. Louis, 1976, The C.V. Mosby Co.

43. Krause, U., Hilne, J., and Frisius, H.: Pseudoexfoliation of the lens capsule and liberation of iris pigment, Acta Ophthalmol. **51:**39, 1973.

44. Laatikainen, L.: Fluorescein angiographic studies of the peripapillary and perilimbal regions in simple, capsular and low-tension glaucoma, Acta Ophthalmol. Suppl. **111:** 3, 1971.

45. Layden, W.E., and Shaffer, R.N.: Exfoliation syndrome, Am. J. Ophthalmol. **78:**835, 1974.

46. Lindberg, J.G.: Kliniska undersokningar over depigmentering av pupillarranden och genomlysbarket av iris vid fall av alderstarr samit i normala ogon hos gamla personer, M.D. thesis, Diss Helsingfors, 1917.

47. Luntz, M.H.: Prevalence of pseudoexfoliation syndrome in an urban South African clinic population, Am. J. Ophthalmol. **74:**581, 1972.

48. Malling, B.: Untersuchungen uber das Verhaltnis zwischen Iridocyclitis und Glaukom, Acta Ophthalmol. **1:** 97, 1923.

49. Malling, B.: Untersuchungen uber das Verhaltnis zwischen Iridocyclitis und Glaukom. II. Klinische Versuche, Acta Ophthalmol. **1:**215, 1923.

50. Mizuno, K., and Muroi, S.: Cycloscopy of pseudoexfoliation, Am. J. Ophthalmol. **87:**513, 1979.

51. Odland, M., and Aasved, H.: Follow-up of initially nonglaucomatous patients with fibrillopathia epitheliocapsularis (so-called senile exfoliation of the anterior lens capsule), XX Meeting of Nordic Ophthalmologists, 1971, p. 77.

52. Olivius, E., and Thorburn, W.: Prognosis of glaucoma simplex and glaucoma capsulare, Acta Ophthalmol. **56:** 921, 1978.

53. Pohjanpelto, P.: The fellow eye in unilateral hypertensive

doexfoliation of the lens capsule, Trans. Ophthalmol. Soc. U.K. **98:**96, 1978.

pseudoexfoliation, Am. J. Ophthalmol. **75:**216, 1973.

54. Pohjanpelto, P.: Argon laser treatment of the anterior chamber angle for increased intraocular pressure, Acta Ophthalmol. **59:**211, 1981.

55. Pohjanpelto, P., and Hurskainen, L.: Studies in relatives of patients with glaucoma simplex and patients with pseudoexfoliation of the lens capsule, Acta Ophthalmol. **50:** 255, 1972.

56. Pohjola, S., and Horsmanheimo, A.: Topically applied corticosteroids in glaucoma capsulare, Arch. Ophthalmol. **85:**150, 1971.

57. Radian, A.B., and Radian, A.L.: Senile pseudoexfoliation in aphakic eyes, Br. J. Ophthalmol. **59:**577, 1975.

58. Ringvold, A.: Electron microscopy of the walls of iris vessels in eyes with and without exfoliation syndrome, Virchow's Arch. [Abt. A Pathol. Anat.] **348:**328, 1969.

59. Ringvold, A.: Electron microscopy of the limbal conjunctiva in eyes with pseudoexfoliation syndrome (p.e. syndrome), Virchow's Arch. [Abt. A Pathol. Anat.] **355:**275, 1972.

60. Ringvold, A.: Light and electron microscopy of the anterior iris surface in eyes with and without pseudoexfoliation syndrome, Albrecht Von Graefes Arch. Klin. Exp. Ophthalmol. **188:**131, 1973.

61. Ringvold, A.: On the occurrence of pseudoexfoliation material in extrabulbar tissue from patients with pseudoexfoliation syndrome of the eye, Acta Ophthalmol. **51:** 411, 1973.

62. Ringvold, A.: A preliminary report on the amino-acid composition of the pseudoexfoliation material, Exp. Eye Res. **15:**37, 1973.

63. Ringvold, A., and Husby, G.: Pseudoexfoliation material—an amyloid-like substance, Exp. Eye Res. **17:**289, 1973.

64. Ringvold, A., and Davanger, M.: Notes on the distribution of pseudoexfoliation material with particular reference to the uveoscleral route of aqueous humor, Acta Ophthalmol. **55:**807, 1977.

65. Ringvold, A., and Vegge, T.: Electron microscopy of the trabecular meshwork in eyes with exfoliation syndrome (pseudoexfoliation of the lens capsule), Virchow's Arch. [Abt. A Pathol. Anat.] **353:**110, 1971.

66. Roth, M., and Epstein, D.L.: Exfoliation syndrome, Am. J. Ophthalmol. **89:**477, 1980.

67. Seland, J.H.: The ultrastructure of the deep layer of the lens capsule in fibrillopathia epitheliocapsularis (FEC),

so-called senile exfoliation or pseudoexfoliation, Acta Ophthalmol. **56:**335, 1978.

68. Simon Tor, J.M.: Glaucoma pigmentario complexus, Arch. Soc. Ophthalmol. Hisp.-Am. **21:**121, 1961.

69. Speakman, J.S., and Ghosh, M.: The conjunctiva in senile lens exfoliation, Arch. Ophthalmol. **94:**1757, 1976.

70. Sugar, H.S.: Das Exfoliations syndrom: Ursache fibrillären Materials auf der Linsenkapsel (English abstract), Klin. Monatsbl. Augenheilkd. **169**(1):1, 1976.

71. Sugar, H.S., Harding, C., and Barsky, D.: The exfoliation syndrome, Ann. Ophthalmol. **10:**1165, 1976.

72. Sunde, O.A.: Senile exfoliation of the anterior lens capsule, Acta Ophthalmol. Suppl. **45:**1, 1956.

73. Sveinsson, D.: The frequency of senile exfoliation in Iceland, Acta Ophthalmol. **52:**596, 1974.

74. Tarkkanen, A.: Pseudoexfoliation of the lens capsule, Acta Ophthalmol. Suppl. **71:**1, 1962.

75. Tarkkanen, A., and Horsmanheimo, A.: Topical corticosteroids and non-glaucomatous pseudoexfoliation, Acta Ophthalmol. **44:**323, 1966.

76. Tarkkanen, A., Voipio, G., and Krivusalo, P.: Family study of pseudoexfoliation and glaucoma, Acta Ophthalmol. **43:**697, 1965.

77. Taylor, H.R., Hollows, F.C., and Mann, D.: Pseudoexfoliation of the lens in Australian Aborigines, Br. J. Ophthalmol. **61:**473, 1977.

78. Tsukahara, S., and Matsuo, T.: Secondary glaucoma accompanied with primary familial amyloidosis, Ophthalmologica **175:**250, 1977.

79. Vannas, A.: Fluorescein angiography of the vessels of the iris in pseudoexfoliation of the lens capsule, capsular glaucoma and other forms of glaucoma, Acta Ophthalmol., Suppl. **105:**37, 1969.

80. Vannas, A., Setala, K., and Rurisuraara, P.: Endothelial cells in capsular glaucoma, Acta Ophthalmol. **55:**951, 1977.

81. Vogt, A.: Ein neues Spaltlampenbild des Pupillargebietes: Hellblauer Pupilearsaumfilz mit Hautchenbildunz aus der Lisenvorderkapsel, Klin. Monatsbl. Augenheilkd. **75:**1, 1925.

82. Weekers, L., Weekers, R., and Dednjaid, J.: Pathogenic du glaucome "capsulaire," Doc. Ophthalmol. **5/6:**555, 1951.

83. Wilson, R.P.: Capsular exfoliation and glaucoma capsulare, Trans. Ophthalmol. Soc. N.Z. **7:**8, 1953.

Chapter 9

LENS-INDUCED OPEN-ANGLE GLAUCOMA

David L. Epstein

Lens-induced glaucoma can occur in several different clinical situations:

1. Swelling of the intact lens may occur as a part of the process of cataract formation and lead to secondary angle-closure glaucoma by increasing relative pupillary block. This is discussed in Chapter 10.

2. Hypermature or mature (rarely immature) cataracts may leak lens proteins into the aqueous humor and obstruct the aqueous outflow channels. This form of lens-induced secondary open-angle glaucoma is classically termed phacolytic glaucoma.

3. Following planned or unplanned extracapsular cataract surgery or after lens injury, a secondary open-angle glaucoma may result from a direct obstruction of the outflow pathways by liberated lens particles and debris. This is sometimes mislabeled phacotoxic or phacoanaphylactic glaucoma because the cellular response to the liberated lens material is incorrectly assumed to be responsible for the obstruction of outflow. A more appropriate term is lens particle glaucoma.

4. When lens material is sequestered in the eye, especially in the vitreous after extracapsular surgery and unplanned vitreous loss, a true phacoanaphylaxis may rarely result in secondary inflammation and occasional glaucoma. Phacoanaphylaxis may also occur as a response to a leaking cataract or free lens material in one eye, following a period of prior sensitization to lens protein antigens in the fellow eye (e.g., after extracapsular surgery).

The different lens-induced reactions are decidedly complex and may have multiple pathophysiologic mechanisms. Classic phacolytic glaucoma (lens protein glaucoma) is the easiest to classify and is the most readily understood entity, whereas certain cases of glaucoma due to retained lens cortex (lens particle glaucoma) and phacoanaphylaxis become progressively more complicated in both classification and understanding of the pathogenesis. Nevertheless, it is useful and important to differentiate these entities in light of our present knowledge.

PHACOLYTIC GLAUCOMA (lens protein glaucoma)
Background

Glaucoma associated with a macrophagic response to lens material leaking from a hypermature cataract was described by Zeeman[27] in 1943. Irvine and Irvine[13] (1952) believed that blockage of the trabecular meshwork by macrophages was the principal mechanism of the glaucoma. Flocks et al.[9] (1955) first defined phacolytic glaucoma as open-angle glaucoma associated with a leaking hypermature cataract; they believed that the mechanism of the glaucoma involved obstruction of the intertrabecular spaces by a combination of macrophages and escaped morgagnian fluid. Goldberg[10] popularized the use of Millipore filtration in identifying the diagnostic macrophages in this condition and agreed that the glaucoma was due to

121

mechanical blockage of the angle by both macrophages and proteinaceous debris. In recent years
the role of macrophages distended with engulfed
lens material has been emphasized in the pathogenesis of this glaucoma, whereas the possible
obstruction of the trabecular meshwork by the liberated lens material itself has been mentioned only
infrequently.[2,11,14,25] However, laboratory investigations have indicated that the soluble lens proteins that leak from hypermature phacolytic lenses
cause a severe obstruction of aqueous outflow.[4-8]

Clinical picture

The term phacolytic glaucoma should be reserved for the sudden onset of open-angle glaucoma caused by a leaking (though relatively intact)
mature or hypermature (rarely immature) cataract.
Lens-induced glaucoma following extracapsular
cataract surgery or penetrating lens trauma should
not ordinarily be classified as phacolytic (see
"Glaucoma Due to Retained Lens Cortex").

Patients typically have an acutely elevated intraocular pressure, often to very high levels, that is
associated with ocular pain and redness. Except in
the most unusual circumstances, the episode is
monocular. Since phacolytic glaucoma usually
occurs in eyes harboring mature or hypermature
cataracts, there is typically a history of gradually
diminished vision over months or years. With the
acute episode of glaucoma, vision may deteriorate
further to inaccurate light projection, but this does
not contraindicate definitive cataract extraction.

Diffuse edema of the corneal epithelium is usually present and may be cleared by topical glycerin. Gonioscopy reveals an open angle with no obvious abnormality; however, concomitant angle
recession is occasionally observed. There is usually a heavy flare in the anterior chamber, with a
variable cellular content. Most often only a moderate number of cells is found in the anterior chamber; these cells are usually larger and slightly more
translucent than typical leukocytes. Commonly,
there are chunks of white material circulating in
the aqueous that perhaps represent small particles
of lens material, cellular aggregates, or insoluble
lens protein aggregates. Crystals of calcium oxalate have been observed in the aqueous humor.[1]
A moderate cellular or particle deposition on the
corneal endothelium may exist, whereas a hypopyon is uncharacteristic except when associated
with a large defect in the lens capsule.

Even though iris blood vessels may be dilated

because of the sudden elevation of intraocular
pressure, new vessels are not ordinarily seen on
the iris.

Typically, white, soft patches are present on the
anterior lens capsule, which probably represent
macrophages attempting to seal leaks in the capsule (Fig. 9-1). The cataract is usually mature
(totally opacified) or hypermature (with a liquid
cortex) and is often frankly morgagnian. Rarely,
an immature cataract may leak, usually through
the posterior capsule.

Despite medical therapy, the pressure may rise
progressively in a short period of time unless cataract surgery is performed. Curiously, following
uncomplicated cataract surgery, intraocular pressure is no longer elevated, and such eyes only
rarely, if at all, develop postoperative alpha-chymotrypsin–associated glaucoma.

Rare cases have been observed in which a hypermature cataract seemed to leak only intermit-
tently, causing recurrent acute episodes of glaucoma. However, most often the onset of phacolytic glaucoma heralds a progressive elevation of
intraocular pressure.

When the cataract is dislocated into the vitreous,
the signs of phacolysis are often subacute, making
it more difficult to achieve the correct diagnosis.
The eye may be only slightly injected, with moderate pressure elevation and anterior chamber reaction. The presence of white patches on the lens
capsule is an important clue to the diagnosis.

Phacolytic glaucoma, as defined, has not been
reported in children. In a recent series of 20 cases
of phacolytic glaucoma, the youngest patient was
35 years old.[24]

Pathophysiology and mechanism of glaucoma

The lens proteins are ordinarily sequestered
within the lens capsule and isolated from the rest
of the eye. In the process of phacolysis, microscopic defects occur in the anterior and posterior
lens capsule, through which soluble lens proteins
enter the aqueous humor. These microscopic leaks
probably reflect an end stage in the process of
cataract formation. A heavy protein flare in the
anterior chamber has been noted in phacolytic
glaucoma and has been attributed to liquid lens
proteins.[11,13,25] There is some evidence that in immature senile cataracts very small quantities of
lens proteins may have already begun to leak into
the aqueous humor.[20]

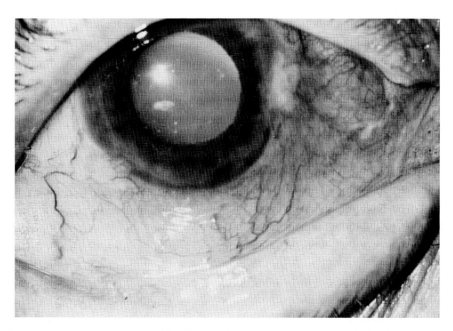

FIG. 9-1. Hypermature cataract with white patches on anterior lens capsule in phacolytic glaucoma.

With age and cataract formation, there occurs an increase in heavy molecular weight protein in the lens.[15,16,21] This heavy molecular weight protein is usually found predominantly in the nucleus rather than in the cortex of the lens. However, in phacolytic lenses high concentrations of this protein are found in the liquid cortex,[7] which may indicate either a process of nuclear disintegration or further aggregation of cortical proteins. Such heavy molecular weight soluble lens protein, by virtue of its size, might be expected to obstruct the trabecular outflow pathway if liberated in sufficient quantities. In patients with phacolytic glaucoma, heavy molecular weight protein has been identified in the aqueous humor in quantities that produce obstruction of aqueous outflow in experimental perfusion studies.[7] The magnitude of lens protein obstruction of outflow increases with the length of the protein perfusion time.[8] This direct protein obstruction of the outflow channels appears to be an important mechanism in phacolytic glaucoma.

Morphologically, eosinophilic proteinlike material and macrophages have been observed in the trabecular meshwork of eyes with phacolytic glaucoma.[12] Accumulation of macrophages is a natural response to the presence of lens material in the anterior chamber, and their presence there does not necessarily result in glaucoma. The macrophages are probably the normal scavenger response to free lens material in the eye; these cells are removing the liberated lens proteins from the trabecular meshwork, as well as sealing lens capsular sites of leakage.

Whether macrophages, having engulfed lens proteins and therefore become bloated, further impair fluid outflow through the trabecular meshwork is not clear. Identical engorged macrophages, although fewer in number than in phacolytic glaucoma, were noted in routine anterior chamber aspirates of children following needling and aspiration of cataracts and were not associated with glaucoma.[26] It can of course be argued that adult lens protein is harder for macrophages to digest and that this somehow results in their immobilization in the trabecular meshwork. Interestingly, Dueker[3] placed large numbers of swollen rabbit macrophages, which had engulfed oil in the peritoneum, into the anterior chamber of rabbits and failed to observe any significant intraocular pressure elevation.

Thus the available evidence suggests that phacolytic glaucoma is due to direct lens protein obstruction of the outflow pathways.[4,7,8] It is remarkable that in excised eyes this protein obstruction cannot be relieved by vigorous irrigation of the anterior chamber or by prolonged perfusion with mock aqueous humor.[8] Yet clinically the glaucoma is rapidly reversible following the removal of the lens. This may indicate that with cessation of the continuous leak of lens proteins, normal cellular processes within the trabecular meshwork, presumably involving macrophages, can alleviate the obstruction to flow. The absence of alpha-chymotrypsin–associated postoperative glaucoma is also surprising[4] and suggests that alpha-chymotrypsin may act on the accumulated lens proteins in the outflow pathways to produce smaller fragments and lessen the obstruction, but this could not be documented experimentally.[8]

Heavy molecular weight protein is almost completely absent in infantile and juvenile lenses.[16,17,21,22] This may explain the lack of classic phacolytic glaucoma in children, but it is also possible that such cataracts do not leak proteins into the aqueous humor.

Insoluble complexes may be formed by the aggregation of heavy molecular weight lens protein.[15] Possibly, the chunky white particles often seen circulating in the aqueous humor of patients with phacolytic glaucoma represent such complexes, or else structural lens fragments may have escaped through larger defects in the lens capsule. Since such lens particles, independent of their protein content, may obstruct trabecular outflow (see "Glaucoma Due to Retained Lens Cortex"), glaucoma in such cases might involve a combination of mechanisms. When a hypermature lens ruptures, either spontaneously or during surgery, glaucoma especially may result from both lens protein and particle obstructions.

In a related entity, certain glaucomas secondary to uveitis may result from direct serum protein obstruction of the outflow pathways.[6,23]

Diagnosis
Special diagnostic techniques

Diagnostic paracentesis will usually reveal the presence of the typical engorged macrophages on microscopic examination (Fig. 9-2). Phase-contrast microscopy is especially useful in this regard, although the Millipore filter technique[10] is the traditional method. Quite often only a few characteristic macrophages are thus identified, and their number does not correlate with the severity of the glaucoma. At times no macrophages are present in the aspirated fluid; this may be more common after topical steroid therapy.

If it is looked for microscopically, almost all cases demonstrate amorphous proteinlike fluid in the anterior chamber aspirate. Biochemical studies have identified the presence of heavy molecular weight protein in phacolytic aqueous humor specimens[7]; such biochemical evaluation of anterior chamber fluid may be useful in identifying cases of phacolytic glaucoma.

Differential diagnosis

Paracentesis and microscopic examination of anterior chamber fluid should be performed, if possible, in suspected cases of phacolytic glaucoma. Yet, as mentioned above, macrophages are occasionally not found on microscopic examination, and the diagnosis can often be made on purely clinical grounds.

The characteristic white patches on the anterior lens capsule (Fig. 9-1) and the unusual circulating cells and chunky particles in the aqueous humor are aids in making the correct diagnosis. When in doubt, one may prescribe medical therapy for glaucoma. If inflammatory signs are minimal, this will consist of routine antiglaucoma therapy. If inflammatory signs are significant, topical steroid therapy in addition to carbonic anhydrase inhibitors and timolol may be tried. While phacolysis is occurring, such treatment will bring about only a temporary control of the glaucoma and high intraocular pressure will recur (except in the very rare case of intermittent lens protein leakage).

Especially in possible cases of phacolysis associated with immature cataract, medical therapy should be tried at first unless diagnostic paracentesis establishes the correct diagnosis. If the glaucoma progressively worsens in the face of treatment, a diagnosis of phacolytic glaucoma should be considered. Then one is justified in removing the lens, since there is a good probability that the uveitis and glaucoma will be relieved.

When the patient first has symptoms, the acute pressure elevation of phacolytic glaucoma must be differentiated from that of primary angle-closure and neovascular glaucoma, and from that of secondary open-angle glaucoma due to uveitis (including glaucomatocyclitic crisis) or trauma (including acute angle-recession glaucoma and ghost cell glaucoma). The history of previous cataract formation and loss of vision in phacolytic glaucoma is helpful.

The typical anterior chamber findings and white patches on the lens may be unique to phacolytic glaucoma. In most inflammatory glaucomas the cellular reaction in the anterior chamber consists

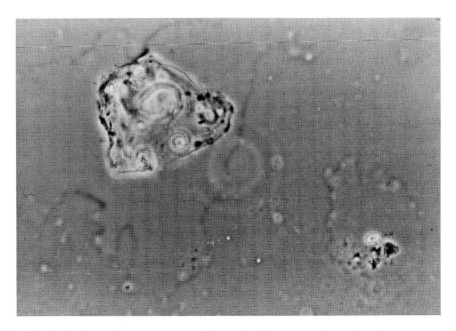

FIG. 9-2. Typical swollen macrophage with engulfed lens material seen by phase-contrast microscopy. (Courtesy Thomas M. Richardson, M.D.)

of smaller leukocytes rather than the larger, more translucent macrophages. Ghost cells are even smaller, off white in color, and usually much more numerous. I have never seen small white patches on the anterior lens capsule in nonphacolytic processes.

Following trauma, a severe secondary open-angle glaucoma with variable inflammatory cells in the anterior chamber may result from insult to the trabecular meshwork associated with the angle recession. The glaucoma may prove to be quite refractory to medical therapy, but the history and physical findings should differentiate this from a phacolytic process. It should be noted, however, that eyes with phacolytic glaucoma occasionally show signs of previous angle recession, suggesting that trauma may have been initially involved in the cataract formation.

When phacolytic glaucoma occurs with a lens that is dislocated into the vitreous, the differential diagnosis is more difficult, since the signs of phacolysis are more subtle and the glaucoma is usually less acute. The differential diagnosis includes primary open-angle glaucoma, angle-recession glaucoma, and an idiopathic type of open-angle glaucoma associated with lens dislocation without angle recession. The latter is not rare, yet the cause is unknown. Whether the lens dislocation and

glaucoma result from remote trauma to the eye (recession glaucoma *sine recession*) or whether the two findings are unrelated is not certain. Unlike phacolytic glaucoma, this glaucoma does not progress rapidly, nor are white patches present on the anterior lens capsule.

Management
Medical therapy

Patients with suspected phacolytic glaucoma should be hospitalized because of the potential for the glaucoma to worsen rapidly. Semiemergent cataract extraction should be planned. As part of the immediate care, the intraocular pressure should be lowered with hyperosmotics, carbonic anhydrase inhibitors (both intravenously and orally), and timolol.[5] Though not fully evaluated, miotics do not seem to be very effective.

The role of topical steroid therapy is uncertain; steroids will quiet the eye preoperatively and may therefore be beneficial. In some cases steroid therapy may act temporarily to lower the pressure, which would indicate some inflammatory cellular component to the glaucoma. More often, however, despite steroid therapy, the pressure returns to high levels and cataract surgery is required, usually within a matter of days. A trial of diagnostic steroid therapy may be useful in differentiating the rare cases of phacolytic glaucoma with immature cataracts from uveitic glaucoma, as mentioned previously.

Surgical therapy

Because of the magnitude of the pressure elevation and its refractoriness to medical therapy, it is often necessary to remove the phacolytic cataract shortly after the patient is diagnosed. Unnecessary delay may result in surgery being performed on the excessively inflamed eye of a patient who may be cerebrally dehydrated and uncooperative from the required osmotic therapy. The pain the patient experiences from acute phacolytic glaucoma is as severe as that from primary angle closure, and this is an additional reason to hasten surgery when intraocular pressure remains elevated.

Retrobulbar anesthesia with epinephrine is preferred because of the inflammation. Digital pressure should be used preoperatively to lower the intraocular pressure further. If the intraocular pressure remains high, either paracentesis or a deliberate, gradual entry into the anterior chamber at the time of cataract section should be employed. A sector iridectomy with the use of alpha-chymotrypsin should be the method for lens delivery. In these phacolytic lenses the capsules are fragile (with microscopic defects), and it is very important to deliver the cataract intracapsularly. If this

"bag of lens protein" is ruptured during delivery, retention of these lens proteins in the eye may result in severe complications (see "Phacoanaphylaxis"). In the event of lens rupture, the anterior chamber should be irrigated to remove the cortical and nuclear lens material. A lens nucleus should not be allowed to remain in the eye (see "Phacoanaphylaxis").

Following uncomplicated cataract surgery, the glaucoma is usually alleviated and the patient in general does quite well. As mentioned, alphachymotrypsin–associated postoperative glaucoma is rare. The postoperative vision is often surprisingly good, and one should keep in mind that the usual poor preoperative vision of inaccurate light projection should not be a deterrent to definitive cataract surgery. Cataract surgery is certainly a better choice than enucleation in patients with questionable preoperative visual potential.

GLAUCOMA DUE TO RETAINED LENS CORTEX (lens particle glaucoma)
Clinical picture

After planned or unplanned extracapsular cataract surgery, or after a penetrating lens injury, cortical lens material may be liberated into the eye and can lead to obstruction of trabecular outflow (Fig. 9-3). The severity of the glaucoma is often correlated with the amount of free cortical

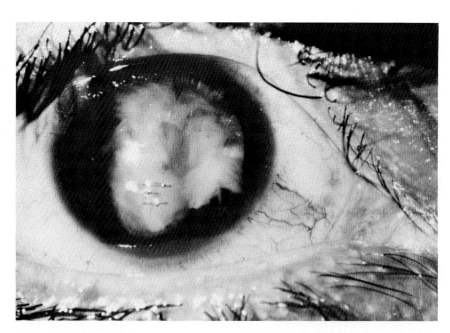

FIG. 9-3. "Fluffed-up" cortical lens material in anterior chamber after penetrating trauma. (Courtesy C. Davis Belcher III, M.D.)

lens material in the anterior chamber. Often there is a delay of several days between the extracapsular surgery or injury and the onset of glaucoma, during which time progressively more cortical material may be "fluffed up" in the anterior chamber.

Significant inflammation may accompany this condition and may be involved in the mechanism of glaucoma. Posterior and anterior synechiae can form, as well as inflammatory pupillary membranes.

In the early stages, there is diffuse corneal edema and the angle is open by gonioscopy. "Fluffed-up" lens cortical material is present in the anterior chamber and in the angle. Cellular reaction and flare are often heavy, and the circulating white cells may include smaller leukocytes and larger, more translucent macrophages. It is uncertain to what degree the leukocyte reaction is a response to the lens material or to the accompanying surgical trauma or injury. Fragments of white cortical lens material may be seen circulating in the aqueous, and there may be deposits of cells and lens debris on the corneal endothelium. If there are large amounts of free lens material, a hypopyon may be observed.

Sometimes a similar form of glaucoma may occur many years after extracapsular cataract surgery when lens material is somehow spontaneously freed into the anterior chamber. Circulating chunks of whitish lens material are then seen in the aqueous, and the cellular reaction is more macrophage-like than in the immediate postoperative condition described above. The onset of such lens particle glaucoma is often associated with the spontaneous dislocation of Soemmering's ring into the anterior chamber (Fig. 9-4).

A previously intact mature or hypermature cataract may spontaneously rupture in the eye, liberating fragments of lens material into the aqueous. To what degree such glaucoma is due to the lens particle obstruction or to a phacolytic process (i.e., lens protein obstruction) is not clear.

Pathophysiology and mechanism of glaucoma

Free particulate lens material readily obstructs the trabecular meshwork,[8] and this mechanism can explain most of the clinical cases of such glaucoma without having to invoke other inflammatory factors. For this reason, such glaucoma has been called lens particle glaucoma.[4] Nevertheless, the inflammatory signs in such eyes may be considerable, and it is not known how much these inflammatory components may also be involved in the pathogenesis of the glaucoma. Some of the inflam-

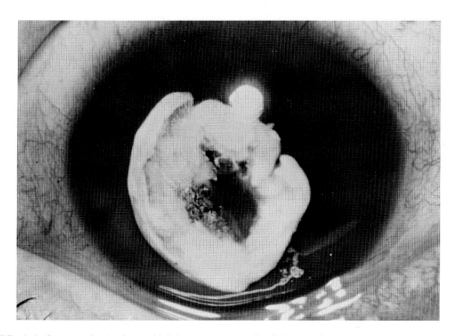

FIG. 9-4. Soemmering's ring, which has spontaneously dislocated into anterior chamber. (From Donaldson, D.D.: Atlas of external disease of the eye, vol. 4, Anterior chamber, iris, and ciliary body, St. Louis, 1973, The C.V. Mosby Co.)

matory signs may be a response to the surgery or trauma itself, rather than a reaction to the lens material.

Free lens material probably leaves the eye mainly via the trabecular outflow pathways. Undoubtedly, cellular processes in macrophages and other phagocytic cells are involved in the "absorption" of such free lens material. It is theoretically possible that such lens material absorption through the outflow channels might result in trabecular dysfunction and open-angle glaucoma many years later.[4,19]

After extracapsular surgery, residual cortical lens material may either be "fluffed up" into the aqueous humor or become sequestered within residual or newly formed lens capsular material. The occurrence of glaucoma in only certain eyes after extracapsular surgery probably relates to the amount of free lens material in the aqueous and the inherent facility of the trabecular outflow pathways. The ability of very small amounts of particulate lens material to cause significant obstruction of outflow in enucleated eyes during perfusion studies[8] suggests that dynamic cellular processes within the meshwork, perhaps involving macrophages, are acting to alleviate rather than aggravate this mechanical, particulate obstruction.

When such glaucoma occurs many years after extracapsular surgery or with spontaneous cataract rupture, the lens capsule has obviously lost its ability to isolate the lens material. Glaucoma in such a setting may be due to either free lens particular material or to heavy molecular weight protein, which is now leaking through the capsular defects (see "Phacolytic Glaucoma"). In addition, it is now possible for an immunologic sensitization to the lens proteins to occur (see "Phacoanaphylaxis").

It is noteworthy that in classic phacolytic glaucoma, described earlier, posterior and anterior synechiae as a rule do not develop. Yet when the lens capsule is violated and free cortical material is liberated into the eye, such synechiae may readily form. It seems that the type of inflammation must be different in the two clinical settings. The association of lens particle glaucoma with coexisting cataract surgery or trauma may explain this difference.

Diagnosis

In the typical postoperative or postpenetrating injury case, the diagnosis is usually correctly made by the clinical findings of significant quantities of free cortical lens material in the aqueous humor. When such lens material is present in small amounts or in atypical clinical settings, an anterior chamber tap and microscopic examination of the fluid may aid in the diagnosis by identifying macrophages and fragments of suspected lens material. Heavy molecular weight protein need not be present in the aqueous humor in lens particle glaucoma, since the glaucoma is due directly to the cortical fragments of lens material and not necessarily to their soluble lens protein content. It must be remembered that macrophages may simply be the normal scavenger response to free lens material in the eye. Therefore if free lens material is present clinically in the aqueous humor, the finding of macrophages is not surprising and does not, by itself, identify the glaucoma as lens related. The clinical response to removal of the lens material may be the best guide.

On the other hand, in those cases occurring many years after extracapsular surgery, examination of the aqueous humor for macrophages, lens particles, or heavy molecular weight protein may aid in identifying the glaucoma as being lens related. Differential diagnosis of such late-onset lens particle glaucoma includes primary open-angle glaucoma, angle-recession glaucoma, and the various uveitic glaucomas.

Management
Medical therapy

If the glaucoma is not too severe, medical therapy consisting of carbonic anhydrase inhibitors, timolol, and perhaps temporary osmotics may be tried.[5] Miotics should be avoided because of the tendency of these eyes toward synechiae formation. Cycloplegics should be employed to dilate the pupil.

The role of topical steroids is not understood. Significant inflammation may occur in such patients (although this is probably not directly related to lens particle glaucoma), and such steroid therapy is useful in quieting the eye. Theoretically, too-frequent steroid administration may delay "absorption" of the lens material. On the other hand, steroid therapy may alleviate a subsequent inflammatory component to the glaucoma and stop secondary complications by preventing synechiae formation. It is probably best to employ moderate steroid administration to such eyes, especially those that are recently postoperative or post-injury.

When the residual lens material is "absorbed," intraocular pressure usually returns to normal unless secondary complications have supervened.

Surgical therapy

If glaucoma due to retained lens cortex does not respond quickly and adequately to the above medical maneuvers, surgical removal of the lens material should be performed without delay. In the early stages of the disorder, this lens material is loose and "fluffy" and easily irrigated out from the anterior chamber, which can dramatically cure the glaucoma. If surgery is undertaken late, lens material may be trapped partially between capsular or inflammatory membranes. Anterior segment microvitrectomy instruments are valuable in removing such lens material through a closed incision, although in selected cases it may be better to use alpha-chymotrypsin and deliver the remaining lens material in toto.

PHACOANAPHYLAXIS
Clinical picture

Glaucoma secondary to phacoanaphylaxis is exceptionally rare and has practically never been correctly diagnosed in a living eye.[4] Most likely, phacoanaphylaxis, even when it occurs, only rarely causes secondary glaucoma.

Phacoanaphylaxis may occur in the following clinical situations, all of which require some latent period for sensitization to previously isolated lens proteins. When lens material is mixed with vitreous as a result of vitreous loss during extracapsular cataract surgery, phacoanaphylaxis may take place by allowing lens proteins to be retained and sequestered in the vitreous, the latter possibly acting as an adjuvant. There is a special risk of phacoanaphylaxis when the free nucleus of the lens has been lost into the vitreous cavity. Phacoanaphylaxis has also been observed when, following extracapsular cataract surgery in the first eye, the second (involved) eye has extracapsular surgery or a leaking mature or hypermature cataract. In addition, phacoanaphylaxis has been noted and should be suspected after penetrating injury to a lens with rupture of the lens capsule and resultant chronic granulomatous inflammation.[18]

Characteristic of phacoanaphylaxis is the persistent, relentless, usually granulomatous inflammation that is centered about liberated lens material. Such chronic inflammation, however, may result in hypotony instead of glaucoma.

Whether a component of phacoanaphylaxis may be involved in certain cases of glaucoma due to retained lens cortex is not clear. In such cases the free cortical lens material, in addition to obstructing trabecular outflow, may serve as a nidus for lens protein sensitization.

Pathophysiology and mechanism of glaucoma

Lens proteins are normally immunologically isolated within the lens capsule. Violation of the lens capsule may allow sensitization to occur after a latent period. This immunologic response to lens protein antigens may be totally separate from other coexisting mechanisms of glaucoma, such as particle obstruction of the meshwork.

The cellular response in phacoanaphylaxis has been well characterized.[18,28] Unlike the simple macrophagic scavenger response seen in straightforward phacolytic and lens particle glaucomas, the complex morphologic response of polymorphonuclear, lymphoid, epithelioid, and giant cells indicate an immunologic response to the lens proteins that persists as long as residual antigen is present. In certain cases this immunologic response may "spill over" to involve the trabecular meshwork and thereby cause or aggravate glaucoma. In other cases, however, this immunologic response may only be coexisting with other, more direct obstructive trabecular processes, including lens proteins or particles. Especially in cases of glaucoma due to retained lens cortex, such multiple pathologic mechanisms may occur simultaneously. What may be the most distinctive feature of pure phacoanaphylaxis is the presence of a residual, sequestered nidus of lens material that serves as the focal point of the immunologic response, along with the lack of great quantities of circulating lens proteins or particles in the aqueous.

Diagnosis

Unfortunately, the correct diagnosis is most often made after enucleation.[18] The above clinical signs should serve as a guide, but when in doubt and faced with relentless uveitis, one should surgically remove and microscopically examine the residual lens material. Diagnostic paracentesis may be useful in identifying this as a lens reaction; however, there is too little data to know exactly what cells are observed in the aqueous humor in phacoanaphylaxis. Macrophages are involved in the granulomatous response,[18] and the observation of these engorged cells might suggest a lens reaction.

Differential diagnosis includes other causes of granulomatous uveitis, in particular, sympathetic ophthalmia, which may coexist with phacoanaphylaxis.

Management

Steroid therapy should be tried initially, but surgical removal of the residual lens material is required to cure the condition.

REFERENCES

1. Bartholomew, R.S., and Rebello, P.F.: Calcium oxalate crystals in the aqueous, Am. J. Ophthalmol. **88:**1026, 1979.
2. Bellows, J.G.: Cataract and abnormalities of the lens, New York, 1975, Grune & Stratton, Inc., pp. 179, 438-441.
3. Dueker, D.K.: Personal communication, 1977.
4. Epstein, D.L.: Lens-induced glaucoma. In Chandler, P.A., and Grant, W.M., editors: Glaucoma, Philadelphia, 1979, Lea & Febiger.
5. Epstein, D.L.: Phacolytic glaucoma. In Fraunfelder, F.T., and Roy, F.H., editors: Current ocular therapy, Philadelphia, 1980, W.B. Saunders Co.
6. Epstein, D.L., Hashimoto, J.M., and Grant, W.M.: Serum obstruction of aqueous outflow in enucleated eyes, Am. J. Ophthalmol. **86:**101, 1978.
7. Epstein, D.L., Jedziniak, J.A., and Grant, W.M.: Identification of heavy molecular weight soluble protein in aqueous humor in human phacolytic glaucoma, Invest. Ophthalmol. Vis. Sci. **17:**398, 1978.
8. Epstein, D.L., Jedziniak, J.A., and Grant, W.M.: Obstruction of aqueous outflow by lens particles and by heavy molecular weight soluble lens proteins, Invest. Ophthalmol. Vis. Sci. **17:**272, 1978.
9. Flocks, M., Littwin, C.S., and Zimmerman, L.E.: Phacolytic glaucoma: a clinicopathological study of one hundred thirty-eight cases of glaucoma associated with hypermature cataract, Arch. Ophthalmol. **54:**37, 1955.
10. Goldberg, M.F.: Cytological diagnosis of phacolytic glaucoma utilizing millipore filtration of the aqueous, Br. J. Ophthalmol. **51:**847, 1967.
11. Greer, C.H.: Ocular pathology, Oxford, 1972, Blackwell Scientific Publications, Ltd., pp. 139-141.
12. Hogan, M.J., and Zimmerman, L.E.: Ophthalmic pathology: an atlas and textbook, Philadelphia, 1962, W.B. Saunders Co., p. 671.
13. Irvine, S.R., and Irvine, A.R.: Lens induced uveitis and glaucoma. III. Phacogenetic glaucoma: lens-induced glaucoma, mature or hypermature cataract; open iridocorneal angle, Am. J. Ophthalmol. **35:**489, 1952.
14. Jaffe, N.S.: Cataract surgery and its complications, ed. 3, St. Louis, 1981, The C.V. Mosby Co.
15. Jedziniak, J.A., Kinoshita, J.H., Yates, E.M., et al.: On the presence and mechanism of formation of heavy molecular weight aggregates in human normal and cataractous lenses, Exp. Eye Res. **15:**185, 1973.
16. Jedziniak, J.A., Kinoshita, J.H., Yates, E.M., and Benedek, G.B.: The concentration and localization of heavy molecular weight aggregates in aging normal and cataractous human lenses, Exp. Eye Res. **20:**367, 1975.
17. Jedziniak, J.A., Nicoli, D.G., Baram, H., and Benedek, G.B.: Quantitative verification of the existence of high molecular weight protein aggregates in the intact normal human lens by light-scattering spectroscopy, Invest. Ophthalmol. Vis. Sci. **17:**51, 1978.
18. Perlman, E.M., and Albert, D.M.: Clinically unsuspected phacoanaphylaxis after ocular trauma, Arch. Ophthalmol. **95:**244, 1977.
19. Phelps, C.D., and Arafat, N.I.: Open-angle glaucoma following surgery for congenital cataracts, Arch. Ophthalmol. **95:**1985, 1977.
20. Sandberg, H.O.: The alpha-crystallin content of aqueous humor in cortical, nuclear, and complicated cataracts, Exp. Eye Res. **22:**75, 1976.
21. Spector, A., Li, S., and Sigelman, J.: Age-dependent changes in the molecular size of human lens proteins and their relationship to light scatter, Invest. Ophthalmol. **13:**795, 1974.
22. Spector, A., Stauffer, J., and Sigelman, J.: The human lens in relation to cataract. In Ciba Foundation Symposium, vol. 19, Amsterdam, 1973, Elsevier, p. 183.
23. Troncosco, M.U.: Recherches experimentales sur la filtration de liquides salins et albumineux à travers la chambre anterieure et son role dans la genese du glaucome, Ann. Ocul. **133:**1, 1905.
24. Volcker, H.E., and Naumann, G.: Zur klinik des phakolytischen Glaukoms, Klin. Monatsbl. Augenheilkd. **166:**613, 1975.
25. Yanoff, M., and Fine, B.S.: Ocular pathology: a text and atlas, New York, 1975, Harper & Row, Publishers, Inc., pp. 378-380.
26. Yanoff, M., and Scheie, H.G.: Cytology of human lens aspirate: its relationship to phacolytic glaucoma and phacoanaphylactic endophthalmitis, Arch. Ophthalmol. **80:**166, 1968.
27. Zeeman, W.P.C.: Zwei Falle von glaucoma phacogeneticum mit anatomischem Befund, Ophthalmologica **106:**136, 1943.
28. Zimmerman, L.E.: Lens induced inflammation in human eyes. In Maumenee, A.E., and Silverstein, A.M., editors: Immunopathology of uveitis, Baltimore, 1964, The Williams & Wilkins Co.

Chapter 10

GLAUCOMA SECONDARY TO LENS INTUMESCENCE AND DISLOCATION

Robert Ritch

Disorders of the lens may be responsible for secondarily inciting both open-angle (see Chapter 9) and angle-closure glaucomas. Angle-closure glaucoma occurs secondary to the intact lens and may result from in situ enlargement of the lens or from subluxation or dislocation.

LENS INTUMESCENCE
Mechanism

Although not generally considered a secondary phenomenon, primary angle-closure glaucoma itself is partially a lens-induced process. The typical patient with angle closure is moderately to severely hyperopic and has a smaller-than-average anterior segment. The iridocorneal angle is usually widely open in youth, and angle-closure glaucoma usually does not occur until the fifth to seventh decade of life. Progressive enlargement of the lens throughout life results in gradual shallowing of the anterior chamber while alterations occur in the anatomic relationships of the structures of the anterior segment. The enlarging lens crowds the iris into a smaller space and, in pushing the iris forward, narrows the iridocorneal angle. Increasing iridolenticular apposition decreases the facility of aqueous flow through the pupillary aperture, leading to an increase in aqueous pressure in the posterior chamber. This in turn distends the peripheral iris (iris bombé), further narrowing the iridocorneal angle (Fig. 10-1, A and B). Various factors causing the pupil to become middilated, such as dim light, emotional stress, or drugs, induce a combination of maximal crowding of the angle by the iris, maximal lens-sphincter contact, and increased bombé. Under these conditions the peripheral iris may balloon against the trabecular meshwork. Iridectomy creates an alternative pathway of aqueous flow between the posterior and anterior chambers.

A gradation exists in the relative proportions of the contributions of peripheral bombé and direct pressure by the lens in inducing the narrowing of the angle. If the lens is large, a correspondingly smaller amount of bombé becomes necessary for the angle to close. In the extreme case, enlargement of the lens pushes the iris forward, mechanically narrowing the space between the iris periphery and the trabecular meshwork (Fig. 10-1, C and D). Two conditions that predispose the eye to this situation are a rapidly developing intumescent senile cataract and a traumatic cataract caused by a perforating injury.[27]

Although it is possible for angle closure due to an intumescent lens to occur in an otherwise normal eye, with the opposite eye having a deep anterior chamber, it is more common when the chamber is smaller to begin with and the angle of the opposite eye is narrow also. Forward lens movement may also be a participatory factor in some cases, because of loosening of the zonules either by trauma or with age.

Diagnostic clues

It is frequently difficult to determine the relative proportions of lens enlargement and iris bombé in angle-closure glaucoma preoperatively. There are certain clues that one can look for in an attempt to distinguish these. Most important is a disparity in

131

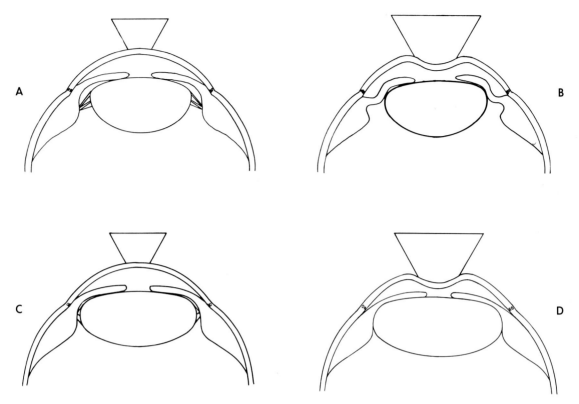

FIG. 10-1. Schematic representation of relationships between structures of anterior segment in angle closure. **A,** Angle closure with significant component of iris bombé resulting from increased iridolenticular contact. **B,** Indentation gonioscopy forces aqueous peripherally, opening angle and causing peripheral iris to become concave. **C,** Angle-closure glaucoma due to intumescent lens. Iris bombé is much less a factor in closure of angle. **D,** Indentation gonioscopy permits only narrow opening into apex of angle, which has triangular conformation.

the depths of the anterior chambers or in the angle configurations between the two eyes. To determine whether a disparity exists and to rule out artifactitious alteration of the angle by bombé, if the eye in question is being treated with miotics, the angles of both eyes should be inspected while they are being treated with the same topical medications. One should remember that miotics may contribute to an increase in iris bombé by constricting the pupil and further increasing iridolenticular contact, and by further shallowing the anterior chamber, despite the fact that they may simultaneously maintain a patent iridocorneal angle.

Unequal cataract formation or progression between the two eyes should alert the examiner to the possibility of a significant contribution to angle closure by the lens even in the absence of chamber depth or angle disparity. In the case of a mature unilateral cataract, this is easy, but in other cases the difference may be evident only by a small inequality of acuity or of anteroposterior lens thick-

ness as determined by slit-lamp examination. Differences might be present on bilateral ultrasonic examination, but this is not useful for routine clinical purposes.

When there is little or no bombé present, the peripheral iris contour closely follows that of the lens, creating a sharp apex to the angle, as opposed to the sense of width one often gets even in a very narrow angle when there is a significant bombé component.

Fortunately, the need to decide preoperatively the proportion of the bombé component is not very great. If the cataract significantly affects acuity, lens extraction solves both problems. When the decrease in acuity does not warrant lens extraction, iridectomy should be performed as the procedure of choice, since in the great majority of cases there is some element of iris bombé and the patient may remain phakic for an extended additional period. In those cases where the criteria for lens extraction are borderline, laser iridectomy is

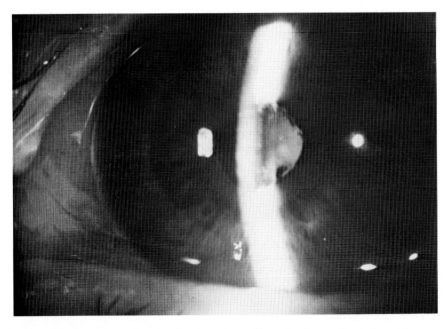

FIG. 10-2. Slit view of anterior chamber in patient with angle closure due to lens intumescence 1 year after successful trabeculectomy.

useful, since one can determine immediately by gonioscopy the success of the procedure in opening the angle and avoid two intraocular operations if lens extraction is necessary.

Postoperative gonioscopy offers a retrospective view of the degree of contribution by the lens to the angle closure. A grade III or IV angle implies a major contribution by bombé, whereas an angle of grade II or less suggests a major contribution by the lens. Patients in whom the angle is narrow postoperatively should be watched for further narrowing as the lens continues to enlarge, and it should not be assumed that once the patient has had an attack of angle closure and has undergone iridectomy, repeated gonioscopy is no longer necessary. Patients who have undergone even a large peripheral iridectomy or filtering procedure may develop angle closure at a later date because of an intumescent lens (Fig. 10-2).

ECTOPIA LENTIS

Berryat (1749), who described a young patient with both lenses in the anterior chamber, was the first to report lens dislocation.[14] Sichel[81] (1846) differentiated between traumatic and spontaneous dislocation, and Arlt (1849) suggested that a congenital factor produced dislocations in children.[14] Stellwag (1856) introduced the term ectopia lentis,[14] and Ringelhan and Elschnig[77] (1931) classi-

fied dislocations as traumatic, secondary, or congenital. The earlier literature was extensively reviewed by Clarke[18] (1939).

The term ectopia lentis refers to displacement of the lens from its normal central position within the posterior chamber. Subluxation implies loosening or breakage of some of the zonules, so that the lens is removed from its normal centration in the optical axis but still remains partially or entirely within the pupillary space and entirely within the posterior chamber. In the case of luxation or dislocation, there are no remaining zonular attachments and, although the lens may remain within the posterior chamber and partially or entirely within the pupillary aperture, it is also susceptible to migration into the anterior chamber or the vitreous.

Numerous entities have been reported to be either causes of or associated with ectopia lentis (see below). In some of these disorders, the lens dislocation is clearly hereditary, whereas in others, it is secondary to trauma or ocular disease. Certain disorders, such as Marfan's syndrome, homocystinuria, and the Weill-Marchesani syndrome, are classically associated with subluxation and/or dislocation of the lens. Others may either be rarely associated, or the association may occur fortuitously. Our present lack of knowledge as to the causes of many of these disorders at the molecular level and our lack of knowledge of the biochemistry of the zonular apparatus frequently precludes precise interpretation of the causative relationships.

Conditions associated with ectopia lentis

A. Heritable disorders
  1. Lens dislocation common
     a. Isolated ectopia lentis[30,46,66,89]
     b. Spontaneous late subluxation of lens[38,63]
     c. Ectopia lentis et pupillae
     d. Isolated microspherophakia
     e. Weill-Marchesani syndrome
     f. Marfan's syndrome
     g. Homocystinuria
     h. Sulfite oxidase deficiency[43]
  2. Lens dislocation reported
     a. Alport's syndrome[83]
     b. Aniridia
     c. Cornea plana[21]
     d. Cotlier-Reinglass syndrome[19]
     e. Craniofacial dysostosis[69]
     f. Cross-Khodadoust syndrome[20]
     g. Ehlers-Danlos syndrome[86]
     h. Familial pseudomarfanism[24]
     i. Focal dermal hypoplasia syndrome[36]
     j. Hyperlysinemia[82]
     k. Klinefelter's syndrome[5]
     l. Klippel-Feil syndrome[47]
     m. Mandibulofacial dysostosis[51,58]
     n. Megalocornea[16]
     o. Persistent hyperplastic primary vitreous[21]
     p. Oxycephaly[26]
     q. Pfändler's syndrome[71]
     r. Pigmentary retinopathy[21]
     s. Polydactyly[18]
     t. Primordial dwarfism[65]
     u. Rieger's syndrome[55]
     v. Sprengel's deformity[26]
     w. Sturge-Weber syndrome[47]
B. Secondary lens dislocations
  1. Extraocular causes
     a. Trauma
     b. Surgical complications
  2. Secondary to ocular disease
     a. Buphthalmos
     b. Exfoliation syndrome[3]
     c. High myopia
     d. Intraocular tumor
     e. Mature or hypermature cataract
     f. Syphilis[45]*
     g. Uveitis

---

*Rather than a direct relationship between syphilis and lens dislocation, it may be that patients with syphilis are more prone to trauma.

Clinical findings

Symptoms

Patients with uncomplicated ectopia lentis experience symptoms that are primarily related to disturbances of visual acuity. Minimal subluxation may be asymptomatic, whereas that of a greater degree results in refractive symptoms. Relaxation of the zonular apparatus permits the lens to assume its natural spherical form, particularly in younger patients, in whom the lens is more pliable because of the absence of nuclear sclerosis. There is a decrease in the equatorial diameter of the lens and an increase in its anteroposterior length. This in turn leads to lenticular myopia, as does anterior displacement of the lens, with or without spherophakia. Tilting or rotation of the lens around any of its axes may result in lenticular astigmatism, which is impossible to correct with lenses. A disparity between the degree of astigmatism found on refraction and that measured by keratometry, as well as a variable amount of astigmatism from one examination to another, should direct the ophthalmologist to rule out an early subluxation. The loss of zonular support also leads to defective accommodation and difficulty with near vision.

If the lens margin is within the pupillary aperture, monocular diplopia results, whereas quadriplopia can occur if the condition is bilateral. Total absence of the lens from the pupil permits an aphakic refraction. A mobile lens results in constantly changing refractive states. Uncorrectable poor visual acuity may lead to amblyopia in children.

Signs

Displacement of the lens may range in severity from a minimal, scarcely noticeable shift in axis to complete dislocation into the anterior chamber or vitreous. In early stages of subluxation, wide dilation of the pupil may be necessary to determine any asymmetry of the lens position. When the zonules are loosened, the lens becomes more or less free to move within the posterior chamber and iridodonesis occurs. When slight, iridodonesis is best detected midway between the pupil and the periphery, where iris support to either the lens or sclera is minimal, and appears as a faint rippling of the iris stroma. One may observe movement of the lens and iris in infants by gently swaying them from side to side or in older patients by firmly jolting the slit-lamp stand while the patient's chin is secure in the chin rest.[47]

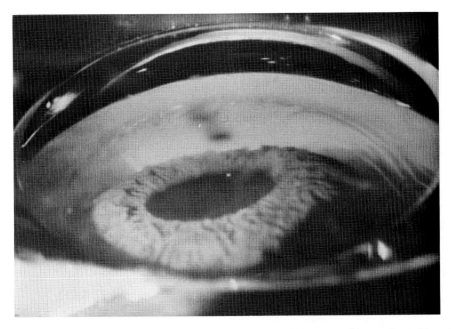

FIG. 10-3. Goniophotograph of angle closure in 28-year-old woman with anterior subluxation of lens. Note conical shape to iris, particularly in region of sphincter, giving structure appearance of "volcano crater."

Careful examination of the anterior chamber may be extremely helpful in detecting early subluxation or in differentiating angle closure due to subluxation of the lens from primary angle closure. Forward movement of the lens results in shallowing of the anterior chamber in the involved eye and a disparity in the depths of the anterior chambers between the two eyes if the condition is unilateral or asymmetric in degree. A difference between anterior chamber depths between the two eyes should always raise the suspicion of ectopia lentis. A mobile lens may also result in variable depths to the anterior chamber between one examination and the next.

When the lens is dislocated posteriorly, a deep chamber with a widely open angle results, similar to that in the aphakic patient. A tilted lens, on the other hand, may result in unequal depths between quadrants in the same chamber, the angle appearing shallow or even closed where the lens is tilted forward, whereas the diametrically opposite quadrants appear deep.

When the lens is subluxed or dislocated anteriorly, gonioscopy reveals a characteristic appearance (Fig. 10-3). The forward movement of the lens, especially when the lens is spherical, frees the peripheral iris from posterior contact with the lens equator and zonules and allows it to fall back-

ward, deepening the angle. The bulk of the lens is in contact primarily with the middle third of the iris, stretching it and creating a bulge that appears to fit the contour of the lens. The region of the sphincter, anterior to this bulge, is angled forward because of the stretching of the middle region of the iris by the lens and appears conical, similar to the crater of a volcano, the lens surface corresponding to the base of the crater. This appearance may sometimes be differentiated from that due to an intumescent, nondislocated lens, in which the entire iris appears to wrap around the lens, and the apex of the angle is sharp, as previously described. Iridodonesis may be present in the former situation but not in the latter. If pupillary block is present, the resultant iris bombé, with or without angle closure and glaucoma, counteracts the tendency for the peripheral iris to fall backward, and the appearance of the angle is then one of angle closure. Because of this, the characteristic gonioscopic appearance is best seen after iridectomy.

On slit-lamp examination, the zonular fibers may appear intact but stretched or thickened. Ruptured zonular fibers may be seen attached to the lens capsule (Fig. 10-4), but more often they are absent, being presumably retracted to the ciliary processes. Vitreous may be present in the pupil-

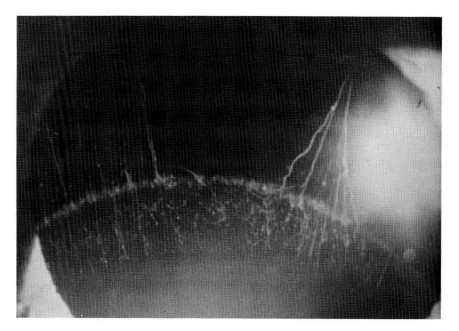

FIG. 10-4. Downward dislocation of lens showing elongated zonules with broken zonules attached to lens surface.

lary space and protrude into the anterior chamber, where it may contribute to pupillary block.

Ophthalmoscopically the edge of the lens appears as a dark crescent because of internal reflection of the light. Two images of the disc may be seen if the examiner is able to focus both through the lens and through the aphakic region of the pupil.

When complications such as uveitis, cataract, glaucoma, or retinal detachment are present, additional symptoms and signs corresponding to these complications are, of course, also present.

Glaucoma associated with ectopia lentis

Several mechanisms can contribute to glaucoma in the presence of a subluxed or dislocated lens (see below). Some of these are coincidental and are not discussed in this chapter. Of those directly related to the lens, the most important are the glaucomas associated with forward movement of the lens. Syndromes whose primary manifestations are lens related are discussed below. Glaucoma secondary to phacolysis is discussed in Chapter 9, angle-recession glaucoma in Chapter 20, and glaucoma secondary to uveitis in Chapter 19.

Causes of glaucoma in the presence of ectopia lentis

A. Lens related
   1. Pupillary block by lens
   2. Pupillary block by lens and vitreous
   3. Pupillary block by vitreous
   4. Lens in anterior chamber
   5. Phacolytic glaucoma
   6. Secondary open-angle glaucoma due to repeated attacks of angle closure
   7. Peripheral anterior synechiae due to chronic angle closure
B. Lens unrelated
   1. Angle recession
   2. Chamber angle anomaly
   3. Coincident primary open-angle glaucoma
   4. Other forms of glaucoma related to an underlying disease process (e.g., ghost cell glaucoma, neovascular glaucoma)

SIMPLE ECTOPIA LENTIS

Several large pedigrees have been reported in which dislocated lenses exist as an isolated autosomal dominant entity and in which pupils are normal.[15,30] The onset of dislocation is unknown, but many cases have been described in which patients were under the age of 10 years. The condition is usually bilateral and symmetric, with the lenses dislocated upward and laterally. Ocular complications include luxation of the lens into the anterior chamber, secondary glaucoma, and retinal detachment. The anterior chamber angles have been reported to be normal.[30] A form with late onset of the dislocation, usually in patients between the ages of 40 and 60, has also been described.[38,63]

ECTOPIA LENTIS ET PUPILLAE

In this autosomal recessive bilateral condition, the lenses and pupils are displaced in opposite directions. The lens tends to be microphakic and often bisects the pupil, resulting in decreased or variable visual acuity or monocular diplopia. In most patients there is some distortion of the pupil also. Patients with lightly pigmented irides and this syndrome have had marked peripheral iris transillumination, poor pupillary dilation, and atrophic sphincters.[57] In a study of patients with densely pigmented irides, there were no transillumination defects, although pupillary dilation was slow, irregular, and incomplete.[22]

Because the iris dilator muscles and zonules are of neuroectodermal origin, it seems likely that this is a neuroectodermal, rather than mesodermal, syndrome. No systemic anomalies are associated with this disorder. There is frequently a family history of consanguinity.[87] Complications are similar to those of simple lens ectopia. The most common cause of secondary glaucoma appears to be dislocation of the lens into the anterior chamber.

MICROSPHEROPHAKIA AND THE WEILL-MARCHESANI SYNDROME

Microspherophakia with ectopia lentis and glaucoma may occur as an isolated familial anomaly in either an autosomal dominant or autosomal recessive pattern[50] and is also occasionally found in association with Marfan's syndrome and homocystinuria,[23] Alport's syndrome,[83] mandibulofacial dysostosis,[58] and Klinefelter's syndrome.[5] The classic associated disorder, however, is the Weill-Marchesani (brachymorphia-brachydactyly) syndrome.

In a 1932 study of Marfan's syndrome, Weill[92] described a patient with brachydactyly and microspherophakia. Marchesani[60] (1939) recognized this combination as a separate entity. Patients with the syndrome exhibit short stature, stubby hands and feet, brachycephaly, and microspherophakia. There is severe limitation of mobility of the fingers and wrists to both active and passive motion. The presence of both microspherophakia and brachydactyly is essential for diagnosis.

Secondary myopia due to the abnormal lens shape occurs early in the second decade. Loss of vision occurs earlier and is more severe among these patients than in other syndromes associated with lens dislocation due to the frequent presence of glaucoma.

The size of the globe is usually normal. On dilated examination, the small lens may be seen situated in the center of the pupil, the equator being visible for 360 degrees (Fig. 10-5). In the undilated eye, the anterior chamber may be shallow because of forward displacement of the lens. Gonioscopy often shows a narrowed angle but is otherwise usually unremarkable. In a pedigree in which one member had the typical syndrome, numerous iris processes bridging the meshwork, fraying of the iris root, and anomalous angle vessels were reported.[33] Posterior segment anomalies have not been described.

Lens dislocation is common and occurs early. In one series, 12 lenses of 10 patients were noted to be dislocated at the initial examination (average age 20 years) and 2 dislocated subsequently.[49] One patient without previous evidence of dislocation had subluxation of both lenses into the anterior chambers after pupillary dilation.

Genetics and pathophysiology

Consanguinity is present in a large proportion of pedigrees in which microspherophakia and brachymorphia are present.[52] Inheritance appears to be recessive in most, but dominant inheritance has been described.[80] Pedigrees exist in which either the brachymorphic habitus[52,56,72,93] or brachydactyly[33,52] occurs in relatives of patients with the complete syndrome. Brachydactyly and spherophakia may also be inherited independently within a pedigree.[72]

In the microspheric lens, the weight and equatorial diameter of the lens is reduced 20% to 25%, whereas the sagittal diameter is increased up to 25%[33,64,67,72] (Fig. 10-6). Zonules have been described as elongated and profuse.[16,64]

Because there is usually no evidence of abnormal zonular development, most authors have considered the defect to be mesodermal, resulting in abnormal ciliary body development.[50] Farnsworth et al.[31] found a decrease of 20% in lens fiber cross-sectional area in a scanning electron microscopic study of a microspherophakic lens. They hypothesized that developmental abnormalities of lens fibers are the primary cause of congenital ectopia lentis in microspherophakia and that the resultant increased circumlental space places an increased strain on the zonule, leading to the lens subluxation. Jensen et al.[49] suggested that both the lens and zonules might be abnormal as a result of a basic metabolic defect. As in other syndromes in which patients are categorized by phenotypic criteria and in which the genetic or molecular causes

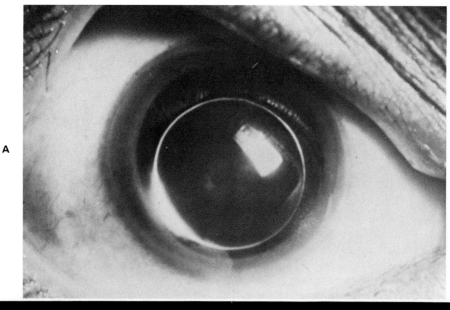

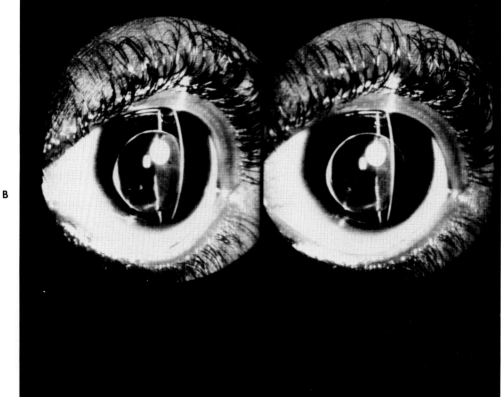

FIG. 10-5. Microspherophakia in Weill-Marchesani syndrome. **A,** Lens periphery is fully visible when pupil is dilated. **B,** Stereoscopic view of microspherophakic lens dislocated anteriorly. (**A** courtesy Maurice Luntz, M.D.; **B** courtesy Anthony Caputo, M.D.)

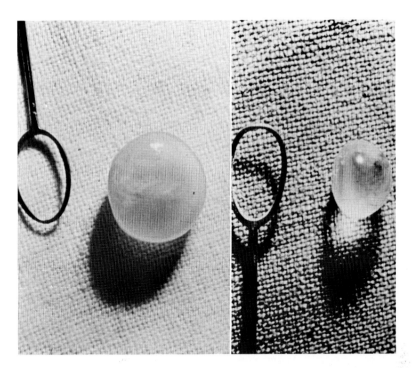

FIG. 10-6. Comparison of normal and microspheric lenses. (From Jensen, A.D., Cross, H.E., and Paton, D. Published with permission from the American Journal of Ophthalmology **77:**261-269, 1974. Copyright by the Ophthalmic Publishing Co.)

are either poorly understood or appear to be variable, more than one mechanism may eventually be discovered.

Mechanism of glaucoma

Glaucoma may occur either by forward movement of the lens or by dislocation of the lens into the anterior chamber. In the first case, loosening of zonules permits the lens to move forward, increasing its area of contact with the iris. This results in pupillary block secondary to which peripheral iris bombé and gradual shallowing of the anterior chamber lead to angle-closure glaucoma. Prolonged or repeated attacks may result in the formation of peripheral anterior synechiae or permanent damage to the trabecular meshwork, after which elevated intraocular pressure may continue even after iridectomy for the pupillary block component. If treatment is delayed, unrestrained motion of the lens may cause a flat anterior chamber, a condition that does not occur in other forms of angle-closure glaucoma, in which the lens is relatively immobile. Once this occurs, surgical treatment becomes hazardous.

Probert[72] noted that glaucoma could occur either

with or without manifest ectopia lentis. In the series by Jensen et al.,[49] two eyes had normally positioned lenses and glaucoma.

Angle closure due to microspherophakia often becomes worse with miotic therapy, and Urbanek[88] (1930) coined the term inverse glaucoma to describe this phenomenon. Parasympathomimetic agents stimulate contraction of the ciliary muscle and further loosen the zonular support, whereas cycloplegics relax the ciliary muscle, tauten the zonules, and pull the lens more posteriorly. This effect appears to occur only in eyes in which zonular attachments are still present.[7] Patients who do not worsen with miotic treatment may be assumed to have fully dislocated lenses or lack of restriction of lens motion by those zonules that do remain.

MANAGEMENT

One should be extremely cautious in treating any patient with angle closure suspected of having an anteriorly subluxed lens. As mentioned, an important clue to the examiner making the diagnosis is asymmetry of the chamber depth and angle width between the two eyes. One should also be suspicious when angle closure occurs in young patients, especially those in whom either the habitus or presence of other congenital anomalies might be suggestive of one of the syndromes associated with lens dislocation.

One should strongly resist the temptation to try to break the attack through the use of multiple instillation of miotics. The cautious use of 2% pilocarpine is reversible by cycloplegics if the anterior chamber shallows further. If this dose of pilocarpine is successful in opening the angle (i.e., does not further shallow the anterior chamber), one should suspect a complete dislocation and use mydriatics cautiously if at all. A reasonable approach to use in these cases would be to place the patient supine and to give oral glycerin and topical timolol. The hyperosmotic effect of the glycerin in shrinking the volume of the vitreous may permit greater motion of the lens in the posterior chamber and relief of the pupillary block. Cautious miosis or cycloplegia as outlined above may be used to supplement this. No hard and fast rule can be applied, and treatment must be individualized.

In one series, patients who had grade I to closed angles after miosis had grade IV angles after mydriasis and after iridectomy.[93] It was suggested that patients refusing iridectomy should be maintained on a regimen of long-term mydriatics. However, this course of treatment seems unwise because of the high incidence of spontaneous dislocation of the lens into the anterior chamber. Mydriatics should also be avoided in a patient known to have a dislocated lens in the opposite eye to minimize the chance of migration into the anterior chamber.

Peripheral iridectomy has been suggested as the safest surgical procedure,[16,17] although Jensen et al.[49] have cautioned that the severe lenticular myopia and subluxation in patients with the Weill-Marchesani syndrome may warrant lens surgery in addition to iridectomy. Surgical complications are common, and vitreous loss more frequent than in routine iridectomy because of loss of protection of the vitreous face by the lens periphery. Laser iridectomy, which does not risk vitreous loss, is probably a safer choice of initial procedure than surgical iridectomy, which can be resorted to if laser iridectomy is unsuccessful. One case has been reported in which a successful surgical iridectomy was blocked because of forward movement of the lens.[7] In performing laser iridectomy in these patients, one should choose as peripheral a location as possible to avoid the later occurrence of lens-iridectomy block due to forward dislocation, particularly since the size of a laser iridectomy is much smaller than that of a surgical one. The fellow eye should receive laser iridectomy prophylactically. After iridectomy, miotics can be used to constrict the pupil to prevent dislocation into the anterior chamber.

Dislocation of the lens into the anterior chamber

Dislocation of the lens into the anterior chamber is a therapeutic emergency, since the complications when this remains untreated are disastrous to the eye (Fig. 10-7). This situation may arise when the iris of a patient with a dislocated lens, particularly a microspherophakic one, is dilated, permitting the lens to float through the pupillary space. Alternatively, a dislocated lens may become wedged in the pupil and held there by the iris sphincter. The consequent buildup of aqueous pressure behind the lens may become sufficient to force the lens through the pupil into the anterior chamber. Alternatively, the chamber may gradually shallow and flatten, the lens remaining within the pupil. Whichever the case, a marked elevation of intraocular pressure ensues because of pupillary block, either by the entrapped lens or by the posterior surface of the lens if it is entirely within the anterior chamber. If the lens remains in the anterior chamber, cataract formation ensues, and adherence between the lens capsule and corneal endothelium result in corneal decompensation. Glaucomatous damage may progress rapidly.

The two options for treatment consist of replacement of the lens into the posterior chamber and lens removal. If the lens is clear, the former of these is the more conservative and safer measure. Relief of the glaucoma with replacement of the lens within the posterior chamber may in some cases be accomplished merely by placing the patient supine with wide dilation of the pupil,[38] since the lens has a tendency to float backward under these conditions. Massage of the cornea may facilitate replacement of the lens.[54] Walton has recommended covering the cornea with a soft contact lens and then pressing with a muscle hook on the contact lens.[17] The use of a spatula inserted through a keratome incision to push the lens backward has been reported[6] and often quoted, but no

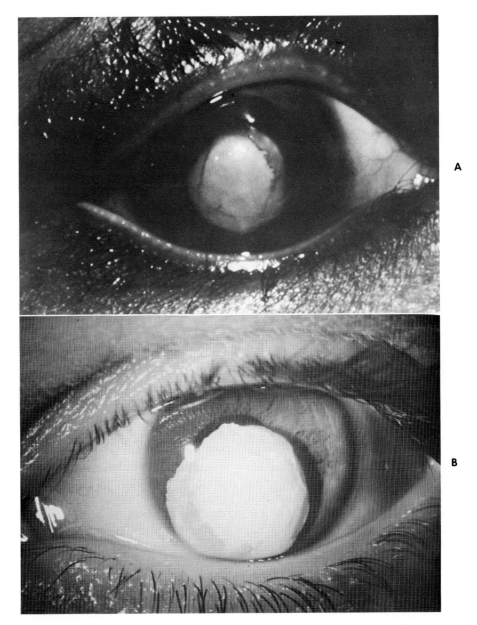

FIG. 10-7. A, Long-standing anterior dislocation of lens in Weill-Marchesani syndrome. Lens has opacified and become adherent to cornea. **B,** Dislocation of hypermature lens nucleus into anterior chamber.

recent reports of the results of this technique exist, and it is not recommended.

If noninvasive measures do not succeed, peripheral iridotomy, iridectomy, or iris transfixation to relieve the pupillary block may deepen the anterior chamber, decrease intraocular pressure, and allow the lens to be reposited more easily.[17] If this option is to be selected, I recommend laser iridectomy, since, being noninvasive, it avoids the possibility of surgical complications.

Once the lens is back in place, the patient is susceptible to future occurrences unless the basis for pupillary block is removed by iridectomy. If the lens is repeatedly incarcerated in the pupil, the formation of extensive peripheral anterior synechiae and permanent glaucoma may result.[16,78] After iridectomy, the patient may be maintained on a regimen of miotics to prevent further dislocation. Anterior dislocation may recur even with the use of miotics if iridectomy is not performed.[29]

Other authors have favored lens extraction as the primary procedure. Iliff and Kramer[42] preferred aspiration for a lens still partially held by zonules and routine incision for a lens completely free in the anterior chamber. They cautioned against attempting to reposit a traumatically dislocated lens. Jaffe[44] has recommended constricting the pupil to trap the lens in the anterior chamber and then removing it by aspiration, phacoemulsification, or limbal incision.

I prefer attempting conservative methods if the lens is clear in cases of simple dislocations into the anterior chamber. If the lens is cataractous, it should be removed. In cases of trauma, if there is additional damage to the eye that requires surgical intervention, the lens should be removed concomitantly, but conservative measures may be used if the dislocation is the only manifestation of the trauma and if the lens is reposited without much difficulty, since lens extraction may always be performed at a later time if cataract formation ensues. If the lens is adherent to the cornea, combined lens extraction and keratoplasty may be required.

Dislocation of the lens into the vitreous

Lenses dislocated into the vitreous cavity may either float free within the vitreous, settle inferiorly, or become attached to the retina. Even when a dense cataract is present, the lens may remain for years without causing difficulty. Conservative treatment is therefore strongly indicated, and extraction of the lens is not warranted unless phacolytic glaucoma supervenes.

Attempts to trap the lens in the anterior chamber by placing the patient in the prone position and then constricting the pupil are rarely successful. If the lens is situated in the posterior vitreous, it may be floated into the pupillary space, where it may be grasped by directing a stream of saline into the vitreous. Jaffe[44] has recommended lens aspiration in patients under 35 years of age.

OTHER HEREDITARY DISORDERS
Marfan's syndrome

Marfan's syndrome is the most common inherited disorder associated with ectopia lentis. The ocular manifestations were first described by Williams (1876).[9] Marfan[61] (1896) described the skeletal abnormalities, and Boerger[8] (1914) associated the systemic and ocular findings.

The disease is characterized by autosomal dominant inheritance with high penetrance. Several clinical varieties exist. Musculoskeletal disturbances consist of arachnodactyly, abnormally long limbs, chest cage deformities, skull anomalies, kyphoscoliosis, hyperextensibility of joints due to defective joint capsules and ligaments, sparsity of subcutaneous fat, and poor muscular development. Cardiovascular anomalies include progressive degenerative changes in the walls of the major vessels, dissecting aortic aneurysm, and cardiac decompensation due to mitral regurgitation. Pedigrees with features of both Marfan's syndrome and the Weill-Marchesani syndrome have been reported.[59]

Ocular abnormalities are numerous. The globe is usually enlarged, often progressively so. Megaloglobus may occur in patients with normal intraocular pressure and is believed to indicate an underlying connective tissue defect of the sclera. High myopia is common and has an axial as well as a lenticular component.[1] Nearly all patients with the classic syndrome have relatively flat corneas, with keratometer readings several standard deviations below the mean.[73]

Transillumination of the iris periphery and hypoplasia of the iris stroma and dilator muscle may be present. Gonioscopy reveals prominent pectinate ligaments, numerous iris processes, peripheral mounds of iris tissue, and vascular anomalies in the angle.[90] Similar gonioscopic findings occur in other systemic connective tissue disorders, such as scoliosis, Legg-Perthes disease, Osgood-Schlatter disease, idiopathic genu varum, and slipped upper femoral epiphysis.[11]

Dislocation of the lens occurs in nearly 80% of patients and is virtually always bilateral.[20] The frequency of dislocation may be greater or less in any one pedigree.[74] Estimates of the age of onset of dislocation range from 50% by 5 years[20] to 70% by 6 years.[41] The lens may dislocate in any direction but characteristically moves superiorly. A small percentage of these dislocate into the anterior chamber or vitreous. Microspherophakia, microphakia, and spherophakia have all been reported and may contribute to anterior dislocation of the lens.

The lens may have an irregular scalloped border, whereas the zonules are often torn and retracted to the lens equator.[21] The zonules are frequently abnormally long.[91] Nevertheless, enough may remain intact to prevent complete dislocation of the lens and to permit normal accommodation. Zonular appearance has been reported normal by light and transmission electron microscopy,[75] in marked contrast to that in homocystinuria; on scanning electron microscopy, however, the zonules have been found to be few and malformed, with loss of their regular parallel orientation, and they are substantially larger in diameter than the zonules of a normal lens.[32] The zonulocapsular attachments are also abnormally narrow.[75,91]

Retinal detachment is common. There does not appear to be an increased incidence of retinal detachment after surgery for dislocated lenses in either Marfan's syndrome or homocystinuria.[23]

Other ocular findings include heterochromia, blue sclerae, keratoconus, megalocornea, strabismus, colobomas of the retina and optic nerve, and pigmentary retinopathy.

Glaucoma is present in about 8% of eyes with ectopic lenses and in one third of these is caused by dislocation of the lens into the pupil. Despite the angle anomalies, all proved cases of glaucoma in the largest series[23] were phacogenic.

Pathologic examination has shown the circumlental space to be 8 to 10 times wider than normal and the distance between the ciliary processes to be 5 to 7 times greater than normal.[91] The ciliary processes are rudimentary, long, and narrow, frequently extending onto the posterior surface of the iris.[75] There is hypoplasia of the circular and oblique ciliary muscles,[10,25] and the longitudinal muscle fibers bypass the scleral spur or pass through it to insert directly onto the trabecular meshwork.[91] The iris root is situated posteriorly, but the presence of masses of mesoderm in the angle recess may give the picture of an anterior insertion on gonioscopy. Schlemm's canal is focally absent and usually discontinuous where present, consisting of small single or multiple endothelium-lined channels bearing a striking resemblance to the chamber angle of the canine eye.[10] Despite the frequency of these anomalies, there is little evidence that they are more than rarely the cause of glaucoma.

Homocystinuria

Homocystinuria, an autosomal recessive disorder, is similar to Marfan's syndrome in that it consists of skeletal, cardiovascular, and ocular abnormalities. It was discovered in 1962,[13,35] and prior series of patients with Marfan's syndrome undoubtedly include cases of homocystinuria. Cross and Jensen[23] (1973) found 142 patients with Marfan's syndrome with urine screening tests negative for homocystinuria and 42 chromatographically documented cases of homocystinuria.

The disease is usually due to a deficiency or abnormality of the enzyme cystathionine synthetase, which catalyzes the condensation of homocysteine and serine to form cystathionine. Excessive homocystine is formed from accumulated homocysteine and is excreted in the urine. Homocysteine reacts with aldehydes to form stable thiazine ring compounds, thus blocking condensation and cross-linking reactions in collagen.[37] Variant forms of homocystinuria are due to blocks in the remethylation of homocysteine to methionine and are associated with reduced levels of serum methionine.

The characteristic clinical triad consists of skeletal, cardiovascular, and ocular abnormalities. Many patients are tall and slender, with abnormal upper to lower segment ratios. However, arachnodactyly is usually less marked than in Marfan's syndrome. Other skeletal anomalies are genu valgum, flat feet, kyphoscoliosis, joint laxity, a deformed sternum, generalized osteoporosis with vertebral collapse, and a high, arched palate.

Thromboembolic phenomena in veins and medium-sized arteries occur in about 50% of patients. Thrombosis may affect multiple areas of the body, including the central retinal artery. Progressive arterial disease may result in thrombosis in a vital organ. Cerebrovascular thromboses, myocardial infarction, pulmonary emboli, and intermittent claudication may occur at a relatively young age. Premature death occurs in about 40% of patients. Disturbances in the peripheral circulation are evidenced by a malar flush. The skin is light, fair, and dry; the hair is fair, coarse, and sparse.

Thromboembolic phenomena are more likely to occur after puncture of a vessel during general anesthesia, and patients with homocystinuria are prone to pulmonary emboli after surgery. Indeed, the first patient with known homocystinuria to require surgery for lens extraction died 2 days later from pulmonary embolism.[53] Increased platelet adhesiveness and secondary adhesiveness induced by high blood levels of homocystine and methionine have been implicated.

The most important ocular finding is lens dislocation, which is present in 90% of cases and is most often downward. In about one third of cases the lens is dislocated completely into the vitreous or anterior chamber.[23] In contrast to Marfan's syndrome, the zonules disintegrate and accommo-

TABLE 10-1
Differential features of Marfan's syndrome and homocystinuria

	Marfan's syndrome	Homocystinuria
Heredity	Autosomal dominant	Autosomal recessive
Skeletal	Arachnodactyly Joint laxity Sternal deformity	Occasional arachnodactyly Osteoporosis Sternal deformity
Vascular	Aortic dissection Aortic and mitral valve disease	Dilation of vessels Frequent thrombosis Livido reticularis Malar flush
Skin	Striae distensae	
Amino acids	Hydroxyprolinuria	Homocystinuria
Mental retardation	Rare	60%
Ectopia lentis	80% First decade Usually superiorly 6% into anterior chamber or vitreous Occasional microspherophakia	90% May occur earlier than in Marfan's syndrome or progress more rapidly Usually inferiorly 33% into anterior chamber or vitreous Occasional microspherophakia
Glaucoma	8% with ectopia lentis 15% with surgical aphakia	23% with ectopia lentis
Angle anomalies	Present	None reported
Retinal detachment	12%	9%

dation is absent.[73] Anterior chamber angle anomalies have not been reported. Whether the zonules are formed abnormally or degenerate more readily because of the metabolic abnormality is unknown.

Histologically Henkind and Ashton[40] noted the presence of a thickened hyaline membrane overlying an atrophic pigment epithelium of the pars plicata and pars plana. Ramsey et al.[76] found this to be composed of disintegrated zonules. The degree of zonular abnormality was apparently age related.

The incidence of retinal detachment is approximately the same as in Marfan's syndrome and does not appear to be influenced by surgical removal of the lens.[23] Pigmentary retinopathy is more common than in Marfan's syndrome.

Glaucoma is due primarily to pupillary block. Lens extraction is frequently complicated by vitreous loss. In addition, increased platelet adhesiveness may produce an occlusive vascular disease leading to optic nerve head atrophy with cupping resembling glaucomatous optic atrophy in the absence of elevated intraocular pressure.[84]

Supplemental pyridoxine and perhaps a low methionine diet may aid in restoring blood levels of the involved metabolites to normal in some patients. Early ambulation after surgery should be encouraged to prevent thrombotic episodes. The use of prophylactic heparin may predispose patients to hemorrhage, and anticoagulants should not be used before surgery.

The sodium nitroprusside test is a simple diagnostic screening test for differentiating homocystinuria from Marfan's syndrome, although false-positive and false-negative reactions may occur. To perform the test, mix 5 ml of urine with 2 ml of sodium cyanide. After 10 minutes, add 2 to 4 drops of 5% sodium nitroprusside. A bright red color develops in the presence of cystine or homocystine. To differentiate cystine, which may be present in the urine in Marfan's syndrome, from homocystine, electrophoresis is necessary.

Other disorders

In the Ehlers-Danlos syndrome, ectopia lentis is not as prominent a feature as in the previously mentioned disorders. Gonioscopy has revealed angle anomalies[68] similar to those in Marfan's syndrome, and at least one patient developed glaucoma.[28] Because extremely thin sclera has been noted during operative procedures[68] and has been noted to rupture following relatively minor trauma to the head or globe,[4] extreme caution should be taken if one is performing filtering procedures on these patients.

Hyperlysinemia is a rare disorder characterized primarily by mental retardation and hypotonia. Dislocated lenses occur.[82]

Pfändler reported a pedigree containing three individuals with mental retardation, ectopia lentis, and keratoconus.[71] Each was the offspring of a different consanguineous marriage between normal parents. One patient had unilateral glaucoma.

Sulfite oxidase deficiency is characterized by muscular rigidity, mental retardation, and bilateral ectopia lentis.[43]

TRAUMATIC DISLOCATION OF THE LENS

Trauma is the most common cause of dislocated lenses, probably accounting for more than all other causes combined.[39] Dislocations secondary to trauma present additional problems not ordinarily encountered with simple subluxations and dislocations. In addition to the lens, any other structure within the eye may be damaged. Hyphema, iridodialysis, angle recession, rupture of the vitreous face, scleral rupture, vitreous hemorrhage, and retinal edema, hemorrhage, or detachment may be present. In these cases treatment of the lens is subordinate to or contingent on treatment of the other injuries. The following discussion pertains to treatment of uncomplicated traumatically dislocated lenses.

After contusion injury, severe ciliary spasm may cause the lens to move forward symmetrically with shallowing of the anterior chamber and narrowing of the angle due to pupillary block. When angle closure occurs, it may be due to pupillary block alone or to a mixed pupillary and lenticulociliary block. There is a disparity in anterior chamber depth between the two eyes on slit-lamp examination and between the angles of the two eyes on gonioscopy. A myopic shift occurs in the involved eye because of forward movement of the lens. These patients are frequently young, probably because younger patients are more prone to this type of trauma. As in pupillary block due to other anterior subluxations, treatment with miotics may fur-

ther shallow the anterior chamber, leading to increased severity of the angle closure and further elevation of intraocular pressure. Mydriatic-cycloplegics in combination with hyperosmotics often reverse the condition, decrease the pupillary block, and cause the anterior chamber to deepen. The former drugs may have to be used on an extended basis to prevent repeated angle closure.

In other cases there may be breakage of zonules but sufficient integrity of the remaining zonular apparatus to maintain the anatomic connection between the lens and ciliary body yet, in the face of ciliary spasm, allow the lens to move forward more than would have occurred were all the zonules intact. One cannot be sure of zonular integrity before dilation, and the examiner should be aware of the possibility of the lens dislocating into the anterior chamber.

If pupillary block persists, laser iridectomy should be attempted. Peripheral iridectomy is more risky in this situation, since there is an increased chance of vitreous loss because of the forward displacement of the lens and exposure of vitreous directly under the peripheral iris, particularly if the vitreous face has been disrupted by the trauma. Laser iridectomy is difficult to perform in the presence of a dilated pupil because of the increased thickness of the iris stroma at any point, and miosis should be cautiously attempted just before the procedure. Sufficient stretch burns should be placed to achieve maximal thinning of the iris stroma at the desired iridectomy site.

An additional problem after trauma is that the lens may be tilted, causing angle and anterior chamber asymmetry. The vitreous may be herniated between the lens and the pupillary margin, and the vitreous face may be either intact or broken. Angle closure may occur on the basis of pupillary block by the vitreous or by a combination of lens and vitreous. In regions of vitreous block, posterior aqueous displacement may occur, so that a mixed type of block results in which pockets of aqueous are interspersed with vitreous posterior to the iris. Both miotics and mydriatic-cycloplegics may give variable responses. Occasionally, particularly if the block has a lenticular component, the glaucoma may be relieved by putting the patient in a supine position. However, if attacks recur or if this does not suffice in curing the problem on the first occasion and medical treatment does not successfully control the glaucoma, peripheral iridectomy becomes necessary.

If the surgeon's preference is to perform a laser iridectomy, this should be done initially over the area of the vitreous to minimize any chance of lens opacity. If a mixed type of block is present, vitreous may be present posterior to the iridectomy, and a second attempt may result in penetration over the aqueous and break the block. If this is unsuccessful, laser iridectomy should then be tried over the area of the lens. If all attempts at laser iridectomy are unsuccessful, or if peripheral iridectomy is the surgeon's first choice, this should be performed over the area of the lens to minimize the chance of vitreous loss. If these measures are insufficient, then open-sky vitrectomy and lens extraction should be performed. It should be evident that these cases may be quite difficult to deal with, and the above guidelines are not absolute.

If the lens is dislocated downward, it is possible for it to adhere to the ciliary body. Conditions of treatment are as above except that caution is indicated during surgery in order to prevent cyclodialysis or hemorrhage. If the lens is firmly adherent, it may be better to do a modified planned extracapsular cataract extraction in which the peripheral equatorial lens capsule is left adherent to the ciliary body and the remainder of the lens removed.

EXTRACTION OF DISLOCATED LENSES

Techniques of lens removal from various positions of dislocation—anterior chamber, posterior chamber, or vitreous—are beyond the scope of this chapter. These techniques are presented elsewhere and include discission,[16] aspiration,[42,44,62] cryoextraction with aspiration,[25] needling the lens to maintain stability of position during surgery,[2,12] and vitrectomy techniques.[70] The rapid development of vitrectomy and ultrasonic fragmentation techniques will undoubtedly contribute to the refinement of procedures for removal of dislocated lenses.

Criteria for removal of a dislocated lens in any eye should be grounded on the potential for improvement of the condition for which extraction is contemplated. Because of the high incidence of operative complications, there is no excuse for removing a dislocated lens merely because it is there. By the same token, a lens in the vitreous should be left alone unless phacolytic glaucoma supervenes.

Legitimate criteria for removal of a dislocated lens include the following:

1. A cataract blocking the visual axis (If the patient is monocular, this is a stronger indication. If the patient is binocular and has a monocular cataract, the mere presence of the cataract is not sufficient unless the patient has difficulty functioning in the absence of binocular vision.)
2. Decreased visual acuity due to the dislocated lens (e.g., lens margin in the pupillary axis) and which is uncorrectable with lenses, mydriasis, or photomydriasis[85]
3. Phacolytic glaucoma
4. Pupillary block glaucoma unresponsive to more conservative measures
5. A dislocated lens in the anterior chamber if conservative measures fail or if the lens is cataractous or adherent to the cornea
6. The necessity for adequate visualization in the presence of a retinal detachment

Retinal detachments are relatively more common in eyes with heritable ectopia lentis. They occur in about 10% of eyes with Marfan's syndrome and homocystinuria. The relationship between the lens displacement and the retinal detachment is unclear. There may be no significant difference in the incidence of retinal detachment between eyes that have undergone surgery for the displaced lens and those that have not.[23]

Jarrett[45] reported that less than 50% of 94 eyes had better vision after the removal of a dislocated lens. The results of lens removal are poorer in traumatic dislocations than in Marfan's syndrome, probably because trauma causes other ocular problems such as contusion deformity and retinal damage. Vitreous loss, in the extraction of dislocated lenses from any cause, is almost the rule after trauma (see below). Forbes[34] has devised a scleral support system that may reduce the incidence of vitreous loss by reducing posterior scleral infolding.

Vitreous loss and extraction of dislocated lenses

1. Marfan's syndrome: 21%[48]
2. Homocystinuria: 24%[48]
3. Trauma: 85%[79]

REFERENCES

1. Allen, R.A., Straatsma, B.R., Apt, L., and Hall, M.O.: Ocular manifestations of the Marfan syndrome, Trans. Am. Acad. Ophthalmol. Otolaryngol. **71:**18, 1967.

2. Barraquer, J.I.: Surgical treatment of lens displacements, Arch. Soc. Am. Oftal. Optom. **1:**30, 1958.

3. Bartholomew, R.S.: Phakodonesis: a sign of incipient lens displacement, Br. J. Ophthalmol. **54:**663, 1970.

4. Beighton, P.: Serious ophthalmological complications in the Ehlers-Danlos syndrome, Br. J. Ophthalmol. **54:**263, 1970.

5. Bessiere, E., Riviere, J., and Leuret, J.P.: An association of Klinefelter's disease and congenital anomalies, captodactyly, microphakia, Bull. Soc. Ophthalmol. Fr. **62:**197, 1962.

6. Bickerton, T.H.: Dislocation of lens: Couching, recovery, Ophthalmol. Rev. **16:**325, 1897.

7. Blaxter, P.L.: Spherophakia, Trans. Ophthalmol. Soc. U.K. **88:**621, 1969.

8. Boerger, F.: Uber zwei Falle von Arachnodaktylie, Z. Kinderheilkd. **12:**161, 1914.

9. Bowers, D.: Williams' prior description of Marfan's syndrome, Am. J. Ophthalmol. **50:**154, 1960.

10. Burian, H.M., and Allen, L.: Histologic study of the chamber angle of patients with Marfan's syndrome, Arch. Ophthalmol. **65:**323, 1961.

11. Burian, H.M., von Noorden, G.K., and Ponseti, I.V.: Chamber angle anomalies in systemic connective tissue disorders, Arch. Ophthalmol. **64:**671, 1960.

12. Calhoun, F.P., Jr., and Hagler, W.S.: Experience with the Jose Barraquer method of extracting a dislocated lens, Am. J. Ophthalmol. **50:**701, 1960.

13. Carson, N.A.J., and Weill, D.W.: Metabolic abnormalities detected in survey of mentally backward individuals in Northern Ireland, Arch. Dis. Child. **37:**505, 1962.

14. Celichowska, J.: Des ectopies et luxations congénitales du cristallin, thesis, Geneva, No. 276, C. Zoellner, 1910.

15. Chace, R.R.: Congenital bilateral subluxation of the lens: report of a family, Arch. Ophthalmol. **34:**425, 1945.

16. Chandler, P.A.: Choice of treatment in dislocation of the lens, Arch. Ophthalmol. **71:**765, 1964.

17. Chandler, P.A., and Grant, W.M.: Glaucoma associated with congenital and spontaneous dislocations of the lens. In Glaucoma, Philadelphia, 1980, Lea & Febiger.

18. Clarke, C.C.: Ectopia lentis: a pathologic and clinical study, Arch. Ophthalmol. **21:**124, 1939.

19. Cotlier, E., and Reinglass, H.: Marfan-like syndrome with lens involvement: hyaloideoretinal degeneration with anterior chamber angle, facial, dental, and skeletal anomalies, Arch. Ophthalmol. **93:**93, 1975.

20. Cross, H.E.: Ectopia lentis in systemic heritable disorders, Birth Defects **10**(10):113, 1974.

21. Cross, H.E.: Differential diagnosis and treatment of dislocated lenses, Birth Defects **12**(3):335, 1976.

22. Cross, H.E.: Ectopia lentis et pupillae, Am. J. Ophthalmol. **88:**381, 1979.

23. Cross, H.E., and Jensen, A.D.: Ocular manifestations in the Marfan syndrome and homocystinuria, Am. J. Ophthalmol. **75:**405, 1973.

24. Dinno, N.D., Shearer, L., and Weisskopf, B.: Familial pseudomarfanism, a new syndrome? Birth Defects **15**(5B):179, 1979.

25. Douvas, N.G.: Management of luxated and subluxated lenses, Trans. Am. Acad. Ophthalmol. Otolaryngol. **73:**100, 1969.

26. Duke-Elder, S.: System of ophthalmology, vol. 3, part 2, Congenital deformities, St. Louis, 1963, The C.V. Mosby Co., pp. 710-715.

27. Duke-Elder, S.: System of ophthalmology, vol. 11, Diseases of the lens and vitreous; glaucoma and hypotony, St. Louis, 1969, The C.V. Mosby Co., pp. 658-663.

28. Durham, D.G.: Cutis hyperelastica (Ehlers-Danlos syndrome) with blue scleras, microcornea, and glaucoma, Arch. Ophthalmol. **49:**220, 1953.

29. Elkington, A.R., Freedman, S.S., Jay, B., and Wright, P.: Anterior dislocation of the lens in homocystinuria, Br. J. Ophthalmol. **57:**325, 1973.

30. Falls, H.F., and Cotterman, C.W.: Genetic studies on ectopia lentis: a pedigree of simple ectopia of the lens, Arch. Ophthalmol. **30:**610, 1943.

31. Farnsworth, P.N., Burke, P.A., Blanco, J., and Maltzman, B.: Ultrastructural abnormalities in a microspherical ectopic lens, Exp. Eye Res. **27:**399, 1978.

32. Farnsworth, P.N., Burke, P., Dotto, M.E., and Cinotti, A.A.: Ultrastructural abnormalities in a Marfan's syndrome lens, Arch. Ophthalmol. **95:**1601, 1977.

33. Feiler-Ofrey, V., Stein, R., and Godel, V.: Marchesani's syndrome and chamber angle anomalies, Am. J. Ophthalmol. **65:**862, 1968.

34. Forbes, M.: Suspension of the globe during intraocular surgery, Trans. Am. Ophthalmol. Soc. **76:**316, 1978.

35. Gerritsen, T., Vaugh, J.G., and Waisman, H.A.: The identification of homocystine in the urine, Biochem. Biophys. Res. Commun. **9:**493, 1962.

36. Goltz, R.W., Henderson, R.R., Hitch, J.M., and Ott, J.E.: Focal dermal hypoplasia syndrome, Arch. Dermatol. **101:**1, 1970.

37. Grieco, A.J.: Homocystinuria: pathogenetic mechanisms, Am. J. Med. Sci. **273:**120, 1977.

38. Harshman, J.P.: Glaucoma associated with subluxation of lens in several members of a family, Am. J. Ophthalmol. **31:**833, 1948.

39. Heath, P.: Secondary glaucoma due to the lens, Arch. Ophthalmol. **25:**424, 1941.

40. Henkind, P., and Ashton, N.: Ocular pathology in homocystinuria, Trans. Ophthalmol. Soc. U.K. **85:**21, 1965.

41. Hindle, N.W., and Crawford, J.S.: Dislocation of the lens in Marfan's syndrome: its effect and treatment, Can. J. Ophthalmol. **4:**128, 1969.

42. Iliff, C.E., and Kramer, P.: A working guide for the management of dislocated lenses, Ophthalmic. Surg. **2:**251, 1971.

43. Irreverre, F., Mudd, S.H., Heizer, W.D., and Laster, L.: Sulfite oxidase deficiency: studies of a patient with mental retardation, dislocated ocular lenses, and abnormal urinary excretion of s-sulfo-L-cysteine sulfite and thiosulfate, Biochem. Med. **1:**187, 1967.

44. Jaffe, N.S.: Subluxation and dislocation of the lens. In Cataract surgery and its complications, ed. 3, St. Louis, 1981, The C.V. Mosby Co.

45. Jarrett, W.H.: Dislocation of the lens: a study of 166 hospitalized cases, Arch. Ophthalmol. **78:**289, 1967.

46. Jaureguy, B.M., and Hall, J.G.: Isolated congenital

ectopia lentis with autosomal dominant inheritance, Clin. Genet. **15:**97, 1979.

47. Jensen, A.D.: Heritable ectopia lentis. In Goldberg, M.F., editor: Genetic and metabolic eye disease, Boston, 1974, Little, Brown & Co.

48. Jensen, A.D., and Cross, H.E.: Surgical treatment of dislocated lenses in the Marfan syndrome and homocystinuria, Trans. Am. Acad. Ophthalmol. Otolaryngol. **76:** 1491, 1972.

49. Jensen, A.D., Cross, H.E., and Paton, D.: Ocular complications in the Weill-Marchesani syndrome, Am. J. Ophthalmol. **77:**261, 1974.

50. Johnson, V.P., Grayson, M., and Christian, J.C.: Dominant microspherophakia, Arch. Ophthalmol. **85:**534, 1971.

51. Kirkham, T.H.: Mandibulofacial dysostosis with ectopia lentis, Am. J. Ophthalmol. **70:**947, 1970.

52. Kloepfer, H.W., and Rosenthal, J.W.: Possible genetic carriers in the spherophakia-brachymorphia syndrome, Am. J. Hum. Genet. **7:**399, 1955.

53. Komrower, G.M., and Wilson, V.K.: Homocystinuria, Proc. R. Soc. Med. **56:**996, 1963.

54. Kravitz, D.: Lens surgery in Marfan's syndrome, Arch. Ophthalmol. **62:**764, 1959.

55. Lemmingson, W., and Riethe, P.: Beobachtungen bei Dysgenesis mesodermalis corneae et iridis in Kombination mit Oligodontie, Klin. Monatsbl. Augenheilkd. **133:**877, 1958.

56. Levy, J., and Anderson, P.E.: Marchesani's syndrome, Br. J. Ophthalmol. **45:**223, 1961.

57. Luebbers, J.A., Goldberg, M.F., Herbst, R., et al.: Iris transillumination and variable expression in ectopia lentis et pupillae, Am. J. Ophthalmol. **83:**647, 1977.

58. Magnasco, A.: Unusual malformation association: mandibulofacial dysostosis and bilateral microspherophakia, Ann. Ottal. **91:**489, 1965.

59. Manfredi, F., Bracciolini, M., Cristallo, E., et al.: Etude clinique (oculaire, cardiovasculaire, constitutionelle) et genetique du syndrome de Marfan, J. Genet. Hum. **25** (suppl. 1), 1977.

60. Marchesani, O.: Brachydaktylie und angeborene Kugellinse als Systemerkrankung, Klin. Monatsbl. Augenheilkd. **103:**392, 1939.

61. Marfan, A.B.: Un cas de deformation congénitale de quatre membres plus prononcée aux extremities characterisée par l'allongement des os avec un certain degré d'amincissement, Bull. Mem. Soc. Hop Paris **13:**220, 1896.

62. Maumenee, A.E., and Ryan, S.J.: Aspiration technique in the management of the dislocated lens, Am. J. Ophthalmol **68:**808, 1969.

63. McCulloch, C.: Hereditary lens dislocation with angle closure glaucoma, Can. J. Ophthalmol. **14:**230, 1979.

64. McGavic, J.S.: Weill-Marchesani syndrome, Am. J. Ophthalmol. **62:**820, 1966.

65. McKusick, V.A.: Primordial dwarfism and ectopia lentis, Am. J. Hum. Genet. **7:**189, 1955.

66. Meyer, E.T.: Familial ectopia lentis and its complications, Br. J. Ophthalmol. **38:**163, 1954.

67. Meyer, S.J., and Holstein, T.: Spherophakia with glaucoma and brachydactyly, Am. J. Ophthalmol. **24:**247, 1941.

68. Pemberton, J.W., Freeman, H.M., and Schepens, C.L.: Familial retinal detachment and the Ehlers-Danlos syndrome, Arch. Ophthalmol. **76:**817, 1966.

69. Pesme, P., Verger, and Montoux: Dysostose craniofaciale avec ectopie du crystallin, Arch. Fr. Pediatr. **7:** 348, 1950.

70. Peyman, G.A., Raichand, M., Goldberg, M.F., and Ritacca, D.: Management of subluxated and dislocated lenses with the vitrophage, Br. J. Ophthalmol. **63:**771, 1979.

71. Pfändler, U.: Une souche du vallon de St. Imier (Suisse), manifestant par consanguinité la transmission récessive de malformations oculaires multiples (ectopie du cristallin, keratocone, cataracte congénitale, atrophie du nerf optique), associées a l'oligophrénie: manifestation d'une achromatopsie totale dans une branche collaterale, Ophthalmologica **119:**103, 1950.

72. Probert, L.A.: Spherophakia with brachydactyly: comparison with Marfan's syndrome, Am. J. Ophthalmol. **36:**1571, 1953.

73. Pyeritz, R.E., and McKusick, V.A.: The Marfan syndrome: diagnosis and management, N. Engl. J. Med. **300:** 772, 1979.

74. Pyeritz, R.E., Murphy, E.A., and McKusick, V.A.: Clinical variability in the Marfan syndrome(s), Birth Defects **15**(5B):155, 1979.

75. Ramsey, M.S., Fine, B.S., Shields, J.A., and Yanoff, M.: The Marfan syndrome: a histopathologic study of ocular findings, Am. J. Ophthalmol. **76:**102, 1973.

76. Ramsey, M.S., Yanoff, M., and Fine, B.S.: The ocular histopathology of homocystinuria: a light and electron microscopy study, Am. J. Ophthalmol. **74:**377, 1972.

77. Ringelhan, O., and Elschnig, A.: Uber die Linsen-Dislokationen, Arch. Augenheilkd. **104:**325, 1931.

78. Rodman, H.I.: Chronic open-angle glaucoma associated with traumatic dislocation of the lens, Arch. Ophthalmol. **69:**445, 1963.

79. Rosenbaum, L.J., and Podos, S.M.: Traumatic ectopia lentis: some relationships to syphilis and glaucoma, Am. J. Ophthalmol. **64:**1095, 1967.

80. Rosenthal, J.W., and Kloepfer, H.W.: The spherophakia-brachymorphia syndrome, Arch. Ophthalmol. **55:**28, 1956.

81. Sichel, J.: Ueber die freiwillige Dislocation und Niedersenkung der Crystalllinse, Z. Gesamte Med. **33:**281, 1846.

82. Smith, T.H., Holland, M.G., and Woody, N.C.: Ocular manifestations of familial hyperlysinemia, Trans. Am. Acad. Ophthalmol. Otolaryngol. **75:**355, 1971.

83. Sohar, E.: Renal disease, inner ear deafness and ocular changes: a new heredofamilial syndrome, Arch. Intern. Med. **97:**627, 1956.

84. Spaeth, G.W.: Glaucomatous changes in homocystinuria. Discussion of Jay, B.: Glaucoma associated with spontaneous displacement of the lens, Br. J. Ophthalmol. **56:** 258, 1972.

85. Straatsma, B.R., Allen, R.A., Pettit, T.H., and Hall, M.O.: Subluxation of the lens treated with iris photocoagulation, Am. J. Ophthalmol. **61:**1312, 1966.

86. Thomas, C., Cordier, J., and Algan, B.: Une étiologie nouvelle du syndrome de luxation spontanée des cristallins: la maladie d'Ehlers-Danlos, Bull. Soc. Belge Ophthalmol. **100:**375, 1952.

87. Townes, P.L.: Ectopia lentis et pupilae, Arch. Ophthalmol. **94:**1126, 1976.
88. Urbanek, J.: Glaucoma juvenile inversum, Z. Augenheilkd. **77:**171, 1930.
89. Vogt, A.: Dislocatio lentis spontanea als erbliche Krankheit, Z. Augenheilkd. **14:**153, 1905.
90. von Noorden, G.G., and Schultz, R.O.: A gonioscopic study of the chamber angle in Marfan's syndrome, Arch. Ophthalmol. **64:**929, 1960.
91. Wachtel, J.G.: The ocular pathology of Marfan's syndrome, Arch. Ophthalmol. **76:**512, 1966.
92. Weill, G.: Ectopie des cristallins et malformations générales, Ann. Ocul. **169:**21, 1932.
93. Willi, M., Kut, L., and Cotlier, E.: Pupillary-block in the Marchesani syndrome, Arch. Ophthalmol. **90:**504, 1973.

Chapter 11

GLAUCOMA ASSOCIATED WITH RETINAL DISORDERS

Charles D. Phelps

This chapter describes glaucoma secondary to retinal disorders and to the treatment of retinal disorders, as well as glaucoma associated with retinal disorders on the basis of common underlying causes. In addition, some associations of glaucoma and retinal disease for which the cause is unknown are described. Retinal disorders secondary to glaucoma and its treatment are not included.

The principal varieties of glaucoma associated with retinal disorders are listed below. Several of these are thoroughly described in other chapters of this textbook; to avoid unnecessary repetition, they are not dealt with in this chapter.

Glaucoma associated with retinal disorders

A. Glaucoma caused by retinal disorders
  1. Open-angle glaucoma apparently caused by retinal detachment (Schwartz's syndrome)
  2. Other types of glaucoma caused by long-standing rhegmatogenous retinal detachment
     a. Angle-closure glaucoma from posterior synechiae and pupillary block caused by detachment-induced iritis (see Chapter 19)
     b. Neovascular glaucoma (see Chapter 12)
  3. Hemolytic, ghost cell, and hemosiderotic glaucoma after vitreous hemorrhage (see Chapter 21)
  4. Neovascular glaucoma associated with retinal ischemic disorders, including diabetic retinopathy and central retinal vein occlusion (see Chapter 12)
  5. Angle-closure glaucoma associated with neonatal retinal diseases: retrolental fibroplasia, persistent hyperplastic primary vitreous, Coats' disease, and retinoblastoma (see Chapters 5 and 13)
  6. Angle-closure glaucoma, uveal effusion, and retinal detachment in nanophthalmos

  7. Transient angle-closure glaucoma following central retinal vein occlusion
B. Glaucoma caused by treatment of retinal disorders
  1. Angle-closure glaucoma following retinal photocoagulation
  2. Angle-closure glaucoma following a scleral buckling operation
  3. Transient glaucoma following an intravitreal injection of gas
  4. Late glaucoma after an intraocular silicone injection
  5. Corticosteroid glaucoma
C. Glaucoma associated with retinal disorders because of a common underlying cause or for unknown reasons
  1. Primary open-angle glaucoma and rhegmatogenous retinal detachment
  2. Pigmentary glaucoma and retinal detachment
  3. Glaucoma and retinitis pigmentosa
  4. Open-angle glaucoma and retinal detachment in Stickler's syndrome
  5. Angle-recession glaucoma and retinal detachment in a contused eye (see Chapter 20)
  6. Glaucoma (developmental, angle closure, angle recession, or phacolytic) and retinal detachment in eyes with displaced lenses (see Chapter 10)
  7. Synechial angle-closure glaucoma and retinal detachment in aphakia (see Chapter 23)
  8. Other types of glaucoma associated with non-rhegmatogenous retinal detachment
     a. Secondary angle-closure glaucoma in eyes with uveitis and exudative retinal detachment (see Chapter 19)
     b. Neovascular glaucoma in diabetics with traction retinal detachment (see Chapter 12)
     c. Glaucoma in eyes with tumors and secondary retinal detachment (see Chapter 13)

GLAUCOMA CAUSED BY RETINAL DISORDERS

Open-angle glaucoma apparently caused by retinal detachment (Schwartz's syndrome)

Rhegmatogenous retinal detachment usually reduces pressure in the affected eye to a level lower than that in the fellow normal eye. The relative hypotony may be marked but more often is slight, so that, on the average, the pressure difference between the two eyes is about two mm Hg.[15]

In 1973 Schwartz[54] described 11 patients with unilateral retinal detachment in whom, contrary to expectations, pressures were much higher in the involved eyes than in the fellow eyes. The involved eyes also had markedly reduced outflow facilities. In all 11 cases the anterior chamber angles were open. With the exception of one patient, who had a recessed angle following trauma, the angles appeared normal. Cells and flare were often present in the anterior chambers. Following surgical reattachment of the retina, intraocular pressures and outflow facilities returned to normal, usually within a few days.

The cause of the outflow obstruction in Schwartz's patients was not readily apparent. Five of the 11 patients had a history of trauma, as did two of four similar patients subsequently reported by Davidorf.[20] Each author found an angle recession in one of his patients. In 18 of our patients who had high intraocular pressures that reverted to normal following surgical reattachment of the retina, my colleagues at the University of Iowa and I found an angle recession in 6 (33%).[48] Thus trabecular damage from previous trauma may be one factor that predisposes an eye to reduced aqueous outflow and high pressure in association with retinal detachment.

Schwartz[54] suggested that another factor is mild iritis secondary to the retinal detachment. He thought that in some eyes the iritis caused enough inflammation of the meshwork to block aqueous outflow. Davidorf[20] interpreted the anterior chamber reaction differently. He thought that the specks floating in the aqueous and vitreous were pigment granules rather than cells and proposed that pigment granules were released from the retinal pigment epithelium into the subretinal space and passed through the retinal hole into the vitreous. Aqueous then carried them into the anterior chamber, where they became trapped in the trabecular meshwork and blocked outflow.

Whatever the mechanism, it is important to remember that unilateral open-angle glaucoma in an eye with cells or pigment granules floating in the aqueous humor may be a sign of unsuspected retinal detachment. (Remember, also, that if the detachment is nonrhegmatogenous, one should think of an underlying choroidal melanoma; see Chapter 13.) The peripheral fundus must be examined carefully through a dilated pupil. If a rhegmatogenous retinal detachment is found and successfully treated, the prognosis for the glaucoma is quite good.

Angle-closure glaucoma, uveal effusion, and retinal detachment in nanophthalmos

Nanophthalmos is a rare developmental ocular anomaly in which the eye is normal in shape but unusually small in size. Most nanophthalmic eyes are markedly hyperopic because of their short axial lengths. They are also susceptible to angle-closure glaucoma, which usually begins acutely during the fourth to sixth decade of life.

In 1974 Brockhurst[13] described five patients with nanophthalmos and angle-closure glaucoma who, after glaucoma surgery or a subsequent cataract operation, were found to have choroidal effusion and nonrhegmatogenous retinal detachment. Calhoun[18] described additional patients with this unusual and severe complication.

Iridectomy in some of the patients in these studies failed to open the anterior chamber angle, suggesting that relative pupillary block was neither the sole nor the initiating pathogenic mechanism. Brockhurst hypothesized that the primary event was the uveal effusion. He suggested that angle closure resulted when the ciliary body detached and swelled sufficiently to rotate its anterior surface forward against the trabecular meshwork. At surgery Brockhurst observed an unusually thick sclera (2.5 mm) in two of his patients, leading Shaffer[56] to suggest that the thick sclera might in some way impede drainage of venous blood through the vortex veins, thus causing the uveal effusion.

Brockhurst could not confirm his hypothesis in his initial group of patients, because in none of them had he noted a choroidal effusion until after the glaucoma surgery, and in some the effusion was not found until several years later. However, Kimbrough et al.[34] described two additional patients with nanophthalmos in whom a peripheral choroidal detachment was identified by ultrasonography before glaucoma surgery. They attempted laser iridotomy as a treatment for the angle-closure glaucoma in these cases. Although it failed to penetrate the iris, the laser energy contracted the peripheral iris and opened the chamber angle, curing the glaucoma. The angles remained open for more than 1½ years after laser treatment.

The relationships of the nanophthalmos, angle-closure glaucoma, and uveal effusion in this unusual syndrome are complex, and we probably have much more to learn about the pathogenesis and treatment. However, the initial results of laser iridoplasty are encouraging, particularly in view of the poor results with conventional glaucoma surgery.

Transient angle-closure glaucoma following central retinal vein occlusion

Rarely, after a central retinal vein occlusion the anterior chamber shallows, the chamber angle narrows, and, if enough of the angle closes, the intraocular pressure rises. After a few weeks the chamber spontaneously returns to a normal depth. Eleven cases of this unusual complication have been reported,[9,19,26,33] and we have observed two others. The chamber shallowing does not occur simultaneously with the vein occlusion. In several cases the chamber depth was normal 1 or 2 days after the vein occlusion and was then found to be shallow several days later. Chamber shallowing has been noted as early as 3 days and as late as 2 years after the onset of blurred vision. The presenting symptom in some patients has been pain, but others have complained only of blurred vision.

This condition must be distinguished, both clinically and conceptually, from two other types of angle-closure glaucoma that more often accompany central retinal vein occlusion. The first type is primary angle-closure glaucoma, in which, as in any type of glaucoma, the high intraocular pressure may occasionally induce a central retinal vein occlusion. In primary angle-closure glaucoma, the patient's other eye also has a shallow anterior chamber and a narrow anterior chamber angle. The second variety of glaucoma included in the differential diagnosis is neovascular glaucoma (see Chapter 12), a devastating secondary glaucoma that frequently occurs several weeks or months after the onset of a central retinal vein occlusion.

Neovascular glaucoma, like the transient angle-closure glaucoma following central retinal vein occlusion, is usually unilateral but is distinguished by the presence of rubeosis iridis. Once the angle-closure stage of neovascular glaucoma occurs, it is permanent.

Most patients with central retinal vein occlusion, of course, do not develop conspicuous alterations of anterior chamber depth. The mechanism of the chamber shallowing in these few unusual cases is obscure. Hyams and Neumann[33] suggested that transudation of fluid from the retinal vessels into the vitreous cavity caused a forward displacement of the lens, pupillary block, and angle-closure glaucoma. However, in two of Grant's patients[26] iridectomy did not immediately relieve the angle closure. Grant wondered if blood or edema fluid in the retina might increase the volume of the posterior segment sufficiently to produce the forward movements of the lens and iris. However, in one of his patients and in another patient we have studied, no thickening of the retina could be measured by echography. Bloome[9] suggested that swelling of the ciliary body due to spasm, edema, or detachment would produce the clinical picture observed, but he was unable to explain how a retinal vein occlusion could cause the ciliary body to swell. None of the above theories explains why the anterior chamber becomes shallow in only these unusual patients and not in the great majority of cases of central retinal vein occlusion.

Whatever the pathogenic mechanism, the prognosis for eventual recovery of normal anterior chamber depth is quite good. In all of the reported cases, the angle gradually widened and the chamber reformed over several weeks. Acetazolamide and pilocarpine in some cases appeared to hasten somewhat the resolution of the angle closure.[26,33] In three cases, treatment with acetazolamide and cycloplegics produced a rapid and dramatic deepening of the chamber.[9,19] Cycloplegics are a logical treatment because the condition resembles malignant glaucoma and angle-closure glaucoma from ciliary body swelling, both of which respond favorably to treatment with cycloplegics.

Although the angle closure eventually resolves, vision is often permanently impaired by retinal damage from the central vein occlusion. In addition, in a few of the reported cases the patients developed typical neovascular glaucoma some weeks to months later.[26,33]

GLAUCOMA CAUSED BY TREATMENT OF RETINAL DISORDERS
Angle-closure glaucoma following retinal photocoagulation

Following retinal photocoagulation, intraocular pressure often rises. At least three pathogenic mechanisms, each occurring at different times after the photocoagulation, may be responsible.

First, the tissue explosion associated with the photocoagulation impact may cause a transient sharp spike of the intraocular pressure. This immediate pressure elevation, which has been thoroughly studied and described by Fraunfelder and Viernstein[24] and McNair et al.,[40] may reach a peak of nearly 900 mm Hg but lasts only about 2 sec. It has been observed in association with ruby laser and xenon arc photocoagulation burns but not with argon laser burns.

Second, modest but more long-lasting pressure elevations have been observed after extensive argon laser photocoagulation treatment of diabetic retinopathy.[8] The pressure goes up during the first hour after treatment and remains elevated for several hours. The anterior chamber angle is open. Studies are in progress to define how often the pressure rises, the time course, and the pathogenic mechanism.

Third, anterior chamber shallowing and in some cases angle closure with high intraocular pressure often develop within a few hours of panretinal photocoagulation for diabetic retinopathy. Mensher[41] observed some shallowing of the anterior chamber in 44 of 45 treated eyes. Fourteen (31%) developed angle closure.

The shallowing of the anterior chamber is accompanied by a temporary myopia[11] that gradually diminishes over several days as the chamber returns to its normal depth. When the chamber is shallow, a detachment or swelling of the choroid and pars plana can usually be observed ophthalmoscopically. Thickening of the ciliary body can be measured by echography.[44]

The intraocular pressure may be as high as 55 mm Hg, yet patients usually have little discomfort. Treatment with miotics is ineffective, and iridectomy in two cases failed to open the chamber angle. Treatment with cycloplegics and corticosteroids may hasten the resolution of the angle closure but has not been proved effective in a controlled therapeutic trial. Timolol, epinephrine, and carbonic anhydrase inhibitors aid in pressure control while the angle is closed. With or without treatment, the angle usually reopens and the pressure returns to a normal level in 2 to 7 days.

Boulton[11] thought that the anterior chamber shallowing was due partly to an outpouring of fluid from the choroid into the vitreous and partly to the annular choroidal detachment. He suggested that these two factors increased the volume in the posterior segment of the eye and pushed the lens-iris diaphragm forward. Mensher,[41] on the other hand, thought that ciliary body swelling was the cause of the chamber shallowing. He hypothesized that photocoagulation damaged the veins returning blood from the ciliary body to the choroidal vortex system. The impedance of venous drainage would cause edema and hyperemia of the ciliary processes.

This complication of retinal photocoagulation rarely causes serious long-term sequelae. We have not observed the formation of peripheral anterior synechiae and permanent angle-closure glaucoma.

Angle-closure glaucoma following a scleral buckling operation

Scleral buckling operations for a detached retina frequently cause the anterior chamber to shallow temporarily.[23,29] After several days the chamber gradually returns to its normal depth. The chamber shallowing in many cases is slight and can be detected only by pachometry. In other patients, however, the shallowing is marked and is accompanied by closure of the anterior chamber angle and elevation of intraocular pressure.[36,47,55,59]

Smith,[59] the first to describe angle closure as a complication of the scleral buckling operation, observed it in 4% of 1000 cases. Sebestyen et al.[55] noted angle closure after 4.4% of 160 scleral buckling operations. We found it in 1.4% of 1558 cases.[47] However, the incidence in our study is probably too low. Angle-closure glaucoma following a scleral buckling operation is often asymptomatic, and its incidence depends on how carefully it is sought. In the first 6 years of our initial study, we found postoperative angle closure in only 0.9% of 1433 cases. In the last 6 months of the study, when we were especially looking for the complication, we observed it in 7.2% of 125 cases. In a subsequent study of 889 additional cases, we detected postoperative angle closure in 7.3%.[17]

Angle-closure glaucoma following a scleral buckling operation may pass unrecognized unless the patient is examined at a slit lamp and his intraocular pressure is measured with an applanation tonometer. Few patients complain of severe pain. In most, the discomfort is no more than that usually produced by the retinal surgery alone. The most common clue to the presence of angle closure is a hazy ophthalmoscopic view of the retina during a bedside examination on the first or second postoperative day. Hazy media should suggest that the cornea is edematous and should not be casually dismissed as a vitreous inflammatory reaction.

When examined at the slit lamp, patients with postoperative angle closure are often found to have mild corneal epithelial edema. The anterior chamber is shallow, intraocular pressure is usually between 25 and 50 mm Hg, and the chamber angle is partially or completely closed. A choroidal detachment is usually present.

The anterior chamber is shallow because the lens is shifted forward from its usual position. The contour of the anterior surface of the iris differs from the midperipheral forward convexity seen in pupillary-block glaucoma (Fig. 11-1). The iris is pushed forward centrally by the lens but in its midperiphery falls away slightly from the cornea. In the angle the root of the iris again comes forward toward the cornea to lie against the trabecular meshwork.

We believe that the chamber shallows and the angle closes when veins draining blood from the ciliary body are obstructed by the scleral buckle. For the most part, blood leaving the ciliary body drains posteriorly into the vortex veins. Experimentally in monkeys, if three or four vortex veins are obstructed, the ciliary body becomes markedly congested and swollen, and the angle closes.[30] Scleral buckling in rabbits also reduces ciliary body blood flow, probably by blocking venous drainage.[21] Capillaries of the ciliary processes have the capacity to enlarge to many times their normal size when their transmural pressure is high.[58] As the ciliary body swells, in cross section it resembles a fan unfolding with its apex attached to the scleral spur and its anterior face rotating toward the trabecular meshwork. If it swells sufficiently, the angle closes.

The frequent finding of peripheral choroidal detachment in eyes with postoperative angle closure supports the above theory. Choroidal detachment in an eye with high intraocular pressure is almost certain evidence of high pressure in the choroidal veins, since transudation of fluid from choroidal capillaries to interstitial spaces requires that the capillary pressure be considerably higher than the intraocular pressure. It seems likely that a scleral buckle over or anterior to the vortex ampullae may obstruct or kink the veins draining the choroid and ciliary body.

Pupillary block is another possible cause of angle closure. However, three observations speak against its playing an exclusive or even an important role in the pathogenesis. First, there is no iris bombé in most cases. Second, we have observed the syndrome in aphakic eyes with an open iridectomy and a vitreous face well behind the pupil. Third, in two cases that we treated with an iridectomy, there was no relief.[47] Nevertheless, it is possible that in some cases pupillary block caused by the forward movement of the lens may be partially responsible for the angle closure.[19]

A third possible mechanism is simple mechanical indentation of the sclera, which, if the buckle is anterior, might rotate the ciliary body forward.[6] This is unlikely to be the sole mechanism, because the chamber shallowing and angle closure resolve with time, even though the buckle seems to maintain its height.

The type of implant may influence how often angle closure occurs after a scleral buckling operation. In our initial study, we observed angle closure following 3.4% of cases in which an episcleral implant was used but in only 0.6% of cases in which an intrascleral implant was used.[47] This difference, however, may only reflect better diagnosis when episcleral implants were used, because we changed our preferred surgical method from intrascleral to episcleral techniques at about the same time that we became especially interested in looking for this type of glaucoma.

In our initial study, we were unable to identify predisposing factors other than the type of surgical technique. However, in a subsequent series of patients, we observed postoperative angle closure more frequently when the buckle was large in circumferential extent, when the patient was elderly, and when the anterior chamber angle was narrow preoperatively. Postoperative angle closure was relatively infrequent in myopic eyes but occurred as often in aphakic eyes as in nonmyopic phakic eyes.[17] Aaberg and Maggiano[1] have observed that postoperative choroidal detachment, a complication related to postoperative angle closure, also occurs more frequently when the patient is elderly and when the buckle is large.

In general, the prognosis for angle-closure glaucoma is good after a scleral buckling operation. If

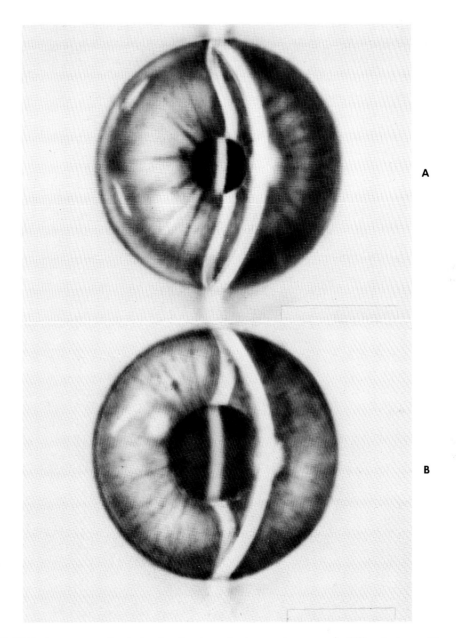

FIG. 11-1. Appearance of anterior chamber in angle-closure glaucoma. **A,** Ciliary body swelling: shallow in center and periphery, with some deepening in midperiphery. **B,** Pupillary block: forward convexity of anterior iris surface. (Courtesy Steven J. Vermillion, M.D.)

left untreated, after several days the chamber gradually deepens, the angle opens, the choroidal detachment flattens, and the intraocular pressure returns to normal. Complete resolution may take from 2 to 4 weeks.

Glaucomatous optic nerve damage from the acute attack is infrequent, because the intraocular pressure is usually not exceptionally high and the pressure elevation usually lasts only 1 to 2 weeks. In some patients, however, peripheral anterior synechiae form, and permanent synechial angle-closure glaucoma may develop.

It is uncertain whether any treatment, other than removal of the buckle, will quickly deepen the chamber and relieve the angle closure. In our experience, iridectomy is of no benefit and miotics worsen the ocular congestion. Some authorities recommend drainage of the choroidal detachment,[19,36,59] and this may sometimes be effective, but in other cases the choroidal detachment immediately recurs.

We prescribe atropine and phenylephrine to relieve ciliary muscle spasm and, perhaps, to flatten the ciliary body. We also give corticosteroids topically in an attempt to reduce the ocular inflammation and to prevent the formation of anterior synechiae. Pressure is lowered with combinations of carbonic anhydrase inhibitors, epinephrine, and timolol.

The favorable experience of Kimbrough et al.[34] using laser iridoplasty for the treatment of angle closure in nanophthalmos, a condition in which the pathogenic mechanism may be similar, has encouraged us to try the same treatment for angle closure following a scleral buckle. In the first two patients we treated, there was immediate and lasting relief of the angle closure. The angle opened only in the treated areas. The iris contraction did not involve the pupillary area, indicating that the treatment was not merely relieving pupillary block.

Other glaucomatous complications of retinal detachment surgery

Patients with complicated cases of retinal detachment are occasionally treated with intravitreal injections of gas to facilitate retinal reattachment.[22,42] Ordinary room air may be used but has the disadvantage of being rapidly absorbed and within a few hours becoming ineffective as a tamponade. Relatively insoluble gases, such as sulfur hexafluoride, maintain their volume for a much longer time. In fact, with sulfur hexafluoride, the gas bubble increases in size for 1 or 2 days and does not return to its original volume for 5 or 6 days. The bubble enlarges because nitrogen from body tissues diffuses into the bubble faster than the relatively insoluble sulfur hexafluoride is absorbed. The enlarging bubble creates a very effective tamponade but may produce a severe temporary form of glaucoma. The glaucoma can be prevented by injecting only a small volume of sulfur hexafluoride, less than 2 ml, or by using a 40:60 mixture of sulfur hexafluoride and air instead of pure sulfur hexafluoride.[42]

Silicone is another substance that is occasionally injected intravitreally in the treatment of desperate retinal detachments.[27,43,65] In some patients silicone is later found in the anterior chamber. Some investigators have observed glaucoma when the anterior chamber becomes filled with silicone[27,43]; others have not.[65] The mechanism of glaucoma, when it occurs, may be direct obstruction of the trabecular meshwork by the silicone oil.

A final type of glaucoma occurs in retinal detachment patients who are given corticosteroids in the treatment of ocular inflammation following detachment surgery. Some patients receiving corticosteroids for 2 to 6 weeks develop an elevation of intraocular pressure. In the general population about 1 of every 3 persons is somewhat corticosteroid sensitive, and about 1 of every 20 will develop a very high pressure with prolonged corticosteroid use (see Chapter 17). In retinal detachment populations the percentages may be higher.[57] Therefore corticosteroids should be prescribed with caution after retinal detachment surgery.

GLAUCOMA ASSOCIATED WITH RETINAL DISORDERS BECAUSE OF A COMMON UNDERLYING CAUSE OR FOR UNKNOWN REASONS
Primary open-angle glaucoma and rhegmatogenous retinal detachment

Primary open-angle glaucoma and retinal detachment afflict the same patient more often than one would anticipate simply from chance concurrence. Open-angle glaucoma was found in 5.8% of 530 retinal detachment patients studied by Becker[5] and in 4% of 817 retinal detachment patients we studied.[48] In contrast, the prevalence of primary open-angle glaucoma in the general population is probably less than 1%.[2,32,39] In addition, ocular hypertension (intraocular pressure of 22 mm Hg or higher) without optic disc damage was found by Baum and Ruiz[3] in 14% of 451 retinal detachment patients and by us in 5.8% of our retinal detachment patients.[48] Other investigators have found a high prevalence of low-outflow facilities in the fellow eyes of patients with unilateral retinal detachment.[5,37] Shammas et al.[57] observed that many of their patients with detached retinas had large cup-to-disc ratios. A large proportion of their patients also developed elevations of intraocular pressure after prolonged topical corticosteroid administration. The high prevalences of all these findings — ocular hypertension, low-outflow facility, large cup-to-disc ratio, and positive corticosteroid provocative test — suggest that retinal detachment patients are unusually susceptible to open-angle glaucoma.

Why should open-angle glaucoma and retinal detachment be associated? It is unlikely that either of the two disorders causes the other. This would fit with none of the current theories of the pathogenesis of either condition. In addition, each condition has been observed to precede the other in certain patients. Thus it seems likely that glaucoma and retinal detachment are linked by a joint underlying predisposition or by some other factor that they share in common.

One possible link between the two diseases is myopia, which occurs frequently in both open-angle glaucoma and retinal detachment patients. However, in our 817 patients with detached retinas, we found glaucoma no more frequently in myopic patients than in nonmyopic patients.[48]

Another possible link between the two diseases is the miotic treatment of glaucoma. Many cases have been reported in which a retinal detachment developed soon after a glaucoma patient began treatment with a miotic or had his prescription changed to a stronger miotic than what he had previously been taking.[4,38,45] These observations have convinced many clinicians that miotics cause retinal detachment. Whether this is true can be determined only by a prospective, controlled, clinical trial. However, even if miotics do cause retinal detachment, they are unlikely to account for more than a small proportion of retinal detachments occurring in patients with open-angle glaucoma, for in many of the patients observed by Becker[5] and by us[48] the glaucoma was unrecognized and thus untreated until the patient sought medical attention for his detached retina. Furthermore, of 30 patients in our series who were using miotics when their retinas detached, only three had recently begun miotic treatment or had their prescription changed to a higher concentration of miotics.[48]

Whatever the reason for the association of retinal detachment and glaucoma, the concurrence of the two conditions creates special diagnostic and therapeutic problems for the ophthalmologist. The signs of one disease may mask those of the other, and the treatment of one may worsen the other. Diagnosis of a retinal detachment is frequently delayed in a patient who is being treated for glaucoma. The loss of peripheral vision may be mistakenly attributed to the progression of glaucomatous optic nerve damage. Pupillary miosis from treatment of the glaucoma may prevent the ophthalmologist from adequately examining the patient's peripheral retina, and the detachment may be overlooked.

Several simple measures facilitate correct diagnosis. First, of course, one must keep in mind the possibility of the two diseases occurring in the same eye. All patients beginning treatment for glaucoma should have careful peripheral retina examinations through a dilated pupil with an indirect ophthalmoscope. This examination should be repeated yearly as well as when detachment symptoms occur. Loss of peripheral vision or a sudden drop in intraocular pressure below customary levels for the patient should suggest a detached retina. A retinal tear should be suspected if a glaucoma patient sees flashing lights or new floaters. Floaters beginning after the start of miotic therapy may represent enhanced entoptic visualization of normal vitreous condensations but sometimes are produced by vitreous hemorrhage from a retinal tear. If permanent miosis or lens opacities prevent adequate fundus examination, echography may help detect a suspected retinal detachment.

Similarly, the diagnosis of glaucoma in an eye with a detached retina may be difficult. Retinal detachment typically lowers intraocular pressure, even in glaucomatous eyes.[15] The optic disc may be difficult to evaluate if the peripapillary retina is detached or if a bullous detachment overhangs the disc. Glaucomatous cupping is easily missed if the fundus is examined only with an indirect ophthalmoscope, particularly if the examiner is concentrating on the detached retina and not on the optic disc. Visual fields are difficult to evaluate for glaucomatous damage if the retina is detached or has previously been detached. One key step in diagnosing open-angle glaucoma in a patient with unilateral retinal detachment, of course, is to examine carefully the optic disc of the fellow eye.

Another is to measure intraocular pressure in both eyes, not only preoperatively, but when the patient returns for his postoperative visits. An applanation tonometer should be used for the pressure measurements because retinal detachment surgery often reduces ocular rigidity.[46,61] Low ocular rigidity will cause a Schiøtz tonometer to give a falsely low estimate of intraocular pressure.

When retinal detachment and glaucoma afflict the same eye, the treatment of each condition often must be modified. Because of the possible role of miotics in the pathogenesis of retinal detachment, these drugs should be used with caution in patients who have had retinal detachment or in patients who are susceptible to retinal detachment because of aphakia, lattice degeneration, or a retinal tear. In these susceptible patients it is prudent to avoid miotics if possible or to begin with a weak concentration and slowly increase the strength until the desired lowering of pressure has been achieved.

If a patient with retinal detachment has open-angle glaucoma, he will probably be sensitive to the intraocular pressure-elevating effects of topical corticosteroids, and these drugs should be used with caution in the postoperative period. Patients who have used miotics for many years may have a small and rigid pupil, which prevents adequate visualization of the fundus. Laser photocoagulation of the iris adjacent to the pupil may enlarge the pupil and allow adequate examination.

The presence of glaucoma in an eye with retinal detachment does not adversely affect the chances for a successful reattachment by a scleral buckling operation.[14] It does, however, reduce the chance for a good visual outcome, because the optic nerve may have been previously damaged by glaucoma.[16]

Pigmentary glaucoma and retinal detachment

The pigment dispersion syndrome (Krukenberg's spindle, midperipheral spokelike iris translucency, and heavy pigmentation of the trabecular meshwork) and pigmentary glaucoma are described in detail in Chapter 7. In this chapter we shall consider only one possible association of pigment dispersion: rhegmatogenous retinal detachment.

In 1974 Brachet and Chermet[12] described 19 patients who had both pigmentary glaucoma and retinal detachment. They suggested that the concurrence of the two conditions represented more than simple chance, but their study provided no information about how often either condition occurred with the other.

Recently, however, Scheie and Cameron[52] reviewed the case histories of 407 patients with the pigment dispersion syndrome and found 26 (6.4%) who also had retinal detachment. The frequency of detachment was the same, whether glaucoma was present (6.0% of 151 patients) or absent (6.6% of 256 patients).

Other studies suggest that the converse is also true, that eyes with rhegmatogenous retinal detachment often have pigment dispersion. Segestyen et al.[55] investigated by gonioscopy 160 cases of retinal detachment and found 11 (6.9%) with marked pigmentation of the angle and glaucoma. Syrdalen[62] found moderate chamber angle pigmentation in 37 (16.7%) and marked pigmentation in 27 (12.1%) of 223 eyes with retinal detachment. Rodriguez-Gonzales[51] found the pigment dispersion syndrome, with or without glaucoma, in 10% of 1532 eyes with detached retinas.

If an association between pigment dispersion and retinal detachment is confirmed by future studies, its cause may be some common degenerative process or, more likely, the high frequency of myopia in both disorders. It is unlikely to be explained by miotic treatment of pigmentary glaucoma since, as is shown in the study by Scheie and Cameron,[52] the frequency of retinal detachment in the pigment dispersion syndrome is the same whether or not glaucoma is present.

Glaucoma and retinitis pigmentosa

An association between glaucoma and retinitis pigmentosa has been described by many investigators during the past century. The reported prevalences of glaucoma in retinitis pigmentosa have ranged from 2% to 12%.[25,35]

These reports are difficult to evaluate. They rarely define clearly whether the retinitis pigmentosa is hereditary or secondary, and, if inherited, whether the transmission is dominant, recessive, or sex linked. The type of glaucoma is usually described as primary, but seldom is a distinction made between angle-closure and open-angle mechanisms. In some cases the glaucoma is described as acute or inflammatory and in others as chronic or simple. Many of the reported case histories and some limited histologic material[25] suggest that the mechanism of glaucoma is often angle closure.

Is this a true association or just the coincidence

of two not uncommon diseases? Little information is available at present to help answer this question. The association, in my experience, is infrequent. I have treated only three patients for both retinitis pigmentosa and glaucoma. In all three, the retinitis pigmentosa was dominantly inherited. Two of the patients had primary angle-closure glaucoma, and the third had congenital glaucoma inherited from the other parent.

Open-angle glaucoma and retinal detachment in Stickler's syndrome

Stickler's syndrome, an inherited connective tissue disease that affects the eyes, ears, face, and skeleton, was first described in 1965[60] and remains unfamiliar to many ophthalmologists. However, the condition is not rare.* In fact, some authorities now think that Stickler's syndrome is the most common of the systemic connective tissue disorders, at least in the North American midwest.[31] The syndrome is inherited by autosomal dominant genetic transmission.

The more frequent ocular manifestations of the syndrome are high myopia, early cataract, vitreoretinal degeneration, and retinal detachment.[7,31,66] In addition, strabismus, amblyopia, and glaucoma are found in some patients. The myopia is usually severe, ranging from 8 to 18 or more diopters, and begins in the first decade of life. The vitreous space in the eyes of patients with Stickler's syndrome is optically empty or is crossed only by sparse strands. Pigment accumulates in clumps in the peripheral retina, avascular preretinal membranes are found in the equatorial region, and the retinal vessels have segmental sheathing. Eventually more than half of the patients with Stickler's syndrome develop a retinal detachment in one or both eyes. Surgical repair of the detachment may be difficult.

The systemic abnormalities in Stickler's syndrome include orofacial anomalies, skeletal malformations, and neurosensory hearing loss. The orofacial anomaly commonly consists of mandibular hypoplasia, glossoptosis, and palatal defects. These features, of course, comprise the well-known Pierre Robin anomaly, which in most cases is probably part of Stickler's syndrome.[31] However, the orofacial anomalies in Stickler's syndrome vary widely in severity from patient to patient, and in some patients the only abnormality may be a bifid uvula, a submucous cleft, or an ab-

normality in motility of the palate. Skeletal manifestations of Stickler's syndrome include hyperextendable fingers, wrists, and knees. Patients often appear marfanoid. Radiographs reveal spondyloepiphyseal dysplasia. Degenerative arthropathy may develop and become debilitating.

The ocular manifestations of Stickler's syndrome are easily confused with those of Wagner's disease. In 1938 Wagner[64] described vitreoretinal degeneration and presenile cataracts in a large family with four affected generations. Two other investigators later reexamined members of the same family.[10,50] Although the vitreoretinal degeneration in the family Wagner studied was very similar in appearance to that occurring in Stickler's syndrome, in other respects the two conditions have differed. The myopia in the families Wagner studied was always less than 4 D until a cataract developed, and no patient developed retinal detachment. No systemic abnormalities were described in the family members. Although subsequent reports have described patients unrelated to the original family studied by Wagner who were thought to have the same syndrome, these patients usually had retinal detachment, and it seems in retrospect that many of them, if not all, had Stickler's syndrome instead.

The glaucoma that occurs in Stickler's syndrome has not been well described and needs further study. The following comments are based on limited personal experience. Several of our patients with Stickler's syndrome have had mild to moderate elevation of intraocular pressure. The anterior chamber angles are open without obvious structural malformation. Some of our patients have had glaucomatous optic nerve damage. This is not always easily determined, because lens opacities and high myopia impair the ophthalmoscopic view of the optic disc. Furthermore, the discs are often tilted, and cupping when present is shallow. Retinal degeneration may cause visual field defects similar to those of glaucoma, and intraocular pressure, measured by applanation tonometry, may be the only reliable criterion on which to base treatment.

Fortunately, the high intraocular pressure in Stickler's syndrome usually responds well to pressure-lowering medications. It is important that miotics be avoided whenever possible. Not only do miotics reduce visual acuity if the eye has an axial lens opacity, but they have the potential of inducing retinal detachment in these highly susceptible patients.

---

*References 7, 28, 31, 49, 53, 63, 66.

REFERENCES

1. Aaberg, T.M., and Maggiano, J.M.: Choroidal edema associated with retinal detachment repair: experimental and clinical correlations, Mod. Probl. Ophthalmol. **20:** 6, 1979.
2. Bankes, J.L., Perkins, E.S., Tsolakis, S., and Wright, J.E.: Bedford glaucoma survey, Br. Med. J. **1:**791, 1968.
3. Baum, A., and Ruiz, R.S.: Intraocular hypertension in retinal detachments, Tex. Med. **68:**104, 1972.
4. Beasley, H., and Fraunfelder, F.T.: Retinal detachments and topical ocular miotics, Ophthalmology **86:**95, 1979.
5. Becker, B.: Discussion of Smith, J.L.: Retinal detachment and glaucoma, Trans. Am. Acad. Ophthalmol. Otolaryngol. **67:**731, 1963.
6. Berler, D.K., and Goldstein, B.: Scleral buckles and rotation of the ciliary body, Arch. Ophthalmol. **97:**1518, 1979.
7. Blair, N.P., Albert, D.M., Liberfarb, R.M., and Hirose, T.: Hereditary progressive arthro-ophthalmology of Stickler, Am. J. Ophthalmol. **88:**876, 1979.
8. Blondeau, P., Pavan, P.R., and Phelps, C.D.: Acute pressure elevation following panretinal photocoagulation, Arch. Ophthalmol. **99:**810, 1981.
9. Bloome, M.A.: Transient angle-closure glaucoma in central retinal vein occlusion, Ann. Ophthalmol. **9:**44, 1977.
10. Böhringer, H.R., Dieterle, P., and Landolt, E.: Zur Klinik und Pathologie der Degeneration hyaloideo-retinalis hereditaria (Wagner), Ophthalmologica **139:**330, 1960.
11. Boulton, P.E.: A study of the mechanism of transient myopia following extensive xenon arc photocoagulation, Trans. Ophthalmol. Soc. U.K. **93:**287, 1973.
12. Brachet, A., and Chermet, M.: Association glaucome pigmentaire et décollement de rétine, Ann. Ocul. **207:**451, 1974.
13. Brockhurst, R.J.: Nanophthalmos with uveal effusion, Arch. Ophthalmol. **93:**1289, 1975.
14. Burton, T.C.: Preoperative factors influencing anatomic success rates following retinal detachment surgery, Trans. Am. Acad. Ophthalmol. Otolaryngol. **83:**499, 1977.
15. Burton, T.C., Arafat, N.T., and Phelps, C.D.: Intraocular pressure in retinal detachment, Int. Ophthalmol. **1:**147, 1979.
16. Burton, T.C., and Lambert, R.W., Jr.: A predictive model for visual recovery following retinal detachment surgery, Ophthalmology **85:**619, 1978.
17. Burton, T.C., and Phelps, C.D.: Unpublished data, 1980.
18. Calhoun, F.P., Jr.: The management of glaucoma in nanophthalmos, Trans. Am. Ophthalmol. Soc. **73:**97, 1976.
19. Chandler, P.A., and Grant, W.M.: Glaucoma, Philadelphia, 1979, Lea & Febiger, pp. 183-186, 190-191.
20. Davidorf, F.H.: Retinal pigment epithelial glaucoma, Ophthalmol. Digest **38:**11, 1976.
21. Diddie, B., and Ernest, T.: Uveal blood flow after 360° constriction in the rabbit, Arch. Ophthalmol. **98:**729, 1980.
22. Fineberg, E., Machemer, R., Sullivan, P., et al.: Sulfur hexafluoride in owl monkey vitreous cavity, Am. J. Ophthalmol. **79:**67, 1975.
23. Fiore, J.V., and Newton, J.C.: Anterior segment changes following the scleral buckling operation, Arch. Ophthalmol. **84:**284, 1970.

24. Fraunfelder, F., and Viernstein, L.J.: Intraocular pressure variation during xenon and ruby laser photocoagulation, Am. J. Ophthalmol. **71:**1261, 1971.
25. Gartner, S., and Schlossman, A.: Retinitis pigmentosa associated with glaucoma, Am. J. Ophthalmol. **32:**1337, 1949.
26. Grant, W.M.: Shallowing of the anterior chamber following occlusion of the central retinal vein, Am. J. Ophthalmol. **75:**384, 1973.
27. Grey, R.H.B., and Leaver, P.K.: Results of silicone oil injection in massive preretinal retraction, Trans. Ophthalmol. Soc. U.K. **97:**238, 1977.
28. Hall, J.G., and Herrod, H.: The Stickler syndrome presenting as a dominantly inherited cleft palate and blindness, J. Med. Genet. **12:**397, 1975.
29. Hartley, R.E., and Marsh, R.J.: Anterior chamber depth changes after retinal detachment, Br. J. Ophthalmol. **57:** 546, 1973.
30. Hayreh, S.S., and Baines, J.A.B.: Occlusion of the vortex veins: an experimental study, Br. J. Ophthalmol. **57:**217, 1973.
31. Herrmann, J., France, T.D., Spranger, J.W., et al.: The Stickler syndrome (hereditary arthro-ophthalmopathy), Birth Defects **11:**76, 1975.
32. Hollows, F.C., and Graham, P.A.: Intraocular pressure, glaucoma, and glaucoma suspects in a defined population, Br. J. Ophthalmol. **50:**570, 1966.
33. Hyams, S.W., and Neumann, E.: Transient angle-closure glaucoma after retinal vein occlusion, Br. J. Ophthalmol. **56:**353, 1972.
34. Kimbrough, R.L., Trempe, C.S., Brockhurst, R.J., and Simmons, R.J.: Angle-closure glaucoma in nanophthalmos, Am. J. Ophthalmol. **88:**572, 1979.
35. Kogbe, O.I., and Follmann, P.: Investigations into aqueous humor dynamics in primary pigmentary degeneration of the retina, Ophthalmologica **171:**165, 1975.
36. Kreiger, A.E., Hodgkinson, B.J., Frederick, A.R., and Smith, T.R.: The results of retinal detachment surgery: analysis of 268 operations with a broad scleral buckle, Arch. Ophthalmol. **86:**385, 1971.
37. Langham, M.E., and Regan, C.D.J.: Circulatory changes associated with onset of retinal detachment, Arch. Ophthalmol. **81:**820, 1969.
38. Lemcke, H.H., and Pischel, D.K.: Retinal detachments after the use of Phospholine Iodide, Trans. Pac. Coast Oto-ophthalmol. Soc. **47:**157, 1966.
39. Leske, M.C., and Rosenthal, J.: Epidemiologic aspects of open-angle glaucoma, Am. J. Epidemiol. **109:**250, 1979.
40. McNair, J., Fraunfelder, F.T., Wilson, R.S., et al.: Acute pressure changes and possible secondary tissue changes due to laser or xenon photocoagulation, Am. J. Ophthalmol. **77:**13, 1974.
41. Mensher, J.H.: Anterior chamber depth alteration after retinal photocoagulation, Arch. Ophthalmol. **95:**113, 1977.
42. Norton, E.D.: Twenty-ninth Edward Jackson Memorial Lecture: intraocular gas in the management of selected retinal detachments, Trans. Am. Acad. Ophthalmol. Otolaryngol. **77:**85, 1973.
43. Okun, E.: Intravitreal surgery utilizing liquid silicone: a long term follow-up, Trans. Pac. Coast Oto-ophthalmol. Soc. **49:**141, 1968.

44. Ossoinig, K.C.: Personal communication, 1980.

45. Pape, L.G., and Forbes, M.: Retinal detachment and miotic therapy, Am. J. Ophthalmol. **85:**558, 1978.

46. Pemberton, J.W.: Schiøtz-applanation disparity following retinal detachment surgery, Arch. Ophthalmol. **81:**534, 1969.

47. Perez, R.N., Phelps, C.D., and Burton, T.C.: Angleclosure glaucoma following scleral buckling operations, Trans. Am. Acad. Ophthalmol. Otolaryngol. **81:**247, 1976.

48. Phelps, C.D., and Burton, T.C.: Glaucoma and retinal detachment, Arch. Ophthalmol. **95:**418, 1977.

49. Popkin, J.S., and Polomeno, R.C.: Stickler's syndrome (hereditary progressive arthro-ophthalmopathy), Can. Med. Assoc. J. **111:**1071, 1974.

50. Ricci, A.: Degeneresence hyaloideo-retienne de Wagner, Bull. Soc. Ophthalmol. Fr. **9:**646, 1961.

51. Rodriguez-Gonzalez, A.: Personal communication of unpublished data presented at the Pan American Congress of Ophthalmology, Santiago, Chile, 1977.

52. Scheie, H.G., and Cameron, J.D.: Personal communication, 1980.

53. Schreiner, R.L., McAlister, W.H., Marshall, R.E., and Shearer, W.T.: Stickler syndrome in a pedigree of Pierre Robin syndrome, Am. J. Dis. Child. **126:**86, 1973.

54. Schwartz, A.: Chronic open-angle glaucoma secondary to rhegmatogenous retinal detachment, Am. J. Ophthalmol. **75:**205, 1973.

55. Sebestyen, J.G., Schepens, C.L., and Rosenthal, M.L.: Retinal detachment and glaucoma. I. Tonometric and gonioscopic study of 160 cases, Arch. Ophthalmol. **67:** 736, 1962.

56. Shaffer, R.N.: Discussion of Calhoun, F.P., Jr.: The management of glaucoma in nanophthalmos, Trans. Am. Ophthalmol. Soc. **73:**97, 1976.

57. Shammas, H.F., Halassa, A.H., and Faris, B.H.: Variations in intraocular pressure, cup:disc ratio, and steroid responsiveness in the retinal detachment population, Arch. Ophthalmol. **94:**1108, 1976.

58. Shimizu, K., and Ujiie, K.: Structure of ocular vessels, New York, 1978, Igaku-Shoin, p. 94.

59. Smith, T.R.: Acute glaucoma after scleral buckling procedures, Am. J. Ophthalmol. **63:**1807, 1967.

60. Stickler, G.B., Gelau, P.G., Farrell, F.J., et al.: Hereditary progressive arthroophthalmopathy, Mayo Clin. Proc. **40:**433, 1966.

61. Syrdalen, P.: Intraocular pressures and ocular rigidity in patients with retinal detachment. II. Postoperative study, Acta Ophthalmol. **48:**1036, 1970.

62. Syrdalen, P.: Trauma and retinal detachment: the anterior chamber angle, with special reference to width, pigmentation, and traumatic ruptures, Acta Ophthalmol. **48:**1006, 1970.

63. Turner, G.: The Stickler syndrome in a family with the Pierre Robin syndrome and severe myopia, Aust. Paeditr. J. **10:**103, 1974.

64. Wagner, H.: Ein bisher unbekanntes Erbleiden des Auges (Degeneratio hyaloideo-retinitis hereditaria) beobachtet in Kanton Zürich, Klin. Monatsbl. Augenheilkd. **100:**840, 1938.

65. Watzke, R.C.: Silicone retinopiesis for retinal detachment: a long-term clinical evaluation, Arch. Ophthalmol. **77:** 185, 1967.

66. Weingeist, T.A., and Judisch, G.F.: Personal communication, 1980.

Chapter 12

NEOVASCULAR GLAUCOMA

Martin Wand

The earlier concepts of neovascular glaucoma were rather confusing. Because of inadequate knowledge of its causes, neovascular glaucoma as we now know it had many different names. The earliest mention of a possible case of neovascular glaucoma occurring after central retinal vein occlusion was made in 1866. In this report, although there was no differentiation beyond *glaucoma,* it was noted that "the arteries of the retina are contracted and pale while the veins are turgid and dark . . . [and] the venous radicles present varicose dilations and ampullae."[163] The term hemorrhagic glaucoma was attributed to Pagenstecher (1871), who described the onset of glaucoma after "apoplexy of the retina," which we now consider to be central retinal vein occlusion.[85] While most physicians subsequently equated hemorrhagic glaucoma with the sequelae of central retinal vein occlusion, confusion understandably soon occurred, because any glaucoma associated with intraocular bleeding was erroneously called by the same name. Referring to a postoperative eye, Fisk[71] (1896) wrote, "On the next day the eye was hard as a stone, the cornea cloudy, the chamber full of blood—hemorrhagic glaucoma."

Salus[165] (1928) first put the diagnosis of neovascular glaucoma on a sound anatomic basis when he described three diabetic patients who had nets of capillaries on the iris near the pupil and larger radial vessels heading into the angle. These patients subsequently developed hemorrhagic glaucoma, and Salus termed this condition rubeosis iridis diabetica. Kurz[119] (1937) correlated gonioscopic findings with histologic examination of the eyes. He found delicate connective tissue associated with the new vessels in the angle, and he believed that the tendency for this tissue to contract was the cause of the synechial angle closure.

Despite this solid foundation, there was still no agreement on a single name. Parsons and Duke-Elder[155] (1948) maintained that "the designation 'hemorrhagic glaucoma' [is] a term which is however best avoided," although no other name was suggested by them. Many different names subsequently appeared in print describing this same condition (e.g., thrombotic glaucoma, congestive glaucoma, hemorrhagic glaucoma, diabetic hemorrhagic glaucoma, and neovascular hemorrhagic glaucoma). In addition, hemorrhagic glaucoma was confused with hemolytic glaucoma, which is now more appropriately called ghost cell glaucoma (see Chapter 21). Weiss et al.[196] (1962) proposed using the term neovascular glaucoma, placing the emphasis where it belonged (i.e., on the new vessel formation rather than on the intraocular hemorrhage, which is not always present). Since then, this term appears to have been universally accepted, and major reviews as well as numerous other articles on this subject have used the term neovascular glaucoma.[77,85]

As is currently accepted, neovascular glaucoma results from the development of a fibrovascular membrane over the trabecular meshwork. This membrane is associated with and results from new vessel formation in the anterior chamber angle. This anterior segment neovascularization is almost always associated with some type of posterior segment disease. Initially, new vessels and a fibrovascular membrane may be present in parts of the angle without any significant increase in the intraocular pressure. As this membrane covers more and more of the angle, thereby obstructing more and more of the trabecular meshwork, increased intraocular pressure may occur without any angle closure. Eventually this membrane contracts, resulting in synechial angle closure and a marked increase in the intraocular pressure with all the accompanying symptoms (see below). These different stages represent the full spectrum of neovascular glaucoma.

CLINICAL PICTURE AND NATURAL HISTORY

Neovascular glaucoma resulting from central retinal vein occlusion had been known long before that associated with diabetic retinopathy, and it initially appeared logical to differentiate these two types of glaucoma.[180] However, it soon became clear that neovascular glaucoma from these two causes were not clinically distinguishable.[129] We now know that many predisposing conditions may lead to neovascular glaucoma but that there appears to be no clinical differentiation of the end results. The rapidity and intensity of onset may vary a great deal with different predisposing causes, but the clinical picture is quite uniform (see Frontispiece).

The earliest detectable stage of neovascular glaucoma is manifested by increased permeability of the blood vessels at the pupillary margin, allowing leakage of fluorescein (Figs. 12-1 and 12-2). On slit-lamp examination, these pupillary vessels may look normal or may not even be visible if the iris is darkly pigmented. The first biomicroscopically detectable findings are tiny tufts of dilated capillaries at the pupillary margin. These can be very subtle and easily mistaken for clumps of pigment frequently seen in the pupillary margin of lightly pigmented irides. High magnification with careful observation is necessary at this stage. If a mirrored contact lens is used for examination of the angle at this stage, the slightest pressure on the lens can cause the dilated pupillary vessels to blanch and be missed.[192]

Contrary to what others have thought,[148] we (my colleagues and I at the Massachusetts Eye and Ear Infirmary) have not seen new vessel formation elsewhere on the iris without seeing pupillary involvement first. Eyes that have seemingly violated this observation have had darkly pigmented irides in which the pupillary vascular tufts were difficult to see on cursory examination. The only true exception to this observation that we have seen was a diabetic patient who had had a peripheral iridectomy previously for narrow angles and in whom the rubeosis occurred initially around

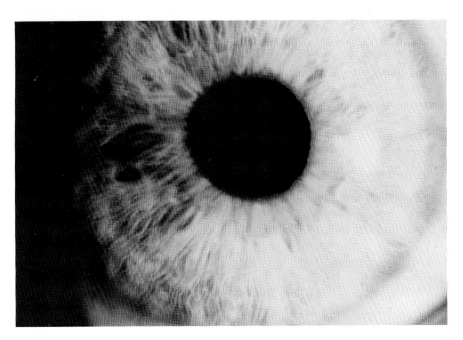

FIG. 12-1. Early rubeosis iridis with normal-appearing pupillary vessels on biomicroscopy. (Courtesy David K. Dueker, M.D.)

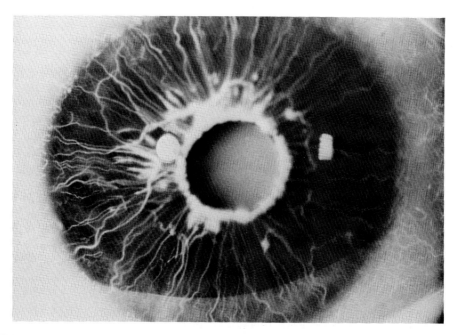

FIG. 12-2. Iris fluorescein angiogram of same eye as in Fig. 12-1 showing marked leakage of fluorescein from new pupillary vessels. Radial iris vessels are normal and show no leakage. (Courtesy David K. Dueker, M.D.)

the iridectomy opening and not at the pupillary margin.[191] However, we view this as the "exception" that strengthens our observations, since this peripheral iridectomy is really the "pupil" through which the aqueous preferentially enters the anterior chamber.

Once begun, new vessel formation extends radially from the pupillary vessels toward the angle. These abnormal new vessels are characterized by their location on the surface of the iris, their variability in size, and their haphazard, irregular meandering pattern toward the angle.[40] The radial vessels tend to join vessels in the collarette, distending these previously present but nonfunctional vessels. These vessels then extend from the collarette toward the periphery in the same haphazard, irregular, but radial direction. When these vessels reach the angle, they cross the ciliary body band and scleral spur. Sometimes new vessels can be seen coming off the circumferential ciliary body artery.

Abnormal angle vessels are easily distinguishable from normal angle vessels. As Chandler and Grant[40] have pointed out, "All normal vessels are located posterior to the scleral spur . . . and the [abnormal vessels] are obviously on the surface of the angle wall or iris, not within the tissues."

Relatively few and relatively large feeder vessels cross the base of the angle, but when they reach the trabecular meshwork, they arborize dramatically into many fine capillaries (Fig. 12-3). These capillaries circumferentially cover an area of up to several clock hours from one feeding vessel and join capillaries from other feeding vessels. At this stage the intraocular pressure may be increased and the facility of outflow decreased, but the angle may still be completely open. As the fibrovascular membrane along the larger-angle vessels contracts, the vessels are pulled taut and stand out from the angle, analogous to the string of a bow. The iris stroma is then tented up along the vessels until synechial angle closure occurs. Ectropion uveae, or (more accurately) ectropion of the posterior pigment layer of the iris, may then occur, generally corresponding to the same meridian where angle closure has occurred. Eventually the areas of closure coalesce, resulting in total sealing of the angle. In the final stage, there is complete closure with iridocorneal attachment, so that usually no angle structures can be seen on gonioscopy. This end stage is almost pathognomonic, since other conditions infrequently produce the totally "zippered-up" appearance of the angle. When the angle is completely closed, there may be very little rubeosis iridis remaining, with only an occasional vessel approaching the angle (Fig. 12-4).

The time sequence of progression is quite vari-

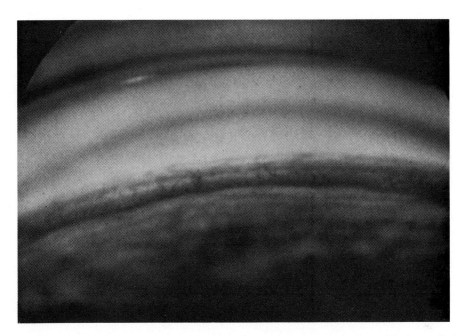

FIG. 12-3. Goniophotograph showing extensive angle neovascularization with large feeder vessels crossing over ciliary body band and scleral spur and arborizing on trabecular meshwork. No synechial angle closure has occurred. (Courtesy Richard J. Simmons, M.D., and David K. Dueker, M.D.)

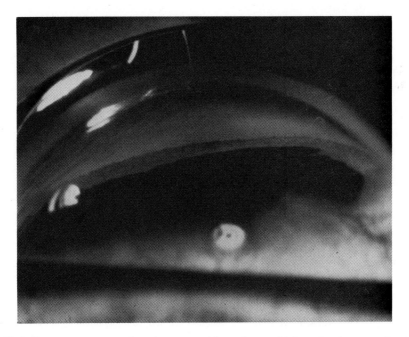

FIG. 12-4. Late-stage neovascular glaucoma with total synechial angle closure and ectropion uveae. No angle structures and no new vessels are visible. (Courtesy Richard J. Simmons, M.D., and David K. Dueker, M.D.)

able. We have seen extensive neovascularization of the angle with early angle closure within days after rubeosis iridis was first noted. We have also seen rubeosis iridis present for years without progression to angle involvement; and we have seen a long quiescent period between the onset of rubeosis iridis and angle involvement that was followed by total angle closure within a few days after the angle involvement. With enough experience, one can almost sense which case of rubeosis iridis is fulminant and which case is "quiet" and unlikely to progress.

Neovascular glaucoma resulting from central retinal vein occlusion seems to have a more rapid and fulminant course than that due to diabetic retinopathy. The progression from no anterior segment involvement to total angle closure can occur within days. Aside from the time sequence, however, the stages of neovascular glaucoma appear to be the same from whatever cause. Although François[74] thought differently, most investigators agree that rubeosis iridis and neovascular glaucoma resulting from diverse causes, including central retinal vein occlusion and diabetic retinopathy, are clinically and histologically indistinguishable.[85,97,151] Recently it has been shown that neovascular glaucoma from different causes is indistinguishable by iris fluorescein angiography as well.[114]

It must be stressed that proliferative diabetic retinopathy, central retinal vein occlusion, and any other predisposing cause of neovascular glaucoma do not inevitably result in anterior segment neovascularization, and rubeosis iridis does not inexorably proceed on to neovascular glaucoma.[135] There are no statistics, but the progression to neovascular glaucoma may be spontaneously halted at any of the already-mentioned stages, and even regression may occur. This variability contributes to the difficulty in comparing the various treatment modalities for neovascular glaucoma.

DIFFERENTIAL DIAGNOSIS

While the underlying disease in neovascular glaucoma usually evolves gradually, the onset of symptoms is frequently precipitous. A patient with neovascular glaucoma will often have a recent onset of severe pain in the eye in association with the typical findings of a markedly increased intraocular pressure, a red eye, and an edematous cornea. Not unexpectedly, acute angle-closure glaucoma figures prominently in the initial differential diagnosis. Peripheral iridectomies have been performed in cases of neovascular glaucoma where the diagnosis was missed. Admittedly, an edematous cornea can make gonioscopy all but impossible despite intensive efforts to lower the intraocular pressure and attempts to clear the cornea transiently with topical glycerin. However, even with a cloudy cornea, it is usually possible to see some engorged new vessels on the surface of the iris in cases of neovascular glaucoma, and that should provide enough of a clue. The past medical and ocular histories are critical here. A long history of diabetes mellitus or the finding of proliferative diabetic retinopathy in the fellow eye are important. Knowledge that vision in the affected eye has been poor for years or that it was suddenly lost in the past few months is very helpful also; the former suggests long-standing retinal detachment, and the later suggests central retinal vein occlusion. Examination of the fellow eye is critical to determine if that angle is narrow, since narrow angles and angle-closure glaucoma are usually bilateral. With a careful history and examination, there should be no problem in differentiating angle-closure glaucoma from neovascular glaucoma.

Heterochromic cyclitis with glaucoma may be confused with neovascular glaucoma. The eye in cyclitis, however, is usually a white and quiet eye in contradistinction to the eye with neovascular glaucoma. Usually only on gonioscopy does the differential diagnosis between these two entities arise. Heterochromic cyclitis has angle neovascularization somewhat like that of neovascular glaucoma, but these vessels are extremely fine, like silk strands, and can easily be missed on gonioscopy. These vessels course over the entire angle, including crossing over the scleral spur onto the trabecular meshwork, signifying that these are pathologic new vessels. However, unlike the vessels in neovascular glaucoma, these do not have an engorged look nor do they arborize over the trabecular meshwork. Rubeosis iridis has not been reported with heterochromic cyclitis, but we have seen one case in which new vessels were present on the iris. These iris vessels were also very fine and similar to the angle vessels. Fortunately, these vessels do not have the tendency to synechiae formation or synechial angle closure.

Any chronic intraocular inflammation can cause or at least be associated with new vessels in the angle, but this is not common. However, these vessels seem to be finer than the new vessels in neovascular glaucoma, and they do not seem to be associated with synechial angle closure. Patients with diabetes mellitus can have prolonged and recurrent episodes of iridocyclitis postoperatively. In a few diabetic patients, prominent vessels on the iris develop after cataract extraction, raising the spectre of neovascular glaucoma. However, once the inflammation is controlled with topical steroids, these vessels disappear as well, suggesting engorgement of already-present iris vessels at least as a contributing cause. Indeed, any intense iridocyclitis can cause congestion of normal iris vessels that can be mistaken for new vessels.

Intraocular hemorrhage with glaucoma must also be considered in the differential diagnosis. Neovascular glaucoma frequently presents with pain, high intraocular pressure, and hyphema. A large hyphema may preclude examination of the rest of the eye to determine the cause of the glaucoma or the bleeding. Any cause of intraocular bleeding with associated glaucoma, including trauma, postoperative bleeding, intraocular tumors,[189,204] cholesterosis bulbi,[193] or other chronic degenerative disorders could be confused with neovascular glaucoma with hyphema. A good history will usually clear up the problem. One recently recognized glaucoma, ghost cell glaucoma,[34,35] deserves special emphasis. This is a transient glaucoma resulting from degenerated red blood cells obstructing the trabecular meshwork. Any cause of vitreous hemorrhage can initiate the degenerative process of changing pliable red blood cells to nonpliable ghost cells. When these cells enter the anterior chamber, they obstruct the trabecular meshwork and cause an increase in the intraocular pressure. The key in diagnosis is seeing, under high magnification of the slit lamp, the extremely tiny (4 to 8 μm) khaki-colored ghost cells in the anterior chamber and covering the angle. The difficulty in diagnosis occurs when a fresh hyphema superimposed on an old vitreous hemorrhage obscures the presence of the ghost cells. In this case the intraocular pressure is high because of the ghost cells, not the hyphema. Anterior chamber aspiration with examination of the aspirate by phase-contrast microscopy will reveal the ghost cells, but one must have a high index of suspicion before performing an aspiration.

FLUORESCEIN STUDIES

The earliest detectable finding in rubeosis iridis is the breakdown in the blood-endothelial barrier, allowing leakage of fluorescein from blood vessels. The blood vessels from the brain, retina, and iris have in common a nonfenestrated endothelium with tight intercellular junctions called zonula occludens. Normally, fluorescein will not pass through these junctions. Damage to the endothelium from any cause will allow passage of fluorescein into the aqueous or vitreous humors. Recent electron microscopic studies on new vessels from diabetic rubeosis iridis have confirmed the presence of fenestration in the endothelial cells, gaps between endothelial cells, as well as changes in the basement membrane.[182] The aqueous protein concentration in patients with neovascular glaucoma has been found to be significantly elevated, supporting this concept of the breakdown of the blood-endothelial barrier in patients with neovascularization.[128]

Two new techniques have been helpful in investigative work, and may prove to be of help in clinical use as well. Vitreous fluorophotometry is probably the most sensitive method for detecting early breakdown of the blood-endothelial barrier. The amount of intravenously administered fluorescein leaking into the vitreous cavity and anterior chamber can be accurately measured through a modified slit lamp. It has been shown that there is a greater concentration of fluorescein in the vitreous of patients with diabetes mellitus than in the vitreous of normal eyes, even when no clinically detectable retinopathy is present.[45,188] The amount of fluorescein present is directly related to the severity of the retinopathy.[45] Of greater significance is the fact that, apparently, the concentration of fluorescein, as measured by vitreous fluorophotometry, is related to and affected by the metabolic control of the diabetes.[46,187] Does this technique have any predictive value? Could this be used to monitor the earlier stages of neovascular glaucoma? Could this technique be used to evaluate the effects of various treatment modalities, including panretinal photocoagulation (PRP) on the development of diabetic retinopathy and neovascular glaucoma? Could this be used to follow patients after central retinal vein occlusion so that treatment with PRP could be initiated at the first signs of increased fluorescein concentration in the vitreous? Further investigations will answer these questions and determine the ultimate usefulness of this technique.

Fluorescein angiography of the iris is the other new technique that has been of great value in our understanding and in our treatment of rubeosis iridis and neovascular glaucoma. Well before any signs of rubeosis iridis can be detected clinically, normal-appearing iris vessels leak fluorescein[106,185] (Figs. 12-1 and 12-2). This leakage may demonstrate mainly the second stage in the breakdown of the blood-endothelial barrier. Vitreous fluorophotometry may measure early, nonvisible diffuse leakage of fluorescein, and iris angiography may measure the more advanced, visible and discrete leakage of fluorescein from the blood vessels. The earliest vascular change detectable by this technique is leakage of fluorescein from the dilated pupillary tufts.[121] It must be stressed that some elderly nondiabetic patients also show leakage of fluorescein from the pupillary vessels.[10] The fact that peripupillary vascular dilation can occur in other conditions, with or without fluorescein leakage, suggests that this finding alone has limited prognostic value.[114,121] The fact that fluorescein leakage occurs before the onset of neovascularization suggests that alteration or damage to the vascular endothelium of preexisting blood vessels must precede new vessel formation.

This early tendency of the pupillary vessels to leak fluorescein is consistent with the clinical finding that dilated pupillary vascular tufts are the first detectable vascular change in the iris as well.[192] Also at this stage, the radial vessels fill irregularly, but no leakage is seen from them (Fig. 12-2). The next stage is neovascularization of the angle with leakage of fluorescein from these new vessels. A method of performing high-power, high-resolution fluorescein goniophotography has recently been described.[111] Fluorescein leakage from newly formed angle vessels was demonstrated in diabetics when these vessels were hardly detectable on routine gonioscopy. This angiographic sequence of pupillary involvement preceding angle involvement is again consistent with clinical findings that, at least in diabetic patients, angle neovascularization occurs after pupillary neovascularization.[192]

As rubeosis iridis progresses, more new vessels are formed elsewhere on the iris, and the large radial vessels begin to leak fluorescein as well. The final stage consists of florid neovascularization with leaking vessels over the entire iris. Laatikainen[121] and Kottow[114] found none of the angiographic changes in rubeosis iridis or neovascular glaucoma to be specific for diabetes mellitus. This is consistent with the hypothesis that anterior segment neovascularization from diabetes and other causes is indistinguishable clinically and histologically.[85,97,151]

Saari et al.[164] have recently found that the fine new iris vessels in Fuchs' heterochromic cyclitis also leak fluorescein. This is in agreement with the understanding that these vessels are truly pathologic vessels and not merely dilated iris vessels already present in response to an inflammatory stimulus. As Chandler and Grant[40] pointed out long before the technique of fluorescein iris angiography was available, any vessel that crosses the scleral spur to the trabecular meshwork, as occurs in neovascular glaucoma and Fuchs' heterochromic cyclitis, must be considered pathologic or anatomically anomalous.

The value of iris angiography is multifold. It allows early detection of neovascularization, often before it becomes otherwise clinically detectable. This may prove to be especially valuable in patients with dark irides, where the early detection of the pupillary tufts can be difficult. Iris angiography may serve as a sensitive monitor of the effectiveness of various treatment modalities.[56] Finally, iris angiography may be of value in predicting the clinical course of eyes at risk.[54] The investigative value of this technique is already well established; the clinical value is in the process of being established.

Fundus fluorescein angiography, while not directly related to rubeosis iridis or neovascular glaucoma, is also of great value in helping to predict which patients with central retinal vein occlusion will develop neovascular glaucoma (see below).

PATHOLOGY

As mentioned, it is not yet possible clinically, angiographically, or pathologically to distinguish between the different causes of neovascular glaucoma.[85,97,114,151] On the basis of a study of a few eyes enucleated for neovascular glaucoma in which liquid silicone rubber was injected into the superior and inferior anterior ciliary arteries, Jocson[107] thought that it might at times be possible to distinguish rubeosis iridis due to central retinal vein occlusion from that due to diabetic retinopathy. He found that new iris vessels that developed after central retinal vein occlusion were larger, coarser, and more irregular than the new iris vessels in cases of diabetic retinopathy. These findings probably correspond to the clinical impression that in rubeosis iridis from central retinal vein occlusion the new vessels frequently appear more engorged and "angry" and the course of the neovascular glaucoma more rapid and fulminant

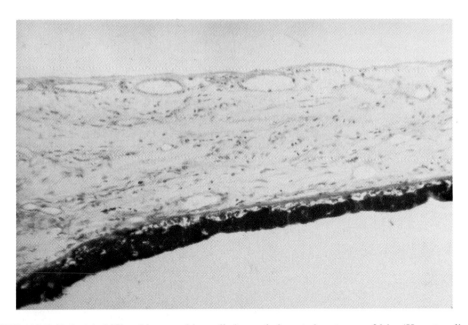

FIG. 12-5. Rubeosis iridis with new, thin-walled vessels in anterior stroma of iris. (Hematoxylin and eosin; ×100.)

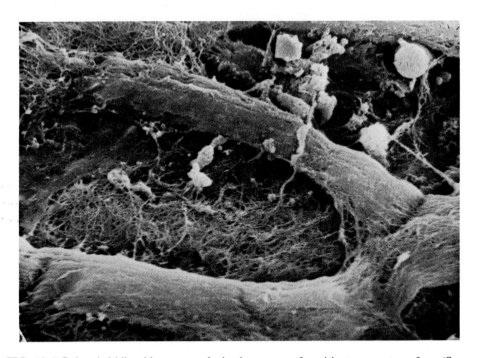

FIG. 12-6. Rubeosis iridis with new vessels that have grown from iris stroma onto surface. (Scanning electron microscope; ×4000.) (Courtesy Thomas M. Richardson, M.D.)

than in that from diabetic retinopathy. A differentiation can be made pathologically only when one sees the vacuolation of the iris pigment epithelium from the accumulation of glycogen, which is a typical finding in diabetic patients.[77]

The newly formed iris vessels tend to be located on the anterior surface of the iris (Figs. 12-5 and 12-6) and tend to be thin walled in comparison with the normal vessels. With time, a fibrovascu-

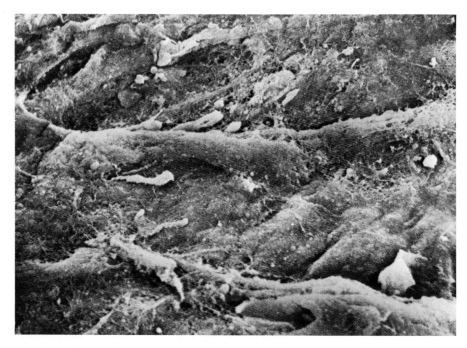

FIG. 12-7. Rubeosis iridis with new vessels on anterior surface of iris; fibrovascular membrane is present along vessel. (Scanning electron microscope; ×2040.) (Courtesy Thomas M. Richardson, M.D.)

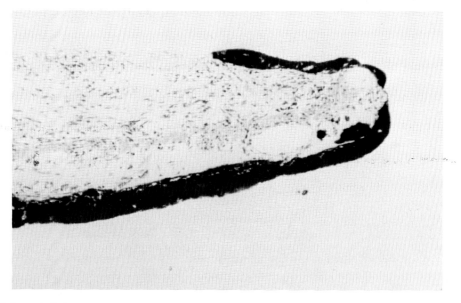

FIG. 12-8. Rubeosis iridis with marked ectropion of iris pigment epithelium. (Hematoxylin and eosin; ×100.)

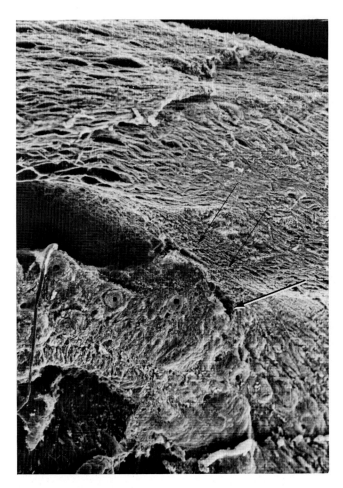

FIG. 12-9. Early synechial angle closure with fibrovascular membrane blocking trabecular mesh-work. True angle, not yet closed, is shown by single arrow; trabecular meshwork, with Schlemm's canal superior to it, is shown by double arrows. (Scanning electron microscope; ×108.) (Courtesy Thomas M. Richardson, M.D.)

lar membrane develops along these vessels (Fig. 12-7). Contraction of this membrane results in radial traction. At the pupil, radial traction on the anterior surface results in distortion of the pupil and in pulling of the posterior iris pigment epithelium over the edge of the pupil and onto the anterior surface (Fig. 12-8). This is really ectropion of the iris pigment epithelium, but by common usage it is called ectropion uveae. At the angle, radial traction results in synechial closure. Ectropion uveae is almost always accompanied by angle closure in the same meridian. Before synechial closure, the connective tissue in the angle can obstruct the trabecular meshwork, resulting in a secondary type of open-angle glaucoma (Fig. 12-9). With angle closure, the iris is pulled up tight against the peripheral cornea to Schwalbe's line,

completely occluding the angle with fibrotic tissue (Fig. 12-10). Occasionally corneal endothelium extends from the cornea onto the iris (Fig. 12-11).[78] This results in a pseudoangle, a finding that is not infrequently confused with an open angle by the unwary gonioscopist (Fig. 12-12). This may be especially misleading, since chronic synechial angle closure may cause new vessels in the angle and on the corresponding radial part of the iris to become inconspicuous. In long-standing synechial angle closure, no new vessels may be visible, and the diagnosis of neovascular glaucoma can be easily missed.

The pathologic changes in the posterior pole will, of course, be dependent on the primary disease process involved. The optic disc changes in neovascular glaucoma are nonspecific.

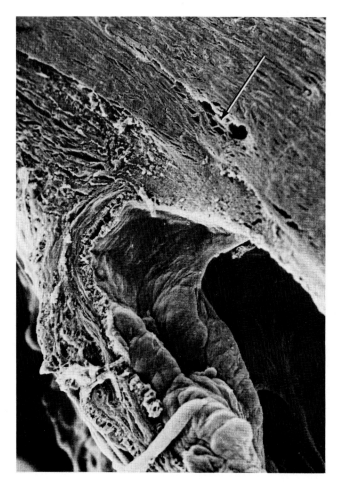

FIG. 12-10. Total synechial closure of angle with atrophic iris pulled anteriorly to Schwalbe's line (not shown). Schlemm's canal is shown by arrow. (Scanning electron microscope; ×172.) (Courtesy Thomas M. Richardson, M.D.)

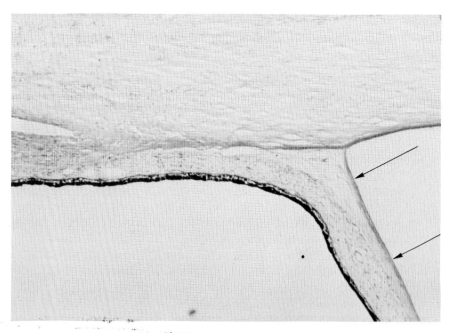

FIG. 12-11. Total synechial closure of angle with corneal endothelium extending onto anterior surface of iris *(arrows)*. (Hematoxylin and eosin; ×40.)

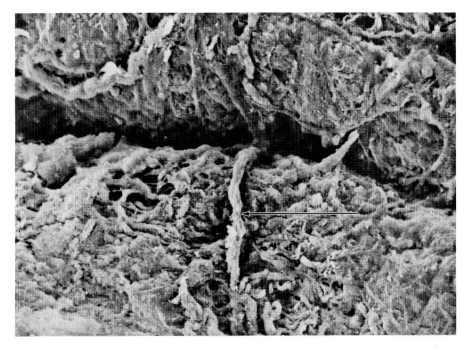

FIG. 12-12. Total synechial closure of angle with formation of pseudoangle. Cornea is on top, and iris is on bottom. There is frequently diminution of new vessels in area of angle closure. One thin vessel is shown here *(arrow)*. (Scanning electron microscope; ×960.) (Courtesy Thomas M. Richardson, M.D.)

CAUSES AND AGGRAVATING FACTORS

There have been many reviews on rubeosis iridis listing the then–currently known causes. Schulze[167] (1967) noted 27 causes, Anderson et al.[3] (1971) noted 28, Yanoff and Fine[203] (1975) noted 25, and Gartner and Henkind[77] (1978) noted 41. Rubeosis iridis and neovascular glaucoma have additionally been reported in Stickler's syndrome.[205] Undoubtedly, other previously reported causes from the literature may not have been cited, and other as yet unreported causes will be published in the future. The list here is based on these previous reviews and reflects our current knowledge.

Disorders associated with rubeosis iridis

A. Vascular disorders
1. Central and branch retinal vein occlusion
2. Central and branch retinal artery occlusion
3. Carotid artery occlusive diseases
4. Aortic arch syndrome
5. Carotid-cavernous sinus fistula
6. Giant cell arteritis
7. Retinal vascular disorders
B. Ocular disorders
1. Diabetic retinopathy
2. Chronic retinal detachment
3. Eales' disease
4. Coats' disease
5. Sickle cell retinopathy
6. Retrolental fibroplasia
7. Persistent hyperplastic primary vitreous
8. Vitreoretinal degeneration
9. Norrie's disease
10. Chronic glaucoma
C. Neoplastic disorders
1. Retinoblastoma
2. Malignant melanoma of the choroid
3. Metastatic carcinoma
D. Inflammatory disorders
1. Chronic uveitis
2. Endophthalmitis
3. Sympathetic ophthalmia
E. Postoperative disorders
1. Cataract extraction
2. Vitrectomy
3. Retinal detachment surgery

It is clear from the above list that almost all the known causes have in common chronic and diffuse posterior segment involvement. According to Smith,[178] "True rubeosis of the iris and angle never occurs in the absence of retinal vascular disease." Perhaps such a statement is dogmatic, but this clinical impression has been borne out by the study by Anderson et al.[3] in which all 70 enucleated eyes with rubeosis iridis were found to have posterior segment disease. As will be seen in the discussion of the theories on pathogenesis, the clinical and pathologic observations are consistent with the present theories on pathogenesis.

Vascular disorders

Central retinal vein occlusion

Central retinal vein occlusion frequently leads to neovascular glaucoma. The frequency seems to increase with the age of the patient,[92] but the reported incidence has varied greatly, from 15% to 65% depending on the study[85]; 30% has been the most commonly accepted figure. However, no one has been able to predict whether any particular individual would develop neovascular glaucoma. Better understanding of the pathogenesis of central retinal vein occlusion has enabled us to predict who is at risk with some accuracy. Hayreh et al.[92] found experimentally that central retinal vein occlusion consisted of two distinct entities, the major difference being the presence or absence of retinal ischemia. When retinal ischemia was absent, venous stasis retinopathy developed; when retinal ischemia was present, hemorrhagic retinopathy developed.

This division of central retinal vein occlusion into ischemic and nonischemic groups had already been known clinically and had been confirmed by fluorescein fundus angiography.[122,123] Using this classification, Tasman et al.[183] showed that rubeosis developed in 60% of eyes with the ischemic type of central retinal vein occlusion and in only 1% of those with the nonischemic type. Elaborating further, Sinclair and Gragoudas[174] found that 86% of patients with central retinal vein occlusion with widespread capillary occlusion, 80% with absent perifoveal network, 75% with 10 or more cotton wool spots, and 75% with an AV transit time of greater than 20 seconds developed rubeosis iridis. Using a multivariate linear discriminant analysis of these data, they were able to prognosticate the fate of central retinal vein occlusion with 91% accuracy. Laatikainen et al.[122] found that 100% of eyes with the ischemic type of central retinal vein occlusion developed leakage of fluorescein from iris vessels versus 24% of eyes with the nonischemic type. However, only 58% of the ischemic group developed neovascularization versus 4% of the nonischemic group. Fundus fluorescein an-

giography appears to be a valuable tool for predicting which patients with central retinal vein occlusion will develop anterior segment neovascularization.

Rubeosis iridis usually develops within 3 months from the onset of central retina vein occlusion[14] (hence the term "100-day glaucoma"). However, there is a great deal of variability, and rubeosis iridis may appear weeks to years after the occlusion. Before it was possible to determine those patients likely to develop rubeosis, it was recommended that patients be examined weekly for neovascularization at around the 3-month period. This is no longer imperative, since angiography within several weeks after the occlusion can show which patients are at risk, and appropriate prophylactic therapy can be initiated early.

An important association between central retinal vein occlusion and preexisting open-angle glaucoma was first noted by Verhoeff[186] in 1913. Since then, some have thought that there is no association between these two entities,[113] but most studies have found a strong association.[18,27,53] Recently it has been found that open-angle glaucoma does not seem to be associated with central retinal vein occlusion in patients younger than 40 years; there has, however, been a positive correlation between central retinal vein occlusion with diabetes mellitus and hypertension in this young population.[162] In patients with central retinal vein occlusion, the percentage of patients who concurrently had or who subsequently developed open-angle glaucoma has varied from 10%[27] to 69%.[18] It is interesting to note that 10%[53] to 16%[18] of the patients with central retinal vein occlusion had normal intraocular pressure in both eyes on the initial examination but subsequently developed increased intraocular pressure in the contralateral eye.

Several investigators have shown that the intraocular pressure is frequently lower immediately after central retinal vein occlusion, with this decrease persisting for several weeks to months.[18,85,91] Thus after central retinal vein occlusion, even if the intraocular pressure is initially normal in both eyes, careful follow-up to detect the appearance of open-angle glaucoma in either eye is mandatory. It may well be that the open-angle glaucoma was the predisposing factor in the development of the central retinal vein occlusion, and the intraocular pressure was only transiently low right after the vascular accident. We have seen a one-eyed man who developed central retinal vein occlusion. His intraocular pressure was normal at the time of the vein occlusion, open-angle glaucoma was not considered a problem then, and no further examinations were made. He was seen many months later with a high intraocular pressure, no signs of neovascularization, and a totally cupped optic disc in his only eye.

It is imperative to detect and treat open-angle glaucoma in the contralateral eye at an early stage, with the hope of preventing central retinal vein occlusion in that second eye. The occurrence of bilateral central retinal vein occlusion is rare, but cases have been reported in the literature,[53,162] and we have seen one case of bilateral central retinal vein occlusion with unilateral neovascular glaucoma. One case of bilateral neovascular glaucoma from bilateral central retinal vein occlusion has been reported.[134] Bilateral occlusion is probably more common than is reported.

Interestingly, retinal neovascularization occurs significantly less frequently than rubeosis iridis after central retinal vein occlusion. Of 50 cases with central retinal vein occlusion confirmed by fluorescein angiography (differentiation was not made between the ischemic and the nonischemic types), 14% developed rubeosis iridis but none developed retinal neovascularization.[39] This was thought to be due to the destruction of the retinal capillary endothelial cells as a result of the central retinal vein occlusion, since endothelial proliferation is thought to be necessary for retinal neovascularization. However, the viable iris capillary endothelium, unaffected by the central retinal vein occlusion, can still respond to the vasoproliferative stimulant.

Branch retinal vein occlusion

Branch retinal vein occlusion is more common than central retinal vein occlusion,[157] but resulting rubeosis iridis and neovascular glaucoma are rarely reported.[87] Sinclair[173] has seen one case of superior angle neovascularization secondary to a superior branch retinal vein occlusion. One case of rubeosis iridis (of five patients with branch retinal vein occlusion) has been reported.[116] Retinal and preretinal neovascularization has been reported to occur in 15%[87] to 33%[110] of patients with branch retinal vein occlusion, indicating that the stimulus for neovascularization is certainly present, as in central retinal vein occlusion. As in central retinal vein occlusion, retinal neovascularization appears to be associated with significant areas of retinal capillary nonperfusion.[5] The difference in the frequency of anterior segment neovascularization between branch retinal vein occlusion and central retinal vein occlusion must have a quantitative rather than a qualitative origin.

Central retinal artery occlusion

Neovascular glaucoma after central retinal artery occlusion is much less common than after central retinal vein occlusion. Most reports are of individual cases without mention of frequency. The only two large series of central retinal artery occlusion addressing the question of neovascular glaucoma report a frequency of less than 1% to 5%.[17,108] The generally accepted incidence is probably around 2%.[77,85] The onset of neovascular glaucoma after central retinal artery occlusion is also significantly different than after central retinal vein occlusion. In the series of Perraut and Zimmerman,[160] the median time interval was 7 weeks. Individual case reports show intervals of 6 weeks[200] to 8 weeks.[195,199]

The histology of rubeosis iridis and neovascular glaucoma due to central retinal artery occlusion is identical to that due to central retinal vein occlusion.[160] Grant[85] (1974) pointed out that "some abnormality of the central retinal artery is regularly associated with occlusion of the central vein." It is now recognized that some degree of arterial obstruction must be present to produce the ischemia that leads to the neovascularization process.[89,92] Perhaps central retinal artery occlusion is associated with such a low incidence of anterior segment neovascularization because the ischemia is usually so complete that there is not enough viable retinal tissue to produce the stimulatory agent (or agents) for neovascularization. This is in agreement with the low incidence of retinal neovascularization in central retinal vein occlusion attributed to the destruction of the retinal endothelial cells.[39] Perhaps the effectiveness of PRP in preventing anterior segment neovascularization results from the conversion of ischemic but viable retinal tissue to nonviable retinal tissue. If this is so, it must be the inner retinal layers that are the source of the vasoproliferative agent (or agents), since these layers are selectively involved in central retinal artery occlusion.[160] Recently Glaser et al.[82] found the first direct evidence of angiogenic activity from the mammalian retina. They have not yet determined which part of the retina contains the angiogenesis factor (AF).

Branch retinal artery occlusion

Only one case of branch retinal artery occlusion with resulting rubeosis iridis has been reported.[29] Apparently, as with branch retinal vein occlusion, there have been no reported cases of secondary neovascular glaucoma. Similar to the difference between branch retinal vein occlusion and central retinal vein occlusion, the difference between branch retinal artery occlusion and central retinal artery occlusion may well be only quantitative rather than qualitative.

Carotid artery occlusive diseases

Decreased blood flow to the eye, from whatever cause, sufficient to result in retinal ischemia may cause anterior segment neovascularization.[85] Unilateral[143] and bilateral[88,109] common carotid artery occlusion, unilateral[99,103,175] and bilateral[63,103] internal carotid artery occlusion, and ophthalmic artery occlusion[132] have been reported to cause rubeosis iridis and neovascular glaucoma. However, this complication is uncommon. It is believed that in most cases of carotid artery disease, enough collateral circulation develops to prevent the critical degree of retinal ischemia necessary for neovascularization to occur.[85] Presumably, other vascular disorders, such as the aortic arch syndrome,[26,144] carotid-cavernous sinus fistula,[196] and giant cell arteritis,[198] have in common decreased ocular blood flow with resulting retinal ischemia.[85]

Ocular disorders

Diabetic retinopathy

Diabetes mellitus is the third leading cause of new blindness in the United States[75] and the leading cause in the 40- to 60-year age group.[176] In the diabetic population, only 5% of the blindness is due to neovascular glaucoma.[176] While this percentage is small, diabetes mellitus is probably the most common cause of neovascular glaucoma today.[85] In a study of 70 consecutive patients with neovascular glaucoma admitted to a Danish hospital over a 5-year span, 43% of the cases were due to diabetes mellitus, followed by 37% due to central retinal vein occlusion.[134] As early as 1939, Fehrmann[67] noted the significant association between rubeosis iridis and diabetic retinal neovascular changes. This association was confirmed in more recent studies where the incidence of rubeosis iridis in unselected diabetic populations ranged from 1%[7] to 5%[184] to 17%,[133] whereas the incidence of rubeosis iridis in patients with proliferative diabetic retinopathy ranged from 33%[133] to 64%.[152] These were clinical studies before the advent of iris fluorescein angiography. Rubeosis iridis is probably even more common than suspected or clinically detectable in the diabetic population. In one histopathologic study of diabetic eyes, a 95% incidence of rubeosis iridis was found.[201] Ninety percent of these eyes had retinal neovascularization as well. There seems to be little question that anterior segment neovascularization in diabetes is directly related to posterior segment disease.

The onset of rubeosis iridis and neovascular glaucoma is also directly related to the duration of diabetes. It is infrequently seen in adult-onset diabetes of less than 15 years' duration. In one study, approximately 14% of the cases occurred in the 15- to 19-year duration group, and 62% occurred in the over-20–year duration group, with the total over-15–year duration group accounting for 76% of the cases.[152] This duration-related incidence has also been shown by Hohl and Barnett,[100] who found that 50% of their patients with rubeosis iridis had diabetes mellitus longer than 20 years. Despite the long duration needed for rubeosis iridis to develop, the average age of patients with neovascular glaucoma from diabetes mellitus is still significantly lower than the average age of patients with neovascular glaucoma from central retinal vein occlusion (45 years versus 67 years).[134]

When a diabetic patient develops neovascular glaucoma in one eye, it is almost inevitable that he will eventually develop it in the other eye.[150] As a corollary, bilateral rubeosis iridis or neovascular glaucoma in an adult almost always implies that the patient has diabetes mellitus.[77] Yet there are still many uncertainties concerning the relationship between diabetes mellitus, rubeosis iridis, and neovascular glaucoma. The time interval between retinal involvement and anterior segment changes is much longer in diabetes than in central retinal vein occlusion. Perhaps it takes a longer time for enough retina to become ischemic from diabetes to approximate quantitatively the retinal injury that results from central retinal vein occlusion. As mentioned, the course of rubeosis iridis is unpredictable, with some cases progressing relatively rapidly to neovascular glaucoma, others slowly, some never progressing to it, and some showing complete regression of the rubeosis iridis.[135] This unpredictable course makes the evaluation of any prophylactic treatment of rubeosis iridis, at least in diabetics, more difficult.

Other ocular disorders

Many other ocular disorders, as noted on p. 173, have been reported to be associated with rubeosis iridis and neovascular glaucoma. Where detailed reports are available, all the cases have been found to be associated with some type of long-standing and widespread retinal disease, such as chronic retinal detachment,[3,206] Eales' disease,[74] Coats' disease,[74,94] sickle cell retinopathy,[24,76] retrolental fibroplasia,[112] and persistent hyperplastic primary vitreous.[167] Chronic primary open-angle glaucoma and other types of chronic glaucoma are occasionally associated with rubeosis iridis and neovascular glaucoma but this association is probably secondary in that increased intraocular pressure predisposes the eye to central retinal vein occlusion.[77,179]

Neoplastic disorders

Retinoblastoma

Walton noted that in 38 of 56 pediatric eyes (68%) with rubeosis iridis, the rubeosis iridis was due to retinoblastoma. This unexpected finding led Walton and Grant[189] to investigate the incidence of rubeosis iridis in cases of retinoblastoma. Of 88 eyes enucleated for retinoblastoma, 39 eyes (44%) had rubeosis iridis. Subsequently, Yoshizumi et al.[204] found an incidence of 30%, and Gartner and Henkind[77] found an incidence of 72%. Walton and Grant found a significant association between rubeosis iridis and choroidal involvement by the tumor. Yoshizumi et al. found the association between rubeosis iridis and involvement of the large retinal vessels by tumor or diffuse intraretinal infiltration by tumor to be so consistent that neovascularization of the iris could be predicted by microscopic examination of sections of the posterior pole. Walton and Grant also found that the duration of the retinoblastoma appeared to be related to the development of rubeosis iridis. Thus it appears that in addition to the retinoblastoma itself being a factor in the neovascularization process, the diffuse and chronic retinal involvement by the tumor may also be a contributing factor.

Malignant melanoma of the choroid

Ellett[59] was apparently the first to note the association between malignant melanoma and rubeosis iridis. Schulze[167] subsequently found that 9% of eyes with rubeosis iridis on microscopic examina-

tion had malignant melanoma. Cappin[37] found malignant melanoma in 15% of eyes with rubeosis iridis and noted that the occurrence of rubeosis correlated with increased tumor size and ocular involvement, tumor necrosis, and extensive retinal detachment. Makley and Teed,[136] studying 212 enucleated eyes with malignant melanoma and opaque media, found that only 0.5% had had rubeosis iridis diagnosed before enucleation. This low incidence is not surprising, since the presence of rubeosis was based on postenucleation review of clinical records, and the anterior segments were not examined histologically. Interestingly, 88% of these eyes had absolute or secondary glaucoma before enucleation. Yanoff[202] also noted a high incidence of glaucoma (30%) in eyes with malignant melanoma but a low incidence of neovascular glaucoma (5%). In none of these studies is there a good histologic examination correlating the extent of rubeosis iridis with the extent of retinal involvement and/or detachment. As with retinoblastoma, it is not clear whether the tumor alone or the tumor in combination with its involvement of the retina is the cause of the new vessel formation.

Other tumors

Of 227 eyes with a tumor metastatic to the eye studied by Ferry and Font,[69] 26 eyes had metastasis to the anterior segment as the predominant feature. Rubeosis iridis was found in 10 of these 26 eyes (38%). The anterior segments in the other 221 eyes with metastatic tumors were not described, and the extent of posterior involvement in the eyes with rubeosis iridis was not described. Rubeosis iridis has been described in four cases of reticulum cell sarcoma.[181]

Inflammatory disorders

As mentioned, chronic low-grade uveitis such as heterochromic cyclytis, is frequently associated with fine new vessels in the angle and rarely on the iris. However, neovascular glaucoma has not been reported with this condition. Inflammation can cause dilation of existing iris vessels, which can be deceptively similar to the engorged vessels of neovascular glaucoma. Many reports suggest that uveitis is associated with rubeosis iridis and neovascular glaucoma, but none provide any more information than the mere listing of iritis as a cause. For example, Hoskins[101] reported 11 of 100 cases of neovascular glaucoma to be due to iritis, Schulze[167] reported 7 of 105 cases of rubeosis iridis to be due to chronic iridocyclitis and 1 case to be due to fungal endophthalmitis, and Gartner and Henkind[77] mentioned endophthalmitis and sympathetic ophthalmia as a cause of rubeosis iridis; however, in none of these reports are sufficient details provided to assess adequately the role of inflammation in the pathogenesis of rubeosis iridis and neovascular glaucoma.

Postoperative disorders
Cataract extraction

Beasley[11] (1970) described two cases of unilateral neovascular glaucoma occurring 6 months and 7 months, respectively, after cataract extraction in diabetic patients. We have had the clinical impression that cataract extractions in diabetics had a higher than expected but seemingly unpredictable incidence of neovascular glaucoma after cataract extraction. We studied 154 diabetic patients who underwent unilateral intracapsular cataract extraction at the Joslin Clinic.[127] Particular attention was paid to the preoperative status of the retinopathy and the postoperative ocular complications within a 6-month period. Of 15 patients with active proliferative diabetic retinopathy who underwent cataract extraction, 6 developed postoperative rubeosis iridis and neovascular glaucoma; rubeosis iridis–neovascular glaucoma did not develop in any of 31 unoperated eyes with active proliferative diabetic retinopathy. In patients with nonproliferative diabetic retinopathy, quiescent diabetic retinopathy, and inactive diabetic retinopathy, there was no statistical difference between the group that underwent cataract extraction and the group that did not. To the best of our knowledge, cataract extraction is not associated with a high incidence of rubeosis iridis or neovascular glaucoma in any other population group. The implication of this study for the diabetic population is clear. In diabetics with active proliferative diabetic retinopathy, plans for performing a cataract extraction should be made cautiously. If a cataract extraction is necessary, careful and frequent postoperative examination is imperative to detect and treat the first signs of rubeosis iridis.

Vitrectomy

Rubeosis iridis and neovascular glaucoma are common complications after vitrectomies in diabetic patients. What is particularly interesting is that if the published results are divided into vitrectomy with and without concurrent cataract extrac-

tion, a startling picture emerges. If only a vitrectomy is performed, rubeosis iridis–neovascular glaucoma develops in 5.5%[81,153] to 8%[126] of patients. If a concurrent cataract extraction or lensectomy is performed, the postoperative complication rate goes up to 12%,[81] 24%,[153] and 36%.[126] There seems to be little disagreement that cataract extraction per se is the main factor leading to the postoperative development of rubeosis iridis and neovascular glaucoma in patients undergoing vitrectomy.[154] The disruption of the anterior hyaloid membrane that occurs with cataract extraction may allow some angiogenesis factor to enter the anterior chamber more readily. There is a clinical impression that rubeosis iridis is a special risk after vitrectomy in eyes with active proliferative diabetic retinopathy,[142] but no studies have confirmed this at the time of writing. In addition, the risks of rubeosis iridis and neovascular glaucoma after vitrectomy in nondiabetic eyes have not been studied adequately. It is not surprising that once rubeosis iridis is present, vitrectomy leads to neovascular glaucoma in 33% of cases within 6 months versus only 17% when vitrectomy is performed in the absence of preoperative rubeosis.[21]

Retinal detachment surgery

Chronic retinal detachment has frequently been mentioned as a cause of rubeosis iridis and neovascular glaucoma.[3,77,167,189] Schulze[167] found retinal detachment, apparently as the only cause, in 24 of 105 enucleated eyes with rubeosis iridis. This was the second most frequent cause in his series (23%), with the most common cause being central retinal vein occlusion (42%). In addition, he found that other ocular diseases that caused rubeosis iridis, such as malignant melanoma, retinoblastoma, retinal degeneration, and Coats' disease, had extensive retinal detachment. Walton and Grant[189] also found retinal detachment to be the second most common cause (32%) of rubeosis iridis in enucleated eyes of children 5 years of age or younger. They found that 5 of 18 eyes with retinal detachment also showed Coats' disease. In one report, laser coreoplasty was followed by rubeosis iridis, but long-standing retinal detachment was also present, and this was probably the cause.[38] It would appear that chronic retinal detachment alone is capable of causing anterior segment neovascularization and is in fact one of the more common causes. In addition, retinal detachment is associated secondarily with other ocular disease, such as retinoblastoma[189,204] and malignant melanoma,[37,136,202] which may contribute to the neovascularization process. Unfortunately, no study has correlated the extent and duration of retinal detachment necessary to stimulate new vessel formation or has even described the course of the rubeosis iridis after the retina is reattached.

THEORIES ON PATHOGENESIS

Because the process of neovascularization is of such great clinical importance to ophthalmology, an enormous amount of basic and clinical research has been generated, and there is no shortage of theories on its pathogenesis. Perhaps the most appealing theory involves the existence of an angiogenesis factor (AF). As early as 1948, Michaelson[141] suggested the presence of a vasoformative substance produced by the retina to stimulate retinal vascular growth. Ashton et al.[9] subsequently suggested that retinal hypoxia, specifically in retrolental fibroplasia, may result in the formation of this substance. Wise[197] then proposed that after retinal capillary obstruction, if the retinal tissue becomes ischemic but not dead, a vasoformative substance is produced that could stimulate new vessel formation. Ashton[8] thought that this vasoformative substance could diffuse forward to stimulate angiogenesis in the iris. In 1971 Folkman et al.[73] isolated a factor from solid neoplasm that was capable of stimulating neovascularization.

This tumor angiogenesis factor (TAF) has not yet been identified, but it has been found to be a soluble and diffusable substance.[79] It is able to stimulate endothelial proliferation in capillary blood vessels in vitro[72] and to induce rabbit corneal neovascularization[80] and rabbit retinal neovascularization in vivo.[70] With the use of a bioassay technique, this TAF has been found in the aqueous of three of five patients with neovascular glaucoma.[15] As mentioned, it has been shown that an AF is present in mammalian retina.[82] In addition, several naturally occurring inhibitors of TAF have been found. A low molecular weight protein component that will inhibit tumor-induced neovascularization has been isolated from cartilage.[124] A similar inhibitor has been isolated from normal vitreous[28] and bovine aorta.[58]

Whether this TAF is a single angiogenic substance or many different substances is still unknown. Whether it is the same substance that produces neovascularization in different parts of the eye or whether there are different substances that are location specific is unknown. Whether this TAF is identical to the substance (or substances)

produced by ischemic retina is also unknown,[93] but at least some biochemical overlap must be present.[124] In any case, it appears that neovascularization requires an AF as well as a diseased ocular bed on which it may act.[90,93] Furthermore, other mediating and/or modifying factors must also be present.

It has been shown that prostaglandins, especially PGE, are capable of inducing neovascularization, at least in corneas.[16,149] It has been suggested that prostaglandins may be the active component in the AF[16] or at least may be the common mediating factor for different AFs. For example, prostaglandins appear to play an active role in ocular trauma,[44] causing increased capillary and ciliary epithelium permeability,[158] as manifested by increased leakage of fluorescein from the iris.[86] Activated macrophages have been shown to induce microvascular proliferation,[161] immunocompetent lymphocytes can induce angiogenesis,[170] and a leukocyte factor has been found in corneal vascularization.[66] Interestingly, activated macrophages and leukocytes, as well as growing tumors, have been shown to produce prostaglandins.[16] Bovine serum albumin[169] and commercial insulin[168] have been shown to produce immunogenic ocular inflammation with characteristics similar to those of proliferative diabetic retinopathy. Further supporting the idea that prostaglandins may play a central mediating role is the finding that indomethacin, a prostaglandin inhibitor, can reduce experimental corneal neovascularization.[51]

Undoubtedly, much new information will add to, change, or perhaps completely refute this present theory on the role of an AF. Regardless of which hypothesis is invoked, presently known clinical facts must be accommodated into this theory. Fundamental to all clinical conditions known to cause neovascularization is the widespread occurrence of retinal capillary closure resulting in chronic tissue ischemia.[156] Presumably, an AF released from the ischemic retina acts on diseased vascular tissue. Conditions that produce total retinal destruction rather than ischemia, such as central retinal artery occlusion, would undoubtedly produce little or no AF and have a low incidence of rubeosis iridis and neovascular glaucoma. The same disease processes that result in retinal ischemia probably cause injury to the iris vessels as well, as manifested, for example, in the leakage of fluorescein from iris vessels in diabetics.[106] The damaged vascular bed allows the AF access to the vascular endothelium to induce neovascularization. This AF diffuses forward and exits through the same passages as the aqueous, accounting for the preferential and sequential involvement of the pupillary margin vessels before the angle vessels. As mentioned before, we have seen one patient who had a peripheral iridectomy before the development of rubeosis iridis. The iris around the iridectomy was involved before the pupillary margin, consistent with a preferential flow of the aqueous and AF through the iridectomy.

It is interesting to note that in 1961 Smith,[178] in discussing various theories of the pathogenesis of neovascularization, said:

With regard to the third theory; the transference of a new-vessel-stimulating substance from the retina by the aqueous humour; I wonder if the invariable sites of the earliest new vessels, namely on the extreme margin of the pupil and on the trabecular meshwork, might validly be considered to be due to these sites being the position of maximum turnover of contact with aqueous humour containing only a very low concentration of the hypothetical substance. I would be particularly interested to hear if any member had a case of rubeosis developing after a peripheral iridectomy. It would be of great significance if the early rubeosis were to develop at the new "pupillary margin" of the iridectomy.

The detrimental effect of cataract extraction in diabetics[127] may be due to the removal of the hyaloid barrier, allowing easier passage of the AF from the posterior segment to the anterior segment.

In addition, the surgical manipulation may further stimulate the angiogenesis process through the resultant inflammation. Increased prostaglandin production may play a critical role here. Clinically inflammation can produce a picture indistinguishable from neovascular glaucoma. We have seen complete resolution of this type of pseudoneovascular glaucoma with the use of only topical steroids. In true neovascular glaucoma, preoperative topical steroids decrease the intensity of the neovascular glaucoma. The detrimental effects of vitrectomy may be due to the removal of a normally occurring vitreous inhibitor.[28] The extra risks of lensectomy at the time of vitrectomy may be due to the already-mentioned removal of the hyaloid barrier.

The beneficial effects of corticosteroids may result from interrupting the production and the actions of the mediating prostaglandins. The beneficial effects of PRP could be due to the conversion of the ischemic retina that produces AF to a totally dead retina that produces no AF. As might be expected, PRP could not possibly destroy all the ischemic retina or eliminate all the AF. Neovascularization must be a quantitative response to the AF, because even in patients successfully treated with PRP before a filtering procedure, we have found a characteristic ring of fine new episcleral and conjunctival vessels around the filtering bleb (Fig. 12-13). Enough AF may still be produced

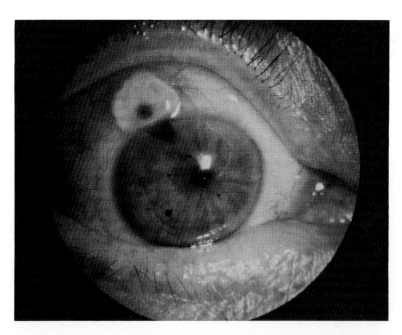

FIG. 12-13. Filtering bleb after filtering procedure in case of neovascular glaucoma. Note ring of episcleral and conjunctival vessels delineating filtering bleb. (Courtesy B. Thomas Hutchinson, M.D.)

to stimulate angiogenesis around the bleb, but there may not be enough AF to stimulate angiogenesis elsewhere in the eye.

If this theory is correct, we may soon see the isolation and identification of the AF (or AFs), as well as its inhibitors and antagonists. Rather than treating rubeosis iridis and neovascular glaucoma with a destructive method such as PRP, it may be possible to therapeutically counteract the effects of the AF with a specific inhibitor. Eventually it may be possible to prevent the original retinal disorders and completely abort the production of the AF.

MANAGEMENT
Medical therapy

Until recently, the prognosis for neovascular glaucoma was essentially hopeless. The only treatment available was medical, since the success of surgery was dismal.[101] In 1974 Grant[85] wrote an exhaustive review of the medical therapy for neovascular glaucoma. This information on medical therapy is essentially still current, since the thrust of treatment is now directed at laser therapy and surgery. Suffice it to say that some of the proposed medical treatment in the past has been characterized more by its diversity than by its effectiveness, having included deferoxamine, streptokinase, fibrinolysin, xanthinol niacinate, heparin, bishydroxycoumarin (Dicumarol), and irradiation.[85] None of these agents have been proved to be of any use in neovascular glaucoma.

Pilocarpine and other miotics, a mainstay in the treatment of open-angle glaucoma, play no significant role in neovascular glaucoma. When neovascularization of the angle is present without synechial closure, the intraocular pressure may be elevated, and miotics can lower the intraocular pressure temporarily. Once angle-closure has occurred, miotics may increase ocular hyperemia and pain[66,176] without significantly lowering the intraocular pressure.[85,194] Epinephrine, another mainstay in open-angle glaucoma, similarly has little role in neovascular glaucoma, causing increased hyperemia without significant lowering of the intraocular pressure.[85,194] The prodrug dipivalyl epinephrine has not been tested on neovascular glaucoma as of this time. It is converted to epinephrine inside the eye and has fewer ocular side effects than standard epinephrine preparations. Its ultimate usefulness remains to be determined, but it is unlikely that it plays a significant role.

As of this time, timolol has not been studied specifically in neovascular glaucoma, but we have found it useful in the preoperative treatment of neovascular glaucoma to temporarily lower the intraocular pressure.[194] Because it decreases the production of aqueous, it can lower the intraocular pressure in neovascular glaucoma with or without synechial angle closure. Therefore it is imperative that its use, especially in early neovascular glaucoma, not give one a false sense of security as the angle relentlessly closes in the face of a relatively normal pressure. We have not found it to increase hyperemia or pain. Before timolol was available, propranolol, another beta-adrenergic blocker, had limited success in lowering the intraocular pressure in neovascular glaucoma.[159]

The carbonic anhydrase inhibitors are effective in lowering the intraocular pressure whether or not synechial angle closure has occurred. Before angle closure occurs, they can have a dramatic effect in lowering the pressure but have no effect on the hyperemia. As with timolol at this stage, it is important not to be lulled into a false sense of security with a temporary normalization of the pressure. This period of grace in early neovascular glaucoma should be used quickly and aggressively to treat the patient definitively. Once synechial angle closure has occurred, the effect of the carbonic anhydrase inhibitors is not as great, but they still provide some relief. Hyperosmotic agents do not have any definitive role in the treatment of neovascular glaucoma, but given either orally or parenterally, they can provide dramatic lowering of the intraocular pressure, at least temporarily. Oral glycerin has been the recommended agent[6,85] except when nausea and vomiting are present. Intravenous 20% mannitol works just as well.

Cycloplegics, such as atropine, would not be expected to lower the intraocular pressure but have been recommended for the relief of pain in late neovascular glaucoma.[36] Topical atropine, 1% twice a day along with topical steroids four times a day in end-stage neovascular glaucoma, frequently decreases the congestion and pain so that alcohol injection or enucleation is not necessary.[85,194] Even more important, this combination is extremely useful in the preoperative preparation of surgically operable eyes.

Although topical steroids do not directly lower the intraocular pressure, they play an important role in the treatment of neovascular glaucoma. As mentioned, chronic iritis can mimic neovascular glaucoma through engorgement of existing iris vessels. This situation is especially common in diabetics after cataract extraction, since they seem to have a significantly higher incidence of postoperative iritis.[31,44] In addition, the course of the postoperative iritis in diabetics is often protracted, persisting up to 6 months after cataract extraction. Since diabetics with active proliferative diabetic retinopathy are at special risk of developing neovascular glaucoma after cataract extraction,[127] it is important to differentiate inflammation-induced pseudoneovascular glaucoma from true neovascular glaucoma. Topical steroids effectively resolve the former but not the latter. In true neovascular glaucoma, topical steroids decrease hyperemia and reduce pain[19,85] but do not eliminate the iris vessels.

In end-stage neovascular glaucoma where relief of pain is the therapeutic end point, atropine 1% twice a day and topical steroids four times a day are very effective. We have made occasional use of a soft-contact bandage lens where extensive microcystic edema is present, but we have not had to resort to retrobulbar alcohol injections or enucleations in many years. Even more important is the use of topical steroids and atropine in the preoperative preparation of the patient for definitive surgery. During this preparation period, PRP is frequently performed, and topical steroids are also helpful in controlling postlaser inflammation. Finally, after filtering surgery, topical steroids are required more frequently and for a longer duration than after routine filtering procedures.

In this discussion on medical therapy, the obvious should be emphasized. Despite our limited knowledge of basic disease processes, every attempt should be made to detect and treat all medical conditions known to contribute to neovascular glaucoma. For example, open-angle glaucoma should be detected and treated early, systemic hypertension and other cardiovascular diseases should be medically controlled, and the erratic control of diabetes mellitus should be avoided.

Cryotherapy

Cryotherapy was introduced in 1950 by Bietti[19] when he demonstrated a decrease in the intraocular pressure after freezing the ciliary body. This mode of therapy did not enjoy widespread clinical popularity until DeRoetth[49,50] presented several large series of glaucoma patients treated with cyclocryotherapy. DeRoetth claimed a high success rate (controlled intraocular pressure) with minor complications, but he did not direct his studies specifically to neovascular glaucoma.

It was not until 1972 that the first studies concerning cyclocryotherapy in neovascular glaucoma were published. Goldstein and Ide[83] treated three patients with diabetic neovascular glaucoma and concluded that relief of ocular pain was good, lowering of the intraocular pressure was transient (months), and rubeosis iridis was aggravated by the freezing. Grant[85] believed that this pain control might be attributed partially to the freezing of sensory nerves. Feibel and Bigger[68] presented the first large series on neovascular glaucoma. They studied 38 patients with neovascular glaucoma and found that 63% (24 of 38 eyes) had a lowering of the intraocular pressure to less than 20 mm Hg. However, the visual acuity results were dismal, with only six patients retaining counting-fingers vision or better, and the complication rate was high. Moderate to severe iritis occurred in 100% of their patients, chronic hypotony occurred in 39%, and postoperative cataracts in 32%. There was no mention of control of ocular pain in their study. Faulborn and Höster[65] found that 94% (17 of 18 eyes) of patients with painful neovascular glaucoma became pain free. In 89% of these nearly blind eyes, pressures of less than 22 mm Hg were achieved. Boniuk[23] reported on 17 patients with neovascular glaucoma treated with cyclocryotherapy, but aside from concluding that pressure and pain control was effective, he gave no data for detailed comparisons of intraocular pressures or complications.

All of the above studies are difficult to compare because of wide variations in the techniques and apparatus employed and in the selection of patients. Bellows and Grant[13] (1973) studied a large series of patients using a protocol designed to allow intelligent comparison of data between studies. In their series of 10 eyes with intractable neovascular glaucoma, only 30% achieved a pressure less than 20 mm Hg and 40% developed posttherapy complications. Bellows and Grant[14] subsequently presented the first long-term follow-up study of patients treated with cyclocryotherapy, but this study was limited to advanced open-angle glaucoma in aphakic eyes. Krupin et al.[118] presented the first long-term (mean of 25 months) follow-up study of patients with neovascular glaucoma. Only 34% of their patients achieved a pressure lower than 25 mm Hg, but 34% developed phthisis, and 59% developed no light perception vision. However, it must be stressed that patients in their study had undergone 360 degrees of cyclocryotherapy. They concluded that a better therapy than cyclocryotherapy was needed for neovascular glaucoma.

Because the complication rate is unacceptably high for the degree of pressure control, cyclocryotherapy is now recommended only when other surgical methods have proved ineffective, the visual prognosis is poor, and pain control is the primary aim.[12]

Our technique is the same as Bellow and Grant's published protocol.[14] We use a cryounit capable of achieving $-60°$ to $-80°$ C and a glaucoma probe of 3.5-mm diameter. The tip is applied with its near edge 2.5 mm from the limbus, in six equidistant points in the inferior 180 degrees of the globe, for 1 minute each. Topical atropine, steroids, and antibiotics are used postoperatively. Increased hyperemia and iritis, transient increased pain and intraocular pressure, and intraocular bleeding are potential risks. Retreatment, if necessary, should be performed in the same inferior 180 degrees of the globe; 360-degree treatment should never be resorted to.

For the sake of completeness, cyclodiathermy deserves mention. DeRoetth[48] reported the use of cyclodiathermy in two cases of neovascular glaucoma in 1946. Pain was relieved, but phthisis resulted in both cases. In 1955 Ellis[60] reported one case in which pressure control was good with no complications. Ando and Kyu[4] reported five cases in which the patients were successfully treated with no complications. Walton and Grant[190] employed a modified penetrating cyclodiathermy technique in 100 operations as a last resort in refractory glaucoma. They had a success rate of only 5% with significant reduction of pressure and had phthisis in 5% of their patients. With this low success–complication ratio and with other better treatments now available, cyclodiathermy is no longer of any clinical significance in neovascular glaucoma.

The effectiveness of PRP in preventing the development and causing the regression of anterior segment neovascularization has already been proved (see below). However, for effective performance of PRP, the ocular media must be clear enough for the transmission of the laser beam. Unfortunately, eyes prone to the development of neovascular glaucoma often have opaque media as well. Panretinal cryotherapy is one of several available methods to overcome this difficulty. It was first reported by Mohan and Eagling[146] in 1978. They treated 10 patients by applying three to four rows of cryotherapy from the limbus back,

in all four quadrants. Three of fi
pretreatment rubeosis iridis had reg
rior segment neovascularization; tv
develop neovascular glaucoma. Thr
tients with pretreatment neovascular g
regression of neovascularization and c̲ ̲ of the
intraocular pressure; two showed progression. The major complication was traction retinal detachment in two cases.

Hilton[98] (1979) used 90 to 120 applications of cryotherapy to the entire retina except the posterior pole. All three eyes with pretreatment rubeosis iridis and opaque media showed regression of the neovascularization. In three eyes with pretreatment neovascular glaucoma and opaque media, one responded to panretinal cryotherapy alone, but two needed additional cyclocryotherapy, and they eventually developed phthisis. May et al.[137] used the same technique in six eyes with pretreatment neovascular glaucoma and opaque media. The intraocular pressure was controlled in all six eyes, with three needing additional medication; all had regression of rubeosis iridis, and no eyes were lost from phthisis.

Panretinal cryotherapy has also been performed in eyes with proliferative diabetic retinopathy and opaque media.[166] The results have been encouraging with regard to cessation or clearing of vitreous hemorrhages, but Schimek and Spencer[166] thought that their data could "not permit any definite conclusion as to the value of retinal [cryo] ablation." The rationale of retinal ablation by cryotherapy is reasonable, and the preliminary results measured by the effects on rubeosis iridis and neovascular glaucoma are encouraging. One inherent difficulty with this technique is that opaque media prevent direct monitoring of the cryotherapy. When the cause of the neovascular glaucoma is unknown, cryotherapy applied to an unsuspected retinoblastoma, for instance, could be disastrous. We personally have not used this technique because of other available methods, but its clinical usefulness must be considered and further investigated.

Photocoagulation

Meyer-Schwickerath[140] introduced photocoagulation and first used it to treat diabetic retinopathy in 1955. In 1967 Beetham and associates started PRP in patients with proliferative diabetic retinopathy. This treatment was based on their observation that there was remarkable similarity in the retinal picture in arrested cases whether they were due to spontaneous remission, pituitary ablation, photocoagulation, choroiditis, optic atrophy, or high myopia. This suggested the possibility that producing chorioretinal lesions with photocoagulation might arrest the progression of diabetic retinopathy.[1] In their pioneering study, they showed that ruby laser PRP improved proliferative diabetic retinopathy.[2] This was subsequently confirmed in a study of 1732 patients by the Diabetic Retinopathy Research Group, which found argon laser PRP to be of benefit in preventing severe visual loss.[52]

Aside from decreasing proliferative changes in the retina, Krill et al.[115] (1971) found that retinal photocoagulation could cause regression of rubeosis iridis in cases of branch retinal vein occlusion as well. Callahan and Hilton[32] (1974) reported one case of central retinal vein occlusion with angle neovascularization that showed regression of the new vessels after PRP, and they suggested that this treatment might be of benefit in neovascular glaucoma.

Bouchon et al.[25] (1976) reported success in treating one case of neovascular glaucoma with PRP. Little et al.[130] (1976) also reported on their success in a retrospective and prospective study. Of 15 treated eyes, 12 showed regression of rubeosis iridis and angle neovascularization after PRP. The three failures occurred in those eyes with 360-degree synechial angle closure. Laatikainen[120] reported regression of rubeosis iridis in 7 of 10 eyes treated postoperatively. In the largest study reported to date, 93 patients received PRP in one eye only for proliferative diabetic retinopathy with the other eye serving as the untreated control.[192] After an average follow-up time of 7.1 years, there was a significantly lower incidence of rubeosis iridis and angle neovascularization (p < 0.025) in the treated eyes versus that in the untreated eyes. Neovascular glaucoma developed in four of the untreated eyes but in none of the treated eyes. This is not statistically significant but is highly suggestive of the prophylactic value of PRP. In an update of Little's 1976 study, Jacobson et al.[104] reported similar success. In eyes with less than 270 degrees of synechial closure, PRP was almost 100% successful in reversing angle neovascularization. None of 15 patients with eyes having greater than 270-degree synechial angle closure showed any improvement with PRP. For reasons that are unclear, Tasman et al.[183] did not find a difference between eyes that received PRP and those that did not.

Because of the success seen in treating diabetics with PRP,[192] as well as the success of Krill et al.[115] with branch retinal vein occlusion, it was thought that PRP could also prevent the development of neovascular glaucoma in central retinal vein occlusion. In several prospective studies, none of the patients (54 patients in four studies) with central retinal vein occlusion who received PRP subsequently developed neovascular glaucoma.[20,102,138,139] As mentioned, patients with the ischemic type of central retinal vein occlusion, as manifested by retinal capillary obliteration on fluorescein angiography, are especially at risk.[20,139,183] No study has been published as of this time, but it would seem reasonable to perform fluorescein angiography routinely on patients with central retinal vein occlusion and prophylactically treat with PRP those with capillary obliteration.

As mentioned, patients prone to the development of neovascular glaucoma also frequently have opaque media, preventing standard PRP. When vitrectomy and/or lensectomy is indicated, either to permit PRP or in conjunction with other surgical procedures, we have performed standard PRP 1 or 2 days after the surgery.

Potentially, a postoperative vitreous rebleed could prevent one from performing PRP, and in such cases, neovascular glaucoma could very well develop while one watched helplessly. Charles[41] has developed a technique of endopanretinal photocoagulation (EPRP). The instrumentation consists of a tiny probe attached to a portable xenon unit, which could then be used to photocoagulate the retina under direct visualization during vitrectomy, so that PRP could be performed without worry about vitreous rebleeding. As of this time, Charles has done 49 EPRP procedures in a heterogeneous group of patients. Approximately 10% of these patients developed postoperative, post-EPRP neovascular glaucoma. In the 11 patients who served as the nontreated (non-EPRP) group, 55% developed neovascular glaucoma after vitrectomy.[4] Interestingly, Goodart and Blankenship,[84] in a large study, found no evidence that previtrectomy PRP prevented postoperative rubeosis iridis. The only question that could be raised concerning their study is that there was no mention of the previtrectomy retinopathy status. Since it is believed that eyes with active proliferative diabetic retinopathy are at special risk after vitrectomy,[21] the patient population must be divided and the results analyzed accordingly. In any case, as more vitrec-

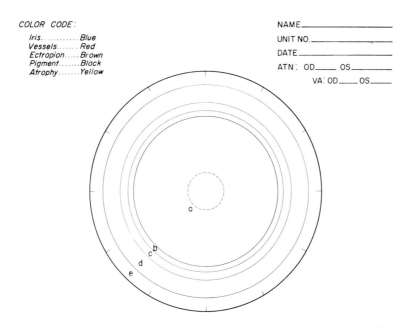

COLOR CODE:

Iris............Blue
Vessels........Red
Ectropion.....Brown
Pigment.......Black
Atrophy.......Yellow

NAME_____
UNIT NO._____
DATE_____
ATN: OD_____ OS_____
VA: OD_____ OS_____

FIG. 12-14. Chart for recording rubeosis iridis and angle neovascularization. *a,* Pupil; *b,* ciliary body band; *c,* scleral spur; *d,* filtration portion of trabecular meshwork; *e,* nonfiltration portion of trabecular meshwork. (From Wand, M., Dueker, D.K., Aiello, L.M., and Grant, W.M. Published with permission from the American Journal of Ophthalmology **86:**332-339, 1978. Copyright by the Ophthalmic Publishing Co.)

tomies are performed, the role of EPRP will undoubtedly be clarified.

Before PRP was conceived, it had been suggested in 1966 that direct laser treatment to the new vessels on the iris might prevent neovascular glaucoma.[64] Theoretically, if angle neovascularization can be eliminated early by direct laser treatment of the vessels, synechial angle closure might not occur and neovascular glaucoma might be avoided. The first published series on this reported mixed results in 10 cases.[47] Direct treatment of the new iris vessels received little further attention until 1977, when Simmons et al.[171,172] introduced the direct laser treatment of angle neovascularization, which they termed goniophotocoagulation (GPC). They treated a total of 88 eyes, some with PRP or pancryotherapy, but most with only GPC. While stressing that their patient population was highly preselected and therefore not comparable to general patient populations, they nevertheless reported remarkable success. They were able to eliminate new vessels from the treated portion of the angle, prevent further synechial angle closure, and maintain the intraocular pressure, with or without medication, at 28 mm Hg or less, in 80% of eyes with angle neovascularization from diabetic retinopathy and 51% of eyes with neovascularization from central retinal vein occlusion.

The technique of GPC is still rather unfamiliar to most ophthalmologists and is therefore described here.[172] A detailed drawing of the angle vessels is made before actual treatment to allow easy identification during treatment (Fig. 12-14), since the visualization of the angle is not as clear through the delivery system as it is with routine slit-lamp gonioscopy. A topical drop anesthetic is almost always sufficient, but an occasional patient may need a retrobulbar anesthetic to tolerate the discomfort from the laser application. An argon laser with slit-lamp delivery and a Goldmann 3-mirror lens are used. The laser is set initially at 0.2 seconds with a 100-μm spot size and 100-mW power. The power may have to be adjusted up or down on an individual basis until definite blanching of the vessels occurs. The beam is aimed at the major vessels on the scleral spur just after they cross over the ciliary body band; the vessels on the trabecular meshwork are avoided, since they will collapse as soon as the major feeding vessel is occluded. Frequently most of the vessels can be treated in one sitting if only part of the circumference is involved. Occasionally, when most of the circumference is involved, treatment may be divided into sessions, 1 day apart, with 180 degrees being treated each time. The treated area should be reexamined at the end of the session, since the initial "occlusion" may be only transient spasm, requiring repeated treatment. Careful observation is necessary to make sure with further treatment that there is no recurrence of the angle neovascularization.

The initial reports are encouraging, but the ultimate role of GPC in our armamentarium remains to be assessed.

Transpupillary cyclophotocoagulation was attempted in one case: Mochizuki[145] treated one eye with neovascular glaucoma secondary to central retinal vein occlusion. Coagulation of one half of the ciliary body was not successful, eventually necessitating 360 degrees of treatment. The intraocular pressure was controlled, the pain was relieved, the ciliary processes were turned to a pigmented band, and the vision was lost because of vitreous hemorrhage and cataract formation. The role of this technique remains to be evaluated.

Surgical therapy

In the past, the surgical success in neovascular glaucoma could be summarized with adjectives such as "hopeless"[85] and "disheartening."[101] Series of surgical cases worldwide almost uniformly had zero success.[55,85,105,116] The only surgical "success" achieved in the past was enucleation for pain. Duke-Elder[55] concluded:

> Any attempt at operative reduction of the ocular tension merely makes matters more acutely worse by inducing profuse and recurrent hemorrhages, and the only practical method of treatment, if a retrobulbar injection of alcohol or cyclodiathermy fails to relieve the pain, is enucleation.

There are essentially two major complications of filtering surgery in neovascular glaucoma: hemorrhages (intraoperative and postoperative) and failure of the filtering bleb. Various modifications of the standard filtering procedures have been tried in an attempt to avoid these complications and to increase the chances for success. The simplest modification has been the use of cautery or diathermy of the sclera and iris to decrease the risk of bleeding. Ellis et al.[61] used a modified Scheie procedure in which the peripheral iridectomy was made with electrocautery applied to the iris scissors to prevent bleeding. Four cases were treated by this method, and in two there was good control of the intraocular pressure, with a follow-up of 1 month and 3 months, respectively. Madsen[135a] used cautery sclerotomy and cautery or diathermy iridotomy and had a 54% (30 of 56 eyes) success rate in controlling the intraocular pressure. The

follow-up ranged from "less than 6 months to greater than 12 months." Hersh and Kass[96] had success in performing iridectomies in eyes with rubeosis iridis by using bipolar microcautery to eliminate the new vessels. Herschler and Agness[95] also used bipolar cautery in trabeculectomies and reported success in 77% (10 of 13 eyes) with 1 year or greater follow-up. Lee et al.[125] modified trabeculectomies by using partial, nonpenetrating cyclodiathermy on the scleral flap and diathermy on the iris vessels. They reported success in all five patients treated by this method with a follow-up of 3 months to 3 years.

Other modifications have included beta-irradiation to prevent postoperative scarring of the filtering bleb.[33] Cameron[33] reported 12 of 13 eyes successfully treated by this method but made no mention of how intraoperative and postoperative hemorrhages were controlled. Christensen and Meyer[42] performed hemiciliary body detachment and hemi-iridectomy with a full-thickness scleral flap in eight eyes. Three eyes achieved a normal intraocular pressure, four developed hypotony, and one had a pressure in the 30s. Suga[179] transplanted a vortex vein into the anterior chamber in five patients with neovascular glaucoma and reported successful control of the intraocular pressure in two cases. It appears that all the reported modified surgical procedures either had mixed results or, if the results were encouraging, it still is too early to analyze them adequately.

One other modification has been tried in an attempt to avoid failure of the filtering bleb: implants for draining aqueous. Ellis[62] reviewed the early history of implants for glaucoma filtering surgery. Horsehair, silk, and other types of sutures; gold, silver, platinum, tantalum, and other metallic wires; sheets and tubes; absorbable gelatin; and various plastics have been used for implants to drain aqueous from the anterior chamber to the subconjunctival space. At best, there have been low rates of success in keeping the filtration site open. Ellis et al.[62] reported success with silicone implants in rabbit eyes, but half of the implants moved into the anterior chamber in 4 to 20 months. MacDonald and Pierce[131] used Silastic setons that were sutured in place to prevent movement, and they were able to maintain filtration in rabbits for up to 8 months. Blumenthal et al.[22] used autogenous cartilege setons in rabbits with success. Molteno et al.[147] used a silicone rubber implant in 12 human eyes, and all were reported to be free of pain with pressures of less than 30 mm Hg.

Postoperative hyphema was present in every case and persisted for up to 3 weeks, but this did not seem to affect the outcome.

Others have used implants clinically and have had good success in maintaining prolonged reduction of the intraocular pressure.[30,57] The largest clinical study to date has been by Krupin et al.,[117] who used a Silastic-Supramid unidirectional pressure-sensitive valve implant in 42 eyes with neovascular glaucoma.[117] They were able to maintain an intraocular pressure of less than 24 mm Hg in 68% of the eyes with a mean follow-up of 13.8 months. External bleb scarring was the most frequent cause of failure in this series (11 cases or 26%).

The problem with all the modified procedures mentioned is that the stimulus for neovascularization has not been eliminated. Cautery and diathermy may eliminate the new vessels at the operative site, but new vessels can recur to scar down the filtration opening. The use of implants may keep the sclerostomy open, but scarring of the conjunctival flap can occur.

While there are undoubtedly many surgical techniques in the treatment of neovascular glaucoma and only time will reveal which is the best technique, it is important to present at least one technique that has been successful. The technique Hutchinson and I have used is based on the premise that once anterior segment neovascularization has been eliminated, the actual surgical technique needs no major modification from the standard external filtering procedure.[194] With the advent of PRP and GPC, this preoperative premise may be fulfilled in many cases. Surgery should be limited to those eyes with useful vision, with one keeping in mind that virtually any vision should be considered useful when the other eye has potential for compromise.

Whenever possible, PRP and/or GPC should be followed by a 1- to 3-week interval before surgery to allow the eye to "quiet" from any acute congestion. Miotics and epinephrine, if being used, should be discontinued. In eyes with a normal disc, an intraocular pressure of up to 50 mm Hg may be tolerated for this period if funduscopy shows adequate perfusion of the disc and no pulsation of the central retinal artery. In any event, one should try to reduce the congestion before surgery to reduce the risk of operative or postoperative hemorrhage.

As already mentioned, immediate preoperative measures include the continuation of topical atropine, steroids, timolol, and oral carbonic anhydrase inhibitors. Osmotic agents may be valuable if the general medical status permits their use, since it is wise to avoid a sudden surgical decompression of a hard eye. Retrobulbar anesthesia with epinephrine is preferred to general anesthesia, since local injection plus orbital massage will further soften the eye and reduce vascular congestion.

We prefer to use full-thickness filtration, such as by trephination or a posterior lip sclerectomy, rather than a trabeculectomy, since the filtering bleb seems to be better maintained with the former. A preplaced paracentesis incision into the anterior chamber is valuable, not only to allow for the slow decompression of a firm eye but, if necessary, to irrigate blood from the anterior chamber and to allow reformation of the chamber and the bleb at the end of the procedure.

Microsurgical techniques are mandatory, with particular emphasis being placed on minimizing tissue trauma and on providing strict hemostasis. The conjunctival flap should be handled gently with either smooth forceps at the incisional edge or by moistened surgical sponges. The conjunctival incision should be made well posterior to the limbus (10 mm+) in the supranasal or supratemporal quadrant so that the future filtration site will be protected by the lid. Dissection is carried to the limbus between conjunctiva and Tenon's fascia to avoid unnecessary bleeding and to provide a thin flap. The final dissection is carried to the peripheral cornea by blunt dissection with a spatula and sharp dissection with a Beaver No. 57 blade. Even the smallest bleeding points are cauterized, with care taken to avoid heating the conjunctival flap, and additional cautery is placed at the limbal incisional site. Tenon's fascia is carefully removed from the episclera with smooth-curved scissors approximately 0.5 mm from the episclera to avoid the episcleral vessels. Prompt cautery should be applied to any bleeding vessels.

The anterior chamber incision is made with a trephine or a knife as close to the flap as possible without buttonholing; this is followed, if needed, by a posterior lip sclerectomy with the Holth punch. The scleral lips of the wound are lightly cauterized to the point of slightest wound retraction. A peripheral iridectomy is performed. If new vessels remain patent on the iris, preiridectomy cautery to the iris is possible when the iris is lifted by forceps. Frequently there is bleeding with iris surgery. Injection of saline via the paracentesis wound will irrigate the anterior chamber and the sclerectomy site. Topical epinephrine may also be used, but iris or ciliary body surface cautery should be avoided after the iridectomy. Should brisk bleeding occur, penetrating diathermy of the ciliary body may be helpful. After hemostasis has been achieved, the conjunctival flap is closed with interrupted 10-0 nylon or 8-0 polyglactin sutures, approximating the anterior conjunctival flap with the posterior Tenon's fascia edge and the posterior cut edge of the conjunctiva. The incision should be anchored well behind the surgical limbus to keep the incisional wound from migrating toward the limbal bleb. The anterior chamber and the bleb are formed through the injection of saline via the paracentesis site. After removal of the superior rectus bridle suture, atropine, topical steroids, and erythromycin ointment are applied. The dressing is covered with a protective shield.

Postoperatively atropine is used two to three times and topical steroids four to six times daily; these medications are gradually tapered off over 3 to 4 weeks. Antibiotics are used on a daily basis indefinitely. The eye may be uncovered during the day early in the postoperative period. Massage is valuable later if the bleb shows evidence of failure, but if used too early, it may accentuate the vascular reaction. A flat chamber is seldom a problem, since lens-cornea apposition (with the potential for increase in either cataract or corneal edema) serves as the only indicator for a choroidal tap and reformation of the anterior chamber. Most hyphemas that develop postoperatively will clear without further surgery.

The intraocular pressure control following filtering surgery for neovascular glaucoma is generally not as good as that for primary open-angle glaucoma. The fibrovascular proliferative reaction is always more severe in the neovascular cases, and the resultant bleb, even when successful, is always more limited, is less succulent, and is often surrounded by a network of delineating conjunctival and episcleral vessels (Fig. 12-13). We have found this network of vessels surrounding the filtration bleb to be unique to operated cases of neovascular glaucoma. Perhaps enough AF (or AFs) is still produced to cause new vessel formation around the filtration bleb. These vessels often limit the size and effectiveness of the filtration bleb. Fortunately, eyes with neovascular glaucoma usually have normal discs, so that postoperative pressures need not be as low as in advanced open-angle glaucoma.

Using these techniques, we have had successful lowering of the intraocular pressure in over 75% of cases. Of greater significance is that no eyes have lost vision from glaucoma alone, but only from the initial disorder that caused the neovascularization process (e.g., diabetic retinopathy, central retinal vein occlusion). Some of these patients have developed cataracts that were successfully removed from below. Several of these patients have achieved vision as good as 20/25 (keep in mind that these same eyes would have been blind and painful only a few years ago).

SUMMARY

Our approach to the patient with incipient neovascular glaucoma is based on the fact that PRP can prevent and cause the regression of anterior segment neovascularization. PRP is routinely performed in eyes with active proliferative diabetic retinopathy and in eyes with central retinal vein occlusion of the ischemic type as shown on fluorescein angiography. Eyes with other predisposing causes of anterior segment neovascularization are followed closely, and at the first signs of rubeosis iridis PRP is performed. When rubeosis iridis is already present but angle involvement has not yet occurred, treatment consists of PRP and closer observation. When angle involvement has occurred, PRP alone is still frequently sufficient to cause regression of new vessels and avoid neovascular glaucoma. If the neovascularization appears to be fulminant and the angle appears to be in imminent danger of closure, GPC is used along with PRP. The primary benefit of GPC appears to be to provide a period of grace so that the PRP may have an effect before angle closure occurs. When rubeosis iridis is present but the media are too opaque to allow PRP, cataract extraction and/or vitrectomy are performed, followed by PRP in the immediate postoperative period. Panretinal cryotherapy and EPRP may also be used when indicated.

When a patient has actual neovascular glaucoma, one should initiate medical therapy as outlined to quiet the eye and lower the pressure as much as possible. During this period, PRP may be performed. When the PRP has reduced the anterior segment neovascularization, a surgical procedure is done. When the media are opaque because of cataract and/or vitreous hemorrhage, we have initiated medical therapy and without preoperative PRP have performed combined cataract extraction–vitrectomy–filtering procedures, followed by

PRP in the immediate postoperative period. With the availability of panretinal cryotherapy and EPRP, we expect success rates to improve.

When end-stage neovascular glaucoma is present in a blind, painful eye, topical atropine and steroids are indicated with a soft contact bandage lens, if necessary, to control the pain. If the eye is still painful, cyclocryotherapy is indicated. Rarely has it been necessary to resort to an alcohol injection or enucleation.

The progress in our understanding and treatment of neovascular glaucoma has been dramatic over the past 7 or 8 years. We can recall formerly seeing patients with neovascular glaucoma and telling them that nothing could be done aside from enucleation. Useful vision can now be restored to many of these same eyes. As rewarding as this progress has been, a realistic appraisal will point out that our present treatment is still analogous to closing the barn door after the horse is out. When the AF (or AFs) is isolated and the exact cause (or causes) of its production is known, then neovascular glaucoma may be preventable, and all the medical and surgical treatment discussed may become, happily, obsolete.

REFERENCES

1. Aiello, L.M., Beetham, W.P., Balodimos, M.C., et al.: Ruby laser photocoagulation and treatment of diabetic proliferating retinopathy. In Goldberg, M.F., and Fine, S.L., editors: Symposium on the treatment of diabetic retinopathy, Pub. No. 1890, Washington, D.C., 1969, U.S. Public Health Service, pp. 437-463.
2. Aiello, L.M., and Briones, J.C.: Ruby laser photocoagulation of proliferating diabetic retinopathy: fifth year follow-up, Int. Ophthalmol. Clin. **16:**15, 1976.
3. Anderson, D.M., Morin, D.J., and Hunter, W.S.: Rubeosis iridis, Can. J. Ophthalmol. **6:**183, 1971.
4. Ando, A., and Kyu, N.: Surgical treatment of hemorrhagic glaucoma (peripheral retinal diathermy), Folia Ophthalmol. Jpn. **24:**113, 1973.
5. Archer, D.B., Ernest, J.T., and Newell, F.W.: Classification of branch retinal vein obstruction, Trans. Am. Acad. Ophthalmol. Otolaryngol. **78:**148, 1974.
6. Ardounin, M.M., Urvoy, M., and Lefranc, J.: Quelques resultats d'utilisation du glycerol par voie buccale comme hypotonisant oculaire, Bull Soc. Ophthalmol. Fr. **64:**330, 1964.
7. Armaly, M.F., and Baloglou, P.J.: Diabetes and the eye. I. Changes in the anterior segment, Arch. Ophthalmol. **77:**485, 1967.
8. Ashton, N.: Retinal vascularization in health and disease, Am. J. Ophthalmol. **44:**7, 1957.
9. Ashton, N., Ward, B., and Serpell, G.: Effect of oxygen on developing retinal vessels with particular reference to the problem of retrolental fibroplasia, Br. J. Ophthalmol. **38:**397, 1954.
10. Bagessen, L.H.: Fluorescein angiography of the iris in diabetics and nondiabetics, Acta Ophthalmol. **47:**449, 1969.
11. Beasley, H.: Rubeosis iridis in aphakic diabetics, J. Am. Med. Assoc. **213:**128, 1970.
12. Bellows, A.R.: Cyclocryotherapy in the management of advanced glaucoma, Harvard Medical School–Massachusetts Eye and Ear Infirmary Glaucoma Course, Boston, April 10, 1980.
13. Bellows, A.R., and Grant, W.M.: Cyclocryotherapy in advanced inadequately controlled glaucoma, Am. J. Ophthalmol. **75:**679, 1973.
14. Bellows, A.R., and Grant, W.M.: Cyclocryotherapy of chronic open-angle glaucoma in aphakic eyes, Am. J. Ophthalmol. **85:**615, 1978.
15. Bellows, A.R., Tapper, D., Langer, R., and Folkman, J.: Personal communication, April 29, 1976.
16. Ben Ezra, D.: Neovasculogenic ability of prostaglandins, growth factors, and synthetic chemoattractants, Am. J. Ophthalmol. **86:**455, 1978.
17. Benedict, W.L.: The clinical significance of closure of the retinal vessels, J. Am. Med. Assoc. **38:**423, 1949.
18. Bertelsen, T.I.: The relationship between thrombosis in the retinal vein and primary glaucoma, Acta Ophthalmol. **39:**603, 1961.
19. Bietti, G.: Surgical intervention on the ciliary body: new trends for the relief of glaucoma, J. Am. Med. Assoc. **142:**889, 1950.
20. Blach, R.K., Hitchings, R.A., and Laatikainen, L.: Thrombotic glaucoma: prophylaxis and treatment, Trans. Ophthalmol. Soc. U.K. **97:**275, 1977.
21. Blankenship, G.: Pre-operative iris rubeosis and diabetic vitrectomy results, Ophthalmology **87:**186, 1980.
22. Blumenthal, M., Harris, L.S., and Galin, M.A.: Experimental study of cartilage setons, Br. J. Ophthalmol. **54:**62, 1970.
23. Boniuk, M.: Cryotherapy in neovascular glaucoma, Trans. Am. Acad. Ophthalmol. Otolaryngol. **78:**337, 1974.
24. Bonuik, M., and Burton, C.: Unilateral glaucoma associated with sickle cell retinopathy, Trans. Am. Acad. Ophthalmol. Otolaryngol. **68:**316, 1964.
25. Bouchon, J.D.G., Ramos, R.G., Oliver, L., and Fuentealba, M.A.: Traitment du glaucome secondaire à neovascularisation de l'iris (rubeose de l'iris), par la photocoagulation, Ann. Ocul. **209:**439, 1976.
26. Bouzas, M.A.: Les manifestations oculaires de la maladie de Takayasu avant et apres l'opération, Bull. Soc. Ophthalmol. Fr. **69:**560, 1969.
27. Braendstrup, P.: Central retinal vein thrombosis and hemorrhagic glaucoma, Acta Ophthalmol. Suppl. **25:**1, 1950.
28. Brem, S., Preis, I., Langer, R., et al.: Inhibition of neovascularization by an extract derived from vitreous, Am. J. Ophthalmol. **84:**323, 1977.
29. Bresnick, G.H., and Gay, A.J.: Rubeosis iridis associated with branch retinal arteriolar occlusions, Arch. Ophthalmol. **77:**176, 1967.
30. Brouillette, G.: Glaucome neo-vasculaire: une technique chirurgicale, Can. J. Ophthalmol. **14:**159, 1979.
31. Caird, F.I., Pirie, A., and Ramsell, T.G.: Diabetes and the eye, Oxford, 1968, Blackwell Scientific Publications, Ltd., p. 127.

32. Callahan, M.A., and Hilton, G.F.: Photocoagulation and rubeosis iridis, Am. J. Ophthalmol. **78:**873, 1974.

33. Cameron, M.E.: Thrombotic glaucoma successfully treated, Trans. Ophthalmol. Soc. U.K. **93:**537, 1973.

34. Campbell, D.G., Simmons, R.J., and Grant, W.M.: Ghost cells as a cause of glaucoma, Am. J. Ophthalmol. **81:**441, 1976.

35. Campbell, D.G., Simmons, R.J., Tolentino, F.I., and McMeel, J.W.: Glaucoma occurring after closed vitrectomy, Am. J. Ophthalmol. **83:**63, 1977.

36. Campinchi, R., and Haut, J.: Traitment exceptionnel de certains glaucomes absolus par l'atropine, Bull. Soc. Ophthalmol. Fr. **66:**10, 1966.

37. Cappin, J.M.: Malignant melanoma and rubeosis iridis, Br. J. Ophthalmol. **57:**815, 1973.

38. Carroll, R.P., and Landers, M.B.: Pinwheel rubeosis iridis following argon laser coreoplasty, Ann. Ophthalmol. **7:**357, 1975.

39. Chan, C.C., and Little, H.: Infrequency of retinal neovascularization following central retinal vein occlusion, Ophthalmology **86:**256, 1979.

40. Chandler, P.A., and Grant, W.M.: Lectures on glaucoma, Philadelphia, 1965, Lea & Febiger, p. 268.

41. Charles, S.: Written communication, Nov. 29, 1979.

42. Christensen, L., and Meyer, S.L.: Neovascular glaucoma: a new surgical approach, Trans. Am. Acad. Ophthalmol. Otolaryngol. **75:**372, 1975.

43. Cole, D.F., and Unger, W.G.: The involvement of prostaglandins in ocular trauma, Exp. Eye Res. **17:**357, 1973.

44. Cramer, F.: Operative complications of cataract extraction in diabetes, Int. Ophthalmol. Clin. **3:**645, 1963.

45. Cunha-Vaz, J.G., Abrew, J.F., Compos, A.J., and Figo, G.M.: Early breakdown of the blood-retinal barrier in diabetes, Br. J. Ophthalmol. **59:**649, 1975.

46. Cunha-Vaz, J.G., Goldberg, M.F., Vygantas, C., and Noth, J.: Early detection of retinal involvement in diabetes by vitreous fluorophotometry, Ophthalmology **86:**264, 1979.

47. DalFiume, E., Saccol, G., and Verzella, F.: Rubeosis iridea trattamento mediante fotocoagulatore laser ad argon, Arch. Rass. Ital Ottal. **3:**19, 1973.

48. DeRoetth, A.: Cyclodiathermy in treatment of glaucoma due to rubeosis iridis diabetica, Arch. Ophthalmol. **35:**20, 1946.

49. DeRoetth, A.: Cryosurgery for the treatment of glaucoma, Am. J. Ophthalmol. **61:**443, 1966.

50. DeRoetth, A.: Cryosurgery for treatment of advanced chronic simple glaucoma, Am. J. Ophthalmol. **66:**1034, 1968.

51. Deutsch, T.A., and Hughes, W.F.: Suppressive effects of indomethacin on thermally induced neovascularization of rabbit corneas, Am. J. Ophthalmol. **87:**536, 1979.

52. Diabetic Retinopathy Study Research Group: Preliminary report on effects of photocoagulation therapy, Am. J. Ophthalmol. **81:**282, 1976.

53. Dryden, R.M.: Central retinal vein occlusions and chronic simple glaucoma, Arch. Ophthalmol. **73:**659, 1965.

54. Dueker, D.K.: Neovascular glaucoma. In Chandler, P.A., and Grant, W.M.: Glaucoma, Philadelphia, 1979, Lea & Febiger, p. 259.

55. Duke-Elder, S.: System of ophthalmology, vol. II, Diseases of the lens and vitreous; glaucoma and hypotony, St. Louis, 1969, The C.V. Mosby Co., p. 667.

56. Editorial: Fluorescein angiography of the iris, Br. J. Ophthalmol. **63:**143, 1979.

57. Egerer, I.: Ein Versuch zur operativen Beherrschung des hämorrhagischen Glaukoms, Klin. Monatsbl. Augenheilkd. **169:**617, 1976.

58. Eisenstein, R., Goren, S.B., Shumacher, B., and Choromokos, E.: The inhibition of corneal vascularization with aortic extracts in rabbits, Am. J. Ophthalmol. **88:**1005, 1979.

59. Ellett, E.C.: Metastatic carcinoma of choroid. III. Rubeosis iridis with melanoma of the choroid and secondary glaucoma, Am. J. Ophthalmol. **27:**726, 1944.

60. Ellis, P.P.: Regression of rubeosis iridis following cyclodiathermy, Am. J. Ophthalmol. **40:**253, 1955.

61. Ellis, P.P., Thompson, R.L., and Tyner, G.S.: A modified filtering operation for hemorrhagic glaucoma, Am. J. Ophthalmol. **54:**954, 1962.

62. Ellis, R.A.: Reduction of intraocular pressure using plastics in surgery, Am. J. Ophthalmol. **50:**733, 1960.

63. Etienne, R., Barut, C., and Ravault, M.: Le glaucome néovasculaire secondaire à la thrombose de l'artère carotide interne, Ann. Ocul. **198:**991, 1965.

64. Farnarier, G., Rampin, S., and Lancon, M.: La rubeose irienne diabetique, Ann. Ocul. **199:**574, 1966.

65. Faulborn, J., and Höster, K.: Erqebnisse der Zyklokryotherapie beim haemorrhagischen Glaukom, Klin. Monatsbl. Augenheilkd. **162:**513, 1973.

66. Federman, J.L., Brown, G.C., Feldberg, N.T., and Felton, S.M.: Experimental ocular angiogenesis, Am. J. Ophthalmol. **89:**231, 1980.

67. Fehrmann, H.: Uber Rubeosis iridis diabetica and ihre allegemein-medizinische Bedeutung; mit anatomischem Befund, Albrecht Von Graefes Arch. Ophthalmol. **140:**354, 1939.

68. Feibel, R.M., and Bigger, J.F.: Rubeosis iridis and neovascular glaucoma, Am. J. Ophthalmol. **74:**862, 1972.

69. Ferry, A.P., and Font, R.L.: Carcinoma metastatic to the eye and orbit, Arch. Ophthalmol. **93:**472, 1975.

70. Finkelstein, D., Brem, S., Patz, A., and Folkman, J.: Experimental retinal neovascularization induced by intravitreal tumors, Am. J. Ophthalmol. **83:**660, 1977.

71. Fisk, A.E.: Diseases of the eye and ophthalmoscopy, Philadelphia, 1896, P. Blakiston, Son & Co., p. 403.

72. Folkman, J.: The vascularization of tumors, Sci. Am. **234:**59, 1976.

73. Folkman, J., Merler, E., Abernathy, C., and Williams, G.: Isolation of a tumor factor responsible for angiogenesis, J. Exp. Med. **133:**275, 1971.

74. François, J.: Rubeose de l'iris et retinopathie diabetique, Ann. Ocul. **205:**1085, 1972.

75. Frank, R.N.: Diabetic retinopathy. In Ryan, S.T., and Smith, R.E., editors: Selected topics on the eye in systemic disease, New York, 1974, Grune & Stratton, Inc., pp. 65-118.

76. Galinos, S., Rabb, M.F., Goldberg, M.F., and Frenkel, M.: Hemoglobin SC disease and iris atrophy, Am. J. Ophthalmol. **75:**421, 1973.

77. Gartner, S., and Henkind, P.: Neovascularization of the iris (rubeosis iridis), Surv. Ophthalmol. **22:**291, 1978.

78. Gartner, S., Taffet, S., and Friedman, A.H.: The association of rubeosis iridis with endothelialization of the anterior chamber, Br. J. Ophthalmol. **61:**217, 1977.

79. Gimbrone, M.A., Leapman, S.B., Cotran, R.S., and

Folkman, J.: Tumor angiogenesis: iris neovascularization at a distance from experimental intraocular tumors, J. Natl. Cancer Inst. **50:**219, 1973.

80. Gimbrone, M.A., Leapman, S.B., Cotran, R.S., and Folkman, J.: Tumor growth and neovascularization: an experimental model using rabbit cornea, J. Natl. Cancer Inst. **52:**413, 1974.

81. Gitter, K.A., and Cohen, G.: Complications of vitrectomy. In Gitter, K.A., editor: Current concepts of the vitreous including vitrectomy, St. Louis, 1976, The C.V. Mosby Co.

82. Glaser, B.M., D'Amore, P.A., Michels, R.G., et al.: The demonstration of angiogenic activity from ocular tissues, Ophthalmology **87:**440, 1980.

83. Goldstein, A.L., and Ide, C.H.: Cyclocryotherapy for secondary glaucoma due to rubeosis iridis, Mo. Med. **69:**736, 1972.

84. Goodart, R., and Blankenship, G.: Panretinal photocoagulation influence on vitrectomy results for complications of diabetic retinopathy, Ophthalmology **87:** 183, 1980.

85. Grant, W.M.: Management of neovascular glaucoma. In Leopold, I.H., editor: Symposium on ocular therapy, vol. 7, St. Louis, 1974, The C.V. Mosby Co.

86. Green, K., and Kim, K.: Patterns of ocular responses to topical and systemic prostaglandin, Invest. Ophthalmol. **12:**752, 1973.

87. Gutman, F.A., and Zegarra, H.: The natural course of temporal retinal branch vein occlusion, Trans. Am. Acad. Ophthalmol. Otolaryngol. **78:**178, 1974.

88. Hart, C.T., and Haworth, S.: Bilateral common carotid occlusion with hypoxic ocular sequelae, Br. J. Ophthalmol. **55:**383, 1971.

89. Hayreh, S.S.: So-called "central retinal vein occlusion." I. Pathogenesis, terminology, clinical features, Ophthalmologica **172:**1, 1976.

90. Hayreh, S.S.: Ocular neovascularization, Arch. Ophthalmol. **98:**574, 1980.

91. Hayreh, S.S., March, W., and Phelps, C.D.: Ocular hypotony following retinal vein occlusion, Arch. Ophthalmol. **96:**827, 1978.

92. Hayreh, S.S., van Heuven, W.A.J., and Hayreh, M.S.: Experimental retinal vascular occlusion. I. Pathogenesis of central retinal vein occlusion, Arch. Ophthalmol. **96:** 311, 1978.

93. Henkind, P.: Ocular neovascularization, Am. J. Ophthalmol. **85:**287, 1978.

94. Henkind, P., and Morgan, G.: Peripheral retinal angioma with exudative retinopathy in adults (Coats' lesion), Br. J. Ophthalmol. **50:**2, 1966.

95. Herschler, J., and Agness, D.: A modified filtering operation for neovascular glaucoma, Arch. Ophthalmol. **97:** 2339, 1979.

96. Hersh, S.B., and Kass, M.A.: Iridectomy in rubeosis iridis, Ophthalmic Surg. **7:**19, 1976.

97. Heydenreich, A., and Schnabel, R.: Zur klinik und pathologie der rubeosis iridis, Klin. Monatsbl. Augenheilkd. **134:**350, 1959.

98. Hilton, G.: Panretinal cryotherapy of diabetic rubeosis, Arch. Ophthalmol. **97:**776, 1979.

99. Hoefnagels, K.L.J.: Rubeosis of the iris associated with occlusion of the carotid artery, Ophthalmologica **148:** 196, 1964.

100. Hohl, R.D., and Barnett, D.M.: Diabetic hemorrhagic glaucoma, Diabetes **19:**994, 1970.

101. Hoskins, H.D.: Neovascular glaucoma: current concepts, Trans. Am. Acad. Ophthalmol. Otolaryngol. **78:**330, 1974.

102. Hövener, G.: Photocoagulation for central retinal vein occlusion, Klin. Monatsbl. Augenheilkd. **173:**392, 1978.

103. Huckman, M.S., and Haas, J.: Reversed flow through the ophthalmic artery as a cause of rubeosis iridis, Am. J. Ophthalmol. **74:**1094, 1972.

104. Jacobson, D.R., Murphy, R.P., and Rosenthal, A.R.: The treatment of angle neovascularization with panretinal photocoagulation, Ophthalmology **86:**1270, 1979.

105. Jayle, G.E., Ourgaud, A.G., and Saracco, J.B.: Problemes operatioires du glaucoma chez le diabetique, Bull. Soc. Ophthalmol. Fr. **67:**255, 1967.

106. Jensen, V.A., and Lundbock, K.: Fluorescein angiography of this iris in recent and long-term diabetes: preliminary communication, Acta Ophthalmol. **46:**584, 1968.

107. Jocson, V.L.: Microvascular injection studies in rubeosis iridis and neovascular glaucoma, Am. J. Ophthalmol. **83:**508, 1977.

108. Karjalainen, K.: Occlusion of the central retinal artery and retinal branch arterioles: a clinical, tonographic and fluorescein angiographic study of 175 patients, Acta Ophthalmol. Suppl. **109:**9, 1971.

109. Kearns, T.P., and Hollenhorst, R.W.: Venous-stasis retinopathy of occlusive disease of the carotid artery, Mayo Clin. Proc. **38:**304, 1963.

110. Kelley, J.S., Patz, A., and Schatz, H.: Management of retinal branch vein occlusion: the role of argon laser photocoagulation, Ann. Ophthalmol. **8:**1123, 1976.

111. Kimura, R.: Fluorescein goniophotography, Glaucoma **2:**359, 1980.

112. King, M.J.: Retrolental fibroplasia, Arch. Ophthalmol. **43:**694, 1950.

113. Kobozeva, O.I.: Tonographic and gonioscopic examinations in retinal vein thrombosis, Oftalmol. Zh. **23:**594, 1968.

114. Kottow, M.W.: Anterior segment fluorescein angiography, Baltimore, 1978, The Williams & Wilkins Co., pp. 129-151.

115. Krill, A.E., Archer, D., and Newell, F.W.: Photocoagulation in complications secondary to branch vein occlusion, Arch. Ophthalmol. **85:**48, 1971.

116. Krüger, K.E.: Beitrag zum Sekundärglaukom bei Rubeosis iridis diabetica, Ophthalmologica **142** (suppl.):604, 1961.

117. Krupin, T., Kaufman, P., Mandell, A., et al.: Filtering valve implant surgery for eyes with neovascular glaucoma, Am. J. Ophthalmol. **89:**338, 1980.

118. Krupin, T., Mitchell, K.B., and Becker, B.: Cyclocryotherapy in neovascular glaucoma, Am. J. Ophthalmol. **86:**24, 1978.

119. Kurz, O.: Zur Rubeosis iridis diabetica, Arch. Augenheilkd. **110:**284, 1937.

120. Laatikainen, L.: Preliminary report on effect of retinal photocoagulation on rubeosis iridis and neovascular glaucoma, Br. J. Ophthalmol. **61:**278, 1977.

121. Laatikainen, L.: Development and classification of rubeosis iridis in diabetic eye disease, Br. J. Ophthalmol. **63:**150, 1979.

122. Laatikainen, L., and Blach, R.K.: Behavior of the iris vasculature in central retinal vein occlusion: a fluorescein angiographic study of the vascular response of the retina and the iris, Br. J. Ophthalmol. **61:**272, 1977.

123. Laatikainen, L., and Kohner, E.M.: Fluorescein angiography and its prognostic significance in central retinal vein occlusion, Br. J. Ophthalmol. **64:**411, 1976.

124. Langer, R., Brem, H., Falterman, K., et al.: Isolation of a cartilage factor that inhibits tumor neovascularization, Science **183:**70, 1976.

125. Lee, P., Shihab, Z.M., and Fu, Y.: Modified trabeculectomy: a new procedure for neovascular glaucoma, Ophthalmic Surg. **11:**181, 1980.

126. L'Esperance, F.A.: Influence of cataract extraction on the outcome of pars plana vitrectomy in eyes with proliferative diabetic retinopathy. In McPherson, A., editor: New and controversial aspects of vitreoretinal surgery, St. Louis, 1977, The C.V. Mosby Co.

127. Liang, G., Aiello, L.M., and Wand, M.: The effects of cataract extraction on anterior segment neovascularization in diabetic patients, manuscript in preparation.

128. Lin, Y.H.Y., Lam, K.W., and Lee, P.: Ascorbate and protein in the eyes with neovascular glaucoma, Association for Research in Vision and Ophthalmology Annual Meeting, Orlando, Fla., May 4-9, 1980.

129. Lisman, J.V.: Rubeosis iridis diabetica, Am. J. Ophthalmol. **31:**989, 1948.

130. Little, H.L., Rosenthal, A.R., Dellaporta, A., and Jacobson, D.R.: The effect of panretinal photocoagulation on rubeosis iridis, Am. J. Ophthalmol. **81:**804, 1976.

131. MacDonald, R.K., and Pierce, H.F.: Silicone setons, Am. J. Ophthalmol. **59:**635, 1965.

132. Madsen, P.H.: Venous-stasis retinopathy in insufficiency of the ophthalmic artery, Acta Ophthalmol. **44:**940, 1966.

133. Madsen, P.H.: Ocular findings in 123 patients with proliferative diabetic retinopathy. I. Changes in the anterior segment of the eye, Doc. Ophthalmol. **29:**331, 1970.

134. Madsen, P.H.: Haemorrhagic glaucoma: comparative study in diabetic and non-diabetic patients, Br. J. Ophthalmol. **55:**444, 1971.

135. Madsen, P.H.: Rubeosis of the iris and haemorrhagic glaucoma in patients with proliferative diabetic retinopathy, Br. J. Ophthalmol. **55:**369, 1971.

135a. Madsen, P.H.: Experiences in surgical treatment of haemmorrhagic glaucoma, Acta Ophthalmol. Suppl. **120:**88, 1973.

136. Makley, T.A., and Teed, R.W.: Unsuspected intraocular malignant melanoma, Arch. Ophthalmol. **60:**475, 1950.

137. May, D.R., Bergstrom, T.J., Parmet, A.J., and Schwartz, J.G.: Treatment of neovascular glaucoma with transcleral panretinal cryotherapy, Ophthalmology **87:**1106, 1980.

138. May, D.R., Klein, M.L., and Peyman, G.A.: A prospective study on xenon arc photocoagulation for central retinal vein occlusion, Br. J. Ophthalmol. **60:**816, 1976.

139. May, D.R., Klein, M.L., Peyman, G.A., and Raichand, X.: Xenon arc panretinal photocoagulation for central retinal vein occlusion: a randomised prospective study, Br. J. Ophthalmol. **63:**725, 1979.

140. Meyer-Schwickerath, G.: Light coagulation, Stuttgart, Germany, 1959, Enke Verlang.

141. Michaelson, I.C.: The mode of development of the vascular system of the retina with some observations of its significance in certain retinal diseases, Trans. Ophthalmol. Soc. U.K. **68:**137, 1948.

142. Michels, R.H., and Ryan, S.J.: Results and complications of 100 consecutive cases of pars plana vitrectomy, Am. J. Ophthalmol. **80:**24, 1975.

143. Michelson, P.E., Knox, D.L., and Green, W.R.: Ischemic ocular inflammation, Arch. Ophthalmol. **86:**274, 1971.

144. Milan, B., and Josip, K.: Manifestations oculaires dans le syndrome de l'arc de l'aorte, Ann. Ocul. **200:**1168, 1967.

145. Mochizuki, M.: Transpupillary cyclophotocoagulation in hemorrhagic glaucoma: a case report, Jpn. J. Ophthalmol. **19:**191, 1975.

146. Mohan, V., and Eagling, E.M.: Peripheral retinal cryotherapy as a treatment for neovascular glaucoma, Trans. Ophthalmol. Soc. U.K. **98:**93, 1978.

147. Molteno, A.C.B., VonRooyen, M.M.B., and Bartholomew, R.S.: Implants for draining neovascular glaucoma, Br. J. Ophthalmol. **61:**120, 1977.

148. Mylius, K.: Rubeosis iridis und Sekundarglaukom, Ophthalmologica **142**(suppl.):605, 1961.

149. Nanziata, B., Smith, R.S., and Weimer, V.: Corneal radiofrequency burns: effect of prostaglandins and 48/80, Invest. Ophthalmol. **16:**285, 1977.

150. Ohrt, V.: Glaucoma due to rubeosis iridis diabetica, Ophthalmologica **142:**356, 1961.

151. Ohrt, V.: Rubeosis iridis diabetica, Dan. Med. Bull. **11:**17, 1964.

152. Ohrt, V.: The frequency of rubeosis iridis in diabetic patients, Acta Ophthalmol. **49:**301, 1971.

153. Okun, E.: Pars plana vitrectomy in advanced diabetic retinopathy. In Gitter, K.A., editor, Current concepts of the vitreous including vitrectomy, St. Louis, 1976, The C.V. Mosby Co.

154. Okun, E., and McMeel, J.W.: Discussion of McMeel, J.W.: Closed vitrectomy in diabetic retinopathy. In Freeman, H., Hirose, I., and Schepens, C., editors: Vitreous surgery and advances in fundus diagnosis and treatment, New York, 1975, Appleton-Century-Crofts.

155. Parsons, J.H., and Duke-Elder, S.: Diseases of the eye, ed. 11, New York, 1948, Macmillan Publishing Co., Inc., p. 283.

156. Patz, A., Lutty, G., and Coughlin, W.R.: Inhibitors of neovascularization in relation to diabetic and other proliferative retinopathies, Trans. Am. Ophthalmol. Soc. **76:**102, 1978.

157. Patz, A., Yassur, Y., Fine, S.L., et al.: Branch retinal venous occlusion, Trans. Am. Acad. Ophthalmol. Otolaryngol. **83:**373, 1977.

158. Pederson, J., and Green, K.: Solute permeability of the normal and prostaglandins E_2 stimulated epithelium and the effect of ultrafiltration on active transport, Exp. Eye Res. **21:**569, 1975.

159. Perpignano, A.: Azione ipotonizzante sull'occhio dell'inderal, Arch. Rass. Ital. Ottal. **36:**245, 1968.

160. Perraut, E., and Zimmerman, L.W.: The occurrence of glaucoma following occlusion of the central retinal artery, Arch. Ophthalmol. **61:**845, 1959.

161. Polverini, P.J., Cotran, R.S., Gimbrone, M.A., and Unanue, E.R.: Activated macrophages induce vascular proliferation, Nature **269:**804, 1977.

162. Priluck, I.A., Roberston, D.M., and Hollenhorst, R.W.: Long-term follow up of occlusion of the central retinal vein in young adults, Am. J. Ophthalmol. **90**:190, 1980.

163. Robertson, C.A., translator: Glaucoma and its cure by iridectomy, from the French of Testelin and Warlomont, Albany, N.Y., 1866, J. Mansel, p. 27.

164. Saari, M., Vuorre, I., and Nieminen, H.: Fuchs' heterochromic cyclitis: simultaneous bilateral fluorescein angiographic study of the iris, Br. J. Ophthalmol. **62**:715, 1978.

165. Salus, R.: Rubeosis iridis diabetica, eine bisher unbekannte diabetische Irisveränderung, Med. Klin. **24**:256, 1928.

166. Schimek, R.A., and Spencer, R.: Cryopexy treatment of proliferative diabetic retinopathy, Arch. Ophthalmol. **97**:1276, 1979.

167. Schulze, R.R.: Rubeosis iridis, Am. J. Ophthalmol. **63**:487, 1967.

168. Shabo, A.L., and Maxwell, D.S.: Insulin-induced immunogenic retinopathy resembling retinitis proliferans of diabetes, Trans. Am. Acad. Ophthalmol. Otolaryngol. **81**:497, 1976.

169. Shabo, A.L., and Maxwell, D.S.: Experimental immunogenic proliferative retinopathy in monkeys, Am. J. Ophthalmol. **83**:471, 1977.

170. Sidkey, Y.A., and Auerbach, R.: Lymphocyte-induced angiogenesis: a quantitative and sensitive assay of the graft-vs-host reaction, J. Exp. Med. **141**:1084, 1975.

171. Simmons, R.J., Depperman, S.R., and Dueker, D.K.: The role of goniophotocoagulation in neovascularization of the anterior chamber angle, Ophthalmology **87**:79, 1980.

172. Simmons, R.J., Dueker, D.K., Kimbrough, R.L., and Aiello, L.M.: Goniophotocoagulation for neovascular glaucoma, Trans. Am. Acad. Ophthalmol. Otolaryngol. **83**:80, 1977.

173. Sinclair, S.M.: Personal communication, June 26, 1976.

174. Sinclair, S.M., and Gragoudas, E.S.: Prognosis for rubeosis iridis following central retinal vein occlusion, Br. J. Ophthalmol. **63**:735, 1979.

175. Smith, J.L.: Unilateral glaucoma in carotid occlusive disease, J. Am. Med. Assoc. **182**:683, 1962.

176. Smith, M.D., and Becker, B.: Ocular complications in diabetes. In Fajans, S.S., editor: Diabetes mellitus, Bethesda, Md., 1976, National Institutes of Health.

177. Smith, R.: Concerning glaucoma and retinal venous occlusion, Trans. Ophthalmol. Soc. U.K. **75**:265, 1955.

178. Smith, R.: Neovascularization in ocular disease, Trans. Ophthalmol. Soc. U.K. **81**:125, 1961.

179. Suga, K.: Transplantation of a vortex vein into the anterior chamber in hemolytic and hemorrhagic glaucoma, Folia Ophthalmol. Jpn. **24**:258, 1973.

180. Sugar, H.S.: Place of hemorrhagic glaucoma in etiologic classification, Arch. Ophthalmol. **28**:587, 1942.

181. Sullivan, S.T., and Dallow, R.L.: Intraocular reticulum cell sarcoma, Ann. Ophthalmol. **9**:401, 1977.

182. Tamura, T.: Electron microscopic study on the small blood vessels in rubeosis iridis diabetica, Jpn. J. Ophthalmol. **13**:65, 1969.

183. Tasman, W., Magargal, L.E., and Augsberger, J.J.: Effects of argon laser photocoagulation or rubeosis iridis and angle neovascularization, Ophthalmology **87**:400, 1980.

184. Turiaskaya, A.M.: Gonioscopy in patients with diabetes mellitus, Oftamol. Zh. **2**:135, 1966.

185. Vannas, A.: Fluorescein angiography of the vessels of the iris in pseudo-exfoliation of the lens capsule, capsular glaucoma, and some other forms of glaucoma, Acta Ophthalmol. Suppl. **105**:9, 1969.

186. Verhoeff, F.H.: Effect of chronic glaucoma on central retinal vessels, Arch. Ophthalmol. **42**:145, 1913.

187. Waltman, S.R.: Early detection of diabetic retinopathy, Sixth National RPB Science Writers Seminar in Eye Research, Los Angeles, California, Oct. 1979.

188. Waltman, S.R., Oestrich, C., Krupin, T., et al.: Quantitative vitreous fluorophotometry: a sensitive technique for measuring early breakdown of the blood-retinal barrier in young diabetic patients, Diabetes **27**:85, 1978.

189. Walton, D.S., and Grant, W.M.: Retinoblastoma and iris neovascularization, Am. J. Ophthalmol. **65**:598, 1968.

190. Walton, D.S., and Grant, W.M.: Penetrating cyclodiathermy for filtration, Arch. Ophthalmol. **83**:47, 1970.

191. Wand, W., and Dueker, D.K.: Unreported observation.

192. Wand, M., Dueker, D.K., Aiello, L.M., and Grant, W.M.: Effects of panretinal photocoagulation on rubeosis iridis, angle neovascularization, and neovascular glaucoma, Am. J. Ophthalmol. **86**:332, 1978.

193. Wand, M., and Gorn, R.A.: Cholesterosis of the anterior chamber, Am. J. Ophthalmol. **78**:143, 1974.

194. Wand, M., and Hutchinson, B.T.: The surgical treatment of neovascular glaucoma, Perspect. Ophthalmol. **4**:147, 1980.

195. Weiss, D.I., and Leopold, I.V.: Prognosis of secondary glaucoma following retinal artery occlusion, Am. J. Ophthalmol. **51**:793, 1961.

196. Weiss, D.I., Shaffer, R.N., and Nehrenberg, T.R.: Neovascular glaucoma complicating carotid-cavernous fistula, Arch. Ophthalmol. **69**:304, 1963.

197. Wise, G.N.: Retinal neovascularization, Trans. Am. Ophthalmol. Soc. **54**:729, 1956.

198. Wolter, J.R.: Secondary glaucoma in cranial arteritis, Am. J. Ophthalmol. **59**:625, 1965.

199. Wolter, J.R.: Double embolism of the central retinal artery and long posterior ciliary artery followed by secondary hemorrhagic glaucoma, Am. J. Ophthalmol. **73**:651, 1972.

200. Wolter, J.R., and Ryan, R.W.: Atheromatous embolism of the central retinal artery, Arch. Ophthalmol. **87**:301, 1972.

201. Yanoff, M.: Ocular pathology of diabetes mellitus, Am. J. Ophthalmol. **67**:21, 1969.

202. Yanoff, M.: Mechanisms of glaucoma in eyes with uveal melanoma, Int. Ophthalmol. Clin. **12**:51, 1972.

203. Yanoff, M., and Fine, B.S.: Ocular pathology: a text and atlas, New York, 1975, Harper & Row, Publishers, Inc., p. 339.

204. Yoshizumi, M.O., Thomas, J.V., and Smith, T.R.: Glaucoma-inducing mechanisms in eyes with retinoblastoma, Arch. Ophthalmol. **96**:105, 1978.

205. Young, N.J.A., Hitchings, R.A., Sehmi, K., and Bird, A.C.: Stickler's syndrome and neovascular glaucoma, Br. J. Ophthalmol. **63**:826, 1979.

206. Zollinger, R.: Klinische Untersuchungen uber Gafassneubildungen auf der Iris, Ophthalmologica **123**:216, 1952.

Chapter 13

GLAUCOMA ASSOCIATED WITH INTRAOCULAR TUMORS

M. Bruce Shields

MALIGNANT MELANOMAS
Uveal melanoma and intraocular pressure

As early as 1896, ophthalmologists were aware that the intraocular pressure can be influenced by the presence of malignant melanomas of the uvea.[30] In five reported studies, totaling 695 eyes with melanoma of the choroid and ciliary body,* the prevalence of elevated intraocular pressure ranged from 27%[9] to 56%,[30] and the number of cases of reduced pressure varied from 3%[31] to 53%.[9] In some studies the elevated pressure occurred more often with melanomas of the choroid as opposed to ciliary body melanomas,[9,30] although other investigators found no correlation between the prevalence of glaucoma and the location of the tumor.[25,31,49]

A more recent study showed an elevated intraocular pressure to be significantly more common in eyes with anterior uveal melanoma as compared with the pressure in eyes with choroidal melanoma.[52] In a histologic study of 96 eyes with malignant melanoma involving one or more portions of the uveal tract, the overall prevalence of glaucoma was 20%, but it was 14% in the eyes with choroidal melanoma and 41% in the eyes with anterior uveal melanoma.[52] Similar observations were made in a clinicopathologic study of 11 consecutive cases of anterior uveal melanoma, in which 5 eyes (45%) had elevated pressures.[44] In the latter two studies, all eyes with anterior uveal melanoma and glaucoma had either primary or

*References 9, 25, 30, 31, 49.

secondary tumor involvement of the iris.[44,52] In contrast, when the melanoma is primarily limited to the ciliary body, the intraocular pressure is often reduced. In a clinicopathologic study of seven eyes with ciliary body melanoma of presumed early diagnosis, the intraocular pressure was equal to the fellow eye in two cases and 2 to 3 mm Hg lower in five.[15]

Diagnosis of uveal melanoma and glaucoma

There is considerable variation in both the clinical and histopathologic findings of patients with uveal melanoma and glaucoma. The clinical presentation may be that of acute glaucoma with either an open or closed angle, whereas the glaucoma in other cases may be more insidious. In some cases diagnosis of the malignant melanoma is difficult, particularly when visualization of a posteriorly located tumor is obscured by opaque media or a retinal detachment.[52] Cases have been reported in which glaucoma surgery was mistakenly performed for acute angle-closure glaucoma secondary to an unsuspected choroidal melanoma.[29,45] In one case studied, a malignant melanoma of the choroid presented as a choroidal detachment after cataract surgery, but later retinal detachment and neovascular glaucoma developed, which finally led to the correct diagnosis.[27] Ocular inflammation or hemorrhage may also occur as an initial finding in eyes with malignant melanoma of the choroid or ciliary body,[18] which could lead to diagnostic confusion.

Anterior uveal melanomas are generally less dif-

194

ficult to recognize, although associated findings may occasionally confuse the diagnosis. The eye may appear to have iritis, which usually represents free tumor cells in the anterior chamber.[44] In other cases the melanoma may be mistaken for a cho-roidal detachment or a cyst of the iris.[44] Cystlike spaces involving the iris and ciliary body occur in some eyes with anterior uveal melanoma due to separation of the two epithelial layers of the uvea by an eosinophilic exudate[22,44] (Fig. 13-1). A third

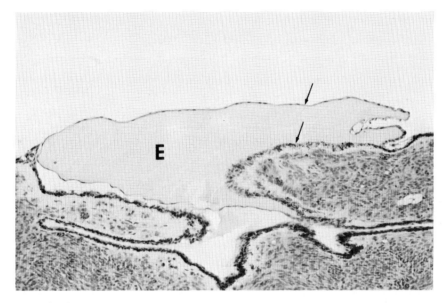

FIG. 13-1. Light microscopic view of epithelial layers *(arrows)* of ciliary body separated by prominent eosinophilic exudate *(E)*. Stroma of ciliary body contains melanoma. (Hematoxylin and eosin; ×100.) (From Shields, M.B., and Klintworth, G.K.: Ophthalmology **87:**503, 1980.)

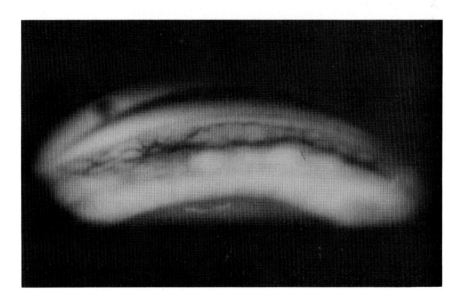

FIG. 13-2. Gonioscopic view of malignant melanoma of ciliary body presenting as multiple, pale tumors on peripheral iris and in anterior chamber angle.

diagnostic problem is distinguishing uveal melanomas from benign and metastatic lesions (Fig. 13-2). The clinical differentiation between a melanoma and a nevus or melanosis of the iris may be particularly difficult, since a melanoma presumably may arise from either of the latter two lesions.[14,36] Furthermore, both nevi and melanosis of the iris may be associated with glaucoma.[16,24,38] Other benign lesions that should be considered in the differential diagnosis of anterior uveal melanomas include leiomyomas of the iris,[5,8] adenomas of the iris pigment epithelium,[34] melanocytomas

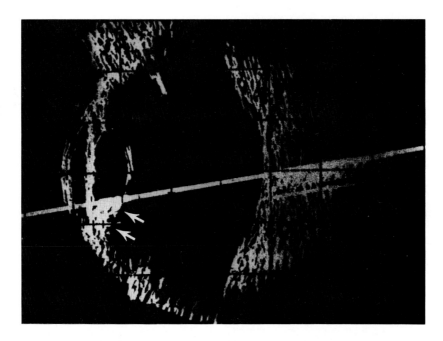

FIG. 13-3. B-scan ultrasonographic view of eye in Fig. 13-2 showing ciliary body mass *(arrows)*.

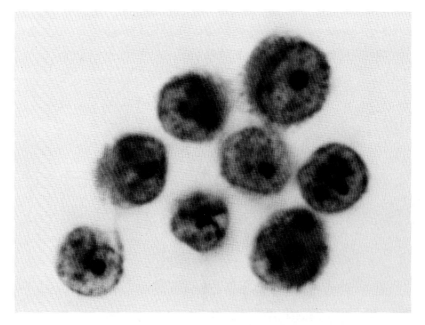

FIG. 13-4. Light microscopic view of melanoma cells aspirated from aqueous of eye in Fig. 13-2. (Papanicolaou; ×400.)

of the ciliary body and iris,[42] and coronal adenomas, or benign epithelial tumors of the ciliary processes.[2]

Several diagnostic procedures are helpful in identifying a malignant melanoma. Ultrasonography may demonstrate the presence of a choroidal or ciliary body melanoma that cannot be directly visualized (Fig. 13-3), although this technique does not with absolute certainty distinguish a neoplasm from other masses of the posterior ocular segment.[21] The radioactive phosphorous (^{32}P) test is reported to be of value in differentiating benign lesions of the choroid and ciliary body from malignant ones, but it is not particularly helpful in lesions of the iris.[40] Fluorescein angiography of the iris, however, is said to be useful in distinguishing melanomas from benign lesions, such as leiomyomas.[5,8] Paracentesis of the anterior chamber with cytologic examination of the aspirate may also be helpful in distinguishing a melanoma from a benign or metastatic tumor (Fig. 13-4).

Mechanism of glaucoma

The mechanism of glaucoma in eyes with choroidal melanoma is usually related to the mass effect of a large posterior tumor associated with total retinal detachment. The resulting forward displacement of the lens leads to a pupillary block with subsequent peripheral anterior synechiae and chronic angle-closure glaucoma (Fig. 13-5).[52] In other cases the large choroidal melanoma and total retinal detachment may cause rubeosis iridis and subsequent neovascular glaucoma.[52]

In eyes with anterior uveal melanoma, the mechanism of glaucoma is usually obstruction of the anterior chamber angle either by direct extension of the tumor (Figs. 13-6 and 13-7) or by seeding of tumor cells (Fig. 13-8) or melanin granules (Fig. 13-9) in the trabecular meshwork.[44,52] One situation has been referred to as melanomalytic glaucoma, because it is postulated that macrophages engulf melanin from necrotic melanomas and subsequently obstruct the anterior chamber angle (Fig. 13-10).[53] An electron microscopic study of melanomalytic glaucoma showed that the melanin granules were within both macrophages and trabecular endothelial cells that were either free or partially detached.[50] Another entity designated "tapioca melanoma," is characterized by low-grade nodular malignant melanomas of the iris that resemble tapioca. This form of melanoma is associated with glaucoma in one third of the

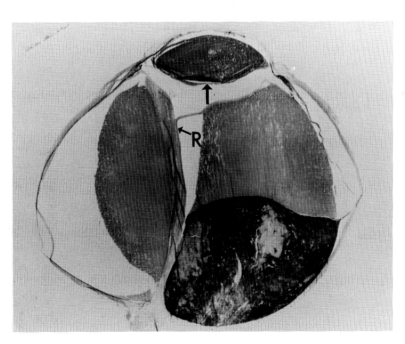

FIG. 13-5. Light microscopic view of large choroidal melanoma with complete retinal detachment *(R)* and anterior displacement of lens *(arrow)* with resultant posterior and anterior synechiae and closure of anterior chamber angle. (Hematoxylin and eosin; ×3.) (From Yanoff, M. Published with permission from the American Journal of Ophthalmology **70**:898-904, 1970. Copyright by the Ophthalmic Publishing Co.)

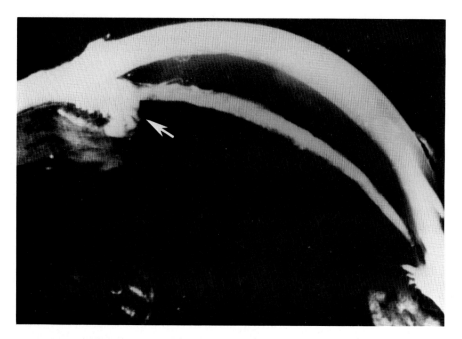

FIG. 13-6. Gross pathology specimen showing ciliary body tumor *(arrow)*.

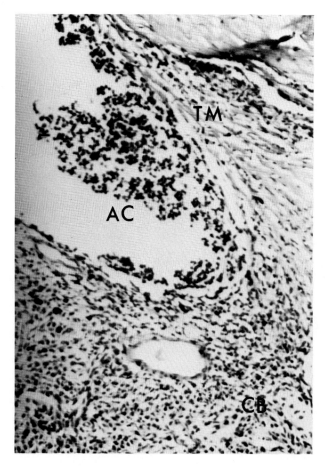

FIG. 13-7. Light microscopic view of eye in Fig. 13-6 showing epithelioid melanoma of ciliary body *(CB)* with tumor cells in anterior chamber angle *(AC)* and trabecular meshwork *(TM)*. (Hematoxylin and eosin; ×250.)

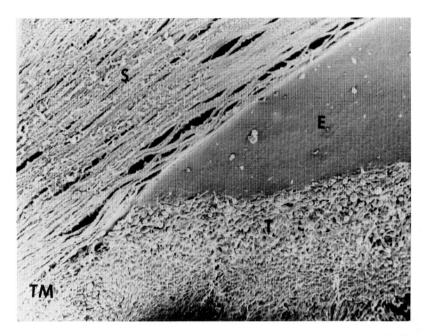

FIG. 13-8. Scanning electron microscopic view of eye with malignant melanoma of ciliary body showing tumor cells *(T)* in anterior chamber and on cornea; corneal endothelium *(E);* corneal stroma *(S);* and trabecular meshwork *(TM).* (×120.) (From Shields, M.B., and Klintworth, G.K.: Ophthalmology **87:**503, 1980.)

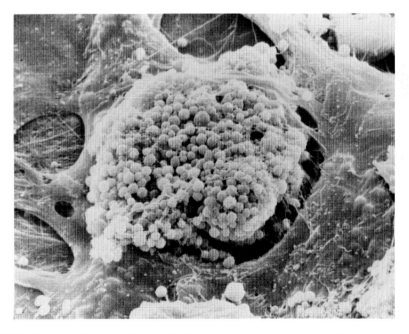

FIG. 13-9. Scanning electron microscopic view of melanin granules in trabecular meshwork of eye with ciliary body melanoma. (×3,800.) (From Shields, M.B., and Klintworth, G.K.: Ophthalmology **87:**503, 1980.)

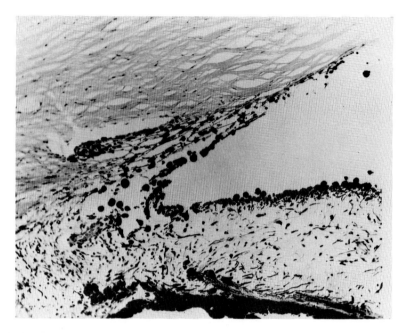

FIG. 13-10. Light microscopic view of eye with necrotic malignant melanoma of ciliary body showing section not containing neoplasm, in which pigment-laden macrophages are on anterior surface of iris, on posterior surface of cornea, in anterior chamber angle, and within trabecular meshwork. (Hematoxylin and eosin; ×100.) (From Yanoff, M., and Scheie, H.G.: Arch. Ophthalmol. **84:**471, 1970. Copyright 1970, American Medical Association.)

cases.[35] Rarely, anterior uveal melanomas produce an angle-closure glaucoma either by the formation of peripheral anterior synechiae from a diffuse melanoma on the anterior surface of the iris[22] or by acute angle-closure glaucoma associated with a melanoma of the ciliary body and anterior choroid.[48]

Management

In nearly all cases eyes with malignant melanoma of the uvea and secondary glaucoma are enucleated. By the time glaucoma has developed, the melanoma is either large and associated with extensive retinal detachment or has spread throughout the anterior chamber angle by direct extension or seeding. In the previously mentioned clinicopathologic study of 11 eyes with anterior uveal melanoma, 3 of the 4 patients with ciliary body melanoma and glaucoma died of metastatic melanoma within 2½ years after enucleation.[44] Histologic examination of these three eyes revealed epithelioid melanoma cells in the anterior chamber angle, occasionally as far into the aqueous outflow system as Schlemm's canal. This is clearly a potential route of metastasis from the eye, and diagnostic and surgical maneuvers that raise the intraocular pressure may accelerate this mode

of tumor spread. Melanomas of the iris have a more benign course than those of the choroid,[36] with reports of long survival rates,[10] suggesting the possibility for more conservative management. However, rarely, metastases have been reported with malignant melanoma limited to the iris,[47] including a tapioca iris melanoma.[55]

The standard technique of enucleation produces a marked elevation of the intraocular pressure, which may cause extraocular dissemination of tumor cells at the time of surgery. This is especially likely when prior glaucoma exists on the basis of tumor cells in the aqueous outflow channels.[44] Suggested measures to reduce this dissemination of melanoma cells at the time of enucleation include cauterization of all episcleral vessels when the cells are thought to be in the filtration angle[44] and stabilization of the intraocular pressure with techniques such as a manometric pressure-regulating system.[26]

BENIGN OCULAR TUMORS

As previously noted, a nevus of the iris may occasionally be confused with a malignant melanoma, especially when it is associated with glaucoma. The iris nevus (Cogan-Reese) syndrome[38] is characterized by the presence of nodular or dif-

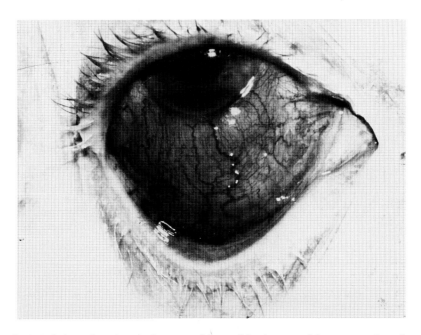

FIG. 13-11. Inferior subconjunctival mass and layered hyphema and hypopyon, obscuring mass of iris and ciliary body in patient with metastatic carcinoma.

fuse pigmented lesions on the surface of the iris. It is thought to be a variation of the iridocorneal endothelial syndrome.[43] The glaucoma in this group of disorders is associated with a membrane across the anterior chamber angle, the contracture of which leads to the formation of peripheral anterior synechiae.[6] Glaucoma has also been observed in association with a necrotic melanocytoma of the iris, and the mechanism of glaucoma in the case studied was thought to be dispersion of pigment into the anterior chamber angle.[41] Secondary glaucoma has been reported in association with a nevus of Ota that was presumably due to the heavy pigmentation of the trabecular meshwork.[16] Cysts of the iris or ciliary body may develop from separation of the epithelial layers, and in rare cases these may be extensive enough to cause forward displacement of the peripheral iris with secondary angle-closure glaucoma.[7] An unusual form of glaucoma has been described in which an epithelial inclusion cyst of the iris with numerous goblet cells ruptured, leading to open-angle glaucoma, presumably due to mucus in the trabecular meshwork.[28]

METASTATIC MALIGNANCIES
Metastatic carcinoma

The prevalence of metastatic carcinoma in the eye and orbit was 12% in one study of 203 patients with autopsy-proved primary carcinoma.[3] The most common primary sites are the breast and lung, and the most common site of ocular metastasis is the posterior uvea.[3,12] In a series of 227 cases of carcinoma metastatic to the eye and orbit, glaucoma was present in 7.5%.[12] In 26 of the 227 eyes, the metastatic carcinoma was primarily in the anterior segment of the eye and the prevalence of glaucoma was 56%.[13] Ocular symptoms in eyes with anterior uveal tumors include reduced visual acuity, redness, and pain; the common signs consist of grayish white, translucent nodules on the iris, iridocyclitis, hypopyon, rubeosis, and hyphema[13,19,32] (Fig. 13-11).

The mechanism of glaucoma in eyes with metastatic carcinoma may be of the open- or closed-angle type. In some cases the trabecular meshwork may be covered by sheetlike plaques of tumor cells or infiltrated by neoplastic cells, whereas other eyes may have angle closure due to the tumor mass or peripheral anterior synechiae.[13] Iridocyclitis, hyphema, and rubeosis iridis may also contribute to the glaucoma.

In the above-mentioned study of 227 eyes, the median survival from the time of ocular surgery (enucleation, iridectomy, cyclectomy, paracentesis, or glaucoma filtering surgery) was 5.4 months when the metastasis was predominantly in the anterior uveal tract and 7.2 months when the metastasis was confined to the posterior ocular segment.[13] Since enucleation would not be expected to prolong survival, it is rarely indicated except for intractable pain. Metastatic carcinomas typically respond well to radiation therapy, and this is the preferred treatment in most cases. Chemotherapy and laser photocoagulation have also been used.[17] Paracentesis of the anterior chamber with cytologic examination of the aspirate is helpful when the diagnosis is in doubt. In some cases the glaucoma may persist after radiation therapy, and this should be managed in the most conservative manner that is sufficient to control the intraocular pressure.

Leukemia

Acute leukemia may also involve the anterior chamber of the eye. In one study of 39 children with acute leukemia (predominately lymphatic or myelocytic), anterior chamber activity was found in 28%,[1] and anterior chamber involvement associated with acute lymphoblastic leukemia is described in another report.[33] Glaucoma may be a complication of leukemic infiltration of the anterior ocular segment and may present in association with hyphema and hypopyon.[37,56] Anterior chamber paracentesis may provide the cytologic diagnosis, and treatment consists of irradiation and chemotherapy. Infiltration of the anterior segment of the eye in a case of histiocytosis-X has also been reported as a cause of secondary glaucoma.[11]

NEOPLASMS IN CHILDREN
Retinoblastoma

Retinoblastoma, the most common intraocular malignancy in children, may be associated with secondary glaucoma. In a histologic study of 149 eyes, evidence of a glaucoma-inducing mechanism was seen in 49.6% of the cases, although an elevated intraocular pressure was recorded in the clinical records in only 22.8%.[54] The most common mechanism of glaucoma in this study was neovascularization of the iris and the formation of peripheral anterior synechiae, which were present in 30% of the eyes. Two additional large histopathologic studies of retinoblastoma also found rubeosis iridis in a high percentage of the cases.[46,51]

Although glaucoma is rarely observed clinically,[46,51] histologic evidence suggests that it is present in many cases.[46] Iris neovascularization carries a more grave prognosis, and the physician should pay close attention to the iris and anterior segment in managing eyes with retinoblastoma.[46] Other causes of glaucoma in eyes with retinoblastoma include invasion of the angle with tumor cells, which may masquerade as uveitis with hypopyon, and

angle-closure glaucoma due to compression by the tumor mass or increased posterior segment volume associated with subretinal exudate and retinal detachment.[51,54] The treatment of most eyes with retinoblastoma, especially when glaucoma is present, is enucleation.

Juvenile xanthogranuloma

Juvenile xanthogranuloma, a benign disease of infancy and childhood, is characterized by yellow, elevated, papular cutaneous lesions most commonly of the head and neck. Involvement of the iris, which is characteristically unilateral, consists of salmon-colored to darkly pigmented lesions, which remain asymptomatic in some eyes and lead to spontaneous hyphema or uveitis in other eyes.[57] Secondary glaucoma may result from infiltration or compression of the angle by the tumor or from the hyphema or uveitis. The diagnosis can be made by paracentesis, which reveals histiocytes and Touton giant cells,[39] although the clinical history and picture is usually sufficient to make the diagnosis. The recommended treatment of juvenile xanthogranuloma with secondary glaucoma is corticosteroids combined with irradiation.[20]

Medulloepithelioma

A medulloepithelioma (diktyoma) is a primary tumor of childhood that arises most often from nonpigmented ciliary epithelium.[4] In a study of 56 cases, glaucoma was observed clinically in 26 eyes, and histopathologic evidence of secondary glaucoma was seen in 18 eyes, 11 of which had rubeosis iridis.[4] Peripheral anterior synechiae and shallow anterior chambers were also commonly observed. In one report, unilateral glaucoma occurred in an infant with two white flocculi floating in the anterior chamber, delicate neovascularization of the iris, and a globular ciliary body mass.[23] The diagnosis of medulloepithelioma was established by electron microscopic examination of the surgically removed flocculi, and the glaucoma was subsequently controlled with cyclocryotherapy and topical epinephrine.

REFERENCES

1. Abramson, A.: Anterior chamber activity in children with acute leukemia, Ann. Ophthalmol. **12:**553, 1980.
2. Bateman, J.B., and Foos, R.Y.: Coronal adenomas, Arch. Ophthalmol. **97:**2379, 1979.
3. Bloch, R.S., and Gartner, S.: The incidence of ocular metastatic carcinoma, Arch. Ophthalmol. **85:**673, 1971.
4. Broughton, W.L., and Zimmerman, L.E.: A clinicopathologic study of 56 cases of intraocular medulloepitheliomas, Am. J. Ophthalmol. **85:**407, 1978.

5. Brovkina, A.F., and Chichua, A.G.: Value of fluorescein iridography in diagnosis of tumours of the iridociliary zone, Br. J. Ophthalmol. **63:**157, 1979.

6. Campbell, D.G., Shields, M.B., and Smith, T.R.: The corneal endothelium and the spectrum of essential iris atrophy, Am. J. Ophthalmol. **86:**317, 1978.

7. Chandler, P.A., and Grant, W.M.: Lectures on glaucoma, Philadelphia, 1965, Lea & Febiger, pp. 208-209.

8. Christiansen, J.M., Wetzig, P.C., Thatcher, D.B., and Green, W.R.: Diagnosis and management of anterior uveal tumors, Ophthalmic Surg. **10:**81, 1979.

9. Dunnington, J.H.: Intraocular tension in cases of sarcoma of the choroid and ciliary body, Arch. Ophthalmol. **20:**359, 1938.

10. Dunphy, E.B., Dryja, T.P., Albert, D.M., and Smith, T.R.: Melanocytic tumor of the anterior uvea, Am. J. Ophthalmol. **86:**680, 1978.

11. Epstein, D.L., and Grant, W.M.: Secondary open-angle glaucoma in histiocytosis X, Am. J. Ophthalmol. **84:**332, 1977.

12. Ferry, A.P., and Font, R.L.: Carcinoma metastatic to the eye and orbit. I. A clinicopathologic study of 227 cases, Arch. Ophthalmol. **92:**276, 1974.

13. Ferry, A.P., and Font, R.L.: Carcinoma metastatic to the eye and orbit. II. A clinicopathological study of 26 patients with carcinoma metastatic to the anterior segment of the eye, Arch. Ophthalmol. **93:**472, 1975.

14. Font, R.L., Reynolds, A.M., Jr., and Zimmerman, L.E.: Diffuse malignant melanoma of the iris in the nevus of Ota, Arch. Ophthalmol. **77:**513, 1967.

15. Foss, R.Y., Hull, S.N., and Straatsma, B.R.: Early diagnosis of ciliary body melanomas, Arch. Ophthalmol. **81:**336, 1969.

16. Foulks, G.N., and Shields, M.B.: Glaucoma in oculodermal melanocytosis, Ann. Ophthalmol. **9:**1299, 1977.

17. Frank K.W., Sugar, H.S., Sherman, A.I., et al.: Anterior segment metastases from an ovarian choriocarcinoma, Am. J. Ophthalmol. **87:**778, 1979.

18. Fraser, D.J., and Font, R.L.: Ocular inflammation and hemorrhage as initial manifestations of uveal malignant melanoma: incidence and prognosis, Arch. Ophthalmol. **97:**1311, 1979.

19. Freeman, T.R., and Friedman, A.H.: Metastatic carcinoma of the iris, Am. J. Ophthalmol. **80:**947, 1975.

20. Gass, J.D.M.: Management of juvenile xanthogranuloma of the iris, Arch. Ophthalmol. **71:**344, 1964.

21. Gitter, K.A., Meyer, D., and Sarin, L.K.: Ultrasound to evaluate eyes with opaque media, Am. J. Ophthalmol. **64:**100, 1967.

22. Hopkins, R.E., and Carriker, F.R.: Malignant melanoma of the ciliary body, Am. J. Ophthalmol. **45:**835, 1958.

23. Jakobiec, F.A., Howard, G.M., Ellsworth, R.M., and Rosen, M.: Electron microscopic diagnosis of medulloepithelioma, Am. J. Ophthalmol. **79:**321, 1975.

24. Jakobiec, F.A., Yanoff, M., Mottow, L., et al.: Solitary iris nevus associated with peripheral anterior synechiae and iris endothelialization, Am. J. Ophthalmol. **83:**884, 1977.

25. Jensen, O.A.: Malignant melanomas of the uvea in Denmark 1943-1952, Acta Ophthalmol. Suppl. **75:**1, 1963.

26. Kramer, K.K., LaPiana, F.G., and Whitmore, P.V.: Enucleation with stabilization of intraocular pressure in the treatment of uveal melanomas, Ophthalmic Surg. **11:**39, 1980.

27. Kraushar, M.F., and Medow, N.B.: Malignant melanoma of the choroid presenting as choroidal detachment following cataract surgery, Ophthalmic. Surg. **10:**68, 1979.

28. Layden, W.E., Torczynski, E., and Font, R.L.: Mucogenic glaucoma and goblet cell cysts of the anterior chamber, Arch. Ophthalmol. **96:**2259, 1978.

29. Levine, D.J.: Surgical reversal of acute angle closure glaucoma due to malignant melanoma: case report, Glaucoma **1:**84, 1979.

30. Marshall, C.D.: On tension in cases of intraocular tumor, Trans. Ophthalmol. Soc. U.K. **16:**155, 1896.

31. Martin-Jones, J.D.: Uveal sarcomata, Br. J. Ophthalmol. **11**(suppl.)**:**27, 1946.

32. Miller, B., Rush, P., and Luntz, M.H.: Metastatic carcinomas of the iris, Ann. Ophthalmol. **12:**514, 1980.

33. Ninane, J., Taylor, D., and Day, S.: The eye as a sanctuary in acute lymphoblastic leukemia, Lancet **1:**452, 1980.

34. Offret, H., and Saraux, H.: Adenoma of the iris pigment epithelium, Arch. Ophthalmol. **98:**875, 1980.

35. Reese, A.B., Mund, M.L., and Iwamoto, T.: Tapioca melanoma of the iris. I. Clinical and light microscopy studies, Am. J. Ophthalmol. **74:**840, 1972.

36. Rones, B., and Zimmerman, L.E.: The prognosis of primary tumors of the iris treated by iridectomy, Arch. Ophthalmol. **60:**193, 1958.

37. Rowan, P.J., and Sloan, J.B.: Iris and anterior chamber involvement in leukemia, Ann. Ophthalmol. **8:**1081, 1976.

38. Scheie, H.G., and Yanoff, M.: Iris nevus (Cogan-Reese) syndrome: a cause of unilateral glaucoma, Arch. Ophthalmol. **93:**963, 1975.

39. Schwartz, L.W., Rodrigues, M.M., and Hallett, J.W.: Juvenile xanthogranuloma diagnosed by paracentesis, Am. J. Ophthalmol. **77:**243, 1974.

40. Shields, J.A.: Accuracy and limitations of the ^{32}P test in the diagnosis of ocular tumors: an analysis of 500 cases, Ophthalmology **85:**950, 1978.

41. Shields, J.A., Annesley, W.H., and Spaeth, G.L.: Necrotic melanocytoma of iris with secondary glaucoma, Am. J. Ophthalmol. **84:**826, 1977.

42. Shields, J.A., Augsburger, J.J., Bernardino, V., et al.: Melanocytoma of the ciliary body and iris, Am. J. Ophthalmol. **89:**632, 1980.

43. Shields, M.B.: Progressive essential iris atrophy, Chandler's syndrome, and the iris nevus (Cogan-Reese) syndrome: a spectrum of disease, Surv. Ophthalmol. **24:**3, 1979.

44. Shields, M.B., and Klintworth, G.K.: Anterior uveal melanomas and intraocular pressure, Ophthalmology **87:**503, 1980.

45. Singer, P.R., Krupin, T., Smith, M.E., and Becker, B.: Recurrent orbital and metastatic melanoma in a patient undergoing previous glaucoma surgery, Am. J. Ophthalmol. **87:**766, 1979.

46. Spaulding, A.G.: Rubeosis iridis in retinoblastoma and pseudoglioma, Trans. Am. Ophthalmol. Soc. **76:**584, 1978.

47. Sunba, M.S.N., Rahi, A.H.S., and Morgan, G.: Tumors of the anterior uvea. I. Metastasizing malignant melanoma of the iris, Arch. Ophthalmol. **98:**82, 1980.

48. Sussman, W., and Weintraub, J.: Acute congestive glaucoma caused by malignant melanoma, Ann. Ophthalmol. **8:**665, 1976.

49. Terry, T.L., and Johns, J.P.: Uveal sarcoma-malignant melanoma: a statistical study of 94 cases, Am. J. Ophthalmol. **18:**903, 1935.

50. Van Buskirk, E.M., and Leure-duPree, A.E.: Pathophysiology and electron microscopy of melanomalytic glaucoma, Am. J. Ophthalmol. **85:**160, 1978.

51. Walton, D.S., and Grant, W.M.: Retinoblastoma and iris neovascularization, Am. J. Ophthalmol. **65:**598, 1968.

52. Yanoff, M.: Glaucoma mechanisms in ocular malignant melanomas, Am. J. Ophthalmol. **70:**898, 1970.

53. Yanoff, M., and Scheie, H.G.: Melanomalytic glaucoma: report of a case, Arch. Ophthalmol. **84:**471, 1970.

54. Yoshizumi, M.O., Thomas, J.V., and Smith, T.R.: Glaucoma-inducing mechanisms in eyes with retinoblastoma, Arch. Ophthalmol. **96:**105, 1978.

55. Zakka, K.A., Foos, R.Y., and Sulit, H.: Metastatic tapioca iris melanoma, Br. J. Ophthalmol. **63:**744, 1979.

56. Zakka, K.A., Yee, R.D., Shorr, N., et al.: Leukemic iris infiltration, Am. J. Ophthalmol. **89:**204, 1980.

57. Zimmermann, L.: Ocular lesions of juvenile xanthogranuloma (nevoxanthoendothelioma), Trans. Am. Acad. Ophthalmol. Otolaryngol. **69:**412, 1965.

GLAUCOMAS ASSOCIATED WITH SYSTEMIC DISEASE AND DRUGS

Chapter 14

GLAUCOMA SECONDARY TO ELEVATED EPISCLERAL VENOUS PRESSURE

Michael E. Yablonski and Steven M. Podos

HISTORICAL BACKGROUND

Ascher[3-5] (1942) first reported that clear aqueous could be observed to flow in the episcleral veins of humans. This finding confirmed previous histologic studies of the human eye that showed connections between Schlemm's canal and the episcleral veins.[5] Previous animal experiments had indicated that aqueous flowed out of the eye into the episcleral veins; Ascher noted that Lauber (1901) showed that the blood of the dog anterior ciliary vein contained a lower erythrocyte concentration than systemic blood and explained this observation on the basis of dilution of the blood with aqueous. Uribe-Troncoso[73] (1921) collected clear fluid from the perilimbal sclera of the in vivo rabbit eye immersed in oil, measured the rate of aqueous flow at 2.1 μl/min, and showed the patent connections between the anterior chamber and the episclera. Seidel[67] (1923) showed that India ink injected into the anterior chamber of the rabbit soon appeared in the episcleral veins. He postulated that the driving force for flow of aqueous out of the eye was the hydrostatic pressure difference between the anterior chamber and the episcleral veins. This concept was further developed by Goldmann[31] (1949).

After Ascher's observation of aqueous veins in humans, it was hoped that the study of these veins might be helpful in the diagnosis and treatment of glaucoma. Ascher believed that there were fundamental differences in the appearance of these veins in glaucomatous eyes as compared with the veins in normal eyes. Several glaucoma medications were reported to alter the appearance of the aqueous veins.[4,5,30] Despite initial enthusiasm, however, the clinical significance of the evaluation of the aqueous veins remains controversial.

Seidel[67] first began measuring episcleral venous pressure using a pressure chamber technique. After Ascher's emphasis on the importance of episcleral veins, the measurement of episcleral venous pressure received renewed interest. Using the pressure chamber technique, Thomassen[71] (1947) studied the effect of pilocarpine on episcleral venous pressure. Linner[48] (1949) showed episcleral venous pressure to be less than intraocular pressure, and Thomassen et al.[72] (1950) and Bain[7] (1954) showed that diurnal changes in episcleral venous pressure preceded similar changes in intraocular pressure. Goldmann[31] (1949) introduced a torsion balance technique for measuring episcleral venous pressure. This technique was used by Minas and Podos[55] and by Podos et al.[62] and was found to be comparable to the pressure chamber method used by Brubaker.[21] A third method of measurement, utilizing a jet of air, was introduced by Krakau et al.[43,44] (1973).

The measurement of the effect of increased episcleral venous pressure on intraocular pressure yielded significant data concerning the phenomenon of pseudofacility.[46] Disappointingly, episcleral venous pressure measurements were of no clinical value in primary open-angle glaucoma[62];

however, in several secondary glaucomas, they were found to be very important. An elevated episcleral venous pressure was found to be the cause of increased intraocular pressure in carotid cavernous fistula.[75] Weiss[76] and Phelps[60] showed most cases of glaucoma in encephalotrigeminal angiomatosis to be due to episcleral venous pressure elevation. Minas and Podos[55] described a familial form of secondary glaucoma due to idiopathic elevation of episcleral venous pressure. Recently we have been impressed with the frequent occurrence of an elevated intraocular pressure due to increased episcleral venous pressure in thyroid ophthalmopathy.

ANATOMY AND PATHOPHYSIOLOGY
Anatomy of the venous system (Fig. 14-1)

The venous drainage of the orbit occurs by three principal routes: the superior ophthalmic vein, the inferior ophthalmic vein, and the facial veins, all of which are interanastomosed. The main route of blood flow from the eye is via the superior ophthalmic vein, which drains intracranially through the superior orbital fissure into the cavernous sinus, from which blood is drained primarily via the superior and inferior petrosal sinuses into the internal jugular vein.[2] A relatively small amount is drained via the external jugular veins and still less via the suboccipital plexus into the vertebral and deep cervical veins.[2,53] The cavernous sinus also has connections with the ipsilateral

pterygoid plexus and the contralateral cavernous sinus.[18,19]

The inferior ophthalmic vein communicates with the larger superior ophthalmic vein and also sends branches through the inferior orbital fissure to the pterygoid plexus, which drains into the deep veins of the neck.

The facial veins communicate with the superior ophthalmic vein via the nasofrontal, lacrimal, and lid veins and communicate with the inferior ophthalmic vein via the infraorbital vein. The facial veins drain mainly in the external jugular veins.

Because of the numerous interconnections between the orbital venous drainage routes and the lack of venous valves, blood can be diverted from one system to the other with blood flow in any direction, depending on the hydrostatic pressure gradient.[25,69]

The venous distribution of the eye itself is divided into several systems: the retinal veins, vortex veins, anterior ciliary veins, and posterior ciliary veins, with variable anastomotic connections existing between them. The retinal veins drain into the central retinal vein, which leaves the eye through the lamina cribrosa and then traverses the optic nerve for a variable distance before exiting to join the orbital veins. The vortex veins are the main venous drainage for the uveal tissue of the eye and are in turn connected to the orbital veins via the posterior ciliary veins.[37] The anterior ciliary veins drain the anterior uvea, emerging from

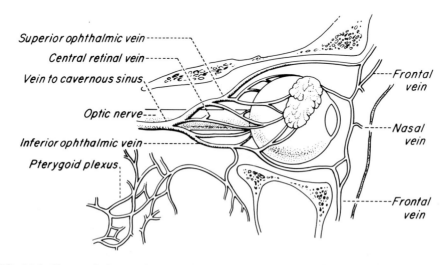

FIG. 14-1. Venous drainage of orbit. Superior ophthalmic vein, inferior ophthalmic vein, and facial veins are three principal routes of orbital venous drainage, all interanastamosed as shown. Superior ophthalmic vein is main route, draining through superior orbital fissure into cavernous sinus. Inferior ophthalmic vein drains mainly into pterygoid plexus. Facial veins drain into external jugular veins.

the eye near the limbus, where they form the circumcorneal ring of episcleral veins, which anastomose with the bulbar conjunctival veins.[5] The episcleral veins are the system into which drain the collector channels of Schlemm's canal. From the episcleral veins blood flows into the orbital veins mainly via the veins of the extraocular muscles. The posterior ciliary veins drain the posterior region of the sclera. Under conditions in which central venous pressure is abnormally high, anastomotic channels are found between the retinal venous system and the vortex system.[6] In humans there are no appreciable connections between the vortex veins and the episcleral veins.

Normal aqueous humor dynamics

Aqueous is normally secreted by the ciliary body at a rate of approximately 2.0 μl/min. Some of this fluid, the exact proportion of which is uncertain, leaves the eye by pressure-independent routes.[13,14] However, the bulk of the aqueous humor leaves the eye across the trabecular meshwork into Schlemm's canal, from which it drains via collector channels into the episcleral veins.[3-5] The rate of aqueous flow by this route, F_s, is given by equation 1, which assumes the flow to be a passive process; hence it is a function of intraocular pressure, P_i, minus episcleral venous pressure, P_e (assumed to equal the hydrostatic pressure in Schlemm's canal),[47,49] and the resistance to flow, R_t, offered by the tissues lying between the anterior chamber and Schlemm's canal.[31]

$$F_s = (P_i - P_e)/R_t \qquad (1)$$

Equation 1 pertains only to the condition in which intraocular pressure exceeds episcleral venous pressure ($P_i - P_e > 0$). Protein colloid osmotic pressure has been omitted from equation 1 because under the usual circumstance of $P_i - P_e > 0$, the values of protein colloid osmotic pressure in the anterior chamber and Schlemm's canal, π_i and π_s respectively, nearly equal zero. Equation 2 takes into account the protein colloid osmotic pressure.

$$F_s = (P_I - P_e + \sigma_s[\pi_s - \pi_i])/R_t \qquad (2)$$

Under the condition of $\pi_s = \pi_i = 0$, equation 2 reduces to equation 1. σ_s is the reflection coefficient for protein of the tissues between the anterior chamber and the canal,[41] probably nearly equal to 1.0, and is therefore omitted from equation 3.

$$F_s = (P_i - P_e + \pi_s - \pi_i)/R_t \qquad (3)$$

It has been shown that when intraocular pressure falls below episcleral pressure ($P_i - P_e < 0$), the apparent resistance, R_t, increases many fold.[59] The cause for this apparent rectification across the trabecular meshwork is not known. However, it seems likely to be due to the oncotic pressure of plasma proteins of the blood in Schlemm's canal, which would be considerable under the condition of $P_i - P_e < 0$. Such oncotic pressure would tend to reach a balance with the hydrostatic pressure gradient, resulting in a negligible net flow across the trabecular meshwork. Since π_i would be essentially zero, equation 3 reduces to equation 4, which gives the value of reverse flow from Schlemm's canal into the anterior chamber.

$$F_s \text{ (reverse)} = (P_e - P_i - \pi_s)/R_t \qquad (4)$$

Only when the value of P_e exceeds P_i by more than the value of π_s would an ultrafiltrate of plasma be expected to flow in the reverse direction into the anterior chamber from Schlemm's canal. However, since the value of π_s is equal to about 25 mm Hg when the canal is filled with blood, it is unlikely that P_e would exceed P_i by more than this amount, except under the most extreme conditions (e.g., when the value of P_i has been reduced to zero during surgery in the face of an elevated episcleral venous pressure). Under such circumstances the magnitude of the reverse flow into the anterior chamber would be given by equation 4.

In the steady state, the rate of aqueous production, F_p, must equal the sum of the rate at which aqueous leaves the eye by pressure-independent routes, F_u, and via the trabecular drainage system, F_s.

$$F_p = F_u + F_s \qquad (5)$$

Combining equations 1 and 5 yields equation 6,

$$P_i = (F_p - F_u) R_t + P_e \qquad (6)$$

which shows that in the steady state, intraocular pressure P_i is determined by F_p, F_u, R_t, and P_e. As can be seen from equation 6, intraocular pressure must always be greater than episcleral venous pressure, except for the unusual circumstance in which pressure-independent flow (uveoscleral flow), F_u, exceeds the rate of aqueous humor production, F_p. This, of course, is impossible in the steady state, since the eye would shrivel.

The mechanism of uveoscleral flow is unknown; however, it seems reasonable to assume that a main driving force for F_u is the imbalance of

Starling's forces between the aqueous and the blood. Thus as F_p fell below F_u, P_i would tend to fall below P_e until F_u were decreased to equal F_p. Thus it seems likely that under these extreme circumstances F_u is not truly pressure independent. In the extreme circumstance in which aqueous production has ceased, P_i would fall, according to Starling's law, to a level given by equation 7, at which time F_u would equal zero.

$$P_i = P_c - \sigma_c \pi_c \qquad (7)$$

In this equation P_c is the mean capillary pressure in the eye, π_c is the protein colloid osmotic pressure of plasma, and σ_c is the reflection coefficient for protein between the capillary lumen and aqueous.[41] As described above, reverse flow across the trabecular meshwork in the steady state is not a factor when P_i falls below P_e, because Schlemm's canal soon fills with blood, at which time the oncotic pressure of the blood prevents any reverse flow into the anterior chamber.

Pathophysiology of venous pressure elevation

Elevation of venous pressure has been used to measure the effect of increased intraocular pressure on aqueous production. A cuff placed around the neck of volunteers caused an increase in episcleral venous pressure. It was found that increased P_e was matched by only about four fifths as much an increase in P_i.[45,46] It was concluded that the lack of equality between the changes in P_i and P_e was due to a coincident decrease in the rate of aqueous production, F_p,[46] or to fluid being forced out of the eye from compartments other than the anterior chamber.[8] This interpretation has recently been confirmed by measuring F_p fluorophotometrically.[82] These findings indicate the presence of pseudofacility, namely, that portion of the total outflow facility, C_{total} (measured tonographically), that is not due to fluid leaving the eye through Schlemm's canal.[8]

$$C_{total} = C_t + C_{ps} \qquad (8)$$

where C_{ps} is the pseudofacility and C_t is the true outflow facility, the inverse of R_t, the resistance to outflow across the trabecular meshwork. Nevertheless, it is important to realize that the neck cuff experiment is very difficult to interpret because the condition of steady state is doubtful, and the effect of changes in P_e and P_i on R_t and F_u in equation 6 must be considered.

Rosen and Johnston[64] reported a prompt rise in intraocular pressure in response to the Valsalva maneuver in 93% of normal subjects. They thought that this was most likely due to vascular engorgement of the uvea. This explanation was supported by a sharp fall in intraocular pressure as soon as the Valsalva maneuver ceased. In contrast, only 25% of patients with uncontrolled glaucoma showed an increase, presumably because of the tamponading effect of the intraocular pressure on the uveal blood volume. Uveal vascular engorgement would not be expected to occur until vortex venous pressure exceeded intraocular pressure, which would be less likely if the intraocular pressure were elevated. Segal et al.[66] showed no significant change in arterial blood pressure during pressure breathing at a level of 29.2 mm Hg above atmospheric pressure. They found the relationship between intraocular pressure and venous pressure to be similar to that described by Rosen and Johnston.[64]

Barany[8] has shown that an elevated episcleral venous pressure results in an increase in the total outflow facility, C. This increase in C has been interpreted as most likely being due to a dilation of Schlemm's canal, a result of the increased intraluminal hydrostatic pressure. In contrast, it has been shown that in patients with chronic elevation of venous pressure, outflow facility is decreased, presumably because of secondary pathologic changes in the aqueous outflow channels.[55]

In view of these considerations, it is difficult to predict the exact relationship between elevations in P_e and the resultant increase in intraocular pressure. Under ordinary circumstances it is reasonable to assume that the value of P_i is greater than that of P_e; however, the resultant change in P_i may be less than, equal to, or threoretically even greater than the change in P_e, depending on the corresponding changes in the components of equation 6.

In addition to the direct effect of an elevated episcleral venous pressure on P_i, as described by equation 6, there are other mechanisms by which an elevated venous pressure may cause increased intraocular pressure. If an elevated venous pressure of the eye results in increased vortex venous pressure, there may be an accumulation of blood in the uveal capacitance vessels, causing swelling of the uvea at the expense of anterior chamber volume.* This process may be further aggravated by

_____
*References 15, 33-36, 68, 80.

the imbalance of Starling's forces causing the accumulation of extracellular fluid in the uvea and hence further swelling. Thus, elevated ocular venous pressure may result in shallowing of the anterior chamber and secondary angle-closure glaucoma. Such attacks are often initially intermittent but may lead to permanent angle-closure glaucoma due to the formation of peripheral anterior synechiae.

Another form of glaucoma associated with venous pressure elevation is neovascular glaucoma. The decreased perfusion pressure to the eye results in relative ischemia. Frank central retinal vein thrombosis may result. These factors may lead to the development of rubeosis iridis and result in neovascular glaucoma.[65,69,77]

Chronic elevation of intraocular pressure due to an elevated venous pressure may cause typical glaucomatous optic disc damage, apparently the result of alterations of the nerve head similar to those produced by primary open-angle glaucoma. Increased venous pressure would decrease the perfusion pressure of the blood supply to the nerve head, thus making it more susceptible to damage according to the vascular hypothesis of glaucomatous nerve head damage. On the other hand, to the extent that increased intracranial venous pressure accompanied increased ocular venous pressure, the resultant increased cerebrospinal fluid pressure would be expected to protect the nerve head, according to the mechanical hypothesis.[81]

Effect of pharmacologic agents on episcleral venous pressure

The effect of pilocarpine on P_e has been studied by several investigators with variable results. Thomassen,[71] using the chamber method, found that pilocarpine caused a decrease in P_e; however, the levels of P_e found in this study (about 30 mm Hg) cast doubt on his method. Bain,[7] in a study with only a small number of subjects, found that topical pilocarpine caused a decrease in episcleral venous pressure, which preceded the fall in intraocular pressure. Others found that pilocarpine yielded an initial rise in P_e, lasting 4 to 8 minutes, followed by a return to normal.[40,79] Linner[48] found pilocarpine and acetazolamide to have no effect on P_e.

Topical epinephrine was found to have no effect on P_e by Wilke[79] and Kupfer et al.[45] Similarly, Wettrell et al.[78] found orally administered beta-adrenergic agonists and antagonists to have no effect on P_e. Clonidine has been found to cause an initial transient decrease in P_e 15 minutes after topical application, followed by a return to normal values after 60 minutes.

CLASSIFICATION

Those forms of glaucoma due to an elevated episcleral venous pressure are caused either by obstruction to venous flow, arteriovenous fistulas, or idiopathic episcleral venous pressure elevation.

Venous obstruction

Venous obstruction may be caused by retrobulbar tumors,[11,57] but this is not a common feature. The orbital congestion of thyroid exophthalmos may cause partial obstruction to orbital venous flow and hence result in an elevated ocular venous pressure. The superior vena cava syndrome results in obstruction to the venous return from the head and, consequently, an elevated venous pressure.

Arteriovenous fistula

Increased venous pressure due to increased blood flow is caused by an arteriovenous fistula of some type. Arteriovenous fistulas rarely occur within the orbit itself[22]; however, because of the numerous connections between the intracranial and orbital venous systems, intracranial fistulas commonly raise the ocular venous pressure. A carotid-cavernous fistula is the most common arteriovenous fistula, due most often to traumatic basal skull fractures and spontaneous artery perforation from ruptured, congenital, or atherosclerotic aneurysms of the internal carotid artery.[18,25] Intracranial vascular shunts can occur elsewhere also.[56] For example, fistulas may occur between the middle meningeal artery and the sphenoparietal sinus. These fistulas result in direct entry of arterial blood into the intracranial dural venous sinuses, causing retrograde flow into the veins of the orbit.[22] The extent of the increase in orbital venous pressure depends on the ability of the extracranial routes to drain the orbital venous system.

Orbital venous varix formations may be congenital or secondary to an arteriovenous fistula either within the orbit itself or, more commonly, within the cranium, resulting in the shunting of blood into the orbit.[51,74] What may begin as an orbital hemangioma may progress to a true venous varix.[50,80] The orbital varix not associated with an arteriovenous fistula is more common in children and does not usually result in a sustained elevated venous pressure.

Weiss[76] postulated that glaucoma in the Sturge-Weber syndrome is often due to an elevated P_e secondary to localized arteriovenous fistulas of an episcleral hemangioma. This theory was confirmed by Phelps,[60] who found 19 of 19 glaucomatous eyes with the Sturge-Weber syndrome to show episcleral hemangiomas with a mean episcleral venous pressure of 18.1 ± 6.4 mm Hg. He noted that the episcleral hemangioma may extend into the sclera itself and even involve Schlemm's canal.

Idiopathic elevation of pressure

Elevation of episcleral venous pressure of unknown cause has also been reported.[12,55,63] Perhaps a localized obstruction to venous drainage exists. Another possibility is a localized arteriovenous fistula.[28,30]

DIAGNOSIS

Other causes of ocular hyperemia may be confused with an elevated ocular venous pressure. Local irritation, conjunctivitis, scleritis, episcleritis, and orbital inflammation can best be differentiated from an elevated venous pressure by the measurement of venous pressure.[61] Thus the sine qua non for the diagnosis of glaucoma due to an elevated episcleral venous pressure is the finding of an elevated value for P_e.

Measurement of episcleral venous pressure

All methods used to measure episcleral venous pressure are based on the principle of applying a measurable pressure external to the vein until the wall collapses. It is assumed that venous walls have little inherent rigidity, so that as soon as the pressure externally exceeds the intraluminal pressure, the wall of the vein will begin to collapse.

There has been considerable discussion in the literature as to which endpoint is most accurate.[43,48,54] Theoretically, using the complete collapse of the vein as an endpoint should give falsely elevated measurements, since such collapse would raise the intravenous pressure, depending on the speed of the measurement and the extent of collateral venous flow bypassing the obstruction.[48] Phelps and Armaly[61] reported a difference of 2 to 3 mm Hg between the pressure required to indent the vein slightly and that required for complete collapse. It has been suggested that the earliest perceptible change in venous caliber or 50% reduction in venous caliber be used as the endpoint[54]; however, both of these are less definite than complete venous collapse. Brubaker[21] found that the end-

point causing complete collapse with the pressure chamber technique resulted in close agreement with cannulation measurements. On the other hand, using the Goldmann torsion balance technique, he found the 50% decrease in caliber to be the better endpoint.

The pressure chamber method (Fig. 14-2) was first described by Seidel[67] in 1923. The device consists of a chamber in which the pressure can be altered to any desired level. One side of the chamber is formed by a thin, transparent elastic membrane, which is the side placed against the eye. The opposite side of the chamber is rigid and transparent, enabling one to view the episcleral vein against which the membrane is applied. The pressure in the chamber required to cause the venous endpoint is taken as the episcleral venous pressure.

Another method of measurement (Fig. 14-3), described by Goldmann,[31] uses a torsion balance to apply a variable force over a constant area of conjunctiva overlying the episcleral vein under study.[21,30] The pressure of the endpoint is determined by dividing the force applied by the area of the probe tip.

In the method of measurement described by Krakau et al.,[43] the pressure needed to collapse the episcleral vein is caused by a jet of air directed against the vessel. The advantage of the method is that local anesthetics are not required. The technique has a reproducibility and accuracy comparable to the other techniques, and it was found that episcleral venous pressure was about 3 to 4 mm Hg higher than conjunctival venous pressure. On the other hand, Linner et al.,[49] using a pressure chamber device, reported conjunctival venous pressure to be 0.74 mm Hg higher than P_e and advised that it is possible to use conjunctival veins when episcleral veins are not readily accessible. Conjunctival veins can be distinguished from episcleral veins by the fact that episcleral veins remain fixed whereas conjunctival veins move when an applicator is applied to the surface of the eye.

Phelps and Armaly,[61] using the chamber technique, took measurements at the location where the veins emerge from the sclera and compared them with measurements taken several mm downstream. Podos et al.,[62] using a modification of the Goldmann device, found no significant difference in episcleral venous pressure between normal eyes (9.0 mm Hg) and eyes with primary open-angle glaucoma (8.6 mm Hg). Mims and Holland,[54] using the chamber device, showed no effect of in-

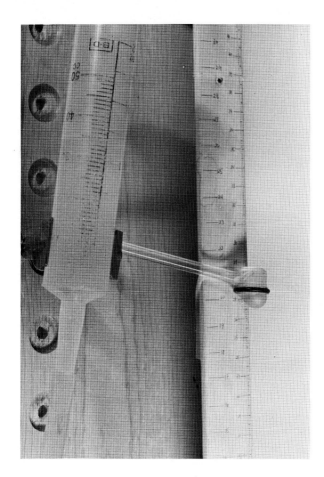

FIG. 14-2. Pressure chamber for measurement of episcleral venous pressure. Plastic chamber, one side of which is formed by thin, transparent elastic membrane that is applied to episcleral veins, is connected by tubing to reservoir, and entire system is filled with water. Height of fluid level in reservoir above chamber determines pressure within chamber.

FIG. 14-3. Torsion balance device for measurement of episcleral venous pressure. (From Podos, S.M., Minas, T.F., and Macri, J.T.: Arch. Ophthalmol. **80:**209, 1968. Copyright 1968, American Medical Association.)

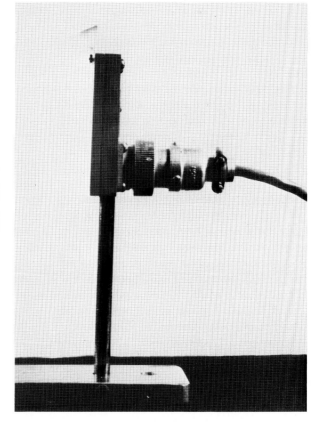

traocular pressure on the value of episcleral venous pressure. Brubaker[21] compared the measurements obtained by the pressure chamber method and the torsion balance method with measurements obtained by direct cannulation in rabbits. He found that cannulation of the vessel wall in the direction of flow yielded measurements that were independent of variations in intraocular pressure, and these measurements were therefore chosen as the standard for comparison. The mean episcleral venous pressure determined by cannulation was 9.3 ± 0.13 mm Hg. The endpoint with the pressure chamber method had better reproducibility than that with the torsion balance method. Total collapse of the episcleral vein with the chamber method gave results not statistically significantly different from those with the cannulation method, whereas this endpoint produced significantly higher values with the torsion bar method.

Certain clinical characteristics are common to most forms of glaucoma due to an elevated episcleral venous pressure. Other characteristics are more specific to individual causes.

General clinical characteristics

Certain clinical characteristics exist in most forms of glaucoma secondary to venous pressure elevation. The episcleral veins are dilated and tortuous.[25] The resultant elevation of intraocular pressure is approximately equal in magnitude to the venous pressure elevation above the normal value of 10 mm Hg.[74] A recumbent posture usually causes a slight rise in episcleral and intraocular pressure. The anterior chamber angle is open and of normal appearance, except that blood is frequently seen in Schlemm's canal, although this is an inconsistent finding and often is seen in normal eyes as well. Tonography usually shows normal values.[74] However, in long-standing cases the outflow resistance is often increased because of damage to the outflow channels.[55] When this occurs, the rise in intraocular pressure may exceed the rise in episcleral venous pressure, and an abnormal elevation of intraocular pressure may persist after the episcleral venous pressure returns to normal. Typical glaucomatous nerve head damage may result, with corresponding glaucomatous visual field loss. An elevated central retinal venous pressure may result in central retinal vein thrombosis and secondary neovascular glaucoma. Extremely dilated retinal veins are usually not seen, because the increase in retinal venous pressure is balanced by the approximately equal increase in intraocular pressure.

Suspicion of an elevated venous pressure as the cause of glaucoma should be aroused whenever glaucoma is accompanied by prominent conjunctival and episcleral vessels. Often the diagnosis is missed because it is assumed that the prominent vessels are due to another cause, such as reaction to glaucoma medications or other causes of external eye inflammation.

Specific clinical characteristics

The individual causes of glaucoma secondary to an elevated ocular venous pressure often have their own distinguishing findings. In some causes of episcleral venous pressure elevation, such as the superior mediastinal syndrome or a severe arteriovenous fistula, the accompanying findings are so striking that the diagnosis is readily apparent. However, in others, such as idiopathic elevation of episcleral venous pressure, the diagnosis is not obvious.

Superior mediastinal syndrome

Superior vena cava obstruction in severe cases is associated with the findings of exophthalmos and a "pumpkin head" appearance due to the edema and cyanosis of the face and neck.[1,2] Patients show dilated veins in the upper extremities, head, neck, and chest. Increased intracranial pressure may cause headache, stupor, vertigo, mental changes, and convulsions. Ocular signs and symptoms include papilledema; prominent veins of the fundus, episclera, and conjunctiva; an elevated P_e; and an elevated intraocular pressure that increases markedly when the patient is in a recumbent position.[9] In one case, the intraocular pressure went from 20 mm Hg to 35 mm Hg when the patient assumed a recumbent position.[20] The optic discs do not usually show glaucomatous cupping, presumably because of the counterbalancing effect of increased intracranial pressure.[81] Mild eye findings may be the earliest manifestations of the syndrome, and the patient may have only eyelid edema.[58] When the syndrome is suspected, pathologic conditions in the upper thorax, such as aortic aneurysm, thoracic neoplasm, and, more rarely, chronic cicatrizing mediastinitis, enlarged hilar lymph nodes, or intrathoracic goiter, must be sought out.

Arteriovenous fistula (Fig. 14-4)

With a carotid-cavernous sinus fistula, the distinguishing clinical features are pulsating exophthalmos with an audible bruit, the subjective sen-

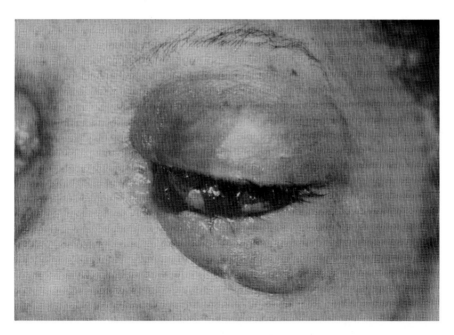

FIG. 14-4. Carotid cavernous fistula: edema of lids, chemosis with protrusion of conjunctiva through palpebral fissure, and proptosis due to raised orbital venous pressure.

sation by the patient of a pulsating sound, and orbital pain.* Because of the low perfusion pressure for blood flow in the eye, vision may be markedly decreased and an ischemic eye syndrome may be present.[18,25,65] Because of intracranial connections between the two cavernous sinuses,[18] a fistula on one side may result in pulsating exophthalmos occurring bilaterally, or it may be alternating.[18,69] The reversal of blood flow into the orbital venous system causes congestion of the orbital veins and soft tissues. Arterial pulsations are transmitted through the shunted blood. Pulsating exophthalmos, edema of the lids and conjunctiva, and dilated tortuous episcleral and conjunctival veins are the result of this pathologic condition.[25,67] In severe cases in which the intraocular pressure rise is not as high as the rise in retinal venous pressure, dilated retinal veins may result. Usually, in cases of an arteriovenous fistula, although the episcleral veins are dilated and tortuous, the intervening tissue retains its normal appearance.[25] Muscle palsy may be associated with an arteriovenous fistula, either because of the trauma causing the fistula or by compression from the orbital edema.[34] Spontaneous choroidal detachments may rarely occur.[34]

The eye findings in an arteriovenous fistula are usually the most prominent findings.[67] Symptoms

of visual impairment and diplopia are present in about half the cases, and ocular pain is present in about one third.[38] Ocular signs are proptosis in nearly all patients and globe pulsations in about 30%.[38] In about 80% of cases one will find conjunctival injection, dilated retinal veins, or an audible bruit heard best by placing the bell of a stethoscope over the closed lids. About 50% of patients have decreased visual acuity and periorbital edema with venous dilation. Papilledema and retinal hemorrhage are rare. Tonography shows large swings in intraocular pressure coincident with the pulse. Outflow facility is usually normal to high if the outflow structures have not been damaged.

Ophthalmodynamometry shows decreased ophthalmic artery pressure in the involved side.[23,38,65] In long-standing cases routine x-ray films may show widening of the superior orbital fissure and pressure erosion of the adjacent sella and sphenoid sinus. The arteriovenous fistula itself is best demonstrated by arteriography.[70] Intraocular pressure is elevated in about 60% of cases; however, glaucomatous nerve head damage is much less common.[69] Madsen[52] reported one case of absolute glaucoma out of 18 patients with an arteriovenous fistula.

An elevated episcleral venous pressure is the most common cause of intraocular pressure elevation in an arteriovenous fistula; however, there are other causes. In cases of long-standing elevation

---

*References 18, 25, 27, 56, 65.

in P_e, the outflow facility may become impaired. The relative ischemia of the eye, due to decreased perfusion pressure, may cause a uveitic reaction with secondary inflammatory angle changes, or frank rubeosis iridis may occur, resulting in neovascular glaucoma.[39,65,77]

Orbital varices

In orbital varices, the most characteristic clinical finding is intermittent exophthalmos, usually brought on by some form of the Valsalva maneuver or by bending over.[42,80] Between episodes the involved eye may actually become enophthalmic.[42] All reported cases have been unilateral. Patients may also show varices of the lids, anterior orbit, forehead, and palate.[50,51,80] Varices elsewhere are sometimes seen also. The conjunctiva may show multiloculated cysts, yielding the erroneous diagnosis of orbital lymphangioma.[80] Orbital x-ray films frequently show orbital phleboliths and an enlarged orbit.[50,51,80] B-scan ultrasound may show retroocular fluid-filled spaces that enlarge during the Valsalva maneuver.[42] Computerized tomography may show the orbital varix as a soft tissue mass.[42] Venography may also reveal the malformation[50,51,80]; however, the abnormality will often be missed on arteriography.

Since venous pressure is usually normal between attacks, glaucoma is not a common feature; however, the outflow facility may decrease, resulting in increased intraocular pressure and glaucomatous nerve head damage.[42] Repeated stress on the nerve due to recurrent proptotic episodes and sometimes actual compression of the optic nerve by the varix may cause optic atrophy to occur; however, usually the vision remains normal throughout life.[42]

Sturge-Weber syndrome

Hemangiomas of the lid without intracranial involvement or with intracranial involvement (Sturge-Weber syndrome) are associated with an elevated episcleral venous pressure and secondary glaucoma, often with buphthalmos in congenital cases.[26,60,76] The glaucomatous eye almost always demonstrates an episcleral hemangioma, the extent of which is proportional to the severity of the glaucoma.[60,76] Usually the glaucomatous eye is associated with a cutaneous hemangioma of the upper lid. Other ocular lesions include a darker iris on the affected side and, occasionally, tortuous retinal vessels. These patients may show a marked eleva-

tion of intraocular pressure when recumbent, presumably because of choroidal hemangioma distention. This is a transient phenomenon, and such a change would not cause a steady-state increase in intraocular pressure unless the lens-iris diaphragm were pushed forward enough to yield angle closure.

In encephalotrigeminal angiomatosis, the characteristic associated findings provide the diagnosis. Nevertheless, the episcleral venous pressure must be measured to establish that the elevated intraocular pressure is due to an elevated P_e. The episcleral hemangiomas may occasionally be difficult to see except by careful biomicroscopic examination.[60] Occasionally the hemangioma is seen only at the time of trabeculectomy, when Tenon's cover is reflected. Other types of glaucoma are also associated with this phakomatosis[23,76] (see Chapter 4), although according to Phelps,[60] by far the most common cause of glaucoma is an elevated P_e. In addition, choroidal hemangiomas may occur that shallow the anterior chamber and compromise the angle.

Idiopathic elevation of P_e (Fig. 14-5)

Idiopathic elevation[12,55,62,63] of episcleral venous pressure tends to run in families. Patients show an elevated episcleral venous pressure that is somewhat less than the elevation of intraocular pressure. Often the outflow facility is abnormally low.[12,62,63] The angle is open with or without blood in Schlemm's canal. The course is similar to that of open-angle glaucoma with the eventual development of glaucomatous nerve head damage and corresponding visual field loss if the intraocular pressure is sufficiently elevated.

Thyroid exophthalmopathy (Fig. 14-6)

In thyroid exophthalmopathy, the intraocular pressure may become elevated. Sometimes this pressure elevation is due to the restriction of extraocular muscles, and the resultant transient elevation of intraocular pressure occurs when the patient attempts to properly position the eyes for tonometry.[16] In severe exophthalmos, the orbital congestion may cause an elevated ocular venous pressure and resultant increased intraocular pressure. The outflow facility, as measured by tonography, may be abnormally high; however, it seems likely that much of this observation is due to an increased pseudofacility caused by the engorged choroid.

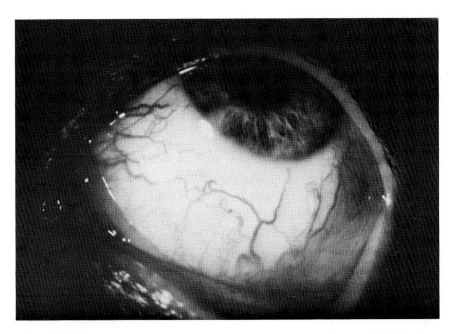

FIG. 14-5. Idiopathic elevation of episcleral venous pressure. Prominent episcleral veins associated with elevated intraocular pressure and elevated episcleral venous pressure is often found in other family members also.

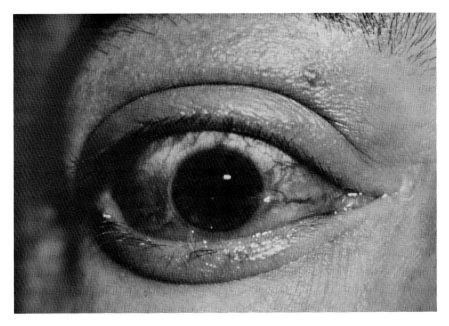

FIG. 14-6. Thyroid exophthalmopathy. Proptosis, lid retraction, and lid edema typical of Graves' disease. Dilated episcleral veins with episcleral venous pressure elevation secondary to orbital congestion.

MANAGEMENT
Management of the underlying cause

The treatment of open-angle glaucoma secondary to an elevated episcleral venous pressure should initially be directed to treating the underlying cause of the venous pressure elevation.

Superior mediastinal syndrome

In the superior mediastinal syndrome, the primary concern is to treat the cause of the superior vena cava obstruction. Once the cause of the obstruction is diagnosed, its successful treatment will usually result in the alleviation of the eye findings as well.

Arteriovenous fistula

Treatment of an arteriovenous fistula has taken several forms: ligation of the ipsilateral internal carotid artery, intentional embolization of the fistula, and intracranial ligation of arteries leading to the fistula.[52,65] On the other hand, without surgical intervention one might expect spontaneous closure of the fistula in 18% of patients and a significant improvement in 43%, with only 33% showing no change and 6% dying of the disease.[52] Strokes are a common complication of surgical intervention, and most cases of neovascular glaucoma associated with arteriovenous fistulas occur only after surgical correction of the fistula,[65,77] whereas the glaucoma due only to the elevation of episcleral venous pressure is seldom of the severe type leading to blindness. Consequently, Sanders and Hoyt[65] have cautioned against surgical intervention unless the course is deteriorating.

Orbital varices

Orbital varices are usually a fairly benign condition. Attempted surgical removal of such a vascular anomaly is likely to do more irreparable damage to vision than would occur from the condition itself if left untreated.[17] The main indication for surgery is cosmetic.[80] If the varices involve the lids and episcleral tissues, removal may yield considerable cosmetic improvement with little risk as long as the orbit behind the equator of the globe is not entered.[80]

Thyroid exophthalmopathy

In cases of glaucoma with an elevated P_e associated with the orbital congestion of thyroid exophthalmopathy, the intraocular pressure will come under better control as the orbital congestion improves. The improvement may occur spontane- ously or may follow treatment of the underlying thyroid disorder. Steroids have been described as successful, and occasionally surgical orbital decompression becomes necessary in order to save the vision of the eye.

Management of the glaucoma
Medical therapy

The treatment of elevated intraocular pressure when it is due to an elevated episcleral venous pressure is similar to the treatment of simple open-angle glaucoma with some notable differences.[42] Drugs that decrease the rate of aqueous formation, such as carbonic anhydrase inhibitors[55] and beta-adrenergic blocking agents, are effective. Drugs that increase the outflow facility, such as topical miotics[1] and epinephrine, may yield a decrease in intraocular pressure, especially if the outflow facility has been compromised.[5,39] However, the elevated episcleral venous pressure presents a limit below which the intraocular pressure may not be decreased despite a marked decrease in the rate of aqueous production and an increased outflow facility, thus limiting the effects of these agents. Although oxygen inhalation has been shown to lower P_e,[29] more practical pharmacologic agents that lower P_e have not been found.

Surgical therapy

If the intraocular pressure cannot be decreased to an acceptable level as determined by the usual criteria used for open-angle glaucoma, namely, progressive deterioration of visual field and optic disc, glaucoma surgery may be necessary. Only by the usual glaucoma filtering operation can intraocular pressure be decreased below episcleral venous pressure; however, the surgery is accompanied by complications not present in simple open-angle glaucoma. Because of an elevated ocular capillary pressure secondary to venous pressure elevation, when intraocular pressure is decreased to atmospheric pressure after the eye is opened, the capillary hydrostatic pressure may exceed the oncotic pressure of plasma proteins, resulting in sustained transcapillary filtration into intraocular tissues.

This is most marked in the choroid and ciliary body, where the capillary filtration coefficient is highest. For this reason Bellows et al.[10] have recommended the routine drainage of the suprachoroid at the time of filtering surgery and have advised leaving the posterior sclerostomy patent after surgery to prevent the postoperative formation of a choroidal effusion.[10] Bigger[12] has pointed out that eye surgery in these patients is associated with a tendency for hemorrhage because of the dilated veins and hyperemic tissues. Christensen and Records[24] reported a case of expulsive hemorrhage during intraocular surgery in the Sturge-Weber syndrome, presumably due to an elevated capillary pressure and choroidal hemangioma.[24]

If neovascular glaucoma occurs, the prognosis is particularly bleak. This type of glaucoma, associated with an elevated episcleral venous pressure, is usually associated with a large AV fistula in which the decreased perfusion pressure results in an ischemic eye and rubeosis iridis. Such an occurrence would lend strong weight in favor of surgical correction of the fistula; however, panretinal photocoagulation was found to be effective in one case of a carotid-cavernous fistula.[36] Usually rubeosis iridis associated with an AV fistula occurs only after surgical correction of the fistula. The medical and surgical treatment of this type of neorvascular glaucoma is otherwise similar to that of other types of neovascular glaucoma as described in Chapter 12.

REFERENCES

1. Alfano, J.E.: Glaucoma following ligation of the superior vena cava, Am. J. Ophthalmol. **60:**412, 1965.
2. Alfano, J.E., and Alfano, P.A.: Glaucoma and the superior vena caval obstruction syndrome, Am. J. Ophthalmol. **42:**685, 1956.
3. Ascher, K.W.: Aqueous veins, Am. J. Ophthalmol. **25:** 31, 1942.
4. Ascher, K.W.: Aqueous veins: local pharmacologic effects on aqueous veins; glaucoma and aqueous veins, Am. J. Ophthalmol. **25:**1301, 1942.
5. Ascher, K.W.: The aqueous veins: physiologic importance of the visible elimination of intraocular fluid, Am. J. Ophthalmol. **25:**1174, 1942.
6. Anderson, D.R.: Vascular supply to the optic nerve of primates, Am. J. Ophthalmol. **70:**341, 1970.
7. Bain, W.E.S.: Variations in the episcleral venous pressure in relation to glaucoma, Br. J. Ophthalmol. **38:**129, 1954.
8. Barany, E.H.: The influence of extraocular venous pressure on outflow facility in Cercopithecus ethiops and Macaca fascicularis, Invest. Ophthalmol. Vis. Sci. **17:** 711, 1978.
9. Bedrosian, E.H.: Increased intraocular pressure secondary to mediastinal syndrome, Arch. Ophthalmol. **47:**641, 1952.
10. Bellows, R.A., Chylack, L.T., Epstein, D.L., and Hutchinson, T.: Choroidal effusion during glaucoma surgery in patients with prominent episcleral vessels, Arch. Ophthalmol. **97:**493, 1979.
11. Bietti, G.B., and Vanni, V.: Glaucoma secondaire à une obstruction veineuse extra-oculaire, Ophthalmologica **142:** 227, 1961.
12. Bigger, J.F.: Glaucoma with elevated episcleral venous pressure, South Med. J. **68:**1444, 1975.
13. Bill, A.: Aspects of the drainage of aqueous humor in cats, Arch. Ophthalmol. **67:**148, 1962.
14. Bill, A.: Early effects of epinephrine on aqueous humor dynamics in vervet monkeys (Cercopithecus ethiops), Exp. Eye Res. **8:**35, 1969.
15. Bloome, M.A.: Transient angle-closure glaucoma in central retinal vein occlusion, Ann. Ophthalmol. **9:**44, 1977.
16. Bock, V.J., and Stepanik, J.: Glaukom bei thyreogenem Exophthalmus, Ophthalmologica **142:**365, 1961.
17. Brauston, B.B., and Norton, E.W.D.: Intermittent exophthalmos, Am. J. Ophthalmol. **55:**701, 1963.
18. Brismar, G., and Brismar, J.: Spontaneous carotid-cavernous fistulas: clinical symptomatology, Acta. Ophthalmol. **54:**542, 1976.
19. Brismar, G., and Brismar, J.: Aseptic thrombosis of orbital veins and cavernous sinus, Acta. Ophthalmol. **55:**9, 1977.
20. Brolin, E.S.: Ocular tension changes imposed by rapid, intentionally varied venous pressure in a case of pulmonary tumor, Acta. Ophthalmol. **27:**394, 1949.
21. Brubaker, R.F.: Determination of episcleral venous pressure in the eye, Arch. Ophthalmol. **77:**110, 1967.
22. Burton, C.V., and Goldberg, M.F.: Exophthalmos from ruptured intracavernous carotid aneurysm without pulsation, bruit or murmur, Am. J. Ophthalmol. **70:**830, 1970.
23. Clay, C.L., Vignaud, J., Lasjaunias, P., and Moret, J.: Problemes actuels poses par les fistules arterioveineuses carotido-caverneuses, Arch. Ophthalmol. (Paris) **35:**639, 1975.
24. Christensen, G.R., and Records, R.E.: Glaucoma and expulsive hemorrhage mechanisms in the Sturge-Weber syndrome, Ophthalmology **86:**1360, 1979.
25. DeKeiyer, R.J.W.: Spontaneous carotico-cavernous fistulas: the importance of the typical limbal vascular loops for the diagnosis, the recognition of glaucoma and the uses of conservative therapy in this condition, Doc. Ophthalmol. **46:**403, 1979.
26. Dunphy, E.B.: Glaucoma accompanying nevus flammeus, Am. J. Ophthalmol. **18:**709, 1935.
27. Elliot, A.J.: Ocular manifestations of carotid-cavernous fistulas, Postgrad Med. **15:**191, 1954.
28. Gaasterland, D.E., Jacson, V.L., and Sears, M.L.: Channels of aqueous outflow and related blood vessels. III. Episcleral arteriovenous anastomoses in the rhesus monkey eye (Macaca mulatta), Arch. Ophthalmol. **84:**770, 1970.
29. Gallin, P.F., Yablonski, M.E., Shapiro, D., and Podos, S.M.: Oxygen effects on aqueous flow and episcleral venous pressure, ARVO Abstracts, p. 82, 1980.
30. Gartner, S.: Blood vessels of the conjunctiva, Arch. Ophthalmol. **32:**464, 1944.
31. Goldmann, H.: Die Kammerwasservenen und das Poiseulle'sche Gesetz, Ophthalmologica **118:**496, 1949.
32. Graffin, A.L., and Corddry, E.G.: Studies of the peripheral blood vascular beds in the bulbar conjunctiva of man, Bull. Johns Hopkins Hosp. **93:**275, 1953.
33. Grant, W.M.: Shallowing of the anterior chamber following occlusion of the central retinal vein, Am. J. Ophthalmol. **75:**384, 1973.
34. Harbison, J.W., Guerry, D., and Wiesinger, H.: Dural arteriovenous fistula and spontaneous choroidal detachment: new cause of an old disease, Br. J. Ophthalmol. **62:**483, 1978.
35. Harris, G.J., and Rice, P.R.: Angle closure in carotid cav-

ernous fistula, Ophthalmology **86:**1521, 1979.

36. Harris, M.J., Fine, S.L., and Miller, N.R.: Photocoagulation treatment of proliferative retinopathy secondary to carotid-cavernous fistula, Am. J. Ophthalmol. **90:**515, 1980.

37. Heyreh, S.S., and Baines, J.A.B.: Occlusion of the vortex veins: an experimental study, Br. J. Ophthalmol. **57:**217, 1973.

38. Henderson, J.W., and Schneider, R.C.: The ocular findings in carotid-cavernous fistula in a series of 17 cases, Am. J. Ophthalmol. **48:**585, 1959.

39. Holman, E., Gerbode, F., and Richards, V.: Communications between the carotid artery and cavernous sinus, Angiology **2:**311, 1951.

40. Kaskel, D., Becker, H., and Rudolf, H.: Fruhwirkungen von Clonidin, Adrenalin, und Pilocarpin auf den Augeninnendruck und Episkleralvenendruck des gesunden menschlichen Auges, Albrecht Von Graefes Arch. Klin. Exp. Ophthalmol. **213:**251, 1980.

41. Kedem, O., and Katchalsky, A.: Thermodynamic analysis of the permeability of biological membranes to non-electrolytes, Biochim. Biophys. Acta **27:**229, 1958.

42. Kollarits, C.R., Gaasterland, D., Di Chiro, G., et al.: Management of a patient with orbital varices, visual loss, and ipsilateral glaucoma, Ophthalmic Surg. **8:**54, 1977.

43. Krakau, C.E., Widakowich, J., and Wilke, K.: Measurement of the episcleral venous pressure by means of an airjet, Acta. Ophthalmol. **51:**185, 1973.

44. Krakau, C.E., and Wilke, K.: Effects of loading of the eye on intraocular pressure and on the episcleral venous pressure, Acta. Ophthalmol. **52:**107, 1974.

45. Kupfer, C., Gaasterland, D., and Ross, K.: Studies of aqueous humor dynamics in man. II. Measurements in young normal subjects using acetazolamide and L-epinephrine, Invest. Ophthalmol. **10:**523, 1971.

46. Kupfer, C., and Ross, K.: Studies of aqueous humor dynamics in man. I. Measurements in young normal subjects, Invest. Ophthalmol. **19:**518, 1971.

47. Linner, E.: Measurement of pressure in Schlemm's canal and in the anterior chamber of the human eye, Experientia **5:**451, 1949.

48. Linner, E.: Further studies of the episcleral venous pressure in glaucoma, Am. J. Ophthalmol. **41:**646, 1956.

49. Linner, E., Rickenbach, C., and Werner, H.: Comparative measurements of the pressure in the aqueous veins and the conjunctival veins using different methods, Acta Ophthalmol. **33:**101, 1955.

50. Lloyd, G.A.S.: Phleboliths in the orbit, Clin. Radiol. **16:**339, 1965.

51. Lloyd, G.A.S., Wright, J.E., and Morgan, G.: Venous malformations in the orbit, Br. J. Ophthalmol. **55:**505, 1971.

52. Madsen, P.H.: Carotid-cavernous fistulae: a study of 18 cases, Acta Ophthalmol. **48:**731, 1970.

53. Meyer, O.: Inflammatory jugular phlebostenosis as the cause of glaucoma exogenicum, Br. J. Ophthalmol. **30:**682, 1946.

54. Mims, J.L., and Holland, M.G.: Applanation and Schiøtz tonometer standardizations for the owl monkey eye with a new technique for measuring episcleral venous pressure, Invest. Ophthalmol. **10:**190, 1971.

55. Minas, T.F., and Podos, S.M.: Familial glaucoma associated with elevated episcleral venous pressure, Arch. Ophthalmol. **80:**201, 1968.

56. Newton, T.H., and Cronqvist, S.: Involvement of dural arteries in intracranial arteriovenous malformations, Radiology **93:**1071, 1969.

57. Nordmann, J., et al.: A propos de 14 cas de glaucome par hypertension veineuse d'origine extraoculaire, Ophthalmologica **142**(suppl.):501, 1961.

58. Pecora, J.L., and Patel, A.J.: Eyelid edema as the presenting sign in superior vena cava syndrome, Ann. Ophthalmol. **12:**1161, 1980.

59. Pederson, J.E., MacLellan, H.M., and Gaasterland, D.E.: The rate of reflux fluid movement into the eye from Schlemm's canal during hypotony in the rhesus monkey, Invest. Ophthalmol. Vis. Sci. **17:**377, 1978.

60. Phelps, C.D.: The pathogenesis of glaucoma in Sturge-Weber syndrome, Trans. Am. Acad. Ophthalmol. Otolaryngol. **85:**276, 1978.

61. Phelps, C.D., and Armaly, M.F.: Measurement of episcleral venous pressure, Am. J. Ophthalmol. **85:**33, 1978.

62. Podos, S.M., Minas, T.F., and Macri, J.T.: A new instrument to measure episcleral venous pressure: comparison of normal eyes and eyes with primary open angle glaucoma, Arch. Ophthalmol. **80:**209, 1968.

63. Radius, R.L., and Maumenee, A.E.: Dilated episcleral vessels and open angle glaucoma, Am. J. Ophthalmol. **86:**31, 1978.

64. Rosen, D.A., and Johnston, V.C.: Ocular pressure patterns in the Valsalva maneuver, Arch. Ophthalmol. **62:**810, 1959.

65. Sanders, M., and Hoyt, W.: Hypoxic ocular sequelae of carotid-cavernous fistulae: study of the causes of visual failure before and after neurosurgical treatment in a series of 25 cases, Br. J. Ophthalmol. **53:**82, 1969.

66. Segal, P., Gebick, L., Janiszewski, S., and Skwierczynska, J.: Intraocular pressure during pressure breathing. I. Healthy adults, Am. J. Ophthalmol. **64:**956, 1967.

67. Seidel, E.: Weitere experimentelle Untersuchungen Uber die Quelle und den Verlauf der intraokularen Saftsrommung. XX. Uber die Messung des Blutdruckes in dem episcleral Venengeflecht, den vorderen ciliar-und den Wirbelvenen normaler Augen, Albrecht Von Graefes Arch. Ophthalmol. **112:**252, 1923.

68. Stolpman, E.: Doppelseitige nicht-traumatische carotis sinus cavernosis fistel, Albrecht Von Graefes Arch. Klin. Exp. Ophthalmol. **185:**83, 1972.

69. Sugar, H.S., and Meyer, S.J.: Pulsating exophthalmos, Arch. Ophthalmol. **23:**1288, 1939.

70. Taniguchi, R.M., Goree, J.A., and Odom, G.L.: Spontaneous carotid-cavernous shunts presenting diagnostic problems, J. Neurosurg. **35:**384, 1971.

71. Thomassen, T.L.: The venous tension in eyes suffering from simple glaucoma, Acta. Ophthalmol. **25:**221, 1947.

72. Thomassen, T.L., Perkins, E.S., and Dobree, J.H.: Aqueous veins in glaucomatous eyes, Br. J. Ophthalmol. **34:**221, 1950.

73. Uribe-Troncoso, M.: Physiologic nature of Schlemm canal, Am. J. Ophthalmol. **4:**321, 1921.

74. Walsh, F.B., and Dandy, W.E.: The pathogenesis of intermittent exophthalmos, Trans. Am. Ophthalmol. Soc. **42:**334, 1944.

75. Weekers, R., and Delmarcelle, Y.: Pathogenesis of intraocular hypertension in cases of arteriovenous aneurysm, Arch. Ophthalmol. **48:**338, 1952.

76. Weiss, D.I.: Dual origin of glaucoma in encephalotrigeminal hemangiomatosis, Trans. Ophthalmol. Soc. U.K. **93:**477, 1971.

77. Weiss, D.I., and Shaffer, R.N.: Neovascular glaucoma complicating carotid-cavernous fistula, Arch. Ophthalmol. **69:**60, 1963.

78. Wettrell, K., Wilke, K., and Pandolfi, M.: Effect of beta-adrenergic agonists and antagonists on repeated tonometry and episcleral venous pressure, Exp. Eye Res. **24:**613, 1977.

79. Wilke, K.: Early effects of epinephrine and pilocarpine on the intraocular pressure and the episcleral venous pressure in the normal human eye, Acta Ophthalmol. **52:**231, 1974.

80. Wright, J.E.: Orbital vascular anomalies, Trans. Am. Acad. Ophthalmol. Otolaryngol. **78:**OP606, 1974.

81. Yablonski, M.E., Ritch, R., and Pokorny, K.: Effect of decreased intracranial pressure on optic disc, ARVO Abstracts, p. 165, 1979.

82. Yablonski, M.E., et al.: Unpublished data, 1980.

Chapter 15

GLAUCOMA ASSOCIATED WITH SYSTEMIC DISEASE

Richard A. Stone

The relationship between glaucoma and systemic disease is complex. A number of systemic disorders have well-defined ocular complications that produce an elevated intraocular pressure. These disorders are emphasized in this chapter. In addition, there is an association of open-angle glaucoma with a variety of systemic conditions. Although a review of these associations is beyond the scope of this book, some are discussed, particularly when the distinction between primary and secondary glaucoma is not clear. Finally, a number of systemic conditions occasionally cause optic nerve cupping and field loss that may be glaucomatous in nature without an elevation of intraocular pressure. These are discussed in the section on low-tension glaucoma.

ENDOCRINE DISORDERS

The possibility that endocrine mechanisms may have a role in the regulation of intraocular pressure in the normal eye and may explain the abnormalities in aqueous humor dynamics that occur in glaucoma has stimulated many investigations. To date, no study has demonstrated convincingly that primary open-angle glaucoma is related to an abnormality in endocrine function.[57] Glaucoma does occur, however, in association with several endocrine disorders through a variety of pathologic processes.

Pituitary disease

Many authors have reported an association of glaucoma with pituitary tumors. The glaucoma occurring in these cases resembles primary open-angle glaucoma.

Several investigators have found an association of glaucoma with acromegaly arising from eosinophilic pituitary adenomas. Howard and English[50] found that 7 of 70 patients with acromegaly had glaucoma, although in one case there was a previous history of fibrinous iritis and peripheral anterior synechiae. The diagnosis of glaucoma was made 6 to 34 years after the onset of acromegaly. These patients had cupping of the optic disc and visual field defects, and tonography showed decreased facilities of outflow. The intraocular pressures of five of these patients were controlled with topical medication, but two required filtering surgery. Forty-five of the 70 patients in this series, however, did not have intraocular pressures recorded in their charts, and Howard and English stressed that the true prevalence of elevated intraocular pressures in this series of patients may well have been higher than that reported. Smaller series also have tended to support the association of an elevated intraocular pressure or glaucoma with acromegaly.

The coexistence of glaucoma and chromophobe pituitary adenomas has also been noted. Van Bijsterveld and Richards[95] found three cases of open-angle glaucoma among 14 patients with chromophobe adenomas. All three of these patients had elevated intraocular pressures, but only one had decreased outflow facility and optic nerve head cupping. Although field loss occurred in all three patients, in one and perhaps both of the patients without frank optic nerve cupping the field loss may have been related to the pituitary tumor rather than to the elevated intraocular pressure. The concurrence of glaucoma and basophilic pituitary adenomas has also been reported.[85]

The above studies indicate that the association of glaucoma with pituitary tumors, while unusual, does appear to occur more frequently than by chance. Although this concurrence may be accidental, a possible causative role for pituitary disease in the development of these glaucomas cannot be excluded at the present time.[36] The strongest clinical evidence for association occurs with acromegaly, and these patients appear to have an increased incidence of low outflow facilities and elevated intraocular pressures. There is as yet no conclusive evidence linking growth hormone with the control of intraocular pressure in normal patients or with the development of primary open-angle glaucoma, but a hormonal mechanism may be present. For instance, although patients with primary open-angle glaucoma have normal baseline plasma growth hormone levels, they show an exaggerated elevation of growth hormone levels after intravenous arginine administration.[43]

The treatment of patients with pituitary disease and elevated intraocular pressures is the same as that for patients with primary open-angle glaucoma. Visual field changes can occur because of the glaucoma or the pituitary disease, and it is important to follow these patients with careful perimetry so that the cause of any progressive field change can be identified. This association of glaucoma with pituitary disease underscores the need for careful scrutiny of the visual fields of all glaucoma patients to detect coexisting disease in the visual pathways, particularly when the pattern of visual field loss is not typical of glaucoma or when the amount of field loss is disproportionate to the degree of cupping. In addition, patients with pituitary disease should be screened for glaucoma.

Cushing's syndrome

Cushing's syndrome is a metabolic disorder caused by a chronic excess of glucocorticoids. It can arise from adrenocortical tumors that autonomously secrete cortisol or from certain nonpituitary tumors that secrete ACTH (adrenocorticotropic hormone) and cause adrenal hyperplasia. In those cases where the pituitary gland secretes excessive ACTH, typically from a basophilic adenoma, the specific term Cushing's disease is applied.

Abnormalities in intraocular pressure have been reported in patients with Cushing's syndrome of either the type with adrenal adenoma or the type with excessive ACTH production. Krasnovid[60] found both elevations of intraocular pressure and increased diurnal variations in intraocular pressure in patients with Cushing's syndrome, and both he and Linnér[66] found decreased diurnal fluctuations in intraocular pressure in patients with adrenal or pituitary insufficiency.

Some patients with Cushing's syndrome develop increased intraocular pressure and may develop optic nerve cupping and visual field loss. In one series, 7 of 29 patients with Cushing's syndrome had intraocular pressures above 23 mm Hg.[72] Three of these patients had visual field defects, but only one had a true glaucomatous defect. The facility of outflow is generally reduced in such cases, and following adrenalectomy, the increased intraocular pressure and the reduced facility of outflow may return to normal.[4,57] Haas and Nootens[44] reported a patient with Cushing's syndrome secondary to a benign adrenal adenoma who had marked bilateral intraocular pressure elevations, reduced outflow facilities, and optic nerve head cupping in one eye. Following adrenalectomy, the patient's intraocular pressure and outflow facility returned to normal. Topical steroid testing showed that the patient, both of his parents, and one sister were high steroid responders. Haas and Nootens postulated that a genetic sensitivity to the intraocular pressure effects of corticosteroids causes the rise in intraocular pressure found in some patients with Cushing's syndrome.

The relationship between corticosteroids, intraocular pressure, and glaucoma is discussed in greater detail in Chapter 17.

Diabetes mellitus

The relationship between diabetes and open-angle glaucoma has been studied extensively. Although not all series are in agreement,[2,3] primary open-angle glaucoma appears to be more prevalent among patients with diabetes,[1,5,57] and the intraocular pressures of both adult and juvenile diabetic patients appear to be higher than in the nondiabetic population.[84,90] In addition, secondary glaucomas can develop as a direct or indirect consequence of diabetes mellitus. These conditions are discussed elsewhere in this text.

Thyroid disease

Graves' disease is characterized by hyperthyroidism with diffuse goiter, dermopathy, and ophthalmopathy. All of these need not occur, and the clinical course of any one of the manifestations may be largely independent of the others. The disorder may occur at any age, but the incidence is highest between the ages of 30 and 50 years. Women are more frequently affected than men. The cause of the ophthalmic manifestations of this disease is uncertain.

A nonuniform and sometimes confusing terminology has been applied to the ophthalmopathy of Graves' disease, but most authors separate the thyrotoxic, or noninfiltrative, form from the thyrotropic, or infiltrative, form. This distinction is useful for purposes of discussion, but clinically there is often overlap.

Thyrotoxic ophthalmopathy occurs in some 50% to 75% of patients with Graves' disease. Affected patients are usually between 20 and 40 years of age, and there is a marked female preponderance. The eye findings consist of a characteristic stare with lid retraction and lid lag that is most marked in downward gaze. Mild exophthalmos, although uncommon, may occur, but the proptosis may be more apparent than real because of the lid retraction. The globe retrodisplaces normally. With correction of the hyperthyroidism, the eye signs generally resolve spontaneously.

Thyrotropic ophthalmopathy (Fig. 15-1) occurs less frequently, but some evidence of infiltrative ophthalmopathy occurs in 10% to 20% of patients with Graves' disease. About 2% develop severe "malignant" exophthalmos. Thyrotropic ophthalmopathy usually occurs with the onset of the hyperthyroidism and subsides with its treatment. However, it may occur in euthyroid patients or may develop after the hyperthyroidism has been treated.

Secondary glaucoma can occur in thyrotropic ophthalmopathy by means of several mechanisms. The retrobulbar inflammatory process can compromise the orbital venous system and raise the episcleral venous pressure. In some instances frank thrombosis of the orbital veins has been documented.[28] An impaired outflow facility can also contribute to intraocular pressure elevation. Contraction of the extraocular muscles against intraorbital adhesions may cause marked variations in intraocular pressure in different positions of gaze. Usually fibrosis affects the inferior muscles, and a significant increase in introcular pressure may occur in upward gaze.[99] Because of these gaze-related changes in intraocular pressure, tonometry should be performed on these patients in several positions of gaze.

Scleral rigidity shows wide fluctuations in patients with thyroid disease.[45] In the management of these patients it is best to use applanation tonometry to avoid this potential problem.

In patients with thyrotropic ophthalmopathy and normal outflow facilities, pressure elevations in isolated fields of gaze usually require no therapy. With significantly impaired outflow facilities, sustained pressure elevations may be present in all fields of gaze but exaggerated in certain gaze positions. Whether this latter condition represents a concurrence of primary open-angle glaucoma and thyrotropic ophthalmopathy or a true secondary glaucoma generally cannot be determined on clinical grounds, but the treatment of such patients is analogous to the treatment of patients with open-angle glaucoma. Visual acuity and visual field studies are important in following these patients. It sometimes can be difficult to determine the cause of visual loss in these patients, however, because the infiltrative optic neuropathy may cause visual field defects similar to those seen in glaucoma. After a period of several years the orbital disease frequently goes into remission with some reduction in orbital congestion, but the glaucoma may persist. The prognosis for vision in many of these patients may be poor.

Corneal exposure and secondary infection also can occur as a result of thyrotropic ophthalmopathy. A severe anterior chamber reaction may develop, leading to peripheral anterior synechiae and secondary glaucoma. In such cases the corneal disease should be treated primarily and glaucoma therapy instituted as necessary.

Efforts to correlate abnormalities of thyroid function with primary open-angle glaucoma have yielded inconclusive findings. Although some studies have reported a high incidence of elevated intraocular pressure in patients with hyperthyroidism,[75] most studies are unable to substantiate such a relationship.[17] Patients with hypothyroidism have been noted to have elevated intraocular pressures as well, and low protein-bound iodine values and low radioiodide uptakes have been reported in open-angle glaucoma.[6] A more recent study, however, has demonstrated that the thyroxine (T_4), thyrotropin (TSH), and triiodothyronine (T_3) resin uptake levels of glaucoma patients do not differ from those of normal controls.[61] In patients with hypothyroidism and elevated intraocular pressures, systemic thyroid medication has been reported to lower the intraocular pressure.[73,75] Although much of the experimental data is contradictory, it ap-

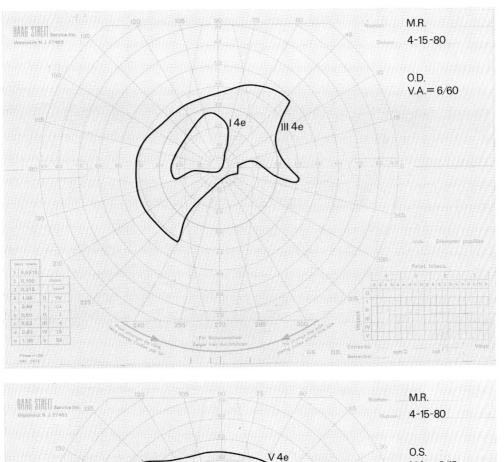

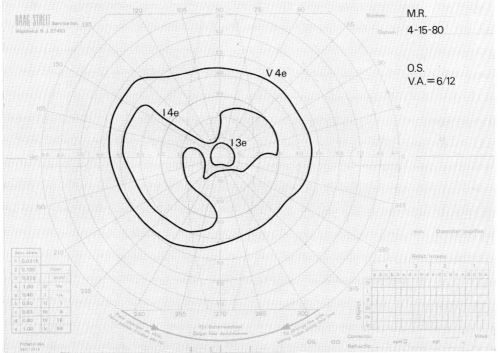

FIG. 15-1. Elevated intraocular pressure secondary to infiltrative thyrotrophic ophthalmopathy. This 53-year-old woman underwent radioactive iodide treatment for hyperthyroidism 1 year before rapid onset of bilateral exophthalmos, motility limitation, and blurred vision. Her visual acuity measured 6/60 OD with marked visual field deficit (**A**) and afferent pupillary defect. Her left eye had visual acuity of 6/12 with less marked visual field defect (**B**). Intraocular pressures measured in mid-20s bilaterally with eyes in primary position and increased to low- to mid-30s on attempted upward gaze. Optic discs showed no significant cupping in either eye. *Continued.*

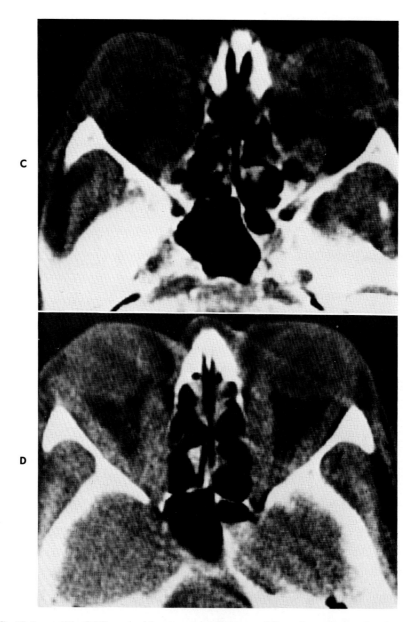

FIG. 15-1. cont'd. CAT scan without contrast illustrates bilateral proptosis **(C).** With contrast, muscles appear thickened and show slight enhancement on CAT scan **(D).** Patient received high-dose oral steroids, resulting in some improvement in motility and some lessening of orbital congestion.

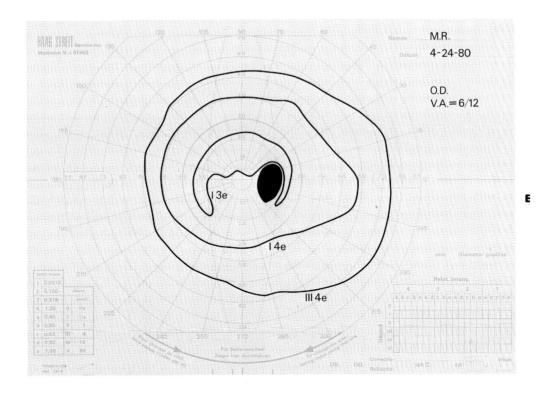

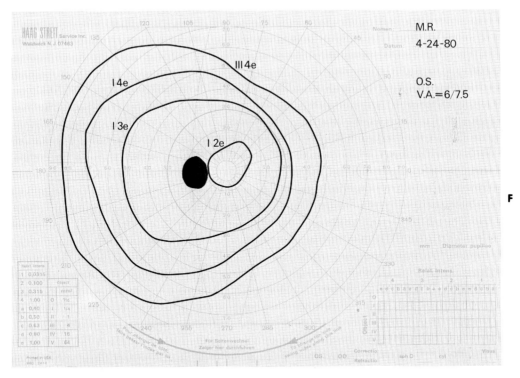

Fig. 15-1 cont'd. Visual acuity improved to 6/12 OD and 6/7.5 OS with corresponding improvement in both right (**E**) and left (**F**) visual fields. Intraocular pressure was normal in primary position but still rose as high as low 30s bilaterally in attempted upward gaze. No specific antiglaucoma therapy was advised. (Courtesy Irving M. Raber, M.D., Scheie Eye Institute.)

pears that pharmacologic doses of thyroid hormone may decrease intraocular pressure by increasing outflow facility,[57] but thyroid hormone currently has no therapeutic role in treating glaucoma.

Thus there is no evidence that abnormalities in thyroid function directly result in an elevated intraocular pressure. Only in thyrotropic ophthalmopathy, where an elevated intraocular pressure occurs from complications of the orbital disease, does a true secondary glaucoma arise from thyroid dysfunction.

VASCULAR DISEASE
Ocular ischemia

Local ocular ischemia, including central retinal vein occlusion and, rarely, central retinal artery occlusion, can lead to the development of rubeosis iridis and hemorrhagic glaucoma. About 25% of patients experiencing central retinal vein occlusion develop rubeosis iridis. This problem is discussed in detail in Chapter 12.

Central retinal vein occlusion
(Figs. 15-2 and 15-3)

In addition to the problem of rubeosis iridis, there is a striking association between preexisting glaucoma and central retinal vein occlusion. Estimates of the prevalence of glaucoma among patients with central retinal vein occlusion vary considerably and have been reported in the broad range of 9% to 69%.[25] Presumably, the elevated intraocular pressure lowers the perfusion pressure in the central retinal artery, permitting mechanical occlusion or thrombosis of the central retinal vein. Typically, there is coexisting atherosclerotic disease in the central retinal artery. Increased intraocular pressure may also cause mechanical distortion of the lamina cribrosa and further compromise flow through the central retinal vein.[8] An eye with a recent vein occlusion often is relatively hypotonous,[81] and the underlying abnormality in intraocular pressure in that eye may not be immediately apparent. Therefore it is imperative to examine the contralateral eye for evidence of an elevated intraocular pressure. Because an elevation of intraocular pressure is a predisposing factor to the development of a retinal vein occlusion and because an elevated intraocular pressure can further compromise the retinal circulation in an eye with a retinal vein occlusion, an elevated intraocular pressure in either eye of such a patient should be treated appropriately.

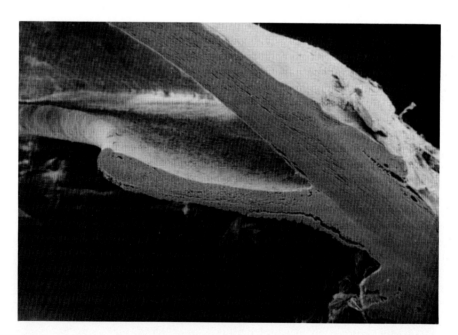

FIG. 15-2. Neovascular glaucoma secondary to central retinal vein occlusion. Broad peripheral anterior synechiae and early ectropion uveae are present. Normal contours of anterior iridic surface are effaced by fibrovascular membrane. (Scanning electron microscope; ×25.) (Courtesy Ralph C. Eagle, Jr., M.D., Scheie Eye Institute.)

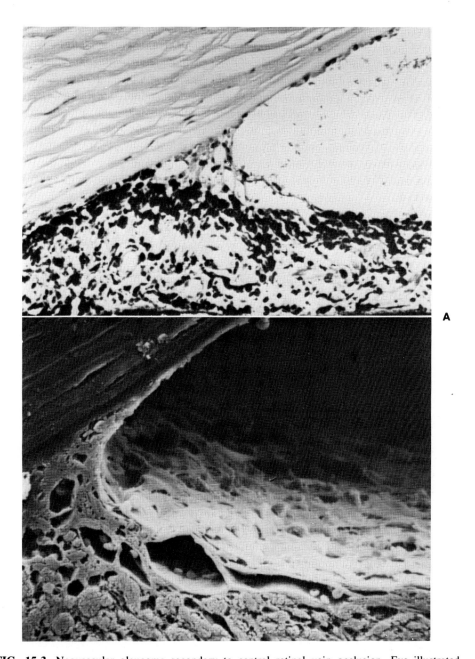

FIG. 15-3. Neovascular glaucoma secondary to central retinal vein occlusion. Eye illustrated in Fig. 15-2 is examined at higher magnification by light *(top)* and scanning electron microscopy *(bottom)*. Peripheral iris is adherent to Descemet's membrane **(A)**. Membrane of fibroblasts covers new blood vessels in pseudoangle and on anterior iridic surface. *(Top:* Hematoxylin and eosin; ×125. *Bottom:* Scanning electron microscope; ×256.)   *Continued.*

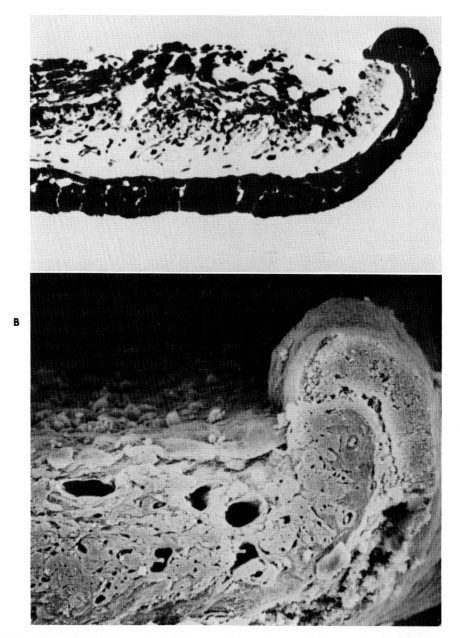

FIG. 15-3 cont'd. Fibrovascular membrane covers and effaces anterior iridic surface **(B).** Contraction of membrane has led to eversion of pigment epithelium and sphincter muscle (ectropian uveae). (*Top:* Hematoxylin and eosin; ×125. *Bottom:* Scanning electron microscope; ×256.) (Courtesy Ralph C. Eagle, Jr., M.D., Scheie Eye Institute.)

Occasionally occlusion of the central retinal vein causes a shallowing of the anterior chamber, presumably because of an abnormal accumulation of blood or edema in the posterior segment that results in anterior displacement of the iris-lens diaphragm. In some cases angle-closure glaucoma develops.[42,51] This glaucoma usually has been noted within 2 to 3 weeks after the occurrence of the vein occlusion. With absorption of the fluid in the posterior segment, the anterior chamber depth returns to normal, often within several weeks.

Gonioscopy of the uninvolved eye may help distinguish this unusual form of secondary angle-closure glaucoma from primary angle-closure glaucoma. If the contralateral eye has an open angle, one must consider a secondary angle-closure mechanism. If the contralateral eye has a narrow, potentially occludable angle, one must consider a primary angle-closure mechanism. The diagnostic distinction is important because of the therapy. In primary angle-closure glaucoma with a pupillary block mechanism, iridectomy is necessary. In this rare form of secondary angle-closure glaucoma associated with central vein occlusion, surgical iridectomy fails to deepen the anterior chamber acutely and may not immediately normalize the intraocular pressure. Because of the self-limited nature of this form of secondary angle-closure glaucoma, medical therapy is the preferred treatment, and iridectomy should be reserved for nonresponsive cases. Pilocarpine controls the intraocular pressure in most patients sufficiently for spontaneous resolution of the chamber shallowing to occur.[42,51] Treatment with cycloplegics to tighten the lens zonules and to displace the iris-lens diaphragm posteriorly, as well as with drugs to suppress aqueous secretion, such as timolol or carbonic anhydrase inhibitors, may produce a more dramatic and consistent therapeutic response[11] and appears to be a rational therapeutic approach at the present time.[15] There is no apparent association between this unusual form of angle-closure glaucoma and the subsequent development of rubeosis iridis.[15]

Cerebrovascular disease

An elevated episcleral venous pressure and secondary glaucoma may arise from arteriovenous malformations or from carotid-cavernous fistulas, as discussed in Chapter 14. Ocular ischemia and rubeosis iridis may develop as a complication of a variety of systemic vascular diseases, including carotid occlusive disease, Takayasu's (pulseless) disease, and temporal arteritis. The occurrence of a central retinal artery occlusion or a central retinal vein occlusion in association with systemic vascular disease can also result in the development of rubeosis iridis and secondary glaucoma.[35] These conditions are discussed elsewhere in this text.

Rapid progression of visual field loss has been noted in some glaucoma patients with low systemic or low ophthalmic artery blood pressures,[21,23,63,83] and occlusive carotid artery disease has been cited as an etiologic factor in low-tension glaucoma. It should be emphasized, however, that these findings are by no means invariable. For instance, Jampol and Miller[53] have reported five patients with occlusive carotid artery disease and untreated intraocular pressure elevations who did not develop glaucomatous disc or field changes over a 3- to 12-year follow-up period.

Blood pressure and intraocular pressure

There tends to be a positive correlation between intraocular pressure readings and blood pressure measurements.[9] The Framingham study furthermore has demonstrated an association between ocular hypertension and systemic blood pressure.[56] The two disorders, however, do not necessarily occur in the same patient, and systemic hypertension does not appear to be an etiologic factor in the development of glaucoma. Sudden lowering of an elevated systemic blood pressure in patients with established glaucoma may precipitate acute visual field loss in susceptible individuals,[32,47,83] presumably because of a sudden drop in the perfusion pressure at the optic nerve head. Considering the large number of glaucoma patients undergoing treatment for systemic hypertension and the small number of these reports, it is not clear whether the visual loss described in these reports is causally or coincidentally related to lowering of the systemic blood pressure. Nevertheless, the high prevalence of both disorders makes the suggestion that sudden blood pressure control in glaucoma patients may result in visual field loss an important concern.

In the absence of controlled prospective clinical studies, it would appear wisest to monitor glaucoma patients carefully when medication for systemic hypertension is given and to recommend gradual control of the systemic blood pressure in glaucoma patients, particularly if the glaucoma is not well controlled.

COLLAGEN VASCULAR DISORDERS

Secondary glaucoma can arise from the uveitis or may occasionally be associated with the episcleritis or scleritis that accompanies some of these disorders. Corticosteroid-induced glaucoma, either from topical or, less frequently, from systemic steroid administration, is another problem in these patients. These disorders are discussed in detail in other chapters of this text.

RENAL DISEASE AND HEMODIALYSIS

Elevated intraocular pressures occur in patients after renal transplantation with a reported incidence as high as 33%.[49,102] Frequently the intraocular pressure elevation appears to be related to the intake of systemic steroids, because the intraocular pressure elevation parallels the steroid use. The intraocular pressures usually respond well to conventional topical antiglaucoma therapy.

During hemodialysis in patients with renal failure, fluctuations in intraocular pressure occur. Ramsell et al.[82] noted that during the first 2 hours of hemodialysis, a small fall in intraocular pressure occurred. After 6 hours of hemodialysis, however, the intraocular pressure rose in 10 of 19 patients. The degree of elevation was quite variable but averaged 6.9 mm Hg in those patients experiencing an intraocular pressure rise. Serum osmolality falls during hemodialysis, and a lag in the equilibration of the osmolality of the intraocular fluids to the changing serum osmolality may result in the osmotic transfer of free water into the eye and contribute to this elevation of intraocular pressure. Additional factors, perhaps related to central nervous system (CNS) mechanisms, might mediate this response.[82] Generally, these swings in intraocular pressure are not of sufficient magnitude or duration to be of clinical significance in patients with normal outflow facilities. In patients with impaired outflow facilities, however, a marked rise in intraocular pressure may occur.

HEMATOLOGIC DISORDERS
Blood composition

Abnormalities in serum protein, chloride, cholesterol, the potassium/calcium ratio, pH, and osmolality in patients with open-angle glaucoma have been reported but have not been found consistently. There is no definite evidence for a relationship between these blood constituents and the development of an elevated intraocular pressure and glaucoma.[26]

Hyperviscosity syndromes

Diseases such as polycythemia and the dysproteinemias are associated with increased serum viscosity and decreased blood flow velocity, resulting in dilation, tortuosity, and possible thrombosis of the retinal veins. If thrombosis of the central retinal vein occurs, neovascular glaucoma may develop.

In hyperviscosity syndromes, an acute rise in intraocular pressure may occur without the presence of rubeosis iridis but with an open angle and blood in Schlemm's canal. Presumably, the glaucoma in these cases develops because of an acute thrombosis within Schlemm's canal. Medical treatment of the increased intraocular pressure is the preferred therapeutic approach, although the intraocular pressure may be difficult to control.[41]

Sickle cell hemoglobinopathies

The sickle cell hemoglobinopathies arise from the substitution of a single amino acid in normal adult hemoglobin A to form hemoglobin S. Erythrocytes containing hemoglobin S may develop a sickle configuration under certain conditions, such as hypoxia. Sickled erythrocytes are less pliable than normal red blood cells and can therefore occlude small blood vessels. Some 10% of North American blacks have hemoglobin S. The hemoglobin mutation is inherited directly from either parent and can occur as the sickle cell trait (AS hemoglobin) or sickle cell anemia (SS disease). Hemoglobin S also can occur in sickle cell thalassemia (SThal) and sickle cell C disease (SC disease). SS disease causes the most severe systemic problems, with chronic anemia and recurrent episodes of hemolysis and painful crises. The SC and SThal hemoglobinopathies cause less severe anemia and milder symptoms. The sickle cell trait causes the least severe symptoms of these disorders.

The predominant ocular complication of the sickle cell hemoglobinopathies is sickle cell retinopathy,[65,101] which can be classified into proliferative and nonproliferative forms.[39] The proliferative retinopathy is characterized by peripheral arteriolar occlusions, peripheral arteriolar-venous anastomoses, peripheral neovascularization, vitreous hemorrhage, and retinal detachment. These ocular complications, particularly retinal neovascularization, vitreous hemorrhage, and retinal detachment, appear to be most prevalent in SC and SThal dis-

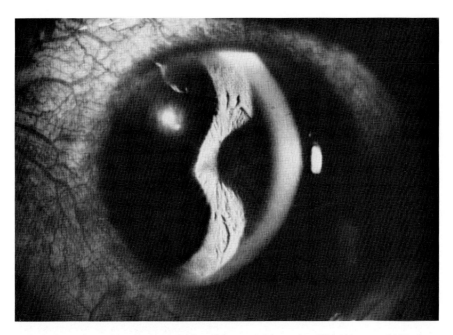

FIG. 15-4. Secondary glaucoma and sickle cell hemoglobinopathy. This 41-year-old black woman with SC disease developed sudden visual acuity drop to 6/12 in left eye. Initial findings included neovascularization of temporal retina extending into vitreous cavity, superior traction retinal detachment, and vitreous and subretinal hemorrhage. Small fibrovascular tuft was also noted temporally in right eye. No retinal therapy was recommended at that time. Over next 4 years, left eye developed uveitis, rubeosis iridis, secluded pupil, and secondary glaucoma. Right eye has maintained good vision, but vision in left eye has deteriorated to no light perception. Photograph illustrates secluded pupil with iris bombé in left eye.

ease. The nonproliferative sickle cell retinopathy has venous tortuosity, "black sunbursts," refractile fundus deposits, "silver wire" changes in the arterioles, and salmon-patch hemorrhages. Central retinal artery occlusions and central retinal vein occlusions have been observed, particularly in patients with SS disease. Patients with the other forms of sickle cell hemoglobinopathies, however, are not immune from the vasoocclusive ocular complications. Angioid streaks have been described in all types of sickle cell hemoglobinopathies.

Secondary glaucoma can occur as a complication of the retinal vascular disease (Fig. 15-4). As in other conditions characterized by ocular ischemia, rubeosis iridis and neovascular glaucoma can develop. Only a small number of cases of rubeosis iridis have been reported as a complication of sickle cell hemoglobinopathies, however, and the association appears strongest with SC disease.[40] The development of rubeosis has been noted in patients with the sickle cell trait, but these patients also had coexisting diabetes mellitus[12] or

central retinal vein occlusion,[105] which may have accounted for the rubeosis.

Vitreous hemorrhage that occurs in sickle cell retinopathy may cause a hemolytic glaucoma analogous to the hemolytic glaucoma occurring after any intraocular hemorrhage, as discussed in Chapter 21.

Shapiro and Baum[88] reported a patient with the sickle cell trait who developed an acute rise in intraocular pressure. The angle was open, but Schlemm's canal was filled with blood. They postulated that a low-grade asymptomatic iritis, which was also present in the contralateral eye, created ocular hypotony and allowed blood to reflux into Schlemm's canal. Then hemostasis with resulting hypoxia and pH alterations may have produced sickling and occlusion of Schlemm's canal. In this patient normalization of the intraocular pressure and outflow facility paralleled the disappearance of the blood from Schlemm's canal. Friedman et al.[33] also reported a patient with the sickle cell trait, spontaneous hemorrhage into the trabecular meshwork, blood in Schlemm's canal, and an elevated intraocular pressure, but no iritis. The elevated intraocular pressure was treated medically. After the trabecular hemorrhage and blood in Schlemm's canal reabsorbed, the intraocular pressure remained normal without medication.

Patients with sickle cell hemoglobinopathies, even the sickle cell trait, may develop significant intraocular pressure elevations in response to the occurrence of relatively small hyphemas.[33,38] Anterior chamber aspirates from SA and SC patients with hyphemas reveal a higher percentage of sickled erythrocytes in the aqueous humor than in the plasma.[37] This sickling may arise from the reducing properties of the high ascorbate in the aqueous humor or perhaps from a drop in aqueous pH and a fall in Po_2 associated with the occurrence of the hyphema, all of which would contribute to increased sickling. The sickled erythrocytes may significantly impair aqueous outflow and cause the intraocular pressure elevation.[37]

The medical treatment for hyphema-induced glaucoma in patients with sickle cell hemoglobinopathies may adversely affect the sickling process or the ocular circulation.[37,38,79] Acetazolamide administration can cause hemoconcentration and systemic acidosis, the latter of which may exacerbate erythrocyte sickling. Methazolamide may be a safer carbonic anhydrase inhibitor to use because it tends to cause less systemic acidosis than acetazolamide and may slightly raise aqueous humor pH. Acetazolamide also increases the aqueous concentration of ascorbic acid, and this may cause further sickling in the aqueous humor. Hyperosmolar agents may increase hemoconcentration and viscosity and thus further compromise the microcirculation in the eye, particularly in the central retinal artery and the small vessels of the optic nerve and perifoveal region. Topical epinephrine, if it induces vasoconstriction, may further compromise the local ocular circulation.[37] Although no clinical or laboratory studies currently exist that can provide clinical guidance, it appears that topical timolol may be the agent of choice in such situations.

Acute intraocular pressure elevations in patients with sickle cell hemoglobinopathies are of concern because of associated retinal vascular complications, particularly central retinal artery occlusions, at normal or moderately elevated intraocular pressures.[37] Although the blood flow in the small vessels of the optic nerve or central retinal artery can be compromised by an elevated intra-ocular pressure in any patient, several reports suggest that patients with sickle cell hemoglobinopathies are particularly susceptible.[79]

Goldberg[37] has emphasized that the clinical management of black patients with hyphemas requires reassessment because of the high incidence of sickle cell hemoglobinopathies among this group. Black patients with hyphemas should be screened immediately for sickle cell hemoglobin, followed by a hemoglobin electrophoresis. In addition, 24-hour monitoring of the intraocular pressure and visual function are important. According to Goldberg, in such circumstances paracentesis may be indicated with only a slight intraocular pressure elevation of "perhaps 25 mm Hg or greater, for more than one day, despite judicious use of anti-glaucomatous medications, and even if the hyphema is less than total." A prospective randomized clinical trial of patients with sickle cell hemoglobinopathy and hyphemas will be necessary to confirm the wisdom of such aggressive surgical management.

INTRAOCULAR NEOPLASTIC DISEASE

Malignant intraocular tumors, such as retinoblastoma, leukemic infiltration of the eye, and neoplastic disease metastatic to the eye, can produce secondary glaucoma. Nonmalignant neoplastic conditions, such as neurofibromatosis or juvenile xanthogranuloma, when they involve intraocular structures, can also result in secondary glaucoma. Such conditions are discussed elsewhere in this text.

PRIMARY FAMILIAL AMYLOIDOSIS

The hereditary systemic amyloidoses are a group of generalized disorders, the systemic manifestations of which include weakness, peripheral neuropathy, and gastrointestinal, cardiovascular, renal, and endocrine abnormalities consistent with the widespread deposition of amyloid. The predominant inheritance pattern is autosomal dominant. Ocular involvement includes the accumulation of characteristic cottonlike amyloid vitreous capacities, bilateral severe secondary open-angle glaucoma, lid abnormalities, extraocular muscle weakness, proptosis, internal ophthalmoplegia, anisocoria, and retinal perivasculitis. The vitreous opacification can progress to impair vision seriously and prevent fundus visualization.[14,58,74]

Patients who develop glaucoma have open angles, pigment in the trabecular meshwork, pigment on the corneal endothelium, and abnormal iris transillumination. Powdery white flakes also may occur on the pupillary margin of the iris and on the anterior lens capsule in patients with glaucoma. Amyloid vitreous opacities also are present in these cases. Although primary familial amyloidosis is a rare disease, it appears that up to one fourth of the patients may be at risk to develop glaucoma. The longer the disease has been present, the greater appears to be the risk of developing glaucoma.[93]

Widespread deposition of amyloid in ocular structures occurs in this condition. Using light microscopy, Paton and Duke[74] demonstrated amyloid deposition within the trabecular meshwork of a glaucomatous eye from a patient with primary familial amyloidosis but found no amyloid deposition within the trabecular meshwork in the contralateral nonglaucomatous eye. Segawa[87] and Tsukahara and Matsuo,[93] using electron microscopy, also demonstrated amyloid accumulation in the trabecular meshwork of trabeculectomy specimens from patients with primary systemic amyloidosis and glaucoma. This trabecular amyloid deposition presumably accounts for the aqueous outflow abnormality.

The exfoliation syndrome clinically has similar deposits in the anterior segment that are composed of an amyloidlike substance.[20,62,69] Patients with primary familial amyloid, however, also have vitreous opacities, systemic manifestations of generalized amyloid deposition, a strong family history, and a greater likelihood of bilateral glaucoma, all of which help differentiate this disorder from the exfoliation syndrome. Other ocular conditions with vitreous opacities, such as asteroid hyalitis, posterior uveitis, and intraocular neoplastic disease, are not likely to be confused with amyloidosis.

Meretoja[68] described another group of patients with familial amyloidosis, cranial neuropathy, and lattice corneal dystrophy who also appeared at risk to develop a secondary open-angle glaucoma. Among these patients, however, no vitreous opacities were present.

The therapy for glaucoma associated with primary systemic amyloidosis should follow the general guidelines for treating primary open-angle glaucoma. Visual fields and optic discs can become difficult to follow in patients with advanced vitreous opacities. Filtering surgery may be necessary, but Chandler and Grant[14] have noted the de-position of what appears to be amyloid within the bleb and a resulting gradual failure of filtration. Digital massage may be of help in such cases. Cyclodialysis also may be effective in controlling intraocular pressure.[14]

IRRADIATION

Ocular radiotherapy may cause difficult-to-control elevations of intraocular pressure by a variety of mechanisms. An iridocyclitis with or without an associated hyphema may produce an elevation of intraocular pressure,[26,27] or peripheral anterior synechiae may obliterate the angle structures.[34] Atrophy and depigmentation of the ciliary processes also may occur, with marked pigment deposition in the outflow channels and a subsequent rise in intraocular pressure.[13] Interstitial keratitis and scleral necrosis have been noted to occur following radiation,[27] and in theory radiation injuries may cause direct obliteration of the outflow channels, although histologic evidence for such a mechanism is currently lacking.

Glaucoma also may develop in response to irradiation-induced changes in the ocular blood vessels. Conjunctival telangiectases can develop after ocular irradiation. When localized, such a conjunctival telangiectasis is of little consequence, but if generalized, it may result in a rise in intraocular pressure.[7] Radiation-induced thrombosis of the iris and ciliary body vessels with degeneration of the ciliary epithelium and an associated glaucoma has been described.[27] Generalized retinal ischemia, central retinal artery occlusions, and central retinal vein occlusions occur as sequelae of high doses of ocular radiation, and rubeosis iridis may develop in this context. Rubeosis iridis with angle neovascularization and secondary glaucoma has also occurred after irradiation in an eye with an ophthalmoscopically normal fundus.[55]

ORBITAL DISEASE

Any orbital condition causing obstruction or thrombosis of the venous system draining the eye can produce a secondary glaucoma. Such conditions include orbital hemorrhage, orbital cellulitis, orbital abscess, orbital tumors and pseudotumors, thyrotrophic ophthalmopathy, and Paget's disease involving the bones of the orbit. This mechanism of secondary glaucoma is discussed in detail in Chapter 14. In some instances aqueous outflow facility may be impaired without an elevation of episcleral venous pressure.

SYSTEMIC VIRAL INFECTIOUS DISEASE IN WHICH GLAUCOMA IS NOT ASSOCIATED WITH FRANK UVEITIS
Hemorrhagic fever with renal syndrome

Hemorrhagic fever with renal syndrome is a viral disease characterized by fever, malaise, nausea and vomiting, hypertension, hematuria, albuminuria, oliguria, and uremia. Hemorrhagic phenomena occur because of capillary dysfunction and the deficiency of multiple blood coagulation factors, suggesting disseminated intravascular coagulation. Mortality is as high as 10%. About the tenth day after the onset of symptoms, a diuresis begins and clinical improvement occurs.

Eye findings during the acute period include lid edema, conjunctival injection and hemorrhage, retinal hemorrhages, and transient myopia. Matti-Saari[67] described three patients with this disease who developed acute bilateral glaucoma characterized by a sudden increase in intraocular pressure and marked shallowing of the anterior chamber. Bilateral iridectomies in one patient did not result in immediate deepening of the anterior chambers, suggesting that pupillary block was not the underlying mechanism. Matti-Saari attributed the chamber shallowing to vascular congestion, edema, and hemorrhage into the ciliary body accompanied by relaxation of the lens zonules, forward displacement of the iris-lens diaphragm, and occlusion of the trabecular meshwork by the peripheral iris. This mechanism explains the myopia as well as the acute glaucoma. Mydriatics and topical steroids resulted in more rapid improvement than treatment with miotics and appeared to be the more suitable therapeutic regimen. The use of systemic antiglaucomatous medications may have to be curtailed because of the severe renal failure in these patients. In all three patients studied, the anterior chambers deepened after the onset of the diuretic phase of the disease. Medical rather than surgical therapy is to be recommended in this condition because of the self-limited nature of the disorder.

Herpes zoster

Two forms of secondary glaucoma can occur with herpes zoster. Glaucoma usually develops as a consequence of acute iridocyclitis. Rarely, an acute unilateral glaucoma, can occur on the affected side, characterized by pupillary dilation, limbal injection, severe pain, and the absence of iridocyclitis. This latter form of glaucoma usually follows the skin eruption but occasionally may precede it. Duke-Elder and Perkins[29] have postulated a mechanism involving the affected ophthalmic division of the trigeminal nerve.

Mumps

Polland and Thorburn[76] noted the occurrence of transient bilateral acute open-angle glaucoma in an adult during convalescence from mumps. Although the superficial periocular tissues were injected, there was no sign of episcleritis or iritis in this patient. Polland and Thorburn attributed the intraocular pressure elevation to trabecular edema and recommended treatment with oral acetazolamide and topical steroids. They suggested that a transient rise in intraocular pressure during convalescence from mumps may be overlooked or misinterpreted as conjunctivitis in a young person and that this complication may be more frequent than is currently appreciated.

Influenza

Acute angle-closure glaucoma has been noted to occur occasionally in association with influenza.[19] It is not certain whether these observations represent the coincidental occurrence of the two disorders or whether influenza causes ocular changes (perhaps vascular congestion of the ciliary body) that further compromise an already narrow angle.

PARASITIC DISEASE

Involvement of the eye by parasitic disease, such as onchocerciasis or river blindness, can cause uveitis and secondary glaucoma (see Chapter 19).

DERMATOLOGIC DISORDERS

Glaucoma occasionally occurs in association with certain dermatologic disorders. For instance, acne rosacea or erythema multiforme may be accompanied by keratitis. An associated uveitis or inflammation of the outflow pathways may result in a secondary glaucoma.[100] Secondary open-angle glaucoma has also been noted in poikilodermatomyositis with uveitis and retinal hemorrhages.[94] Heterochromia and pigmentary glaucoma may occur in association with periocular linear scleroderma (morphea).[89] A unilateral secondary glaucoma, presumably on a vascular basis, has also been noted with generalized scleroderma.[46] The phakomatoses are discussed in Chapter 4, and juvenile xanthogranuloma is discussed in Chapter 13.

NEUROLOGIC DISORDERS

Mechanisms that control intraocular pressure are currently poorly understood, but a possible CNS role has been extensively studied, and a possible CNS origin for glaucoma has occasionally been proposed. Electroencephalographic abnormalities in patients with glaucoma have been used as evidence for possible diencephalic dysfunction, and autonomic dysfunction also has been postulated. At the present time such hypotheses are speculative.[96] Ocular hypotony frequently occurs in patients with myotonic dystrophy, but the aqueous flow rate appears normal as measured by fluorophotometry,[97] and the mechanism for this hypotony is uncertain at the present time.

LOW-TENSION GLAUCOMA

A small number of patients develop characteristic glaucomatous optic atrophy and visual field defects in the absence of an elevated intraocular pressure. It has been suggested that those cases in which an underlying disorder has been identified as being different from open-angle glaucoma be classified as pseudoglaucoma.[10] An underlying cause is often difficult to identify in the clinical setting, however, and the term low-tension glaucoma is widely used to classify these disorders. The syndrome may be subdivided into true glaucoma, conditions associated with stable visual field abnormalities, and conditions associated with progressive visual field abnormalities.

True glaucoma

Well over 90% of all patients with glaucomatous optic atrophy and visual field defects but with normal intraocular pressures have true glaucoma. Because of diurnal fluctuations, the intraocular pressure may be normal at the time of examination but elevated at other times during the day. In conditions associated with reduced scleral rigidity, such as high myopia, Schiøtz tonometry may result in artifactually low intraocular pressure measurements. Certain cases of "burned-out" glaucoma, with marked outflow impairment but also with decreased aqueous secretion, may also fall into this category.

Stable disc and visual field abnormalities

Congenital optic disc anomalies, such as colobomas or pits of the optic nerve,[71] may simulate glaucomatous optic atrophy and can be associated with a visual field defect. Previous episodes of true secondary glaucoma, such as steroid-induced glaucoma, resolved uveitic glaucoma, or repeated episodes of glaucomatocyclitic crises, may have left the patient with optic disc cupping and glaucomatous visual field defects. A large proportion of patients with low-tension glaucoma, perhaps over 25%, have a well-documented history of major hemodynamic crises with a fall in blood pressure and a shocklike state occurring before the routine observation of the asymptomatic field changes.[21-24,86] Gastrointestinal and uterine hemorrhage, cardiac arrest, and anesthetic-induced hypotension have been implicated. The disc changes and field abnormalities detected in these patients have tended to remain stable.[18,21,22] Prospective studies of patients experiencing systemic hypotension, however, have been unable to document the subsequent development of glaucomatous optic atrophy and field changes.[52,64] If glaucomatous optic disc and field changes occur as a consequence of systemic hypotension, this complication must be relatively infrequent, and additional factors may be required.

Optic disc cupping may develop after episodes of ischemic optic neuropathy. These patients have an acute decrease in vision associated with disc swelling, with or without disc hemorrhages. Some of these patients may develop excavation of the optic nerve head during the succeeding months. The development of such cupping occurs more frequently in ischemic optic neuropathy secondary to temporal arteritis,[31,48,70] but a small proportion of patients with idiopathic ischemic optic neuropathy also may develop an abnormal cup size or shape.[48,78] The optic atrophy that typically occurs after ischemic optic neuropathy is characterized by pallor. Usually the remaining disc rim in these patients is significantly paler than the remaining disc rim in glaucomatous discs with similar cup sizes,[78,91,92] and the visual loss in patients with ischemic optic neuropathy is often greater than the degree of cupping.

Nonglaucomatous cupping may occur in congenital optic atrophy and after episodes of trauma, central retinal artery occlusion, and demyelinating or inflammatory disease of the optic nerve.[91] In many instances associated findings help distinguish such cupping from glaucoma. For instance, trauma, central retinal artery occlusions, and ischemic optic neuropathy frequently show generalized ateriolar attenuation.[91] Generalized disc pallor is also commonly noted in these ischemic conditions. Segmental disc pallor is also occasionally seen. As discussed above, such pallor is not characteristic of the remaining disc rim in glaucomatous optic nerve heads. Peripapillary hard retinal exudates can be seen in eyes with papillitis after resolution of the swollen nerve head.[91] The clinical history will often distinguish these patients from those with glaucoma or low-tension glaucoma. In a nonmasked study, Radius and Maumenee[80] studied 112 cases of nonglaucomatous optic atrophy from a variety of causes, including ischemia, trauma, demyelinating or inflammatory disease, pressure necrosis, and congenital optic atrophy. Although there was a small increase in optic nerve cupping in these eyes as compared with that in contralateral eyes and a control series, Radius and Maumenee concluded that few if any of the optic nerves in this study showed characteristic glaucomatous changes.

Methanol poisoning also has been noted to be associated with the development of cupping.[16,80] The patient's history of rapid visual loss with a severe reduction in central visual acuity will distinguish this condition from progressive low-tension glaucoma.

Progressive disc and visual field abnormalities

An extensive and often contradictory literature has addressed the problem of why some patients develop progressive glaucomatous cupping and visual field defects in the presence of normal intraocular pressure. Numerous studies have attempted to relate these findings to circulatory or hematologic disorders. Many patients with low-tension glaucoma have low systemic blood pressures or low ophthalmic artery pressures as measured by ophthalmodynamometry,[21,23] frequently on the basis of carotid occlusive disease. It has been proposed that low-tension glaucoma may represent a slowly progressive ischemic optic neuropathy.[21] On the other hand, some patients with low-tension glaucoma have elevated systemic blood pressures, and many patients with carotid artery disease fail to develop glaucomatous disc or field changes.[53] Calcification of the intracranial portion of the carotid artery pressing the optic nerve was once thought to be responsible for some cases of low-tension glaucoma.[59] This finding, however, is so prevalent in elderly people with no evidence of cupping that it has been hard to substantiate such an association.[21] Degenerative changes in the

small vessels supplying the optic nerve may accompany such large-vessel disease, but such an association is not well documented. Optic nerve cupping and arcuate visual field defects have been noted to occur in association with syphilitic optic atrophy.[10] Optic disc cupping and nasal field defects have been noted in a case of the subclavian steal syndrome.[30]

An association of low-tension glaucoma with hyperlipoproteinemia has been noted,[103,104] but another study found an even higher incidence in the control group.[98] Drance[21] found either increased platelet adhesiveness or an abnormally prolonged euglobulin lysis time in some patients with low-tension glaucoma, but Joist et al.[54] failed to detect a difference in blood coagulability, fibrinolysis, and platelet function between patients with low-tension glaucoma and a control group. Anemia has been noted in some patients with progressive low-tension glaucoma, although the evidence for a true association is scant. Although a possible relationship between low-tension glaucoma and diabetes has been proposed, most studies of patients with low-tension glaucoma find that the incidence of diabetes does not differ from that in controls.[24,103]

Disease of the chiasm,[10] such as pituitary tumors, aneurysms near the chiasm,[77] or opticochiasmatic arachnoiditis, and also optic nerve tumors have been reported in association with optic nerve cupping. Usually, however, such neurologic abnormalities produce optic nerve changes and visual field defects that are quite different from the abnormalities found in glaucoma.

Although some of the associations discussed above may be noted, no clear cause can be found for most patients with progressive low-tension glaucoma. Patients with idiopathic low-tension glaucoma may have an unusual sensitivity of the optic nerve head even to normal levels of intraocular pressure, and the disorder may represent a multifactorial disease.

Clinically patients with idiopathic low-tension glaucoma tend to be older individuals, and the disease is frequently bilateral (Fig. 15-5). Often the intraocular pressure is in the high-normal range, and the outflow facility is low normal or mildly impaired. With time, some of these patients may develop frank elevations of intraocular pressure.

The treatment of low-tension glaucoma may be difficult and disappointing. A thorough evaluation

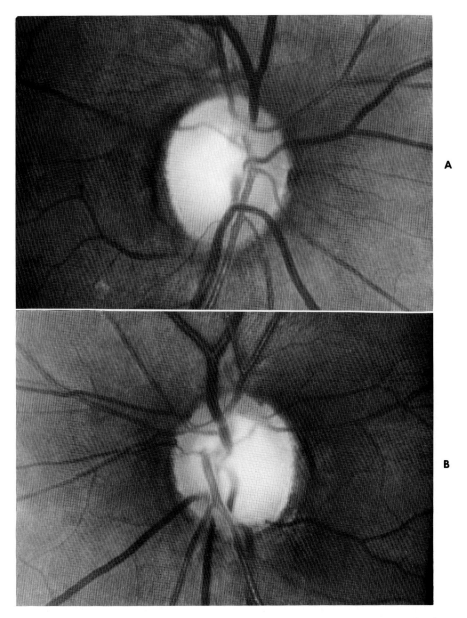

FIG. 15-5. Low-tension glaucoma. This 62-year-old woman was noted 5 years previously to have 0.2 cup/disc ratio OD and 0.3 cup/disc ratio OS. Cupping increased over subsequent years in both eyes, so that there is now prominent vertical elongation to OD cup (**A**) and marked inferior extension of OS cup (**B**).   *Continued.*

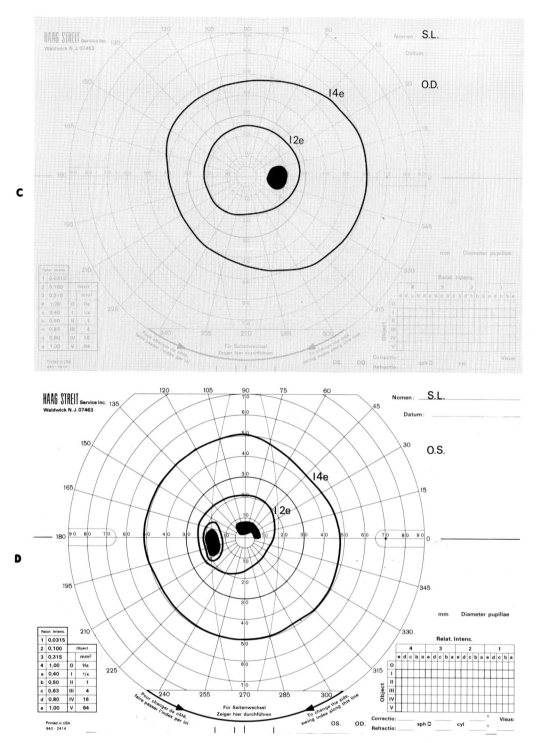

FIG. 15-5 cont'd. Visual field in right eye has remained full **(C),** but an early arcuate defect has developed superiorly in left eye **(D).** Multiple intraocular pressure measurements have never been above 21 mm Hg. Tonography yielded outflow values of 0.11 OD and 0.04 OS. Except for hypertension and borderline diabetes, complete medical, neurologic, and radiologic evaluation was negative. Patient is currently receiving topical timolol, which lowers her intraocular pressure approximately 4 to 5 mm Hg.

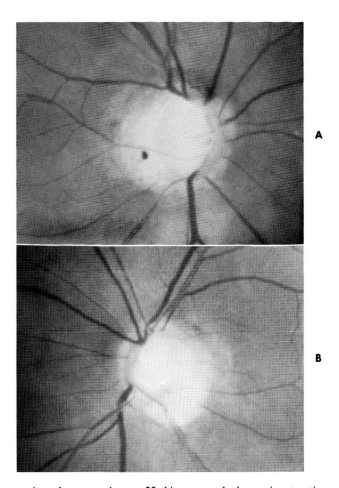

FIG. 15-6. Low-tension glaucoma. At age 55 this woman had prominent optic nerve cupping bilaterally, 6/6 vision bilaterally, and bilateral arcuate visual field defects. Her angles were wide open, outflow facility measured 0.25 OD and 0.27 OS by tonography, and water provocative test was negative. Skull x-ray and neurologic evaluations have been negative. Many intraocular pressure measurements at different times of day have never yielded value above 20 mm Hg. Past treatment included epinephrine and carbachol, but over ensuing years her optic disc cupping and visual field loss have progressed in both eyes. Fundus photos show marked optic disc cupping in both right (**A**) and left (**B**) eye with corresponding visual field defects in right (**C**) and left (**D**) eye. Nerve fiber layer shows wedge-shaped defect in superotemporal region of right eye (**E**). Patient is currently being treated with topical timolol, which maintains her intraocular pressure in range of 10 in both eyes. (Courtesy Edwin U. Keates M.D., Scheie Eye Institute.)   *Continued.*

for underlying glaucoma, including diurnal intraocular pressure measurements, visual fields, and gonioscopy, should be initiated. Tonography or certain provocative tests also may be helpful. If underlying glaucoma is found, it should be treated appropriately. If an underlying neurologic problem is found, which is unusual, it also should be treated with appropriate therapy. In idiopathic low-tension glaucoma, one should attempt to lower the intraocular pressure as much as possible (Fig. 15-6). In initiating topical therapy, it is best to treat one eye first so that comparison with the contra-lateral untreated eye can be used to assess the intraocular pressure response. Despite maximum medical therapy, visual field loss may progress, and filtering surgery may be attempted to further lower the intraocular pressure. In such cases surgical procedures that result in low postoperative intraocular pressures, such as trephinations, are frequently recommended. Despite "successful" lowering of intraocular pressure by medical and surgical means, however, a number of these patients will continue to have visual field loss.[18]

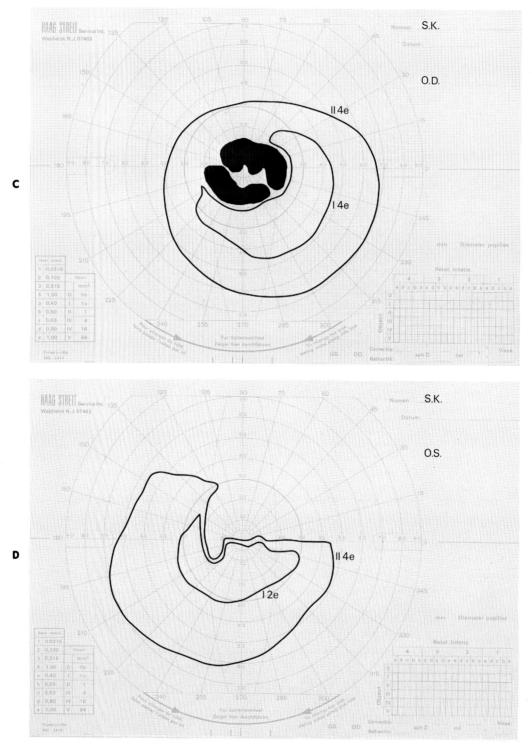

FIG. 15-6 cont'd. For legend see p. 241.

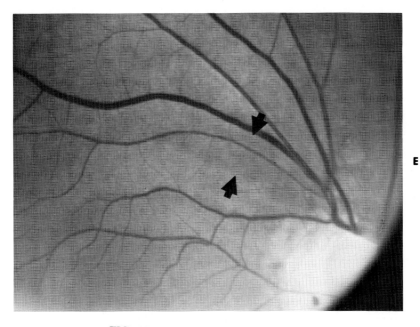

FIG. 15-6 cont'd. For legend see p. 241.

REFERENCES

1. Armaly, M.F., and Baloglou, P.J.: Diabetes mellitus and the eye. II. Intraocular pressure and aqueous outflow facility, Arch. Ophthalmol. **77:**493, 1967.
2. Armstrong, J.R., Daily, R.K., Dobson, H.L., and Girard, L.J.: The incidence of glaucoma in diabetes mellitus: a comparison with the incidence of glaucoma in the general population, Am. J. Ophthalmol. **50:**55, 1960.
3. Bankes, J.L.K.: Ocular tension and diabetes mellitus, Br. J. Ophthalmol. **61:**557, 1967.
4. Bayer, J.M., and Neuner, H.P.: Cushing-Syndrom und erhohter Augeninnendruck, Dtsch. Med. Wochenschr. **92:**1792, 1967.
5. Becker, B.: Diabetes mellitus and primary open-angle glaucoma, Am. J. Ophthalmol. **71:**1, 1971.
6. Becker, B., Kolker, A.E., and Ballin, N.: Thyroid function and glaucoma, Am. J. Ophthalmol. **61:**997, 1966.
7. Bedford, M.A.: The corneal and conjunctival complications following radiotherapy, Proc. R. Soc. Med. **59:** 529, 1966.
8. Behrman, S.: Retinal vein obstruction, Br. J. Ophthalmol. **46:**336, 1962.
9. Bengtsson, B.: Some factors affecting the distribution of intraocular pressures in a population, Acta Ophthalmol. **50:**33, 1972.
10. Blazar, H.A., and Scheie, H.G.: Pseudoglaucoma, Arch. Ophthalmol. **44:**499, 1950.
11. Bloome, M.A.: Transient angle-closure glaucoma in central retinal vein occlusion, Ann. Ophthalmol. **9:**44, 1977.
12. Boniuk, M., and Burton, G.L.: Unilateral glaucoma associated with sickle-cell retinopathy, Trans. Am. Acad. Opthalmol. Otolaryngol. **68:**316, 1964.
13. Bothman, L.: Glaucoma following irradiation, Arch. Ophthalmol. **23:**1198, 1940.
14. Chandler, P.A., and Grant, W.M.: Amyloidosis and open-angle glaucoma. In Glaucoma, ed. 2, Philadelphia, 1979, Lea & Febiger.
15. Chandler, P.A., and Grant, W.M.: Angle closure glaucoma secondary to occlusion of the central retinal vein. In Glaucoma, Philadelphia, 1979, Lea & Febiger.
16. Chandler, P.A., and Grant, W.M.: Progressive low-tension glaucoma. In Glaucoma, ed. 2, Philadelphia, 1979, Lea & Febiger.
17. Cheng, H., and Perkins, E.S.: Thyroid disease and glaucoma, Br. J. Ophthalmol. **51:**547, 1967.
18. Chumbley, L.C., and Brubaker, R.F.: Low-tension glaucoma, Am. J. Ophthalmol. **81:**761, 1976.
19. Daniele, S.: Primary closed-angle glaucoma and influenza: report of three cases, Ann. Ottal. **95:**961, 1969.
20. Dark, A.J., Streeten, B.W., and Cornwall, C.C.: Pseudoexfoliative disease of the lens: a study in electron microscopy and histochemistry, Br. J. Ophthalmol. **61:** 462, 1977.
21. Drance, S.M.: Some factors in the production of low tension glaucoma, Br. J. Opthalmol. **56:**229, 1972.
22. Drance, S.M., Morgan, R.W., and Sweeney, V.P.: Shock-induced optic neuropathy: a cause of nonprogressive glaucoma, N. Engl. J. Med. **228:**392, 1973.
23. Drance, S.M., Sweeney, V.P., Morgan, R.W., and Feldman, F.: Studies of factors involved in the production of low tension glaucoma, Arch. Ophthalmol. **89:**457, 1973.
24. Drance, S.M., Sweeney, V.P., Morgan, R.W., and Feldman, F.: Factors involved in the production of low tension glaucoma, Can. J. Ophthalmol. **9:**399, 1974.

25. Dryden, R.M.: Central retinal vein occlusions and chronic simple glaucoma, Arch. Ophthalmol. **73:**659, 1965.

26. Duke-Elder, S.: System of opthalmology, vol. 11, Diseases of the lens and vitreous; glaucoma and hypotony, St. Louis, 1969, The C.V. Mosby Co., p. 405-406, 675.

27. Duke-Elder, S., and MacFaul, P.A.: Injuries, part 2, Non-mechanical injuries. Vol. 14 in Duke-Elder, S.: System of ophthalmology, St. Louis, 1972, The C.V. Mosby Co., pp. 964-985.

28. Duke-Elder, S., and McFaul, P.A.: The ocular adnexa, part 2, Lacrimal, orbital and paraorbital diseases. Vol. 13 in Duke-Elder, S.: System of ophthalmology, St. Louis, 1974, The C.V. Mosby Co., p. 948.

29. Duke-Elder, S., and Perkins, E.S.: Diseases of the uveal tract. Vol. 9 in Duke-Elder, S.: System of ophthalmology, St. Louis, 1966, The C.V. Mosby Co., p. 347.

30. Dwyer-Joyce, P.: The fields in subclavian steal, Trans. Ophthalmol. Soc. U.K. **92:**819, 1972.

31. Eagling, E.M., Sanders, M.D., and Miller, S.J.H.: Ischaemic papillopathy: clinical and fluorescein angiographic review of forty cases, Br. J. Ophthalmol. **58:**990, 1974.

32. François, J., and Neetens, A.: The determination of the visual field in glaucoma and the blood pressure, Doc. Ophthalmol. **28:**70, 1970.

33. Friedman, A.H., Halpern, B.L., Friedberg, D.N., et al.: Transient open-angle glaucoma associated with sickle cell trait: report on four cases. Br. J. Ophthalmol. **63:** 832, 1979.

34. Fry, W.E.: Secondary glaucoma, cataract and retinal degeneration following irradiation, Trans. Am. Acad. Ophthalmol. Otolaryngol. **56:**888, 1952.

35. Gartner, S., and Henkind, P.: Neovascularization of the iris (rubeosis iridis), Surv. Ophthalmol. **22:**291, 1978.

36. Godtfredsen, E.: Glaucoma and pituitary tumour, Acta Ophthalmol. **46:**600, 1968.

37. Goldberg, M.F.: The diagnosis and treatment of sickled erythrocytes in human hyphemas, Trans. Am. Ophthalmol. Soc. **76:**481, 1978.

38. Goldberg, M.F.: The diagnosis and treatment of secondary glaucoma after hyphema in sickle cell patients, Am. J. Ophthalmol. **87:**43, 1979.

39. Goldberg, M.F.: Sickle cell retinopathy. In Duane, T.D., editor: Clinical ophthalmology, vol. 3, Diseases of the retina, New York, 1979, Harper & Row, Publishers, Inc.

40. Goldberg, M.F., and Tso, M.O.M.: Rubeosis iridis and glaucoma associated with sickle cell retinopathy: a light and electron microscopic study, Ophthalmology **85:**1028, 1978.

41. Gorin, G.: Clinical glaucoma, New York, 1977, Marcel Dekker, Inc., p. 337.

42. Grant, W.M.: Shallowing of the anterior chamber following occlusion of the central retinal vein, Am. J. Ophthalmol. **75:**384, 1973.

43. Greco, A.V., Ricci, B., Altomonte, L., et al.: GH secretion in open-angle glaucoma, Ophthalmologica **179:** 168, 1979.

44. Haas, J.S., and Nootens, R.H.: Glaucoma secondary to benign adrenal adenoma, Am. J. Ophthalmol. **78:**497, 1974.

45. Haddad, H.H.: Tonography and visual fields in endocrine exophthalmos, Am. J. Ophthalmol. **64:**63, 1967.

46. Halmay, V.O., Bajan, O.M., and Felden, E.: Halbese-

itiges mit Skleroderma assoziiertes Glaukom. Klin. Monatsbl. Augenheilkd. **152:**558, 1968.

47. Harrington, D.O.: The pathogenesis of the glaucoma field, Am. J. Ophthalmol. **47**(part 2):177, 1959.

48. Hayreh, S.S.: Pathogenesis of cupping of the optic disc, Br. J. Ophthalmol. **58:**863, 1974.

49. Hovland, K.E., and Ellis, P.P.: Ocular changes in renal transplant patients, Am. J. Ophthalmol. **63:**283, 1967.

50. Howard, G.M., and English, F.P.: Occurrence of glaucoma in acromegalics, Arch. Ophthalmol. **73:**765, 1965.

51. Hyams, S.W., and Neumann, E.: Transient angle closure glaucoma after retinal vein occlusion, Br. J. Ophthalmol. **56:**353, 1972.

52. Jampol, L.M., Board, R.J., and Maumenee, A.E.: Systemic hypotension and glaucomatous changes, Am. J. Ophthalmol. **85:**154, 1978.

53. Jampol, L.M., and Miller, N.R.: Carotid artery disease and glaucoma, Br. J. Ophthalmol. **62:**324, 1978.

54. Joist, J.H., Lichtenfeld, P., Mandell, A.I., and Kolker, A.E.: Platelet function, blood coagulability, and fibrinolysis in patients with low tension glaucoma, Arch. Ophthalmol. **94:**1893, 1976.

55. Jones, R.F.: Glaucoma following radiotherapy, Br. J. Ophthalmol. **42:**636, 1958.

56. Kahn, H.A., Leibowitz, H.M., Ganley, J.P., et al.: The Framingham eye study. II. Association of ophthalmic pathology with single variables previously measured in the Framingham heart study, Am. J. Epidemiol. **106:** 33, 1977.

57. Kass, M.A., and Sears, M.L.: Hormonal regulation of intraocular pressure, Surv. Ophthalmol. **22:**153, 1977.

58. Kaufman, H.E.: Primary familial amyloidosis, Arch. Ophthalmol. **60:**1036, 1958.

59. Knapp, A.: On the association of sclerosis of the cerebrobasal vessels with optic atrophy and cupping, Trans. Am. Ophthalmol. Soc. **30:**343, 1932.

60. Krasnovid, T.A.: A new hypothesis on the mechanism of diurnal variations in intraocular tension, Oftalmol. Zh. **21:**185, 1966.

61. Krupin, T., Jacobs, L.S., Podos, S.M., and Becker, B.: Thyroid function and the intraocular pressure response to topical corticosteroids, Am. J. Ophthalmol. **83:**643, 1977.

62. Layden, W.E., and Shaffer, R.N.: Exfoliation syndrome, Am. J. Ophthalmol. **78:**835, 1974.

63. Leighton, D.A., and Phillips, C.I.: Systemic blood pressure in open-angle glaucoma, low tension glaucoma, and the normal eye, Br. J. Ophthalmol. **56:**447, 1972.

64. Levy, N.S., and Rawitscher, R.: The effect of systemic hypotension during cardiopulmonary bypass on intraocular pressure and visual function in humans, Ann. Ophthalmol. **9:**1547, 1977.

65. Lieb, W.A., Geeraets, W.J., and Guerry, D. III.: Sickle-cell retinopathy: ocular and systemic manifestations of sickle-cell disease, Acta Ophthalmol. Suppl. **58:**1, 1959.

66. Linnér, E.: The rate of aqueous flow and the adrenals, Trans. Ophthalmol. Soc. U.K. **79:**27, 1959.

67. Matti Saari, K.: Acute glaucoma in hemorrhagic fever with renal syndrome (nephropathia epidemica), Am. J. Ophthalmol. **81:**455, 1976.

68. Meretoja, J.: Comparative histopathological and clinical findings in eyes with lattice corneal dystrophy of two different types, Ophthalmologica **165:**15, 1972.

69. Meretoja, J., and Tarkkanen, A.: Occurrence of amyloid in eyes with pseudo-exfoliation, Ophthalmic Res. **9:**80, 1977.

70. Miller, S.: Doyne Memorial Lecture: The enigma of glaucoma simplex: optic disc cupping in normal eyes, Trans. Ophthalmol. Soc. U.K. **92:**563, 1972.

71. Neame, H.: Congenital hole at optic disc: report of 10 cases with especial reference to visual field defects, Trans. Ophthalmol. Soc. U.K. **67:**109, 1948.

72. Neuner, H.P., and Dardenne, U.: Augenveränderungen bei Cushing-Syndrom, Klin. Monatsbl. Augenheilkd. **152:**570, 1968.

73. Pantieleva, V.M., Klyachko, V.R., and Barkman, S.M.: Ocular hydrodynamics in primary hypothyroidism, Vestn. Oftalmol. **3:**18, 1971.

74. Paton, D., and Duke, J.R.: Primary familial amyloidosis (ocular manifestations with histopathologic observations), Am. J. Ophthalmol. **61:**736, 1966.

75. Pohjanpelto, P.: The thyroid gland and intraocular pressure (tonographic study of 187 patients with thyroid disease), Acta Ophthalmol. Suppl. **97:**9, 1968.

76. Polland, W., and Thorburn, W.: Transient glaucoma as a manifestation of mumps, Acta Ophthalmol. **54:**779, 1976.

77. Portney, G.L., and Roth, A.M.: Optic nerve cupping caused by an intracranial aneurysm, Am. J. Ophthalmol. **84:**98, 1977.

78. Quigley, H., and Anderson, D.R.: Cupping of the optic disc in ischemic optic neuropathy, Trans. Am. Acad. Ophthalmol. Otolaryngol. **83:**755, 1977.

79. Radius, R.L., and Finkelstein, D.: Central retinal artery occlusion (reversible) in sickle trait with glaucoma, Br. J. Ophthalmol. **60:**428, 1976.

80. Radius, R.L., and Maumenee, A.E.: Optic atrophy and glaucomatous cupping, Am. J. Ophthalmol. **85:**145, 1978.

81. Raitta, C., Vannas, S., and Aurekoski, H.: Aqueous humor dynamics after central retinal vein occlusion, Acta Ophthalmol. **46:**26, 1968.

82. Ramsell, J.T., Ellis, P.P., and Paterson, C.A.: Intraocular pressure changes during hemodialysis, Am. J. Ophthalmol. **72:**926, 1971.

83. Reese, A.B., and McGavic, J.S.: Relation of field contraction to blood pressure in chronic primary glaucoma, Arch. Ophthalmol. **27:**845, 1942.

84. Safir, A., Paulsen, E.P., Klayman, J., and Gerstenfeld, J.: Ocular abnormalities in juvenile diabetics: frequent occurrence of abnormally high tensions, Arch. Ophthalmol. **76:**557, 1966.

85. Schmelzer, H.: Hypophyse und Glaukomgenese, Klin. Monatsbl. Augenheilkd. **129:**114, 1956.

86. Schwartz, B.: Shock and low-tension glaucoma, N. Engl. J. Med. **288:**417, 1973.

87. Segawa, K.: The fine structure of the iridocorneal angle tissue in glaucomatous eyes. V. Glaucoma secondary to primary familial amyloidosis, Jpn. Clin. Ophthalmol. **30:** 1375, 1976.

88. Shapiro, A.L., and Baum, J.L.: Acute open-angle glaucoma in a patient with sickle cell trait, Am. J. Ophthalmol. **58:**292, 1964.

89. Stone, R.A., and Scheie, H.G.: Periorbital scleroderma associated with heterochromia iridis, Am. J. Ophthalmol. **90:**858, 1980.

90. Traisman, H.S., Alfano, J.E., Andrews, J., and Gatti, R.: Intraocular pressure in juvenile diabetics, Am. J. Ophthalmol. **64:**1149, 1967.

91. Trobe, J.D., Glaser, J.S., and Cassidy, J.C.: Optic atrophy: differential diagnosis by fundus observation alone, Arch. Ophthalmol. **98:**1040, 1980.

92. Trobe, J.D., Glaser, J.S., Cassidy, J.C., et al.: Nonglaucomatous excavation of the optic disc, Arch. Ophthalmol. **98:**1046, 1980.

93. Tsukahara, S.M., and Matsuo, T.: Secondary glaucoma accompanied with primary familial amyloidosis, Ophthalmologica **175:**250, 1977.

94. Tuovinen, E., and Raudasoja, R.: Poikilodermatomyositis with retinal hemorrhages and secondary glaucoma, Acta Ophthalmol. **43:**669, 1965.

95. van Bijsterveld, O.P., and Richards, R.D.: Pituitary tumors and intraocular pressure, Am. J. Ophthalmol. **57:**267, 1964.

96. Waitzman, M.B.: Hypothalamus and ocular pressure, Surv. Ophthalmol. **16:**1, 1971.

97. Walker, S.D., and Brubaker, R.F.: Aqueous humor dynamics in myotonic dystrophy, Invest. Ophthalmol. **19**(suppl.):140, 1980.

98. Walker, W.M., Walton, K.W., Magnani, H.N., et al.: Glaucoma and ischaemic vascular disease risk factors, Trans. Ophthalmol. Soc. U.K. **96:**237, 1976.

99. Weekers, R., Prijot, E., and Lavergne, G.: Mesure de la pression oculaire, de la résistance à l'ecoulement de l'humeur aqueuse et de la rigidité dans les exophthalmies endocriniennes, Ophthalmologica **139:**382, 1960.

100. Weiss, D.I.: Glaucoma and systemic disease. In Duane, T.D., editor: Clinical ophthalmology, vol. 5, New York, 1979, Harper & Row, Publishers, Inc.

101. Welch, R.B., and Goldberg, M.F.: Sickle-cell hemoglobin and its relation to fundus abnormality, Arch Ophthalmol. **75:**353, 1966.

102. Wilson, D.M., and Martin, J.H.S.: Raised intraocular tension in renal transplants recipients, Med. J. Aus. **1:** 482, 1973.

103. Winder, A.F.: Circulating lipoprotein and blood glucose levels in association with low-tension and chronic simple glaucoma, Br. J. Ophthalmol. **61:**641, 1977.

104. Winder, A.F., Paterson, G., and Miller, S.J.H.: Biochemical abnormalities associated with ocular hypertension and low-tension glaucoma, Trans. Ophthalmol. Soc. U.K. **94:**518, 1974.

105. Yanoff, M., and Fine, B.S.: Ocular pathology: a text and atlas, New York, 1975, Harper & Row, Publishers, Inc., pp. 340-341.

Chapter 16

EFFECTS OF NONSTEROIDAL DRUGS ON GLAUCOMA

Robert M. Mandelkorn and Thom J. Zimmerman

The subject of this chapter is not true secondary glaucoma but drugs that can precipitate angle-closure attacks, cause elevation of intraocular pressure in patients with open-angle glaucoma, or worse, quietly promote the development of chronic angle closure. The ophthalmologist and the nonophthalmic physician should be aware that many commonly used drugs can secondarily cause or aggravate glaucoma. Drugs prescribed for such diverse conditions as depression, allergy, and hypertension can cause elevation of intraocular pressure, pupillary dilation, and lens swelling. The patient with narrow angles or previously undiagnosed angle-closure glaucoma is in particular danger. Since he is not likely to bring the range of his complaints to the attention of a specialist, it is necessary that his physician be alert to the dangers.

Cautions regarding specific drugs that have been associated with attacks of angle-closure glaucoma or aggravation of open-angle glaucoma are given in the *Physicians' Desk Reference (PDR)*. For a list of these drugs, refer to Tables 16-1 through 16-8. These drugs produce their unwanted effects through a variety of mechanisms, an understanding of which will help the physician anticipate problems.

Through the mechanism of lens swelling (i.e., the sulfa drugs), narrow angles can be further compromised and precipitate an episode of angle-closure glaucoma. Systemically used agents that can dilate the pupils (e.g., agents for biliary spasm or gastrointestinal overactivity) may also precipitate acute angle closure in susceptible patients. There are several classes of medication that may elevate intraocular pressure even in the controlled or not previously diagnosed open-angle glaucoma patient (see Tables 16-1 through 16-8). The mechanism of this latter pressure elevation is poorly understood.

For the ophthalmologist, prevention of these problems lies in identifying patients at risk. Gonioscopy should be performed on all patients with glaucoma, shallow anterior chambers, or hyperopia. It is crucial that the ophthalmologist be aware of the association between the glaucoma he is treating and the patient's drug regimen. Patients with narrow angles that are judged occludable should be warned about the use of these medications. The ophthalmologist should routinely ask the patient about every drug, prescribed or purchased over the counter, that he has taken in the recent past.

For the nonophthalmic physician, the penlight or flashlight test is the simplest test available. Hold a penlight at the limbus of the eye (where the sclera joins the cornea) and note whether the light shines across the anterior chamber, fully illuminating the iris, or is partly blocked by forward bowing of the iris and therefore unable to illuminate the nasal side of the iris, as in patients with shallow anterior chambers. After this test ask if the patient has seen colored halos around bright lights or if he has blurred vision or eye pain. Any of these symptoms should raise suspicion of subacute attacks of angle-closure glaucoma.

Factors such as the small size of a hyperopic eye,[20,47] disproportion between the size of the lens and the size of the anterior segment of the eye,[13] and an abnormal insertion of the iris into the ciliary body[47] may predispose the patient to angle-closure glaucoma. The event itself is usually precipitated by placing the pupil in the middilated range. When the pupil is in the 3- to 5-mm range,[53] the possibility of angle-closure is greatest. Obviously, very little effect is required by either a weak mydriatic agent, such as dicyclomine (Bentyl), or a moderate miotic agent, such as a weak concentration of pilocarpine, to place the pupil, either previously constricted or dilated, in such a position. Dim light or darkness, emotional disturbance, shock, physical illness, and accident may lead to pupillary dilation.[20]

DRUGS AND GLAUCOMA
Phenothiazines

The adverse ocular effects of phenothiazine compounds are well documented.[32] These agents exhibit both alpha-adrenergic and cholinergic blocking action, and either action may predominate in any one drug.[30] The former is seen with chlorpromazine, with which miosis occurs, and the latter occurs with most phenothiazines. However, the anticholinergic action of these agents is rather weak in comparison with that of atropine.[73] In-

deed, only mepazine[66,72] has been shown to produce clinically observed mydriasis and cycloplegia. The weak effect of these agents on the eye is confirmed by the fact that only triflupromazine (Vesprin) is listed in the *PDR* as an agent that should be used with caution in patients with glaucoma[62] (Table 16-1).

Precipitation or aggravation of glaucoma by these drugs has not been documented. A word of caution, however: when these agents are used together or in combination with other agents, especially the monoamine oxidase (MAO) inhibitors[29] and the tricyclic antidepressants,[30] their actions may be enhanced. In addition to their effects on the autonomic innervation of the eye, the phenothiazines (in particular, prochlorperazine [Compazine][87] and promethazine hydrochloride [Phenergan][3]) may produce idiopathic lens swelling. Theoretically, this can precipitate angle closure in a susceptible patient. Although such attacks with the use of phenothiazines are not documented, these problems are mentioned in the literature in connection with the use of sulfa compounds. This effect is probably attributable to a toxic reaction to the drug and has been reported only rarely (see section on sulfa drugs).

Two new major classes of tranquilizers with

TABLE 16-1
Antipsychotic phenothiazine agents and their derivatives

Generic (brand)	*PDR* warning	Case reports of glaucoma
Phenothiazines		
Chlorpromazine hydrochloride (Thorazine)	No	No
Triflupromazine hydrochloride (Vesprin)	Yes	No
Thioridazine hydrochloride (Mellaril)	No	No
Perphenazine (Trilafon)	No	No
Prochlorperazine (Compazine) edisylate	No	Yes[87]
Prochlorperazine (Compazine) maleate	No	Yes[87]
Fluphenazine hydrochloride (Permitil, Prolixin)	No	No
Fluphenazine (Prolixin) enanthate	No	No
Fluphenazine (Prolixin) decanoate	No	No
Acetophenazine maleate (Tindal)	No	No
Trifluoperazine hydrochloride (Stelazine)	No	No
Promethazine hydrochloride (Phenergan)	No	Yes[3]
Thioxanthenes		
Chlorprothixene (Taractan)	No	No
Thiothixene hydrochloride (Navane)	No	No
Butyrophenones		
Haloperidol (Haldol)	Yes	No
Dibenzoxephines		
Doxepin (Sinequan)	Yes	No

anticholinergic action are represented by doxepin (Sinequan) and haloperidol (Haldol). Doxepin is a dibenzoxepine, a modification of the phenothiazine structure. Its anticholinergic effect is much stronger than that of the phenothiazines.[73] Haloperidol is a butyrophenone.[30] The use of both classes of drugs in patients with glaucoma is cautioned against in the *PDR*, but neither has actually been documented to exacerbate or precipitate glaucoma.

Tricyclic antidepressants

The tricyclic antidepressants are a closely related group of agents that also have anticholinergic action.[30] However, theirs is much stronger than that of the phenothiazines.[73] Indeed, amitriptyline (Elavil, Amitril), imipramine (Tofranil), and protriptyline (Vivactil) have all been shown to cause mydriasis in normal use[22,79] and when taken in overdoses.[74] Amitriptyline, the strongest anticholinergic agent,[73] has been associated with attacks of angle-closure glaucoma.[51] All of these agents carry warnings about their use in patients with glaucoma, and it should be noted that their actions may be augmented by the MAO inhibitors.[29]

Monoamine oxidase inhibitors

The MAO inhibitors are antidepressants with extremely weak anticholinergic action, comparable to that of the phenothiazines.[73] The major risk is that they may potentiate the effects of other drugs,[29] such as phenothiazines, tricyclic antidepressants, antiparkinsonian drugs, and sympathomimetic agents (amphetamines and ephedrine).

These drug interactions are poorly understood, but several theories have been suggested.[29] The enzyme MAO may itself be necessary to inactivate these other agents; the blockage of an enzyme other than MAO that is vital to the inactivation of metabolites of these drugs may take place; or the MAO inhibitor may alter the action of other drugs unrelated to enzyme inhibition. This drug interaction is mentioned in the *PDR* under the specific agent headings, and a warning is given cautioning against the use of these agents in patients with glaucoma (Table 16-2), although no cases of aggravation of glaucoma have been reported in the literature.

Antihistamines

The antihistamines (Table 16-3) are a diverse group of drugs that have in common the ability to

TABLE 16-2
MAO inhibitors that may potentiate the adverse effects of drugs from Tables 16-1, 16-4, and 16-7

Generic (brand)	PDR warning	Case reports of glaucoma
Phenelzine sulfate (Nardil)	Yes	No
Pargyline hydrochloride (Eutonyl)	Yes	No
Tranylcypromine sulfate (Parnate)	Yes	No

block the action of histamine. The H_1-antihistamines[30] block the action of histamine on capillary permeability, and vascular, bronchial, and other smooth muscles. The H_2 antihistamines[30] also block the effect of histamine on the smooth muscles of peripheral blood vessels and, in addition, the secretion of gastric acid. H_1 antihistamines also have a sedative effect, an anticholinergic effect, and local anesthetic properties.[30] The anticholinergic action is usually weak[30]; however, an acute overdose may precipitate an atropine-like toxic state[30,31] with fever, flushed face, and dilated pupils, which could exacerbate glaucoma. Only one case of precipitation of angle-closure glaucoma by one of these drugs, orphenadrine citrate (Norgesic), has been reported.[32] Another antihistamine, promethazine hydrochloride has been documented to cause an idiopathic swelling of the lens.[3] Even though glaucoma did not result from this case, similar incidents with other agents (sulfa)[52] have precipitated attacks of angle-closure glaucoma and should be carefully watched.

The H_2 blocking agents (burimamide, metiamide, and most recently cimetidine) limit their effect to H_2 receptors and are not known at the present time to have any effect on the eye.

Antiparkinsonian drugs

The antiparkinsonian drugs can be divided into two groups: (1) agents that replenish the diminished stores of dopamine in the corpus striatum (caudate nucleus and putamen) and (2) agents that improve clinical symptoms through a strong anticholinergic action. Of the first group of agents used today, the classic drug is levodopa. Because dopamine is the precursor of epinephrine and norepinephrine, the administration of levodopa increases sympathetic tone and dilates the pupils.

TABLE 16-3
Antihistamines

Generic (brand)	PDR warning	Case reports of glaucoma
Ethanolamines		
Diphenhydramine hydrochloride (Benadryl)	Yes	No
Dimenhydrinate (Dramamine)	No	No
Orphenadrine citrate (Norgesic)	Yes	Yes[32]
Ethylenediamines		
Tripelennamine citrate (Pyribenzamine)	Yes	No
Antazoline phosphate (Vasocon-A)	Yes	No
Methapyrilene hydrochloride (Histadyl)	No	No
Alkylamines		
Chlorpheniramine maleate (Chlor-Trimeton)	No	No
Brompheniramine (Dimetane)	Yes	No
Piperazine		
Cyclizine hydrochloride (Marezine)	Yes	No
Phenothiazine		
Promethazine hydrochloride (Phenergan)	Yes	Yes[3]

This action by itself is usually not enough to aggravate glaucoma. However, when used with MAO inhibitors,[30] the sympathomimetic action of levodopa may be increased, so that an eye with narrow angles is at greater risk.

The remaining agents act through strong anticholinergic action.[73] Several of these drugs have been reported to precipitate or aggravate angle-closure glaucoma (Table 16-4), and they should be used cautiously in all patients with glaucoma.

Minor tranquilizers

The minor tranquilizers do not appear to have autonomic activity. However, there has been one report of an attack of angle-closure glaucoma in a patient taking diazepam (Valium).[42] The cause is not clear, as evidenced by the subsequent debate in the literature.[12]

Sedatives and stimulants

The sedatives,[64] including barbiturates, paraldehyde, morphine, meperidine, reserpine, mephenesin and phenytoin, appear to have no significant ill effects on the eye; they may even lower the intraocular pressure (see section on anesthetic agents). However, the stimulants, including amphetamines, caffeine, and methylphenidate (Ritalin), do cause a transient rise in intraocular pressure in patients with glaucoma.[32] The significance of these findings is uncertain. In addition, MAO inhibitors will potentiate the actions of amphetamines.[29] It should also be mentioned that the

TABLE 16-4
Antiparkinsonian agents

Generic (brand)	PDR warning	Case reports of glaucoma
Benztropine mesylate (Cogentin)	No	No
Trihexyphenidyl hydrochloride (Artane)	Yes	Yes[62]
Biperiden hydrochloride (Akineton)	Yes	No
Cycrimine hydrochloride (Pagitane)	Yes	No
Procyclidine hydrochloride (Kemadrin)	No	No

amount of caffeine given orally or intravenously in the experiments was considerably more than the amount in a cup of coffee.

Antispasmolytic agents

The ability of the antispasmolytic agents (Table 16-5) to reduce both gastric secretion and motility of the stomach is directly related to their anticholinergic actions. Herxheimer[41] compared these agents with atropine and showed their potency to range from oxyphenonium, which has 50% the potency of atropine, to propantheline, which has 22% the potency of atropine. Ironically, the weakest anticholinergic agents, dicyclomine and propantheline (Pro-Banthine),[41] which do not dilate

TABLE 16-5

Antispasmolytic agents

Generic (brand)	PDR warning	Case reports of glaucoma
Methscopolamine bromide (Pamine)	Yes	No
Propantheline bromide (Pro-Banthine)	Yes	Yes[58]
Oxyphenonium bromide (Antrenyl)	Yes	No
Tridihexethyl chloride (Pathilon)	Yes	No
Diphemanil methylsulfate (Prantal)	Yes	No
Hexocyclium methylsulfate (Tral)	Yes	No
Dicyclomine hydrochloride (Bentyl)	Yes	Yes[58]
Oxyphencyclimine hydrochloride (Daricon, Vistrax)	No	No

TABLE 16-6

Agents that cause idiopathic lens swelling

Generic (brand)	PDR warning	Case reports of glaucoma
Spironolactone (Aldactone)	No	No
Ethoxzolamide (Ethamide, Cardrase)*	No	No
Dichlorphenamide (Daranide, Oratrol)	No	No
Phenformin (DBI)*	No	No
Hydrochlorothiazide (Hydro-Diuril, Esidrix)*	No	No
Chlorothiazide (Diuril)*	No	No
Chlorthalidone (Hygroton)*	No	No
Polythiazide (Renese)*	No	No
Promethazine (Phenergan)	No	No
Sulfanilamide (AVC Cream, Vagitrol)*	No	Yes[52]
Tetracycline	No	No
Acetylsalicylic acid (aspirin)	No	Yes[68]
Trichlormethiazide (Metahydrin)	No	No
Acetazolamide (Diamox)*	No	No

*Sulfa agents.

the pupil, have actually been found to raise the intraocular pressure as high as 10 to 14 mm Hg when given to patients with open-angle glaucoma.[58] This transient pressure elevation is believed to be due to their anticholinergic action. No cases of precipitation of angle-closure glaucoma due to these agents have yet been documented.

Sulfa drugs

The sulfa drugs, in particular, acetazolamide (Diamox), are known to be capable of lowering intraocular pressure by reducing aqueous formation, and they are commonly used in the medical treatment of glaucoma.

In addition, an idiosyncratic response has been documented, consisting of acute myopia due to swelling of the lens, associated with elevated intraocular pressure, retinal edema, and shallowing of the anterior chamber.[52] This phenomenon was believed to be due to a toxic reaction of the ocular tissues, specifically lens and retina, to the chemical. Significant myopia is observed with a shallowing of the anterior chamber and possible precipitation of angle-closure glaucoma. Because these episodes do not respond to cycloplegic drugs and because the pupils are not affected in these cases, we believe that contraction of the iris and the ciliary body is not involved. This leads us to assume that this phenomenon is due to an idiopathic swelling of the lens or to an alteration of the lens position.[32] This phenomenon has been associated not only with sulfa drugs used as antibiotics, but also those in other forms, such as antihypertensive agents (hydrochlorothiazide [HydroDiuril],[4] chlorthalidone [Hygroton],[23,57] and most recently trichlormethiazide [Metahydrin][4]), and as antiglaucoma medication (acetazolamide,[59] dichlorphenamide [Daranide, Oratrol],[60] and ethoxzolamide [Ethamide, Cardase][36]). This same phenomenon has also been seen with tetracycline,[21] prochlorperazine,[87] promethazine,[3] hydralazine (Apresoline) and hexamethonium in combination,[35] spironolactone (Aldactone),[8] phenformin (DBI),[69] corticotrophin,[4] and acetylsalicylic acid (aspirin).[68] Obviously, those eyes with increased risk factors, such as those with shallow anterior chambers (e.g., the hyperopic patient), are at greater risk of an attack of angle-closure glaucoma than those eyes with deeper anterior chambers (e.g., the myopic patient). Table 16-6 lists the drugs that can cause idiopathic lens swelling.

Cardiac agents for the treatment of arrhythmias

Cardiac agents used to control arrhythmias comprise a diverse group of drugs. Digitalis, through the reduction of the Na-K ATPase activity in the ciliary processes, has been shown to reduce aqueous formation[9] and intraocular pressure[18] in humans and in animals when given intravenously. Unfortunately, toxic side effects limit its use in glaucoma.

Quinidine does not appear to have any effect on intraocular pressure. However, disopyramide phosphate (Norpace), a new agent used for cardiac arrhythmias, does have some anticholinergic action (0.06% as strong as atropine)[62] and has been documented[80] to precipitate an attack of angle-closure glaucoma.

Vasodilator agents

The vasodilator agents include the nitrates and tolazoline. Before the advent of gonioscopy, it was believed that acute glaucoma was caused by dilation of intraocular blood vessels, especially those of the ciliary body and the iris, and that the resultant swelling of the lens pushed the iris forward, obstructing the trabecular meshwork and aqueous outflow.[20] This led to the belief that these agents may precipitate angle-closure glaucoma in susceptible eyes. The nitrates, especially nitroglycerin (glyceryl trinitrate), have been shown to produce a transient partial blackout of vision. However, this is believed to be due to a fall in blood pressure and the associated temporary loss of perfusion to the eye.[32]

The nitrates have also been shown to cause pupillary dilation.[32] However, when nitroglycerin[85] was taken by mouth and amyl nitrate[5] was inhaled by glaucoma patients with narrow angles, acute angle-closure glaucoma could not be precipitated. Tolazoline (Priscoline), another vasodilator, was reported to have precipitated an attack of angle-closure glaucoma.[25]

The results are less clear regarding open-angle glaucoma. Oral nitroglycerin has been reported to decrease[85] the intraocular pressure transiently in both normal and glaucomatous eyes and to increase[88] the intraocular pressure in glaucomatous eyes. The inhalation of amyl nitrate has also been reported to cause both a transient increase[46] and a lowering[15] of the intraocular pressure in glaucomatous individuals. In all cases, however, the intraocular pressure change was not believed to be significant, nor did it last for more than several minutes.

Retrobulbar tolazoline has not been found to elevate intraocular pressure.[89] When given subconjunctivally as a provocative test for open-angle glaucoma, it has been found to cause a transient increase in intraocular pressure that is greater in patients with glaucoma than in normal patients.[75] This effect was not confirmed by Gandolfi[26] when he gave the drug topically. It has been claimed that tolazoline given subcutaneously lowers the intraocular pressure in normal and glaucomatous eyes.[88] However, further studies have questioned its ability to do so when given intravenously.[61]

Interestingly, additional studies done with dibenzylchlorethamine (Dibenamine), a weak vasoactive drug given intravenously, showed a transient lowering of the intraocular pressure.[61] However, because of its side effects, it was not studied further. Overall, except for one reported case of precipitation of angle-closure glaucoma[25] and the possible loss of medical control in one patient with open-angle glaucoma after tolazoline was given subconjunctivally,[75] the use of vasodilator agents appears to be safe for normal patients with narrow angles and open-angle glaucoma.

Vasoconstricting agents

The vasoconstricting agents, in turn, are alpha-adrenergic agonists. Because the pupillary dilating fibers respond to these agents, pupillary dilation is possible. Table 16-7 summarizes the effects of these agents on intraocular pressure.

Sympathomimetic agents

On the whole, the sympathomimetic agents (Table 16-7) lower the intraocular pressure. This effect has been well documented with epinephrine,[49] phenylephrine,[37,49] and ephedrine[37] in patients with open-angle glaucoma and with dopamine in rabbits.[70] In the case of epinephrine, two combinations of actions are well documented. At low concentrations epinephrine reduces aqueous formation, and at higher concentrations the coefficient of outflow is increased and mydriasis occurs.[49] The former effect is believed to be due to stimulation of beta receptors and the latter effect to stimulation of alpha receptors.[49] This is confirmed by the actions of norepinephrine,[49] a pure alpha agent, and of isoproterenol, a pure beta agonist. It should also be noted that protriptylene was found to accentuate the effect of norepinephrine.[49]

However, in spite of these results, it should be noted that a paradoxical elevation of intraocular pressure has been reported with these agents in patients with open angle glaucoma.[50] Further study of these patients has documented that this effect is due to an associated lowering of outflow facility. In addition to the effect on open-angle glaucoma,

TABLE 16-7
Sympathomimetic agents

Generic (brand)	*PDR* warning	Case reports of glaucoma
Epinephrine (E-Carpine, E-Pilo, Mytrate, Epitrate, Epifrin, Glaucon, Epinal, Eppy N)*	Yes	Yes: a[50]; b[39]
Ephedrine (Collyrium with ephedrine)	No	Yes: b[27]
Norepinephrine	No	No
Dopamine	No	No
Metaraminol	No	No
Phenylephrine (Prefrin, Vasocidin, AK-Cide, Blephamide, Efricel, Murocoll, Neo-Synephrine, Vasosulf, Zincfrin, Vernacel)	Yes	Yes: a[50]; b[39]
Amphetamine (Delcobese, Obetrol)	Yes	Yes[32]
Naphazoline (AK-Con, Albalon, Clear Eyes, Degest-2, Naphcon, Vasoclear, Vasocon)	Yes	No
Tetrahydrozoline hydrochloride (Murine, Soothe, Tetracyn, Visine)	Yes	No
Pheniramine maleate (Naphcon-A, Vernacel)	Yes	No
Methoxamine (Vasoxyl)	No	No
Hydroxyamphetamine (Paredrine)	Yes	Yes: b[27]

*This pupillary dilation may be exacerbated by timolol.[7]
a, Open-angle glaucoma; b, angle-closure glaucoma.

the dilation of the pupil is also known to precipitate attacks of angle-closure glaucoma in predisposed patients with narrow anterior chamber angles.[27]

Parasympathomimetic agents

On the other hand, the parasympathomimetic agents, including pilocarpine and carbachol, while indicated in the treatment of open-angle glaucoma[13] and to break attacks of angle-closure glaucoma,[13] have to be used with caution in patients with narrow angles. These agents can cause congestion of the iris and ciliary body, relaxation of the zonules, and shallowing of the anterior chamber[47] (shown by ultrasound to be due to an increase in the sagittal width of the lens and a net forward movement of the lens)[1] and can precipitate angle-closure glaucoma in susceptible patients.

Moderate concentrations of pilocarpine (2% and 4%) have been reported to precipitate rare attacks of angle-closure glaucoma.[13] Mapstone[53] believed this to be due to several mechanisms in addition to those mentioned above. First, pilocarpine opens the anterior chamber angle[33] and increases trabecular meshwork outflow,[39] at the same time reducing uveoscleral outflow.[10] The net result is an increase in the pressure differential from the posterior to the anterior chamber, allowing the iris to bow forward, further shallowing an anterior chamber that is already shallow. Second, pupils that were previously constricted will begin to redilate when pilocarpine begins to wear off, placing the

pupil in the middilated position. According to Mapstone, this is the critical pupillary position for precipitation of acute glaucoma. Therefore, eyes with narrow angles are theoretically at risk of an attack of angle-closure glaucoma when affected by miotic agents. Certainly, in these patients a fine balance exists between the risk factors and the benefit of pulling the iris out of the anterior chamber angle, opening the trabecular meshwork, and reducing the intraocular pressure.

Obviously, the parasympathomimetic agents must be used carefully in the treatment of patients with narrow angles. It should also be noted that pilocarpine may exacerbate several types of glaucoma. These situations include glaucoma secondary to uveitis, malignant glaucoma, neovascular glaucoma, lens- and vitreous-induced pupillary-block glaucoma,[13] and recently a case of angle-recession glaucoma.[11]

Parasympatholytic agents

The parasympatholytic agents appear to pose the same threats to the eye with both open-angle and angle-closure glaucoma as do the sympathomimetic agents. Indeed, atropine, homatropine, scopolamine, cyclopentolate, and tropicamide (Mydriacyl) all produce an elevated intraocular pressure in patients with open-angle glaucoma (23% versus 2% of normal patients).[38] Only eucatropine, a weak agent, shows no effect.

In addition, these agents, as is the case with the

sympathomimetic agents, have been well documented to precipitate angle-closure glaucoma in eyes anatomically predisposed (Table 16-8).

It should also be repeated that anticholinergic agents given systemically, including phenothiazines, tricyclic and MAO antidepressants, and antispasmolytic and antiparkinsonian agents, either alone or in combination, may also be strong enough to move the pupil into the critical mid-dilated position and precipitate an attack of angle-closure glaucoma.

Anesthetic agents

The general anesthetic agents are believed to lower the intraocular pressure. This has been demonstrated with halothane[48] and methoxyflurane (Penthrane).[77] However, two agents—succinylcholine[14] and ketamine[16] elevate intraocular pressure. This effect may be related to the increased tone of the extraocular[44] and orbital muscles seen when these agents are administered. With ketamine,[16] these findings were not related to age, depth of anesthesia, arterial blood pressure, or amount of ketamine administered, whereas, with succinylcholine,[14] the deeper the anesthesia, the lesser the effect. It was also noted that the preanesthetic use of either a barbiturate or a narcotic (morphine sulfate or meperidine) lowered the intraocular pressure in one patient. Crossen and Hoy[16] attributed this to the patient's relaxed state and reduced muscle tension.

Other observers have noted that the intraocular pressure elevation seen in those patients given succinylcholine intravenously, in bolus or dilute drip form, wears off after 4 to 5 minutes.[44] Therefore if succinylcholine is given intravenously in bolus or continuous drip form at least several minutes before intraocular surgery, the eye is at less risk than if the drug is given once the eye is opened. Certainly, extreme care should be taken in selecting anesthesia for open or potentially open globes.

Most topical anesthetic agents have no effect on intraocular pressure. One exception is cocaine, which can augment the response of sympathetically innervated organs to epinephrine, norepinephrine, and sympathetic nerve stimulation.[30] Thus when cocaine is applied topically to the eye, there is increased sensitization of the sulfa-adrenergic terminals in the dilator muscle fibers of the iris to circulating catecholamines, resulting in mydriasis.[39] This same mydriasis may be observed when cocaine is given systemically or in cases of poisoning.[30]

TABLE 16-8
Mydriatic agents

Generic (brand)	PDR warning	Case reports of glaucoma
Cyclopentolate hydrochloride (Cyclogyl)	Yes	Yes: a[38]; b[27]
Tropicamide (Mydriacyl)	Yes	Yes: a[38]; b[32]
Hydroxyamphetamine (Paredrine)	Yes	Yes: b[27]
Atropine (Atropisol)	Yes	Yes: a[38]; b[39]
Homatropine hydrobromide	Yes	Yes: a[38]; b[39]
Scopolamine (Hyoscine)	Yes	Yes: a[38]; b[39]

a, Open-angle glaucoma; b, angle-closure glaucoma.

The basis for this increased sympathetic tone is that cocaine acts by preventing the reuptake of norepinephrine at the adrenergic nerve terminals, thereby prolonging its action at the adrenergic receptor site. Cocaine apparently has no direct action on the adrenergic receptors. This fact is confirmed by the drug's lack of effect on sympathetically denervated eyes, as in Horner's syndrome.[82]

Because of the mydriasis that results from topical application of cocaine, it should be used with caution in patients with potential angle-closure glaucoma. Indeed, cases have been reported in the older literature in which cocaine precipitated angle-closure glaucoma in predisposed patients.[34] The initial reports of patients with open-angle glaucoma suggested that there was a lowering of the intraocular pressure.[34] However, subsequent reports on the use of cocaine in rabbits have shown no effect on intraocular pressure or outflow facility when the drug is given systemically.[63] This medication should be used with caution in all patients with glaucoma.

Antihypertensive agents

Antihypertensive agents usually have no effect on the eye, although clonidine (Catapres), a new alpha-adrenergic sympathomimetic agent, increases the pupillary diameter by approximately 0.9 mm.[76] Even though clonidine lowers the intraocular pressure when given topically to patients with open-angle glaucoma, one should still be cautious about administering it to patients with narrow angles.

Several other agents (including chlorthiazide,[40] hydrochlorothiazide,[4] polythiazide,[28] chlorthalidone,[23,57] hydralazine and hexamethonium,[35] spironolactone,[8] and trichlormethiazide[4]) used to treat hypertension have been documented to cause idiopathic swelling of the lens, which might induce attacks of angle-closure glaucoma in those patients anatomically predisposed.

Hormonal agents

The effect of hormonal agents is unclear. The intraocular pressure in women varies during the menstrual cycle.[67] Dalton[17] stated that the intraocular pressure was highest during the progestational phase of the menstrual period, including the 4 days preceding menstruation and the first 4 days of menstruation. However, Becker and Friedenwald[6] showed that during the progestational phase of the menstrual cycle and during pregnancy, there is an increased facility of outflow and a low intraocular pressure. In Becker and Friedenwald's study, the intraocular pressure increased and the coefficient of outflow decreased during the subsequent estrogenic postpartum and postmenopausal periods. They later confirmed their observations on the effects of progesterone on intraocular pressure by noting a reduction of intraocular pressure in several glaucoma patients treated with oral, intramuscular, and subconjunctival progesterone.

The role of estrogen is less clear. When given systemically, it has been found to increase intraocular pressure,[54] and when given to rats in one study, an accumulation of mucopolysaccharides was found in the region of the angle of the anterior chamber.[65]

On the basis of Becker and Friedenwald's work, Meyer et al.[56] gave an estrogen-progesterone combination to patients with open-angle glaucoma and documented a fall in their intraocular pressure. However, Weinstein et al.[84] reported that three patients aged 26 to 36 years developed visual field and optic nerve changes while taking contraceptives. In all three patients these changes were associated with increased serum cortisol levels. One patient had a family history of glaucoma. A prospective study by Deufrains and Hempel[19] found a small increase in the intraocular pressure over the 2 years that their patients took contraceptive pills.

Several points can be raised regarding angle-closure glaucoma. Acute attacks of glaucoma occur more commonly in women during the menstrual periods.[83] According to Duke-Elder,[20] this exacerbation of angle-closure glaucoma is due to "fluid retention," which is often produced by estrogens. These properties, in combination with the mydriasis seen with these hormones,[24] may be enough to precipitate an attack of angle-closure

glaucoma, as documented recently in one patient taking oral contraceptives.[86]

Alpha-chymotrypsin

Alpha-chymotrypsin, which lyses zonules, is now rather commonly used in routine intracapsular cataract surgery even though the agent causes a significant rise in intraocular pressure in the first week after surgery.[45] Preoperative glaucoma or surgical technique does not appear to be as important in causing this transient rise. Scanning and transmission electron microscopic studies have shown that when owl monkey zonules were exposed to this agent, they disintegrated into small particles that obstructed the openings into the trabecular meshwork overlying Schlemm's canal.[2] The lysed zonules are believed to obstruct the trabecular meshwork, leading to a transient rise in intraocular pressure after cataract surgery. Dilution of the normal solution of 1:5000 to 1:10,000 in combination with irrigation of the anterior chamber after its injection into the eye may prevent the elevation of pressure.[43]

Hyaluronic acid (Healon)

Hyaluronic acid has recently been isolated from rooster combs and produced artificially. It is now being clinically tested for use in eyes after anterior segment surgery to maintain the anterior chamber during the first days. It apparently dissolves after several weeks and exits by the trabecular meshwork. A report of one patient after combined cataract extraction–trabeculectomy, has revealed the following: during the first days after surgery the intraocular pressure was noted to be in the 60s, with a formed anterior chamber (Dr. Kenneth Haik, personal communication). After medical treatment, the pressure was noted to come down within a few days and as of this time is within normal limits. Many factors, including pupillary block or malignant glaucoma, may have been involved, complicating the possible role of hyaluronic acid in this episode of elevated intraocular pressure.

Acetylsalicylic acid (aspirin)

Aspirin itself appears to pose no threat to the patient with open-angle glaucoma. Indeed, in cases of salicylate poisoning, the intraocular pressure may be lowered[81] because of a generalized acidosis.[30] Diminished pupillary reaction to light, as well as edema of the optic nerve head and retina with diminished visual acuity, leading to optic atrophy, have also been observed in cases of salicylate poisoning.[32] Because of observed mydriasis, patients with narrow angles should be carefully observed. However, patients with narrow angles are also at risk because of an idiopathic reaction that can occur, producing lens swelling, myopia, shallowing of the anterior chamber, and intraocular pressure elevation.[68] Certainly, one should be cautious with patients who complain of a sudden onset of blurred vision after ingesting aspirin even in the prescribed fashion. This effect is not mentioned in the *PDR*.

CONCLUSION

Many drugs can aggravate glaucoma or precipitate an attack of angle-closure glaucoma. The physician's defense lies in awareness of this fact, thorough drug histories, and suspicion. Patients should be routinely questioned about the entire range of physical disorders, including subclinical complaints, for which they may be taking medication. These medications should then be evaluated for their possible effects on intraocular pressure and pupil size both alone and in combination with other drugs. Patients with diagnosed glaucoma and those judged susceptible to it should then be watched carefully and warned of the danger.

EPIDEMIC DROPSY

Another interesting condition, related to drug-induced glaucoma, is epidemic dropsy.

Epidemic dropsy is an acute disorder occurring primarily in India. It results from ingestion of an alkaloid, sanguinarine, which is found in the seeds of the Mexican poppy, *Argemone mexicana*. These seeds outwardly resemble the seeds of the mustard plant and may be accidentally mixed in with them, producing mustard oil that is contaminated with sanguinarine. Epidemics have occurred following consumption of other oils also, and the possibility of intentional contamination exists.

The disease derives its name from a rapid onset of pitting edema of the legs and feet. The overlying skin is tender, warm, and erythematous. Other symptoms include diarrhea, hair loss, fever, malaise, exertional dyspnea, hepatomegaly, and hyperpigmentation. Sanguinarine may be found in the serum and urine early in the disease process.[71,78]

A chronic bilateral open-angle glaucoma occurs in approximately 10% of patients with epidemic dropsy. All ages may be affected, but young adults have been the most commonly so. Intraocular pressures are usually over 50 mm Hg. There is an elevation of protein in the aqueous humor and a marked dilation of the small vessels of the uveal tract without evidence of inflammation.[20]

Elevated concentrations of histamine in the plasma and erythrocytes of patients with open-angle glaucoma who had had epidemic dropsy 20 years previously have been reported.[55] The controls consisted of normal subjects rather than patients who had had epidemic dropsy without glaucoma.

The disease appears to have gradually disappeared from the literature in the past few years, perhaps because of better regulation of mustard oil production in India.

REFERENCES

1. Abramson, D.H., Coleman, D.J., Forbes, M., and Franzen, L.A.: Pilocarpine, effect on the anterior chamber and lens thickness, Arch. Ophthalmol. **87:**615, 1972.
2. Anderson, D.R.: Experimental alpha chymotrypsin glaucoma studied by scanning electron microscopy, Am. J. Ophthalmol. **71:**470, 1971.
3. Bard, L.A.: Transient myopia associated with promethazine (Phenergan) therapy: report of a case, Am. J. Ophthalmol. **58:**682, 1964.
4. Beasley, F.J.: Transient myopia during trichlormethiazide therapy, Ann. Ophthalmol. **12:**705, 1980.
5. Becker, B.: In Conference on glaucoma, transactions of first conference, New York, 1955, Josiah Macy, Jr., Foundation, p. 32.
6. Becker, B., and Friedenwald, J.S.: Clinical aqueous outflow, Arch. Ophthalmol. **50:**557, 1963.
7. Becker, B., Goldberg, I., Ashburn, F., et al.: Timolol and epinephrine: a clinical study of ocular interactions, Arch. Ophthalmol. **98:**484, 1980.
8. Belci, C.: Miopia transitoria in corso di terapia con diuretici, Boll. Ocul. **47:**24, 1968.
9. Berggren, L.: Effect of composition of media and of metabolic inhibitors on secretion in vitro by the ciliary processes of the rabbit eye, Invest. Ophthalmol. **4:**83, 1965.
10. Bill, A., and Wälinder, P.: The effect of pilocarpine on the dynamics of aqueous humor in a primate (Macaca Irus), Invest. Ophthalmol. **5:**170, 1966.
11. Bleiman, B., and Schwartz, A.L.: Paradoxical response to pilocarpine, Arch. Ophthalmol. **97:**1305, 1979.
12. Bowden, C.L., and Giffen, M.B.: Psychotropics and glaucoma, Am. J. Psychiatry **134:**1314, 1977.
13. Chandler, P.A., and Grant, W.M.: Glaucoma, ed. 2, Philadelphia, 1979, Lea & Febiger, pp. 82, 131-132, 140, 150, 175, 214, 231, 238, 266.
14. Craythorne, N.W.B., Rothenstein, H.S., and Dripps, R.D.: The effect of succinylcholine on intraocular pressure in adults, infants and children during general anesthesia, Anesthesiology **21:**59, 1960.
15. Cristini, G., and Pagliarani, N.: Amyl nitrate test in primary glaucoma, Br. J. Ophthalmol. **37:**741, 1953.
16. Crossen, G., and Hoy, J.E.: A new parenteral anesthetic—C1581: its effect on intraocular pressure, J. Pediatr. Ophthalmol. **4:**20, 1967.

17. Dalton, K.: Influence of menstruation on glaucoma, Br. J. Ophthalmol. **50:**557, 1963.

18. Desvignes, P., Amar, L., and Regnault, F.: Etude des effects de la digoxine sur les hypertensions oculaires, Bull. Soc. Ophthalmol. Fr. **63:**832, 1963.

19. Deufrains, A., Hempel, E., and Klengic, G.: Results of a prospective ophthalmologic study with reference to hormonal contraction, Dtsch. Gesundhestsw. **30:**901, 1975.

20. Duke-Elder, S.: System of ophthalmology, vol. 11, Diseases of the lens and vitreous; glaucoma and hypotony, St. Louis, 1969, The C. V. Mosby Co., pp. 404-405, 572-577, 684-687.

21. Edwards, T.S.: Transient myopia due to tetracycline, J.A.M.A. **186:**69, 1963.

22. English, H.L.: An alarming side effect of Tofranil, Lancet **1:**1231, 1959.

23. Ericson, L.A.: Hygroton-induced myopia and retinal edema, Acta Ophthalmol. **41:**538, 1963.

24. Fraunfelder, F.T.: Drug-induced ocular side effects and drug interactions, Philadelphia, 1976, Lea & Febiger, p. 188.

25. Gallois, J.: Glaucoma aigu apres Priscol, Bull. Soc. Ophthalmol. Fr., p. 131, 1951.

26. Gandolfi, C.: L'azione del Priscol sulla pressione arteriosa retinica (P.A.R.), Ann. Ottal. **73:**336, 1947.

27. Gartner, S., and Billet, E.: Mydriatic glaucoma, Am. J. Ophthalmol. **43:**975, 1957.

28. Gastaldi, G.M.: Considerazioni sulla miopia transitoria dopo somministrazione di diuretici saluretici, Rass. Ital. Ottal. **34:**178, 1965-1966.

29. Goldberg, L.T.: Monoamine oxidase inhibitors: adverse reactions and possible mechanisms, J.A.M.A. **190:**456, 1964.

30. Goodman, L.S., and Gilman, A.: The pharmacological basis of therapeutics, ed. 5, New York, 1975, MacMillan Publishing Co., Inc., pp. 161, 166, 177, 179, 182, 234, 238, 329, 387, 602-606, 608, 611, 616.

31. Gott, P.H.: Cyclizine toxicity—intentional drug abuse of a proprietary antihistamine, N. Engl. J. Med. **279:**596, 1968.

32. Grant, W.M.: Toxicology of the eye, ed. 2, Springfield, Ill., 1974, Charles C Thomas, Publisher, pp. 132, 134, 213-214, 702, 769, 812-813, 890-892, 951, 1067-1068.

33. Grierson, I., Lee, R., and Abraham, S.: Effects of pilocarpine on the morphology of the human outflow apparatus, Br. J. Ophthalmol. **62:**302, 1978.

34. Groenouw, A.: Uber die Anwendung des Cocains bei glaucoma-tosen Zustanden, Ber. 25 Vers. Ophthalmol. Ges. Heidelb., p. 198, 1896; J. Ber. Ophthalmol. **27:**369, 1896.

35. Grossman, E.E., and Hanley, W.: Transient myopia during treatment for hypertension with autonomic blocking agents, Arch. Ophthalmol. **63:**853, 1960.

36. Halpern, A.E., and Kulvin, M.M.: Transient myopia during treatment with carbonic anhydrase inhibitors, Am. J. Ophthalmol. **65:**212, 1961.

37. Hardesty, J.F.: Control of intraocular hypertension by systemic medication, Trans. Am. Ophthalmol. Soc. **32:**497, 1934.

38. Harris, L.S.: Cycloplegia-induced intraocular pressure elevations: a study of normal and open-angle glaucomatous eyes, Arch. Ophthalmol. **79:**242, 1968.

39. Havener, W.H.: Ocular pharmacology, ed. 4, St. Louis, 1979, The C.V. Mosby Co., pp. 75-78, 227, 244-253, 275-276.

40. Hermann, M.P.: Myopia spasmodique au cours des traitements diuretique, Bull. Soc. Ophthalmol. Fr. **63:**719, 1963.

41. Herxheimer, A.: A comparison of some atropine-like drugs in man, with particular reference to their end-organ specificity, Br. J. Pharmacol. **13:**184, 1958.

42. Hyams, S.W., and Keroub, C.: Glaucoma due to diazepam, Am. J. Psychiatry **134:**447, 1977.

43. Jaffe, N.S.: Cataract surgery and its complications, ed. 2, St. Louis, 1976, The C.V. Mosby Co., p. 243.

44. Katz, R.L., and Eakins, K.B.: Mode of action of succinylcholine on intraocular pressure, J. Pharmacol. Exp. Ther. **162:**1, 1968.

45. Kirsch, R.E.: Glaucoma following cataract extraction associated with use of alpha chymotrypsin, Arch. Ophthalmol. **72:**612, 1964.

46. Kochman, M., and Romer, P.: Experimental investigation of pathologic fluid exchange in the eye, Arch. Ophthalmol. **8:**528, 1914.

47. Kolker, A.R., and Hetherington, J.: Becker-Schaffer's diagnosis and therapy of the glaucomas, ed. 4, St. Louis, 1976, The C.V. Mosby Co., pp. 184, 197, 223, 326.

48. Krupin, T., Feitl, M., Roshe, R., et al.: Halothane anesthesia and aqueous humor dynamics in rabbit eyes, Invest. Ophthalmol. Vis. Sci. **19:**518, 1980.

49. Langham, M.E., Kitazawa, Y., and Hart, R.W.: Adrenergic responses in the human eye, J. Pharmacol. Exp. Ther. **179:**47, 1971.

50. Lee, P.F.: The influence of epinephrine and phenylephrine on intraocular pressure, Arch. Ophthalmol. **50:**863, 1958.

51. Lowe, R.F.: Amitryptiline and glaucoma, Med. J. Aust. **2:**509, 1966.

52. Maddalena, M.D.: Transient myopia associated with acute glaucoma and retinal edema following vaginal administration of sulfanilamide, Arch. Ophthalmol. **80:**186, 1968.

53. Mapstone, R.: Closed-angle glaucoma: theoretical considerations, Br. J. Ophthalmol. **58:**46, 1974.

54. Medgyaszay, A.: Intraokularer Druck und Hormonbehandlung, Ophthalmologica **114:**168, 1947.

55. Mehra, K.S., Prasad, B.B., Gambhir, S.S., et al.: Histamine in relation to epidemic dropsy glaucoma, Ann. Ophthalmol. **6:**367, 1974.

56. Meyer, E.J., Leibowitz, H., Christman, E.H., and Niffenegger, J.A.: Influence of norethynodrel with mestranol on intraocular pressure in glaucoma. II. A controlled double-blind study, Arch. Ophthalmol. **75:**771, 1966.

57. Michaelson, T.T.: Transient myopia due to Hygroton, Am. J. Ophthalmol. **54:**1146, 1962.

58. Mody, M.V., and Keeney, A.H.: Propantheline (Probanthine) bromide in relation to normal and glaucomatous eyes; effects on intraocular tension and pupillary size, J.A.M.A. **159:**1113, 1955.

59. Muirhead, J.F., and Scheie, H.G.: Transient myopia after acetazolamide, Arch. Ophthalmol. **63:**315, 1960.

60. Neuschler, R.: Miopia transitoria in corso di terapia con dichlorofenamide, Boll. Ocul. **43:**507, 1964.

61. Newell, F.W., Ridgway, W.L., and Zeller, R.W.: The treatment of glaucoma with Dibenamine, Am. J. Ophthalmol. **34:**527, 1951.

62. Oradell, N.J.: Physician desk reference, ed. 34, Litton, Indiana, 1980, Medical Economics Co., pp. 973, 1586, 1695.

63. Paterson, C.A.: The effect of sympathetic nerve stimulation on the aqueous humor dynamics of the cocaine pretreated rabbit, Exp. Eye Res. **5:**37, 1966.

64. Peczon, J.D., and Grant, W.M.: Sedatives, stimulants and intraocular pressure in glaucoma, Arch. Ophthalmol. **72:**178, 1964.

65. Polgar, J., Vass, Z., and Tiboldi, T.: Histochemical changes in the rat's eye after prolonged administration of estrone acetate, Szemeszet **106:**178, 1969.

66. Reboton, J., Weedly, R.D., Bylenga, N.D., and May, R.H.: Pigmentary retinopathy and iridocycloplegia in psychiatric patients, J. Neuropsychiatry **3:**311, 1961-1962.

67. Salvati, M.: L'influence de la menstruation sur la tension oculaire, Ann. Ocul. **160:**568, 1923.

68. Sanford-Smith, J.H.: Transient myopia after aspirin, Br. J. Ophthalmol. **58:**698, 1974.

69. Scialdone, D., and Artifoni, E.: Miopia transitoria in corso di terapia con Debinyl, G. Ital. Oftal. **16:**92, 1963; Zentralbl. Ges. Ophthalmol. **91:**107, 1964.

70. Shannon, R.P., Mead, A., and Sears, M.L.: The effect of dopamine on the intraocular pressure and pupil of the rabbit eye, Invest. Ophthalmol. **15:**371, 1976.

71. Shenolikar, I.S., Rukmini, C., Krishnamachari, K.A.V.R., and Satyanarayana, K.: Sanguinarine in the blood and urine of cases of epidemic dropsy, Food Cosmet. Toxicol. **12:**699, 1974.

72. Sigg, E.B.: Autonomic side effects induced by psychotherapeutic agents. In Etron, D.N., editor: Psychopharmacology, a review of progress 1957-1967, proceedings of the Sixth Annual Meeting of the American College of Neuropsychopharmacology, San Juan, Puerto Rico, Dec. 12-15, 1967, PHS Pub. No. 1836, Washington, D.C., 1968, American College of Neuropsychopharmacology, pp. 581-588.

73. Snyder, S.H., and Yamamura, H.I.: Antidepressants and the muscarinic acetylcholine receptor, Arch. Gen. Psychiatry **34:**236, 1977.

74. Steele, C.M., O'Duffy, J., and Brown, S.S.: Clinical effects and treatment of imipramine and amitriptyline poisoning in children, Br. Med. J. **3:**663, 1967.

75. Sugar, S., and Santos, R.: The Priscoline provocative test, Am. J. Ophthalmol. **40:**510, 1955.

76. Tahnke, R., and Iham, H.W.: The effect of Clonidine on intraocular pressure and pupillary diameter, Klin. Monatsbl. Augenheilkd. **161:**78, 1972.

77. Tammisto, T., Hämäläinen, L., and Tarkkanen, L.: Halothane and methoxyflurane in ophthalmic anesthesia, Acta. Anaesthesiol. Scand. **9:**173, 1965.

78. Tandon, R.K., Singh, D.S., Arora, R.R., et al.: Epidemic dropsy in New Delhi, Am. J. Clin. Nutr. **28:**883, 1975.

79. Tolle, R., and Porksen, N.: Thymoleptic mydriasis in the course of treatment, Int. Pharmacopsychiatry **2:**86, 1969.

80. Trope, G.E., and Hind, V.M.D.: Closed-angle glaucoma in patient on disopyramide, Lancet **1:**329, 1978.

81. Varady, J., and Jahn, F.: Uber die Bulbushypotonie bei Vergiflungen mit Salizylsaurepräparaten, Dtsch. Med. Wochenschr. **66:**322, 1940.

82. Walsh, F.B., and Hoyt, W.F.: Clinical neuro-ophthalmology, vol. 1, ed. 3, Baltimore, 1969, The Williams & Wilkins Co., p. 520.

83. Weinstein, P.: Relation of glaucoma to blood pressure, Arch. Ophthalmol. **13:**181, 1935.

84. Weinstein, P., Ahi, D., and Anda, L.: Oral contraceptives and glaucoma, Klin. Monatsbl. Augenheilkd. **162:**798, 1973.

85. Whitworth, C.G., and Grant, W.M.: Use of nitrate and nitrite vasodilators by glaucomatous patients, Arch. Ophthalmol. **71:**492, 1964.

86. Wood, R.: Ocular complications of oral contraceptives, Ophthalmol. Sem. **2:**371, 1977.

87. Yasuna, E.: Acute myopia associated with prochlorperazine (Compazine) therapy, Am. J. Ophthalmol. **54:**793, 1962.

88. Zahn, K.: The effect of vasoactive drugs on the retinal circulation, Trans. Ophthalmol. Soc. U.K. **86:**529, 1966.

89. Zarrabi, M.: Quelques observations sur le Priscol en ophthalmologie, Ophthalmologica **122:**76, 1951.

Chapter 17

CORTICOSTEROID-INDUCED GLAUCOMA

Elizabeth A. Hodapp and Michael A. Kass

In 1950 McLean[53] described the occurrence of elevated intraocular pressure in uveitis patients treated with ACTH injections. The ocular hypertensive effect of glucocorticoid therapy in some patients with uveitis was confirmed by Lijo-Pavia,[50] Francois,[29] and Laval and Collier.[48] Stern[75] and Covell[25] noted that systemic corticosteroid treatment led to increased intraocular pressure in some individuals without ocular disease. Francois[29] (1954) and Goldmann[36] (1962) reported patients with elevated intraocular pressures, optic nerve cupping and atrophy, and visual field loss following prolonged use of corticosteroid eyedrops. Subsequently, hundreds of reports and investigations have confirmed that topical, systemic, and periocular corticosteroid administration can produce increased intraocular pressure and secondary open-angle glaucoma.*

Large-scale prospective studies of the effects of topical corticosteroid administration on intraocular pressure have been performed on normal volunteers,† glaucoma patients,[4,19,20,49] glaucoma suspects,[49] senior citizens,[11] American Indians,[66] Africans,[28] and prison inmates.[45] Marked ocular hypertensive responses have occurred occasionally in normal individuals and commonly among both patients with primary open-angle glaucoma[4,19,20] and their first-degree relatives* (Tables 17-1 and 17-2). Both Armaly[7,8] and Becker[15] postulated three levels of intraocular pressure response to topical corticosteroid administration. They further proposed that such responses were inherited and related to the inheritance of primary open-angle glaucoma.

These theories have been placed in doubt by recent studies indicating a relatively low concordance of corticosteroid testing results in monozygotic twins.[69,70] Other investigators have noted relatively poor reproducibility of the intraocular pressure response to topical dexamethasone, except in the high-responder group.[58] The poor reproducibility and lack of concordance may be explained by variable compliance among subjects being corticosteroid tested.[56]

Regardless of the heritability of the corticosteroid response or its relationship to primary open-angle glaucoma, two clinical points deserve emphasis. First, a substantial percentage of the general population will develop elevated intraocular pressure when treated with prolonged topical, systemic, or periocular glucocorticoid therapy. Second, certain individuals, particularly patients with primary open-angle glaucoma,[4,19,20] first-degree relatives of these patients,[15,18,26,59] myopes,[62] and diabetics,[16] are at greater risk of developing in-

---

*In this chapter corticosteroid-induced glaucoma refers to elevated intraocular pressure, optic nerve cupping, and visual field loss due to glucocorticoid administration; corticosteroid-induced pressure elevation refers to elevated intraocular pressure without glaucomatous damage.

†References 3, 4, 6-8, 15, 49, 71.

*References 17, 18, 26, 31, 59.

TABLE 17-1

Intraocular pressure response to topical corticosteroids

	Becker[15]	Armaly[6-8]
Frequency of administration	4 times daily	3 times daily
Duration of administration	6 weeks	4 weeks
Parameter for classification	Final intraocular pressure	Change in intraocular pressure
Classification system		
Low responder	Ta* < 20 mm Hg	Δ Ta† < 6 mm Hg
Intermediate responder	Ta 20 to 31 mm Hg	Δ Ta 6 to 15 mm Hg
High responder	Ta > 31 mm Hg	Δ Ta > 15 mm Hg

*Final intraocular pressure by applanation measurement.
†Change in intraocular pressure by applanation measurement.

TABLE 17-2

Topical corticosteroid testing in glaucoma patients and normal volunteers

	Low responders (%)	Intermediate responders (%)	High responders (%)
Normal volunteers			
Armaly[3]	66	29	5
Becker[15]	58	36	6
Patients with primary open-angle glaucoma			
Armaly[4,7,8]	6	48	46
Becker[15,19,20]	0	8	92

creased intraocular pressure when treated with corticosteroids.

Several excellent reviews have been published on the relationship of corticosteroid responsiveness and the inheritance of primary open-angle glaucoma*; a thorough discussion of this subject is beyond the scope of this chapter.

Even though corticosteroid-induced glaucoma has been described for many years, it remains a common cause of visual loss. Many cases are not properly diagnosed or managed. The purposes of this chapter are to acquaint the reader with the different clinical presentations of corticosteroid-induced glaucoma and to discuss management of the various forms of this entity.

CLASSIFICATION

Either endogenous or exogenous corticosteroids may produce elevated intraocular pressure (see outline below). Patients with Cushing's syndrome secondary to adrenal adenoma, carcinoma, or

hyperplasia may develop an increased intraocular pressure that then decreases after adrenalectomy.[13,14,37,64] Bayer and Neuner[13,14] described nine patients with Cushing's syndrome secondary to adrenocortical hyperplasia whose intraocular pressures decreased 5 to 12 mm Hg soon after adrenal surgery. The facilities of outflow, diminished preoperatively, returned to normal in the postoperative period. Haas and Nootens[37] reported a patient with Cushing's syndrome secondary to an adrenal adenoma. The patient had a marked elevation of intraocular pressure and diminished tonographic facility of outflow. Following adrenal surgery, the aqueous humor dynamics became normal. The patient, his parents, and one sister were all high responders to topical corticosteroid testing. Haas and Nootens concluded that the increased intraocular pressure encountered in some cases of Cushing's syndrome is due to the response of genetically predisposed individuals to the high levels of endogenous cortisol. This interpretation would explain the normal aqueous humor dynamics in many patients with pituitary-adrenal disorders.

*References 8, 9, 18, 21, 55, 68.

Corticosteroid-induced glaucoma

A. Endogenous corticosteroids
    1. Adrenal hyperplasia (inappropriate secretion of ACTH by the pituitary)
    2. Adrenal adenoma or carcinoma
    3. Ectopic ACTH syndrome (ACTH production by a carcinoma of the lung or pancreas, a thymoma, etc.)
B. Exogenous corticosteroids
    1. Ocular
       a. Eyedrops
       b. Ocular ointments
       c. Inadvertent administration to the eye from the lids or face
    2. Periocular injection
    3. Systemic
       a. Oral
       b. Topical (to the skin)
       c. Injection (repeated injection of glucocorticoid or ACTH)

The vast majority of cases of corticosteroid-induced glaucoma result from exogenous glucocorticoids: topical, periocular, or systemic. (A classification of corticosteroid-induced glaucoma by route of administration is purely organizational and does not imply any difference in the basic clinical presentation or the pathogenesis.) Topical corticosteroids include not only eyedrops and ocular ointments used purposely on the eye, but also creams, lotions, and ointments applied to the eyelids or face for various dermatologic conditions.[77,82] These glucocorticoid preparations may reach the eye in sufficient quantity to produce increased intraocular pressure. In addition, corticosteroids applied to the skin remote from the eyes may be absorbed in sufficient quantity to raise the intraocular pressure in susceptible individuals.[72]

Periocular glucocorticoid injections (subconjunctival, sub-Tenon's, retrobulbar) may produce increased intraocular pressure.* Persistent elevations of intraocular pressure are more common after injection of repository or "depo" corticosteroid preparations.[38]

Systemic glucocorticoid administration may produce elevated intraocular pressure.† Most commonly, this occurs in individuals receiving chronic, suppressive corticosteroid treatment, such as renal transplant recipients, patients with collagen vascular diseases, and patients with severe atopy

and/or asthma. These patients may also have ocular disorders (e.g., iritis, blepharitis) that are treated with topical corticosteroid therapy. The intraocular pressure effects of topical and systemic glucocorticoid administration may be additive.[35]

CLINICAL PICTURE

The route of glucocorticoid administration does not affect the basic clinical picture of corticosteroid-induced glaucoma. Elevated intraocular pressure may occur as early as 1 to 2 weeks or as late as months to years after corticosteroid therapy has been initiated. The duration of therapy necessary to elevate the intraocular pressure depends on the specific drug, the route of administration, the dose, the frequency of administration, other ocular diseases that may be present (e.g., uveitis), and, most important, the susceptibility of the patient.

The age of the patient affects the clinical picture of corticosteroid-induced glaucoma. Infants who develop corticosteroid-induced glaucoma resemble closely patients with primary infantile glaucoma.[2,41,67,78] Frequently they are being treated with combined glucocorticoid-antibiotic preparations prescribed by pediatricians or family practitioners for presumed lacrimal obstruction. The family may describe tearing, photophobia, blepharospasm, and large eyes. Physical findings include buphthalmos, an enlarged corneal diameter, a cloudy and edematous cornea, breaks in Descemet's membrane, elevated intraocular pressure, and abnormal optic disc cupping. The drainage angle of these infants appears normal rather than typically glaucomatous, although this distinction may be exceedingly subtle. Both eyes are involved if the child has been exposed to systemic corticosteroids or bilateral topical glucocorticoid administration.

In older children and adults an uncomplicated case of corticosteroid-induced glaucoma usually presents with a picture closely resembling primary open-angle glaucoma.* The eye is quiet, the intraocular pressure is elevated, the anterior chamber angle is open, the optic disc is cupped, and the visual field demonstrates typical glaucomatous loss. In some cases corneal edema may be present, and the patient may note haloes or complain of discomfort. However, most cases of corticoste-

---

*References 33, 38, 40, 57, 61.
†References 1, 22, 25, 34, 39, 43, 48, 51, 60.

---

*References 25, 29, 36, 61, 64, 68, 72, 77, 82.

roid-induced glaucoma, like most cases of primary open-angle glaucoma, are asymptomatic. If topical corticosteroids have been administered to both eyes, or if the patient is being treated with systemic glucocorticoids, the intraocular pressure is elevated in both eyes; uniocular corticosteroid administration leads to uniocular pressure elevation. Unfortunately, many cases of corticosteroid-induced glaucoma result from the use of glucocorticoids for relatively minor conditions such as eye irritation, mild blepharitis, or contact lens discomfort.

Corticosteroid-induced glaucoma may present as low-tension glaucoma.[76] Patients who were treated with glucocorticoids in the past may have normal intraocular pressure, normal outflow facility, cupping and atrophy of the optic nerve, and glaucomatous visual field loss. Only by a careful history can the physician relate the past corticosteroid treatment to the present ocular condition. Generally, such patients do not develop further glaucomatous damage unless corticosteroid therapy is reinstated.

Any abnormality of the eye may coexist with corticosteroid-induced glaucoma, and thus complicate the clinical picture. A patient with narrow angles who develops corticosteroid-induced glaucoma may appear initially to have subacute or chronic angle-closure glaucoma. An individual with an angle recession who develops corticosteroid-induced glaucoma may appear to have post-traumatic angle-contusion glaucoma.

Signs of underlying ocular disease or other effects of glucocorticoid administration may further alter the clinical picture of corticosteroid-induced glaucoma. Thus the examiner may find evidence of active or resolved inflammation such as anterior chamber reaction, peripheral anterior synechiae, or posterior synechiae. Patients may, in addition, display sequelae of corticosteroid use besides elevated intraocular pressure: (1) posterior subcapsular cataract[39,51,68]; (2) skin atrophy, especially of the eyelids, which occurs after chronic application of fluorinated corticosteroid preparations[77]; (3) ptosis[54]; (4) mydriasis[5,54]; and (5) ocular infection with herpes simplex or various fungi.[77] Individuals receiving systemic corticosteroid therapy may appear Cushingoid with moon facies, truncal obesity, cutaneous striae, plethora, hirsutism, easy bruising, hypertension, diabetes, and osteoporosis.

PATHOPHYSIOLOGY

The mechanism by which corticosteroids elevate intraocular pressure has not been determined fully. There is general agreement in the literature that topical corticosteroids increase intraocular pressure and decrease facility of outflow as measured by tonography.[3,47,54,79] Some investigators have noted that systemic corticosteroids increase aqueous humor production.[27,32, 52]

The pathophysiology of decreased outflow facility in corticosteroid-induced glaucoma has been the subject of intense speculation and investigation. The most commonly postulated mechanism involves an accumulation of mucopolysaccharides (glycosaminoglycans) in the outflow channels.[3,4,30] Mucopolysaccharides are present in the drainage angle,[10,30,81] contribute to the normal resistance to aqueous humor outflow,[12,30] and are subject to depolymerization by lysosomal enzymes.[10,30] Glucocorticoids stabilize lysosomal membranes and thus could produce an accumulation of mucopolysaccharides in the outflow channels and a secondary mechanical obstruction of outflow.[30]

While this theory has been the most widely accepted explanation for corticosteroid-induced glaucoma, several problems remain unresolved. The level of glucocorticoid necessary to stabilize lysosomal membranes may be greater than that present in the aqueous humor of eyes with corticosteroid-induced ocular hypertension.[74] Moreover, the available histologic specimens of trabecular tissue from eyes with corticosteroid-induced intraocular pressure elevations do not demonstrate an unequivocal increase in mucopolysaccharides.[42,72] Finally, the mucopolysaccharide theory does not explain the differential intraocular pressure sensitivity of individuals to corticosteroid administration. Presumably, glucocorticoids stabilize lysosomal membranes in eyes of high-corticosteroid responders and in those of low-corticosteroid responders. To explain the differential sensitivity of individuals to corticosteroid administration, one may postulate a differential penetration of the glucocorticoid into the eye, a differential metabolism of the corticosteroid, a differential sensitivity of the tissues in the outflow channels, or a preexisting difference in the outflow channels. There is no evidence to support any of these theories.

Bill[23] has postulated that corticosteroids may inhibit phagocytosis by the trabecular endothelium. This could lead to an accumulation of debris sufficient to clog the outflow channels.

Pathologic studies of human eyes with elevated intraocular pressures secondary to topical corticosteroid administration have shown thinning of the endothelial cells lining Schlemm's canal[42] and increased density of the cribriform areas of the trabecular meshwork.[65] These findings may not be related specifically to corticosteroids; the exact mechanism by which glucocorticoids affect the outflow channels remains uncertain.

DIAGNOSIS

Patients with elevated intraocular pressures should be questioned carefully regarding the use of corticosteroid eyedrops, ointments, skin preparations, and pills. Physicians and other health care professionals must be questioned with particular care. The patient's medications should be examined and identified. Similarly, a careful history of medication use must be obtained for patients whose clinical pictures resemble infantile glaucoma or low-tension glaucoma.

The crucial test for diagnosing corticosteroid-induced intraocular pressure elevation is the clinical response to discontinuation of glucocorticoids. The majority of patients respond promptly (a few days to several weeks) with decreased intraocular pressure and increased outflow facility.

A number of investigators have reported persistent elevations of intraocular pressure (months to years) following cessation of glucocorticoid therapy.[31,72,73] It is possible that prolonged elevations of intraocular pressure may produce permanent alterations in the outflow channels. However, the possibility that underlying glaucoma was unmasked or aggravated by corticosteroid administration must also be kept in mind.

Differential diagnosis may be difficult when corticosteroid therapy is employed to treat an eye disease that itself alters intraocular pressure (e.g., iridocyclitis). Diagnosis of corticosteroid-induced glaucoma in a patient with iridocyclitis depends on an intraocular pressure fall after glucocorticoid administration has been discontinued. Should the ocular inflammation increase after corticosteroid therapy has been stopped, the intraocular pressure may increase or decrease irrespective of a corticosteroid effect. If it is impossible to withdraw glucocorticoid therapy because of ocular inflammation, it may be impossible to reach a firm diagnosis of corticosteroid-induced glaucoma. If the iridocyclitis is limited to one eye, useful information may be gained by corticosteroid testing of the normal fellow eye.

MANAGEMENT

When corticosteroid therapy is being employed, a baseline intraocular pressure measurement and close observation are mandatory. Although a marked ocular hypertensive response may occur rarely within the first several days of treatment, it is reasonable to remeasure the intraocular pressure after 2 weeks of glucocorticoid therapy. If the intraocular pressure has not risen, and if further corticosteroid therapy is needed, the ophthalmologist should reexamine the patient every 2 to 3 weeks for the first few months and every 2 to 3 months thereafter. At no point does a patient become immune from developing corticosteroid-induced glaucoma.

Discontinuing glucocorticoid therapy is the most effective management of corticosteroid-induced glaucoma. In almost all cases the intraocular pressure elevation resolves promptly. While one is awaiting resolution, treatment with standard antiglaucoma medications may be required to control the intraocular pressure. If corticosteroid therapy must continue despite an elevated intraocular pressure, a weaker glucocorticoid,[63] a lower concentration of the drug,[63] or a drug with less tendency to elevate intraocular pressure may be helpful.[24] Both medrysone and fluorometholone are thought to cause less intraocular pressure elevation for a given antiinflammatory effect than some other steroid compounds.[24] This conclusion is based on in vitro lymphocyte transformation inhibition and is not a direct measure of antiinflammatory potency. Both medrysone and fluorometholone can produce elevated intraocular pressure. If changing or decreasing corticosteroid therapy does not reduce the intraocular pressure, or if such changes in therapy are contraindicated, the ophthalmologist may institute routine antiglaucoma treatment.

Patients with glaucoma may appear refractory to medical treatment during glucocorticoid therapy. Glaucoma patients often use corticosteroid eyedrops to alleviate irritation caused by topical miotic or epinephrine therapy. Stopping glucocorticoid therapy generally allows the intraocular pressure to be controlled by standard antiglaucoma treatment.

Persistently elevated intraocular pressure related to periocular corticosteroid injections is treated by standard medical means. However, if the intraocular pressure cannot be controlled, and if injected material is present beneath the conjunctiva, residual glucocorticoid material may have to be excised.[38]

Corticosteroid-induced glaucoma resistant to medical management should be treated by a standard filtering procedure. It is reasonable to temporize in cases in which optic nerve damage is absent or minimal and in cases in which corticosteroids can be discontinued, even if the intraocular pressure cannot be controlled fully. However, such patients must be followed carefully to establish that the elevated intraocular pressure declines and that the ocular damage stabilizes. If progressive optic nerve or visual field damage occurs or seems very likely to occur, surgical intervention is indicated.

Following filtering surgery, the ophthalmologist can use topical, subconjunctival, or even oral corticosteroids as needed to control inflammation and scarring. (If systemic glucocorticoids are administered, the intraocular pressure of the fellow eye must be monitored carefully.) Although reports exist of possible corticosteroid-induced intraocular pressure elevation despite functional filtering surgery,[80] such reports are not conclusive, and most data indicate that a functional drainage operation precludes a corticosteroid-induced pressure elevation.[44-46]

The overwhelming criterion for identification of corticosteroid-induced glaucoma is suspicion. Once identified, most cases of corticosteroid-induced glaucoma respond promptly to cessation of the drug. The failure of physicians to recognize corticosteroid-induced glaucoma may lead to needless visual loss and difficult medical-legal problems. The recognition and management of corticosteroid-induced glaucoma should be familiar to all ophthalmologists.

REFERENCES

1. Alfano, J.E.: Changes in the intraocular pressure associated with systemic steroid therapy, Am. J. Ophthalmol. **56:**345, 1963.
2. Alfano, J.E., and Platt, D.: Steroid (ACTH) induced glaucoma simulating congenital glaucoma, Am. J. Ophthalmol. **61:**911, 1966.
3. Armaly, M.F.: Effect of corticosteroids on intraocular pressure and fluid dynamics. I. The effect of dexamethasone in the normal eye, Arch. Ophthalmol. **70:**482, 1963.
4. Armaly, M.F.: Effect of corticosteroids on intraocular pressure and fluid dynamics. II. The effect of dexametha-
sone in the glaucomatous eye, Arch. Ophthalmol. **70:**492, 1963.
5. Armaly, M.F.: Effect of corticosteroids on intraocular pressure and fluid dynamics. III. Changes in visual function and pupil size during topical dexamethasone application, Arch. Ophthalmol. **71:**639, 1964.
6. Armaly, M.F.: Statistical attributes of the steroid hypertensive response in the clinically normal eye. I. The demonstration of three levels of response, Invest. Ophthalmol. **4:**187, 1965.
7. Armaly, M.F.: The heritable nature of dexamethasone-induced ocular hypertension, Arch. Ophthalmol. **75:**32, 1966.
8. Armaly, M.F.: Inheritance of dexamethasone hypertension and glaucoma, Arch. Ophthalmol. **77:**747, 1967.
9. Armaly, M.F.: Genetic factors related to glaucoma, Ann. N.Y. Acad. Sci. **151:**861, 1968.
10. Ashton, N.: The role of the trabecular structure in the problem of simple glaucoma, particularly with regard to the significance of mucopolysaccharides. In Newell, F.W., editor: Glaucoma: transactions of the 4th Conference, vol. 4, New York, 1960, Josiah Macy, Jr., Foundation, p. 89.
11. Ballin, N., and Becker, B.: Provocative testing for primary open-angle glaucoma in "senior citizens," Invest. Ophthalmol. **6:**126, 1967.
12. Barany, E.H., and Southbrook, S.: Influence on testicular hyaluronidase on the resistance to flow through the angle of the anterior chamber, Acta Physiol. Scand. **33:**240, 1953.
13. Bayer, J.M.: Ergebnisse und Beurteilung der subtotalen Adrenalektomie beim hyperfuncktions-Cushing, Langenbecks Arch. Klin. Chir. **291:**531, 1959.
14. Bayer, J.M., and Neuner, N.P.: Cushing-Syndrom und erhöhter Augeninnendruck, Dtsch. Med. Wochenschr. **92:**1791, 1967.
15. Becker, B.: Intraocular pressure response to topical corticosteroids, Invest. Ophthalmol. **4:**198, 1965.
16. Becker, B.: Diabetes mellitus and primary open-angle glaucoma: the XXVII Edward Jackson Memorial Lecture, Am. J. Ophthalmol. **77:**1, 1971.
17. Becker, B., and Chevrette, L.: Topical corticosteroid testing in glaucoma siblings, Arch. Ophthalmol. **76:**484, 1966.
18. Becker, B., and Hahn, K.A.: Topical corticosteroids and heredity in primary open-angle glaucoma, Am. J. Ophthalmol. **57:**543, 1964.
19. Becker, B., and Mills, D.W.: Corticosteroids and intraocular pressure, Arch. Ophthalmol. **70:**500, 1963.
20. Becker, B., and Mills, D.W.: Elevated intraocular pressure following corticosteroid eye drops, J.A.M.A. **185:**884, 1963.
21. Becker, B., and Podos, S.M.: Hypersensitivity to glucocorticosteroids and primary open-angle glaucoma. In Etienne, R., and Patterson, G.D., editors: International Glaucoma Symposium Albi, 1974, Lyon, France, 1975, Imprimerie, p. 291.
22. Bernstein, H.N., and Schwartz, B.: Effects of long-term systemic steroids on ocular pressure and tonographic values, Arch. Ophthalmol. **68:**742, 1962.
23. Bill, A.: The drainage of aqueous humor, Invest. Ophthalmol. **14:**1, 1975.

24. Cantrill, H.L., Palmberg, P.F., Zink, H.A., et al.: Comparison of in vitro potency of corticosteroids with ability to raise intraocular pressure, Am. J. Ophthalmol. **79:**1012, 1975.

25. Covell, L.L.: Glaucoma induced by systemic steroid therapy, Am. J. Ophthalmol. **45:**108, 1954.

26. Davies, T.G.: Tonographic survey of the close relatives of patients with chronic simple glaucoma, Br. J. Ophthalmol. **52:**32, 1968.

27. Drager, J.: Der Einfluss lokaler Steroidgaven auf den Augeninnendruck, Klin. Monatsbl. Augenheilkd. **147:**386, 1965.

28. Easty, D.L., and Luntz, M.H.: Influence of topical corticosteroids on intraocular pressure in Africans, Am. J. Ophthalmol. **68:**640, 1969.

29. Francois, J.: Cortisone et tension oculaire, Ann. Ocul. **187:**805, 1954.

30. Francois, J.: The importance of the mucopolysaccharides in intraocular pressure regulation, Invest. Ophthalmol. **14:**173, 1975.

31. Francois, J., Heintz-deBree, C.H., and Tripathi, R.C.: The cortisone test and the heredity of primary open-angle glaucoma, Am. J. Ophthalmol. **62:**844, 1966.

32. Frandsen, E.: Glaucoma and posterior subcapsular cataract following prednisolone (ultracorticol therapy), Acta Ophthalmol. **42:**108, 1964.

33. Garber, M.I.: Methylprednisolone in the treatment of exophthalmos, Lancet **1:**958, 1966.

34. Godel, V., Feiler-Ofry, V., and Stein, R.: Systemic steroids and ocular fluid dynamics. I. Analysis of the sample as a whole: influence of dosage and duration of therapy, Acta Ophthalmol. **50:**655, 1972.

35. Godel, V., Feiler-Ofry, V., and Stein, R.: Systemic steroids and ocular fluid dynamics. II. Systemic versus topical steroids, Acta Ophthalmol. **50:**664, 1972.

36. Goldmann, H.: Cortisone glaucoma, Arch. Ophthalmol. **68:**621, 1962.

37. Haas, J.S., and Nootens, R.H.: Glaucoma secondary to benign adrenal adenoma, Am. J. Ophthalmol. **78:**497, 1974.

38. Herschler, J.: Intractable intraocular hypertension induced by repository triamcinolone acetonide, Am. J. Ophthalmol. **74:**501, 1972.

39. Hovland, K.R., and Ellis, P.P.: Ocular changes in renal transplant patients, Am. J. Ophthalmol. **63:**283, 1967.

40. Kalina, R.E.: Increased intraocular pressure following subconjunctival corticosteroid administration, Arch. Ophthalmol. **81:**788, 1969.

41. Kass, M.A., Kolker, A.E., and Becker, B.: Chronic topical corticosteroid use simulating congenital glaucoma, J. Pediatr. **81:**1175, 1972.

42. Kayes, J., and Becker, B.: The human trabecular meshwork in corticosteroid-induced glaucoma, Trans. Am. Ophthalmol. Soc. **67:**354, 1969.

43. Kitazawa, Y.: Acute glaucoma due to systemic corticosteroid administration, Acta Soc. Ophthalmol. Jpn. **70:**2179, 1966.

44. Kolker, A.E.: Discussion of Wilensky, J.T., Snyder, D., and Gieser, D.: Steroid-induced ocular hypertension in patients with filtering blebs, Ophthalmology **87:**243, 1980.

45. Kolker, A.E., Stewart, R.M., Alton, E., and LeMon, L.: Dexamethasone testing in prison inmates, Invest. Ophthalmol. **10:**198, 1971.

46. Kronfeld, P.C.: The effects of topical steroid administration on intraocular pressure and aqueous outflow after fistulizing operations, Trans. Am. Ophthalmol. Soc. **62:**375, 1964.

47. Kupfer, C.: Pseudofacility in the human eye, Trans. Am. Ophthalmol. Soc. **69:**383, 1971.

48. Laval, J., and Collier, R., Jr.: Elevation of intraocular pressure due to hormonal steroid therapy in uveitis, Am. J. Ophthalmol. **39:**175, 1955.

49. Levene, R., Wigdor, A., Edelstein, A., and Bauma, J.: Topical corticosteroid in normal patients and glaucoma suspects, Arch. Ophthalmol. **77:**593, 1967.

50. Lijo-Pavia, J.: Cortisona y tonus ocular, Rev. Otoneuromol. **27:**14, 1952.

51. Lindholm, B., Linner, E., and Tengroth, B.: Effects of long-term systemic steroids on cataract formation and aqueous humor dynamics, Acta Ophthalmol. **43:**120, 1965.

52. Linner, E.: Adrenocorticol steroids and aqueous humor dynamics, Doc. Ophthalmol. **13:**210, 1959.

53. McLean, J.M.: Discussion of Woods, A.C.: Clinical and experimental observation on the use of ACTH and cortisone in ocular inflammatory disease, Trans. Am. Ophthalmol. Soc. **48:**293, 1959.

54. Miller, D., Peczon, J.D., and Whitworth, C.G.: Corticosteroids and functions in the anterior segment of the eye, Am. J. Ophthalmol. **59:**31, 1965.

55. Miller, S.J.H.: Genetic aspects of glaucoma, Trans. Ophthalmol. Soc. U.K. **86:**25, 1966.

56. Mindel, J.S., Goldberg, J., and Tavitian, H.O.: Similarity on the intraocular pressure response to different corticosteroid esters when compliance is controlled, Ophthalmology **86:**99, 1979.

57. Nozik, R.A.: Periocular injection of steroids, Trans. Am. Acad. Ophthalmol. Otolaryngol. **76:**695, 1972.

58. Palmberg, P.F., Mandell, A., Wilensky, J.T., et al.: The reproducibility of the intraocular pressure response to dexamethasone, Am. J. Ophthalmol. **80:**844, 1975.

59. Paterson, G.: Studies of the response to topical dexamethasone of glaucoma relatives, Trans. Ophthalmol. Soc. U.K. **85:**295, 1965.

60. Paterson, G.P., and Owen, R.: Further studies on systemic steroids. In Paterson, G., Miller, S.J.H., and Paterson, G.D., editors: Drug mechanisms in glaucoma, Boston, 1966, Little, Brown & Co., p. 249.

61. Perkins, E.S.: Steroid-induced glaucoma, Proc. R. Soc. Med. **58:**531, 1965.

62. Podos, S.M., Becker, B., and Morton, W.R.: High myopia and primary open-angle glaucoma, Am. J. Ophthalmol. **62:**1039, 1966.

63. Podos, S.M., Krupin, T., Asseff, C., and Becker, B.: Topically administered corticosteroid preparations, Arch. Ophthalmol. **86:**251, 1971.

64. Radnot, M.: Der Augenbefund bei Cushinger Krankheit, Ophthalmologica **104:**301, 1942.

65. Rohen, J.W., Linner, E., and Witmer, R.: Electron microscopic studies on the trabecular meshwork in two cases of corticosteroid glaucoma, Exp. Eye Res. **17:**19, 1973.

66. Rosenbaum, L.J., Alton, E., and Becker, B.: Dexamethasone testing in Southwestern Indians, Invest. Ophthalmol. **9:**325, 1970.

67. Scheie, H.G., Rubenstein, R.A., and Albert, D.M.: Congenital glaucoma and other ocular abnormalities with idio-

pathic infantile hypoglycemia, J. Pediatr. Ophthalmol. **1:** 45, 1964.

68. Schwartz, B.: Corticosteroids and the eye, Int. Ophthalmol. Clin. **6:**753, 1966.

69. Schwartz, J.T., Reuling, F.H., Feinleib, M., et al.: Twin study on ocular pressure after topical dexamethasone. I. Frequency distribution of pressure response, Am. J. Ophthalmol. **76:**126, 1973.

70. Schwartz, J.T., Reuling, F.H., Feinleib, M., et al.: Twin study on ocular pressure following topically applied dexamethasone. II. Inheritance of variation in pressure response, Arch. Ophthalmol. **90:**281, 1973.

71. Spaeth, G.L.: Effects of topical dexamethasone on intraocular pressure and the water drinking test, Arch. Ophthalmol. **76:**772, 1966.

72. Spaeth, G.L., Rodrigues, M.M., and Weinreb, S.: Steroid-induced glaucoma: A. Persistent elevation of intraocular pressure. B. Histopathologic aspects, Trans. Am. Ophthalmol. Soc. **75:**353, 1977.

73. Spiers, F.: A case of irreversible steroid-induced rise in intraocular pressure, Acta Ophthalmol. **43:**419, 1965.

74. Starka, L., and Obenberger, J.: Steroids and intraocular pressure, J. Steroid Biochem. **7:**979, 1976.

75. Stern, J.J.: Acute glaucoma during cortisone therapy, Am. J. Ophthalmol. **36:**389, 1953.

76. Sugar, H.S.: Low tension glaucoma: a practical approach, Ann. Ophthalmol. **11:**1155, 1979.

77. Tukey, R.B.: Glaucoma following the application of corticosteroid to the skin of the eyelid, Br. J. Dermatol. **95:** 207, 1976.

78. Turner, J.B.: A clinical review of congenital glaucoma, South. Med. J. **64:**1362, 1971.

79. Weekers, R., Grieten, J., and Collignon-Brach, J.: Contribution à l'etude de l'hypertension oculaire provoquee par la dexamethasone dans le glaucoma à angle ouvert, Ophthalmologica **152:**81, 1966.

80. Wilensky, J.T., Snyder, D., and Gieser, D.: Steroid-induced ocular hypertension in patients with filtering blebs, Ophthalmology **87:**240, 1980.

81. Zimmerman, L.: Demonstration of hyaluronidase-sensitive acid mucopolysaccharide, Am. J. Ophthalmol. **44:**1, 1957.

82. Zugerman, C., Saunders, D., and Levit, F.: Glaucoma from topically applied steroids, Arch. Dermatol. **112:** 1326, 1976.

GLAUCOMAS ASSOCIATED WITH INFLAMMATION AND TRAUMA

Chapter 18

GLAUCOMA SECONDARY TO KERATITIS, EPISCLERITIS, AND SCLERITIS

Peter G. Watson

Glaucoma associated with inflammation of the cornea, sclera, and episclera is sufficiently common that one should obtain some assessment of the intraocular pressure, not only in every patient with these conditions, but also every time the patient is seen. It is a tragic experience for one to have spent weeks or months treating an inflamed eye, eventually obtaining an optically clear medium, only to find the disc cupped and pale and the patient without useful vision. Even if such an event cannot always be prevented, it is inexcusable not to have considered the possibility and to have attempted to counteract the effects of elevated intraocular pressure.

Many of the problems arise because of a reasonable reluctance to measure the intraocular pressure with an applanation or Schiøtz tonometer in a patient with active keratitis, either because of the possibility of damaging an already unhealthy epithelium or because of the very real danger of cross infection. Unfortunately, even the most elaborate apparatus for sterilizing Goldmann tonometer heads is ineffective against such viruses as the adenovirus group, and vigorous rubbing with a sterile swab is essential before each use. Digital tonometry can occasionally be an acceptable alternative and is certainly better than nothing. If the pressure is very high, this assessment will be sufficient to determine that treatment needs to be given. If one is in doubt, then the small risks of tonometry probably need to be taken. The Mac-Kay-Marg tonometer with disposable rubber covers is probably the best instrument to use, but

the corneal epithelium can still be damaged with this instrument.

There are as many causes of raised intraocular pressure in these conditions as there are causes for glaucoma. It is often assumed that the rise in pressure is directly related to the inflammatory condition of the eye, but this is often not the case. It is also often assumed that because the disc is pale and cupped, the rise in intraocular pressure is the sole reason for the change, yet many inflammatory diseases are accompanied by or associated with active vasculitis, and there may be other reasons for vascular insufficiency and capillary closure at the optic nerve head. The cause of the raised intraocular pressure in each patient must be considered in terms of what is known to produce it. Is the angle closed? Is there a predisposition to angle-closure glaucoma, and does the fellow eye need treatment? Is the patient already suffering from primary open-angle glaucoma? Is the rise in pressure due to an elevated episcleral venous pressure, to edema of the meshwork, or to obstruction by synechiae? Motzu, in the fourth century BC, said "The physician . . . has to know the course of the ailment before he can treat it." This is as true today as ever it was in the past.

Unfortunately, the investigation is hampered by the possibility of damaging an already diseased cornea or rupturing a very thin sclera or cornea. Gonioscopy is often difficult or impossible in patients with severe keratitis, in which case one may attempt to assess the width of the angle by comparing one eye with the other and noting the position of the iris in relation to the cornea at the limbus. Although by no means foolproof, this method will often indicate whether the glaucoma is due to a narrow angle. Gonioscopy in scleritis rarely presents a problem unless the sclera or limbus is very thin. It is, however, essential to use a three-mirror lens because, as will be seen later, a narrow angle may be due to either a granuloma behind the iris overlying the ciliary body or a granuloma in the posterior sclera itself.

Visual field examination can be extremely confusing if it is attempted in patients with keratitis. It is often valuable, however, if open-angle glaucoma is suspected, if there is segmental atrophy of the optic nerve head, or if a vascular occlusion is suspected. In patients with posterior scleritis with a localized lesion, optic nerve head edema, or exudative detachment, the visual field examination can be invaluable in assessing the progress of the disease and the effect of treatment.

While almost any variety of glaucoma can occur in this group of conditions, some are much more common than others, and others are quite specific for one particular condition. It is useful, therefore, to consider these specific types under separate headings, the most common being mentioned first.

Classification of glaucoma mechanisms

I. Episcleritis
   A. Steroid-induced glaucoma
   B. Acute open-angle glaucoma associated with conjunctival chemosis and elevated episcleral venous pressure
   C. Acute angle-closure glaucoma
   D. Preexisting open-angle glaucoma
II. Anterior scleritis
   A. Open-angle glaucoma
      1. Secondary open-angle glaucoma
         a. Associated with uveitis
         b. Associated with active limbal scleritis resulting in trabecular destruction in severe cases
         c. As a result of vasculitis of the episcleral vessels
         d. Steroid-induced
      2. Preexisting primary open-angle glaucoma
   B. Angle-closure glaucoma
      1. Primary angle-closure glaucoma
         a. Induced by anterior segment edema; no peripheral anterior synechiae (PAS) formation
         b. Predisposition to angle-closure glaucoma precipitated by inflammation
      2. Secondary angle-closure glaucoma with uveitis and PAS formation
   C. Pupillary block glaucoma
   D. Neovascular glaucoma
III. Posterior scleritis
   A. Angle-closure glaucoma due to forward movement of the lens-iris diaphragm
   B. Secondary angle-closure glaucoma with PAS formation
   C. Neovascular glaucoma
IV. Keratitis with little or no anterior uveitis
   A. Open-angle glaucoma
      1. Acute inflammatory changes associated with bacterial, viral, or fungal keratitis
      2. Destructive changes in connective tissue and degenerative diseases
      3. Chronic degenerative changes associated with chronic keratitis
   B. Primary angle-closure glaucoma
      1. Associated with acute inflammation
      2. Chemical injury
   C. Secondary angle-closure: associated with acute and chronic inflammatory disease and PAS formation

EPISCLERITIS
Simple episcleritis

Simple episcleritis is a benign, recurrent condition that, although uncomfortable, never causes permanent harm. The condition is twice as common in men as in women, has its peak incidence in the fourth decade of life, and may affect one eye or both simultaneously or at different times.

The clinical presentation is the same in all the various types. Without prior warning, the eye becomes prickly, red, and slightly tender. These symptoms increase in intensity over the next 24 hours, often accompanied by tearing but never discharge. The symptoms can range from a mild pricking and discomfort with slight redness of the eye to a very red, inflamed eye accompanied by intense conjunctival and episcleral chemosis, swelling of the lids, and a temporary miosis and myopia. Having reached a peak, the symptoms gradually decline again over the next several days, after which there is a short respite before the inflammation recurs either at the same or at another site. In some 60% of patients, this pattern will persist for 3 to 5 years. The intervals between the attacks then increase until no further attacks occur. In a few patients the attacks may last up to 30 years.

The cause remains unknown. The initial attack frequently follows a viral infection, and many patients give a definite history of an exogenous antigen. Seven percent of the patients have clinical gout, but more often than not, no specific etiologic agent can be found. In many patients the disease behaves as a type I hypersensitivity reaction.

Nodular episcleritis[34]

The symptoms, course, age, and sex distribution of nodular episcleritis are the same as for simple episcleritis, but this condition runs a much more protracted course, and the episcleral inflammation, instead of spreading throughout the tissue, localizes in one or several spots with the formation of a nodule within the episcleral tissue. This nodule can be moved under the conjunctiva, and the underlying sclera is not edematous. If the tissues are very inflamed, a drop of 1% epinephrine or 10% phenylephrine will blanch the tissues sufficiently to enable one to observe the underlying sclera.

Glaucoma associated with episcleritis
Steroid-induced glaucoma

Patients with episcleritis have been treated with topical steroids for as long as these have been in use.[6,7] Consider, however, that these patients develop recurrences and may be treated at intervals from as short a period as 2 weeks to as long as 30 years for a benign condition. Fifteen percent of patients treated this way develop posterior subcapsular cataracts.[33] Sixteen percent develop a rise in intraocular pressure.[21] Considering the period of time over which these patients are liable to be given topical steroids, their chances of developing intractable glaucoma and cataracts are very high indeed. A double-masked trial of placebo versus betamethasone versus oxyphenbutazone ointments in this condition showed that betamethasone gave symptomatic relief, oxyphenbutazone was equally effective, and neither shortened the course of the condition.[35] Similar results have been obtained in a recent trial using clobetasone butyrate drops and placebo drops.[18]

Occasionally, in a patient who has attacks that are incapacitating because of watering eyes, swollen lids, and conjunctiva, it is both permissible and necessary to use intensive, strong topical steroids within minutes of the start of an attack. This will sometimes abort the attack. In all other situations, if the patient demands treatment, some nonsteroidal antiinflammatory drops or even placebo drops should be used. If the attacks are severe, frequent, and incapacitating, systemic oxyphenbutazone or indomethacin will usually bring relief.

There is no hereditary tendency to develop episcleritis, but it has been suggested that the normal population can be divided into three groups regarding pressure response to topical steroids: (1) marked responders with rises in intraocular pressure above 30 mm Hg (homozygous [gg]), (2) responders with moderate rises in intraocular pressure to between 20 and 30 mm Hg (heterozygous [ng]), and (3) homozygous (nn) nonresponders who have no rise in intraocular pressure after 6 weeks of topical steroid application.[1,2] Four percent of the normal population are homozygous (gg), 32% heterozygous (ng), and 64% homozygous (nn) nonresponders.

Although 16% of the patients with episcleritis in one study showed transient rises in intraocular pressure of more than 20 mm Hg during the course of local steroid treatment, only 9 of 301 eyes (3%) developed glaucoma (i.e., permanent rises in intraocular pressure with disc and field changes, requiring medication or surgery for control).[33] During treatment of the episcleritis, four of these eyes were known to have open-angle glaucoma before treatment started, and one eye developed the type of glaucoma that is described in the section on acute open-angle glaucoma. The remaining four eyes could be regarded as having definite steroid-induced glaucoma (1.3%). It is probable that these patients were homozygous (gg) responders in whom the changes in the trabecular meshwork had become irreversible, but there was no evidence to show that the two conditions of episcleritis and glaucoma were otherwise linked.

Fortunately, the majority of patients who experience an intraocular pressure rise after using steroids recover completely once the steroids are withdrawn. Recurrent episcleritis may need to be controlled by systemic medication, or the glaucoma may recur. If simple antiglaucomatous medication fails, trabeculectomy must be performed.

Acute open-angle glaucoma

Acute open-angle glaucoma is an unusual but apparently quite specific entity that arises in those patients who develop markedly infiltrated, edematous episclera and swollen lids (Fig. 18-1). In addition to the signs of episcleritis, the patient has an extremely painful eye and deteriorating vision.[16,20] As neither pain nor reduced vision are features of episcleritis, additional problems should be suspected. In this case the intraocular pressure is found to be markedly raised, the cornea mod-

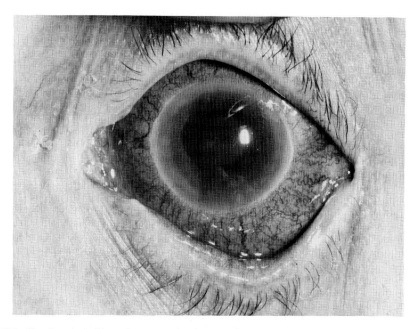

FIG. 18-1. Simple episcleritis and open-angle glaucoma in 60-year-old woman. Onset of pain, discomfort, and misty vision was very sudden. Episcleral and conjunctival tissue was edematous, and there was slight edema of cornea. Angle was wide open.

erately edematous, and the pupil miotic. The angle can be seen to be open, but there is no reflux of blood into Schlemm's canal.

The cause would seem to be simply edema of the trabecular meshwork. The episcleral venous pressure may also be somewhat raised, but the venous congestion usually associated with glaucoma of this cause is absent.

The two patients whom my colleagues and I have seen with this condition responded well to treatment with acetazolamide, dilation of the pupil with short-acting mydriatics (1% tropicamide), and intensive treatment of the episcleral inflammation with hourly application of 0.3% prednisolone drops, which was continued until the inflammation disappeared. Recurrent attacks have been controlled by starting the treatment as soon as the symptoms commence, and this has reduced the inflammatory response sufficiently to prevent the onset of the glaucoma.

Acute angle-closure glaucoma

We have seen two patients subject to attacks of episcleritis who also developed acute angle-closure glaucoma. Both patients responded to the standard therapy for acute angle-closure glaucoma, and peripheral iridectomies were performed through a corneal incision without complication.

Preexisting open-angle glaucoma

Since up to 80% of patients with open-angle glaucoma are (gg) or (ng) steroid responders, it is important to determine whether they have this condition or a family history of it before starting treatment. If a positive history exists, steroids should be avoided and the episcleritis treated with either local oxyphenbutazone ointment or systemic anti-inflammatory agents. If antiglaucomatous therapy is required, pilocarpine should be used but not the beta blockers. Pilocarpine enhances aqueous flow through the trabecular meshwork and disperses the abnormal accumulation of mucopolysaccharides in the inner wall of Schlemm's canal.[15] Beta blockers, on the other hand, result in underperfusion of the meshwork and further accumulation of abnormal substances and thus may fail to control the glaucoma. Trabeculectomy, if necessary, should be performed through an area of unaffected sclera.

SCLERITIS

In contradistinction to episcleritis, scleritis is a severe, painful, potentially destructive eye disease requiring vigorous therapy for its control, sometimes with extremely toxic and dangerous drugs. It is therefore very important to distinguish between these two conditions, which are quite distinct,[4] and which can almost always be recognized when the patient is first seen. This is achieved by taking a careful history and by observing the depth of the inflammation.[33,34] In 1830 Mackenzie[19] gave this exact description:

> The pain is at its onset of the stinging kind extending from the eyeball to the orbit and neighbouring parts of the head. These parts feel hot to the patient and even to the hand of the observer. The pain is strikingly augmented by warmth. It often extends to the forehead, cheekbone and the teeth; . . . pulsating . . . and particularly round the orbit, it consists rather in an agonizing kind of feeling which distresses and wearies out patience of the person affected. It never ceases entirely so long as the disease continues but it varies much in degree, coming on with severity about four or six or eight o'clock in the evening; continuing during the night becoming most severe about midnight and aborting towards five or six in the morning till then totally preventing sleep and occasioning great distress.''

With such severe pain, it is surprising that photophobia and tearing are not prominent features.[31,33] The pain is a consequence of swelling and/or destruction of the scleral tissue. Clinically this gives rise to scleral edema if the disease is anterior to the equator or to choroidal swelling and secondary retinal detachment if the disease is posterior to the equator. Destruction of the sclera (necrotizing scleritis) is a late feature and is almost always preventable if the disease is detected early enough.

Forty-six percent of patients with scleritis have some other systemic disease—usually connective tissue disease. The mortality is also high: between 30% and 45% of patients die within 5 years, largely of cardiovascular disease related to the systemic cause of the scleritis.[21,33] Several clinically distinct varieties of scleritis can be identified:

A. Anterior scleritis
   1. Diffuse
   2. Nodular
   3. Necrotizing
      a. With inflammation
      b. Without inflammation (scleromalacia perforans)
B. Posterior scleritis

Anterior scleritis

Diffuse and nodular anterior scleritis[34]

The onset of diffuse scleritis and of nodular anterior scleritis is often insidious, pain being the prominent feature and the redness of the eye becoming completely ignored. Examination reveals edema of the deep scleral tissue and an overlying episcleral congestion (Figs. 18-2 and 18-3). In nodular scleritis, the scleral inflammation is localized to one or more nodules, which can become immense. These nodules, which are often full of pultaceous material and extremely tender, should not be biopsied, because they fail to heal. One feature that helps distinguish these varieties from the less important episcleritis is that the vascular plexuses lose their regular arrangement, and large bypass channels form. Treatment is with systemic antiinflammatory agents, such as oxyphenbutazone 100 mg four times a day or indomethacin 25 mg four times a day, until the inflammation disappears.

Necrotizing anterior scleritis[34]

Necrotizing anterior scleritis, which is always accompanied by severe inflammation, is much to be feared (Fig. 18-4). Although only 10% of patients with scleral inflammation have necrotizing scleritis, the diagnosis must be considered at all times. Failure to treat it adequately leads to irreparable loss of tissue and the onset of glaucoma and uveitis, which may lead to loss of the eye.

Fortunately, it is almost always possible to detect the necrotizing type of scleritis at the outset; the patient has the condition initially rather than as a progression from the more benign scleritis. The pain is intense, exactly as MacKenzie described it, and the eye is congested up to but usually not including the equator of the globe. In contrast to nodular scleritis, the congestion is more to the edges of the swollen area (representing the site of the active granuloma), and the episclera and sometimes the conjunctiva may be avascular over the center of the lesion, which may break down, leading to loss of tissue. The course of the lesion is insidiously progressive and, if not stopped, will progress both around the globe and backward to involve the posterior segment. Treatment is with systemic steroids in high dosage.[33,34]

Necrotizing scleritis without inflammation (scleromalacia perforans)

The term scleromalacia perforans[29] should be reserved for patients with this condition who are almost always female, with long-standing rheumatoid arthritis, and who develop obliterative vasculitis of the episcleral vasculature. This inevitably leads to avascular necrosis and sequestration of the underlying sclera. The prominent feature is that there is little or no inflammation surrounding the necrotic tissue, and treatment is rarely indicated

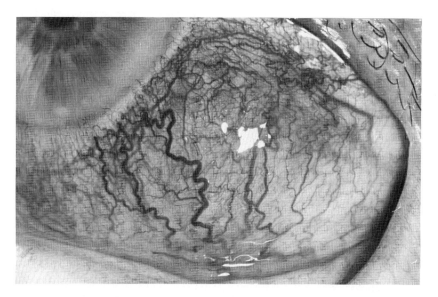

FIG. 18-2. Diffuse anterior scleritis. Intraocular pressure was raised in this patient. Angle was found to be narrow and congested in area of scleral inflammation. There were some cells in anterior chamber. This is possibly clinical counterpart of Fig. 18-13.

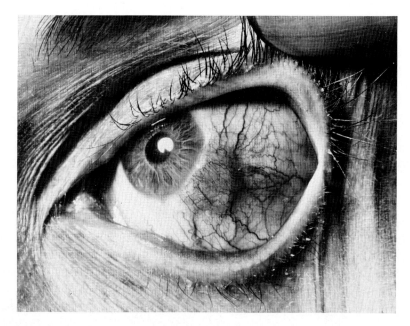

FIG. 18-3. Nodular anterior scleritis. Intraocular pressure was raised, angle was wide open, and trabecular band was prominent. Outflow was reduced. Other eye was normal. This is possibly clinical counterpart of Fig. 18-6.

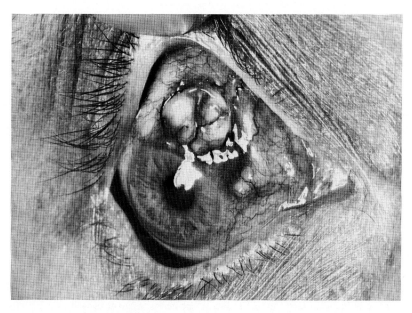

FIG. 18-4. Necrotizing anterior scleritis. Angle was open but narrow and congested in area adjacent to scleral inflammation. This probably is appearance of Fig. 18-8. (From Watson, P.: Diseases of the sclera and episclera. In Duane, T.D., editor: Clinical ophthalmology, vol. 4, New York, 1980, Harper & Row Publishers, Inc.)

unless other complications supervene. Subconjunctival steroids are contraindicated in this disease, since they may induce necrosis leading to perforation of the globe.

Posterior scleritis

Posterior scleritis is a much underdiagnosed condition and is present in three fourths of the eyes that require enucleation. Some 45% of these eyes have never had the diagnosis made before enculeation.[12] The site of the granuloma determines the symptoms and signs. Thus if the inflammation affects the area adjacent to the pars plana, cyclitis and pars planitis will result (Fig. 18-5). If the inflammation overlies the midchoroid, an exudative retinal detachment will be produced; if the inflammation is at the disc, papilledema will result; and, if there is a large posterior granuloma, proptosis will result.[5] The diagnosis often depends on considering the possibility and, if necessary, giving a trial of steroid therapy. Ultrasonography and computed tomographic (CT) scanning can be helpful. Treatment is with systemic steroids.

Glaucoma associated with anterior scleritis

In 301 eyes of patients attending the scleritis clinic at Moorfields Eye Hospital, the intraocular pressure was found to be raised in 12% of the pa-

tients with scleritis, but only 3% required surgery for its control (Table 18-1). However, in a histopathologic study of 92 eyes removed because of scleral disease, 49% had glaucoma.[36] The most common reason for enucleation was intractable glaucoma and uveitis, so the presence of glaucoma must be regarded as having sinister import in patients with scleral inflammation.

Clinically, 90% of the patients with scleritis had inflammation anterior to the equator, and no inflammatory signs could be detected in the posterior segment, even on the closest examination. However, of the eyes that were removed and that also had glaucoma, inflammation was limited to the anterior segment in only 13 (26%) and to the posterior segment in only 6 (12%); the rest (62%) had a combination of both anterior and posterior disease. This underlines the importance of detecting and treating the condition early if irreversible changes are not to supervene.

Further analysis of both the clinical and histopathologic data indicate that different mechanisms are at work in the production of the glaucoma.

Open-angle glaucoma

PRIMARY OPEN-ANGLE GLAUCOMA. Five percent of the patients with scleritis in the above clinical study also had what must be regarded as pri-

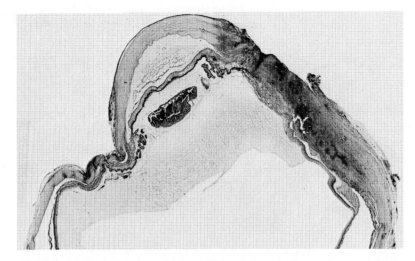

FIG. 18-5. Clinical diagnosis was anterior necrotizing scleritis complicated by cataract, uveitis, and glaucoma. Eye was removed because of intractable pain and intolerance of steroid therapy. It can be seen that inflammation has spread to involve posterior segment as well as angle structures. (From Watson, P.: Diseases of the sclera and episclera. In Duane, T.D., editor: Clinical ophthalmology, vol. 4, New York, 1980, Harper & Row, Publishers, Inc.)

TABLE 18-1
Glaucoma in scleritis

Type of scleritis	Total eyes	Total with glaucoma	Primary open-angle glaucoma	Primary angle-closure glaucoma	Secondary glaucoma	Steroid-induced glaucoma
Diffuse anterior	119	12	6	0	6	0
Nodular anterior	134	11	6	0	5	0
Necrotizing	29	8	2	0	5	1
Scleromalacia perforans	13	4	0	0	4	0
Posterior	6	0	0	0	0	0
TOTAL	301	35	14	0	20	1

Of the patients with secondary glaucoma, nine had no abnormality other than scleritis, seven had keratitis, and six had uveitis. Sclerokeratitis coexisted in some patients. Five patients with episcleritis developed steroid-induced glaucoma.

mary open-angle glaucoma in that they had raised intraocular pressure, field loss, disc changes, and a wide-open angle that did not appear to be abnormal in any way. These patients had not been taking topical steroids, but most had had systemic steroids at some time or another. This incidence, which is twice what might be expected in the population as a whole, might be accounted for either by the presence of a mild degree of inflammation in a trabecular meshwork already compromised by glaucoma or perhaps by an abnormal steroid response. Treatment with miotics or trabeculectomy

was successful. Again, trabeculectomy must be performed in an area where the conjunctiva and sclera appear normal.

SECONDARY OPEN-ANGLE GLAUCOMA. Secondary open-angle glaucoma is an extremely difficult diagnosis to make clinically because the intraocular pressure sometimes rises to very high levels, but the angles appear normal and the disc and field changes are variable. Its presence, however, can be implied from a very rapid response to treatment of the scleritis and from the somewhat congested appearance of the trabecular band when

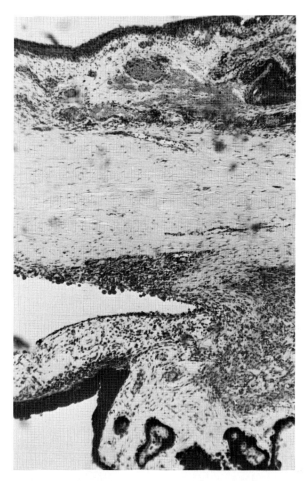

FIG. 18-6. Open angle with inflammatory cells concentrated within outflow system. Intense inflammatory reaction involves episcleral and conjunctival vessels. (From Wilhelmus, K., Grierson, I., and Watson, P.G. Published with permission from the American Journal of Ophthalmology **91:** 697-705, 1981. Copyright by the Ophthalmic Publishing Co.)

viewed gonioscopically. This appearance is not a constant feature, but while it is independent of the presence of uveitis, it does seem to be related to an adjacent area of scleritis. In the histopathologic study, 80% of the glaucomatous eyes had a focus of scleritis overlying the angle structures as opposed to 25% of the nonglaucomatous eyes (p < 0.005)[36] (Fig. 18-6).

GLAUCOMA ASSOCIATED WITH UVEITIS. Of the 14 eyes with open-angle glaucoma, 9 had severe anterior uveitis, and all of these patients had evidence of active trabecular inflammation on histology without any evidence of peripheral anterior synechiae (PAS) formation[36] (Fig. 18-7). Uveitis is a very common feature of eyes removed because of scleritis, being present in 84% of the glaucomatous ones, but it is not a common feature clinically. The combination of both uveitis and glau-

coma must therefore be regarded with deep suspicion, and active measures taken to counteract it. Certainly, severe uveitis occurs only in the most severely affected eyes and seems to arise only when the inflammation has progressed circumferentially around the globe or has extended backward beyond the equator (Table 18-2). It is possible, therefore, that the glaucoma is a result of a combination of severe trabecular damage, damage to the episcleral outflow channels, anterior segment ischemia, and involvement of the uveal tract by the granulomatous reaction (Fig. 18-8).

Treatment is difficult, but it is essential to control both the glaucoma and the concomitant uveitis. Systemic medication with steroids or, in less severe cases, topical antiinflammatory agents, will usually control both the scleritis and the intraocular pressure. However, it may also be necessary to

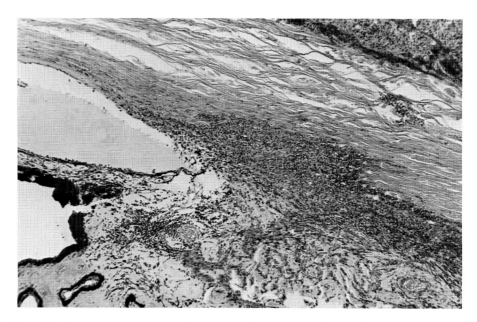

FIG. 18-7. Partially closed angle with intense inflammatory infiltrate within trabecular tissues. (From Wilhelmus, K., Grierson, I., and Watson, P.G. Published with permission from the American Journal of Ophthalmology **91:**697-705, 1981. Copyright by the Ophthalmic Publishing Co.)

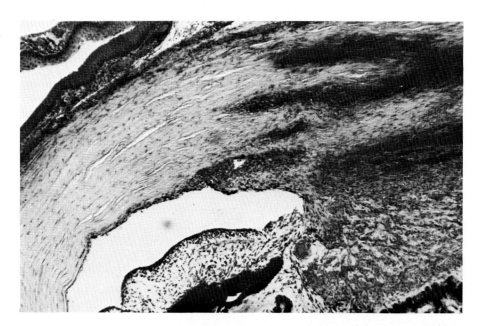

FIG. 18-8. Open angle with many inflammatory cells within outflow system. Deep scleral, interscleral, episcleral, and subconjunctival vessels are foci of inflammation. (From Wilhelmus, K., Grierson, I., and Watson, P.G. Published with permission from the American Journal of Ophthalmology **91:**697-705, 1981. Copyright by the Ophthalmic Publishing Co.)

TABLE 18-2
Percentage of anterior uveitis in scleritis

Type of scleritis	Total eyes	Anterior uveitis (%)
Anterior		
Diffuse	119	35
Nodular	134	17
Necrotizing	29	37
Scleromalacia perforans	13	100
Posterior	6	66

Only two patients developed uveitis in the opposite, apparently unaffected eye.

give mydriatic-cycloplegics and carbonic anhydrase inhibitors. Miotics are rarely effective in the presence of uveitis. Provided there is some relatively normal area of sclera and episcleral tissue, trabeculectomy undertaken at this site is almost always effective. If it fails, however, treatment becomes extremely difficult. Cyclocryotherapy is a poor procedure in an already inflamed eye. Tube implants need to be avoided if at all possible, because the presence of foreign material stimulates further inflammation.

GLAUCOMA IN THE PRESENCE OF ACTIVE LIMBAL SCLERITIS. Although scleritis involves the anterior segment, the inflammatory reaction is maximal about 3 to 5 mm from the limbus. If the inflammation does reach the limbus, it is rarely over more than an area of 45 degrees and, provided the trabecular tissue is otherwise healthy, the remaining meshwork is sufficient to maintain the intraocular pressure at a normal level. However, particularly in patients with diffuse anterior scleritis, the whole circumference of the anterior segment can be involved, and very occasionally the scleritis is most active in the limbal area, in which case the intraocular pressure will rise (Fig. 18-9). In certain patients with long-standing circumferential necrotizing scleritis, the trabecular tissue becomes directly involved. In the histopathologic study, active limbal scleritis was more common in eyes with glaucoma than in those without glaucoma ($p < 0.005$)[36] (Fig. 18-10).

Because the inflammation causing the scleritis is the cause of this type of glaucoma, treatment of the scleral inflammation will reduce the intraocular pressure. In the acute phase of the inflammation, the intraocular pressure tends to rise to very high levels. During this period, carbonic anhy-

drase inhibitors are usually necessary to control the pressure. There is, however, a long period of up to many weeks after the scleritis has disappeared clinically before the intraocular pressure normalizes. Carbonic anhydrase inhibitors can usually be discontinued when the inflammation subsides, but it may be necessary to continue treatment with pilocarpine or timolol during this period. Trabeculectomy is rarely necessary but is effective (Fig. 18-11). The delay in restoration of the intraocular pressure to normal is probably due to damage to the proteoglycan matrix of the trabecular tissue, which requires time to return to normal.[32]

GLAUCOMA RESULTING FROM VASCULITIS OF THE EPISCLERAL VESSELS.[36] This is a condition that cannot be proved to exist except by biopsy of episcleral tissue—a procedure not to be recommended unless it is part of a trabeculectomy procedure. It occurs in eyes with an open angle without anterior chamber inflammation or trabecular meshwork abnormality and where the scleritis is away from the limbus. On gonioscopy, the angle is wide open, but the response to miotics is poor. Tonography reveals a very poor outflow.[14] Histologically the intrascleral outflow channels are surrounded by cuffs of lymphocytes, and there is often perivasculitis in the anterior uveal tissues (Figs. 18-8, 18-10, and 18-12). Vasculitis is a common feature of many of the connective tissue diseases associated with scleritis,[34] the generalized vasculitis and scleral necrosis often occurring simultaneously, and it is possible that the changes observed in the outflow channels are a manifestation of the systemic condition. The glaucoma usually resolves with the treatment of the scleritis or systemic disease.

STEROID-INDUCED GLAUCOMA. Because scleritis needs to be treated with systemic medication, steroid-induced glaucoma is much less of a problem in scleritis than in episcleritis. In a large series, only one case was definitely proved to be caused by steroids alone, although it is almost certain that some of the patients with open angles, many of whom must have been homozygous (gg) responders, had their glaucoma worsened by the use of steroids.[33] McGavin found raised intraocular pressure from this cause in 16% of the eyes that he treated for scleritis and rheumatoid arthritis, but many of these patients also had used local steroids as well.[21] Because of the possibility of steroid-induced glaucoma, we now rarely prescribe local steroids for patients with scleral disease and, if

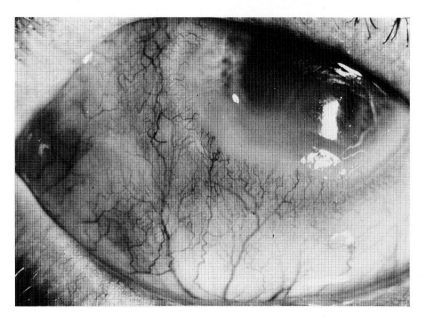

FIG. 18-9. Active limbitis in patient with severe anterior scleritis following herpes zoster and accompanied by keratitis and raised intraocular pressure. Angle was open.

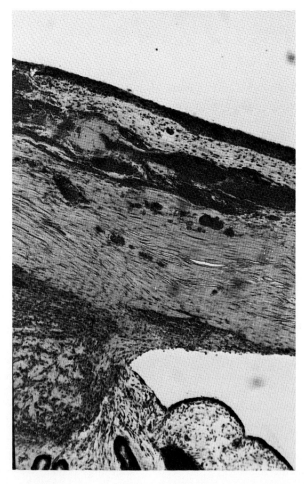

FIG. 18-10. Open-angle glaucoma with intense inflammatory infiltrate within outflow system. Inflammatory cuffing of limbal vessels is evident. (From Wilhelmus, K., Grierson, I., and Watson, P.G. Published with permission from the American Journal of Ophthalmology **91**:697-705, 1981. Copyright by the Ophthalmic Publishing Co.)

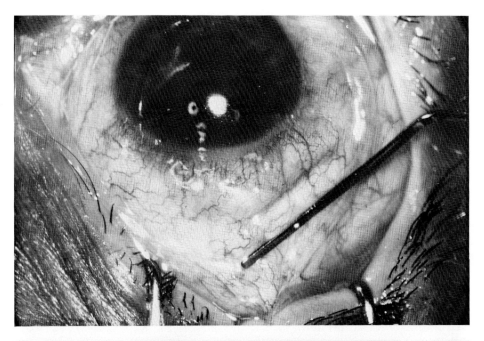

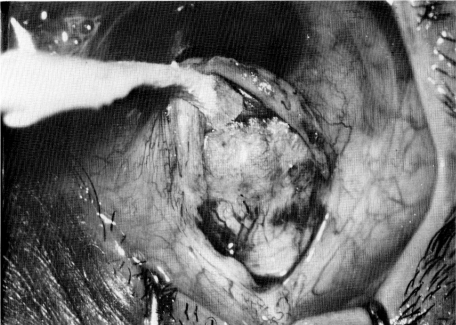

FIG. 18-11. Active limbitis and scleritis with open angle in patient in whom intraocular pressure could not be controlled. Trabeculectomy was successfully performed, and pressure has remained controlled for 5 years. Note gross episcleral and scleral edema.

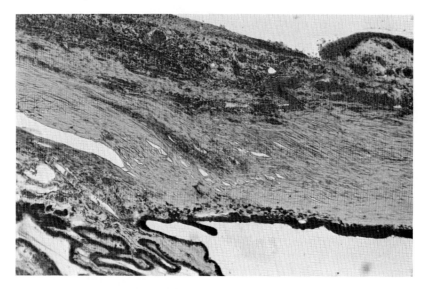

FIG. 18-12. Closed angle with atrophic thin iris and outflow system obliterated. Example shows clear evidence of scleritis and limbal vasculitis. (From Wilhelmus, K., Grierson, I., and Watson P.G. Published with permission from the American Journal of Ophthalmology **91:**697-705, 1981. Copyright by the Ophthalmic Publishing Co.)

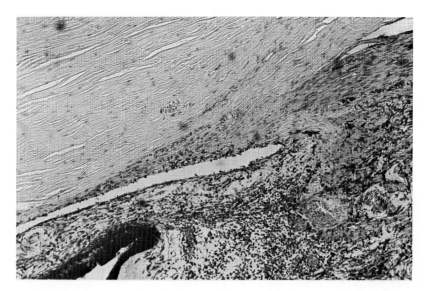

FIG. 18-13. Narrow angle with inflammatory reaction in anterior uvea. Schlemm's canal is closed; inflammatory cells are present within a hyalinized trabecular meshwork.

they are deemed essential, clobetasone butyrate, which has much less of a pressure-elevating effect, is used. Fortunately, most steroid-induced glaucomas resolve on withdrawal of the steroids, but again many patients must be given an antiglaucomatous medication for a prolonged period while the trabecular tissue returns to normal. Occasionally, however, the changes are irreversible, and trabeculectomy has to be undertaken.

GLAUCOMA DUE TO OTHER CAUSES. If scleritis occurs in patients who already have the exfoliation syndrome or phacolytic glaucoma, the scleritis does not appear to alter the course or treatment of the glaucoma. Histologically we have seen one example in which the exfoliation syndrome and scleritis occurred together. The angle of one eye, although wide open, was completely obstructed by a hyaline membrane. The cause of this is obscure but is probably a result of inflammation, fibrin exudation, and secondary hyaline formation from proliferation of the endothelium of the cornea or Schlemm's canal.[9]

Angle-closure glaucoma

PRIMARY ANGLE-CLOSURE GLAUCOMA. Primary angle-closure glaucoma accompanying anterior scleritis is rare, but we have seen two patients whose attacks seemed to have been precipitated by the onset of the scleral inflammation. Whether the combination of a narrow angle with simple dilation of the pupil, ciliary edema, partial obstruction of the outflow channels, or a combination of these factors caused the attack is uncertain. They responded well to antiglaucoma medication, systemic oxyphenbutazone, and peripheral iridectomy performed through the cornea. Two eyes in the histopathologic study, however, showed occluded angles without any evidence of synechiae formation or uveitis, and it is possible that the presence of the acute angle-closure glaucoma was not recognized, the pain being considered a concomitant part of the scleral inflammation (Fig. 18-13).

SECONDARY ANGLE-CLOSURE GLAUCOMA. This is the least common (but most fearsome) type of glaucoma associated with scleral inflammation. The raised intraocular pressure invariably follows a prolonged uveitis that may or may not be severe. Fortunately, anterior uveitis occurs in only a third of the patients with anterior scleritis. It is usually mild and can easily be controlled by dilation of the pupil and treatment of the scleritis. In some

patients, particularly those with severe necrotizing disease, the uveitis is persistent and, although rarely very acute, continues for months while the scleritis is poorly controlled. This gives rise to anterior synechiae formation and eventual occlusion of the angle (Fig. 18-14). In these patients it is most important to treat any acute attacks vigorously because severe "plastic" uveitis inevitably leads to broad anterior synechiae formation and eventually to a false angle. Once this has occurred and the intraocular pressure becomes persistently raised, weak areas of sclera affected by the scleritis will start to bulge and staphyloma formation will result (Fig. 18-15). Staphyloma and spontaneous perforation is a rare event in scleritis and occurs (apart from accidental injury) only in eyes in which the intraocular pressure has been persistently raised.

Treatment is difficult and unrewarding. In the early stages, suppression of the uveitis and scleritis combined with antiglaucoma medication will prevent the continuation of the process, but once the angle has been occluded totally, it is very difficult to control the intraocular pressure. Trabeculectomy is sometimes successful. This should be performed behind the scleral spur so that, after the scleral spur has been dissected from the underlying ciliary muscle, the synechiae can be dissected under direct vision. It is important to replace the superficial flap, since otherwise staphyloma formation can result if the pressure remains high. If this fails, some success can sometimes be obtained from Krasnov's iridocycloretraction procedure, in which two strips of sclera 2 mm wide and 8 mm long are inserted into the anterior chamber to hold open the area of the trabecular tissues between and at the site of both incisions. Success is dependent on a strict antiinflammatory postoperative regimen and a relatively normal area of episcleral and conjunctival tissue through which the aqueous can drain.

Pupillary block glaucoma

Although posterior synechiae are found in 70% of patients who develop uveitis with scleritis and in 40% of those who lose an eye from this disease, pupillary block glaucoma as the sole reason for the rise in intraocular pressure is rare. The one patient we have seen with this complication responded well to a broad iridectomy with division of the synechiae followed by intensive antiinflammatory therapy.

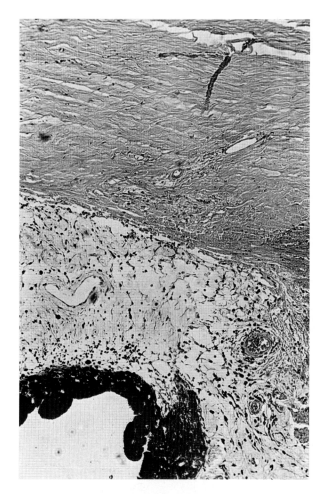

FIG. 18-14. Closed angle with thickened trabecular meshwork; inflammatory cells are present at site of iridotrabecular adhesion. (From Wilhelmus, K., Grierson, I., and Watson, P.G. Published with permission from The American Journal of Ophthalmology **91**:697-705, 1981. Copyright by the Ophthalmic Publishing Co.)

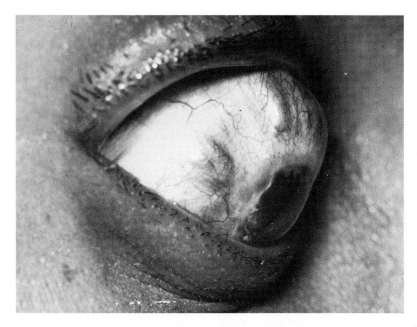

FIG. 18-15. Staphyloma formation in patient with anterior scleritis and persistently raised intraocular pressure. (From Watson, P.: Diseases of the sclera and episclera. In Duane, T.D., editor: Clinical ophthalmology, vol. 4, New York, 1980, Harper & Row, Publishers, Inc.)

Neovascular glaucoma

Although we have never seen this complication clinically in over 600 patients with scleral disease, it was found to be present in 31% of eyes removed presumably for the intractable pain often associated with this condition.[12] Scleritis was not even suspected as the diagnosis in 45% of these eyes, and it is possible, therefore, that neovascular glaucoma associated with anterior scleritis resulted from vasoobliteration but was diagnosed as secondary glaucoma and uveitis. These patients all had deeply cupped discs, vascularization of the iris, and a neovascular membrane in the angle. Molteno[22] implants have been successful in secondary glaucoma following retinal venous occlusion, and it is possible that they might work here also.

Glaucoma associated with posterior scleritis

Angle-closure glaucoma due to choroidal effusion

Angle-closure glaucoma due to choroidal effusion is a specific entity in posterior scleritis. If the cause is not recognized, the patient may be given inappropriate treatment and even submitted to unnecessary surgery.[24,26]

Scleral inflammation usually involves the anterior segment because it is the distribution of the anterior ciliary vessels that is primarily affected, but because these vessels do supply the eye back to the equator, the granuloma can either start in this region or spread backward to it. If this happens, there is an inflammatory reaction in the region of the ciliary body and swelling of the adjacent tissue, which gives rise to an anterior choroidal effusion, which can be circumferential. This results in an anterior rotation of the ciliary body at the scleral spur and closure of the angle of the anterior chamber. A similar cause has been cited in other cases of anterior choroidal effusion[3,13,30,34] (Fig. 18-16).

The diagnosis is relatively simple if the patient has had anterior scleritis (usually of the diffuse type). Concomitant with the onset of the scleritis, the intraocular pressure rises and the anterior chamber shallows to the extent that it appears gonioscopically entirely occluded, whereas the opposite angle remains wide open. The diagnosis is much more difficult if the anterior scleritis is limited in extent or if the patient does not have a past history. Nevertheless, if a unilateral shallow anterior chamber is noted, this diagnosis should always be kept in mind.

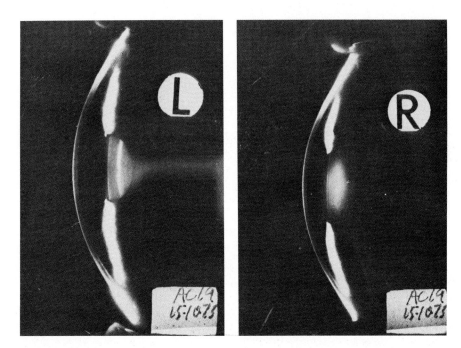

FIG. 18-16. Slit-lamp photograph of normal anterior chamber depth of left eye contrasted with very shallow anterior chamber of right eye in patient who experienced acute angle-closure attack in right eye. Angle closure was found to be due to anterior shift in lens-iris diaphragm caused by posterior scleritis. (From Watson, P.G., and Hazleman, B.L.: The sclera and systemic disorders, London, 1976, W.B. Saunders Co., Ltd.; Courtesy Nicholas P. Brown.)

Treatment with pilocarpine is contraindicated. Apart from not working, it actually will make the anterior chamber shallower,[25] thus making the condition worse. Treatment should be directed to the treatment of the scleritis with systemic oxyphenbutazone (or occasionally steroids) and dilation of the pupil with cycloplegics, together with carbonic anhydrase inhibitors if necessary. This course of treatment has been universally successful in resolving the acute attack and enables close observation of the posterior scleritis.

Secondary angle-closure glaucoma with PAS formation

Although we have not observed this situation clinically, in two of the eyes examined histologically, the scleritis was entirely posterior and the angle was occluded. It is probable that these patients had ciliary body effusions that were caused by the posterior scleritis but that were not recognized as such. Aided by concomitant mild uveitis, the angle became completely occluded and intractable glaucoma resulted.

Neovascular glaucoma

Neovascular glaucoma has also not been observed clinically as a complication of posterior scleritis but has been observed in histologic specimens.[36] In the eyes studied, the granulomatous changes were all posterior to the equator and around the disc. Vasculitis was associated with the scleritis, so that it is reasonable to assume that this could have led to the vascular occlusion. There was no histologic evidence that the new vessel formation was due to a generalized ischemia of the posterior segment. Although glaucoma may manifest itself in many forms, it is almost always preventable and certainly treatable, provided care is taken in detection and the scleral inflammation treated early and energetically.

KERATITIS

Glaucoma induced by keratitis unaccompanied by uveitis is a rare event resulting from either direct involvement of the trabecular meshwork by the disease, which affects the cornea, or from the toxic results of the damage to the corneal stroma.

Chemical burns to the cornea

The most common corneal injury from chemicals is deliberate assault in which ammonia or lye is thrown at or squirted into the recipient's eyes and face. Caustic soda is widely used in industrial processes, and injuries still occur in spite of regulations requiring the use of protective goggles and clothing. Among other effects, these chemicals, together with chloroform, formalin mechlorethamine hydrochloride, and nitrogen mustards cause a marked rise in intraocular pressure.

The severity of the injury and type of response is dependent on the concentration of the chemical and the length of time it is in contact with the cornea.[23] A patient who has been sprayed is immediately afflicted by intense pain, which subsides after 10 to 15 minutes only to be replaced within the hour by more severe pain and a clinical syndrome resembling acute angle-closure glaucoma.

This biphasic response has been thoroughly investigated in chemical burns in rabbits, and it has been shown that as soon as the alkali strikes the cornea, the epithelium is denatured and the collagen contracts, causing a rapid transient rise in intraocular pressure. As the chemical penetrates the cornea, there is an intense generalized ocular inflammatory response with miosis, ocular vasodilation, breakdown of the blood aqueous barrier, and a rise in intraocular pressure that reaches its maximum after 20 to 40 minutes. This pressure rise can be inhibited by polyphloretin and phenylephrine and has been shown to be a direct result of prostaglandin E and F release. The transient rise in intraocular pressure is also present to a lesser extent in the opposite, uninjured eye. Where exactly the prostaglandins act to produce the intraocular pressure rise is uncertain.

If the injury is very severe, the uveitis and damage to the trabecular meshwork may lead to a late secondary open-angle glaucoma[10]; unfortunately, the ciliary processes are also frequently damaged, and as a result profound hypotension supervenes.

A similar type of secondary open-angle glaucoma has been observed in the few survivors of the mustard gas attacks of World War I. These have all been seen in those who have delayed mustard gas keratitis and peripheral corneal aneurysmal dilation of the vessels and corneal opacities. We have a trabeculectomy specimen from one of these patients in whom the trabecular tissue was well within the specimen, but its structure was almost indistinguishable because of excessive hyalinization.

Glaucoma associated with infections of the cornea

The intraocular pressure will rise in any severe stromal infection whether it be due to bacteria, virus, or fungus, and more so if the infection is accompanied by uveitis. If the infection is acute, it is possible that the rise in pressure is due to prostaglandin release and the production of plasmoid aqueous. Generalized corneal and limbal edema will add to the problem through direct involvement of the trabecular meshwork, but it appears that the usual cause is obstruction of the meshwork by cellular exudate combined with some degree of local inflammation.[17]

The most common cause of raised intraocular pressure with keratitis is herpes simplex. Falcon and Williams[11] found that 28% of 183 patients with herpetic keratouveitis were found to have an intraocular pressure of more than 25 mm Hg or a difference of 7 mm Hg in either eye (average 33; range 25 to 50). They found that the intraocular pressure never became raised during the initial attack of herpes simplex, glaucoma being found exclusively in those with stromal disease, with 80% having either disciform keratouveitis or herpetic stromal keratouveitis. Five of their patients developed a glaucomatous field defect, and they concluded that the patients with limbitis were more liable to develop glaucoma than the others. They did not find an abnormal steroid response to be the cause of the raised intraocular pressure and as a consequence recommended that treatment with steroids and antiviral cover not be varied because of the glaucoma; rather, the glaucoma should be treated with the usual antiglaucomatous and antiinflammatory agents (such as oxyphenbutazone or indomethacin) as required.

Syphilitic interstitial keratitis has in the past been a potent cause of secondary glaucoma leading to buphthalmos in the infant, limbitis and scleritis in the juvenile, and secondary open- or closed-angle glaucoma as age advances.[8]

Glaucoma secondary to systemic syndromes with corneal manifestations

The trabecular meshwork occasionally becomes involved in syndromes that affect the cornea. The most common of these is Scheie's syndrome (mucopolysaccharidosis V),[27,28] in which the abnormal mucopolysaccharides have been shown to extend to the angle.

REFERENCES

1. Armaly, M.F.: Effect of corticosteroids on intraocular fluid dynamics. I. Effect of dexamethasone in the normal eye, Arch. Ophthalmol. **70**:482, 1963.
2. Becker, B., and Mills, B.W.: Corticosteroids and intraocular pressure, Arch. Ophthalmol. **70**:500, 1965.
3. Brockhurst, R.J., Schepens, C.L., and Okamura, I.D.: Uveitis. II. Peripheral uveitis: clinical description, complications and differential diagnosis, Am. J. Ophthalmol. **49**:1257, 1960.
4. Campbell, D.M.: Episcleritis, Ophthalmic Rec. **12**:517, 1903.
5. Cleary, P.E., Watson, P.G., McGill, J.I., and Hamilton, A.M.: Visual loss due to posterior segment disease in scleritis, Trans. Ophthalmol. Soc. U.K. **95**:297, 1975.
6. Duke-Elder, S.: The clinical value of cortisone and ACTH in ocular disease, Br. J. Ophthalmol. **35**:637, 1951.
7. Duke-Elder, S.: A series of cases treated locally by cortisone (report to Medical Research Council), Br. J. Ophthalmol. **35**:672, 1951.
8. Duke-Elder, S.: System of ophthalmology, vol. 11, Diseases of the lens and vitreous; glaucoma and hypotony, St. Louis, 1969, The C.V. Mosby Co.
9. Duke-Elder, S., and Leigh, A.G.: Diseases of the outer eye. Vol. 8, part 2, in Duke-Elder, S.: System of ophthalmology, St. Louis, 1965, The C.V. Mosby Co.
10. Duke-Elder, S., and MacFaul, P.A.: Injuries. Vol. 14 in Duke-Elder, S.: System of ophthalmology, St. Louis, 1972, The C.V. Mosby Co.
11. Falcon, M.G., and Williams, H.P.: Herpes simplex, kerato-uveitis and glaucoma, Trans. Ophthalmol. Soc. U.K. **98**:101, 1978.
12. Fraunfelder, F.T., and Watson, P.G.: Evaluation of eyes enucleated for scleritis, Br. J. Ophthalmol. **60**:227, 1976.
13. Gass, J.D.M.: Retinal detachment and narrow angle glaucoma secondary to pseudo tumour of the uveal tract, Am. J. Ophthalmol. **64**:612, 1967.
14. Givner, I.: Uncommon complications of scleritis, Eye, Ear, Nose and Throat Mon. **32**:515, 1953.
15. Grierson, I., Lee, W.R., and Abraham, S.: Effects of pilocarpine on the morphology of human outflow apparatus, Br. J. Ophthalmol. **62**:302, 1978.
16. Harbin, T., and Pollack, J.: Glaucoma in episcleritis, Arch. Ophthalmol. **93**:948, 1975.
17. Hogan, M.J., Kimura, S.T., and Thygeson, P.: Pathology of herpes simplex kerato-iritis, Am. J. Ophthalmol. **57**:551, 1964.
18. Lloyd-Jones, D., Tokarewicz, A., and Watson, P.G.: Clinical evaluation of clobetasone butyrate eye drops in episcleritis, Br. J. Ophthalmol. **65**:641, 1981.
19. Mackenzie, W.: A practical treatise on the diseases of the eye, London, 1830, Longman, p. 409.
20. Mann, W.A., and Markson, D.E.: A case of recurrent iritis and episcleritis on a rheumatic basis: treated with A.C.T.H., Am. J. Ophthalmol. **33**:459, 1950.
21. McGavin, D.D., Williamson, J., Forrester, J.V., et al.: Episcleritis and scleritis: a study of the clinical manifestations and association with rheumatoid arthritis, Br. J. Ophthalmol. **60**:192, 1976.
22. Molteno, A.C.B., Straughan, J.L., and Ancker, E.: Long tube implants in the management of glaucoma, South Afr. Med. J. **50**:1062, 1976.

23. Paterson, C.A., and Pfister, P.R.: Intraocular pressure changes after alkali burns, Arch. Ophthalmol. **91:**211, 1974.

24. Philips, C.D.: Angle closure glaucoma secondary to ciliary body swelling, Arch. Ophthalmol. **92:**287, 1974.

25. Poinoswarny, D., Nagasubramanian, S., and Brown, N.A.P.: The effects of pilocarpine on the visual acuity and on the dimensions of the cornea and anterior chamber, Br. J. Ophthalmol. **60:**678, 1976.

26. Quinlan, M.P., and Hitchings, R.A.: Angle closure glaucoma secondary to posterior scleritis, Br. J. Ophthalmol. **62:**330, 1978.

27. Rasteiro, A.: Scheie's syndrome, Exp. Ophthal. Coimbra. **3:**62, 1977.

28. Scheie, H.G., Hambrick, G.W., and Barness, L.A.: A newly recognised "forme fruste" of Hurler's disease (gargoylism), Am. J. Ophthalmol. **53:**753, 1962.

29. van der Hoeve, J.: Scleromalacia perforans, Ned. Tijdschr. Geneeskd. **75:**4733, 1931.

30. Vogt, F.: Scleritis in connection with choroidal detachment in rheumatic patients, Szemeszet **115:**217, 1978.

31. Wardrop, J.: An account of the rheumatic inflammation of the eye with observation on the treatment of the disease, Medico Chir. Trans. **10:**1, 1818.

32. Watson, P.G., and Grierson, I.: The place of trabeculectomy in the treatment of glaucoma, Ophthalmology **88:** 175, 1981.

33. Watson, P.G., and Hayreh, S.S.: Scleritis and episcleritis, Br. J. Ophthalmol. **60:**163, 1976.

34. Watson, P.G., and Hazleman, B.L.: The sclera and systemic disorders, London, 1976, W.B. Saunders Co., Ltd.

35. Watson, P.G., McKay, D.A., Clemett, R.S., et al.: Treatment of episcleritis: a double blind trial comparing betamethasone 0.1%, oxyphenbutazone 10% and placebo eye ointments, Br. J. Ophthalmol. **57:**866, 1973.

36. Wilhelmus, K., Grierson, I., and Watson, P.G.: Histopathologic and clinical associations of scleritis and glaucoma, Am. J. Ophthalmol. **91:**697, 1981.

Chapter 19

GLAUCOMA ASSOCIATED WITH UVEITIS

Theodore Krupin

Glaucoma secondary to uveitis presents a number of problems to the ophthalmologist. While some forms of uveitis may be classified into clinical entities, most intraocular inflammations are nonspecific and can be broadly described only as anterior or posterior, granulomatous or nongranulomatous. Medical therapy is usually directed at relieving the resulting inflammation and elevated intraocular pressure and rarely at eliminating the underlying cause of the uveitis. The chronic and recurrent nature of the inflammation may produce permanent structural changes that in turn alter aqueous humor dynamics. It may be difficult to pinpoint the actual cause for the pressure elevation or to determine whether it results from active inflammation, insufficient antiinflammatory therapy, corticosteroid therapy, insufficient antiglaucoma therapy, or permanent changes in ocular structure. Secondary glaucoma can present itself as either open- or closed-angle glaucoma or as a combination of the two. Proper diagnosis and management of the glaucoma must take into account all of these possibilities.

PATHOPHYSIOLOGY OF ELEVATED INTRAOCULAR PRESSURE
Inflammation
Trabecular block-dysfunction

Uveitis is usually associated with ciliary body inflammation and hyposecretion of aqueous humor. This may mask the effects of uveitis on aqueous outflow channels, and intraocular pressure may vary depending on the predominance of outflow obstruction or hyposecretion. The obstruction of outflow channels can be caused by swelling or dysfunction of trabecular sheets or endothelial cells or by the accumulation of inflammatory material in the outflow channels. Even though endothelial cells lining the trabeculum and the juxtacanalicular tissue can be mobilized to remove inflammatory products from the outflow channels, they themselves can cause obstruction. Fibrin, white blood cell aggregates, and macrophages can also block outflow channels. In addition, normal serum components may become adsorbed or entrapped in the aqueous outflow system and obstruct the channels.[16] The trabecular endothelial cells can be replaced, but each bout of recurrent inflammation may reduce the effectiveness of the trabecular meshwork as a biologic filter and permanently damage the system.

Prostaglandins

Prostaglandins, a group of naturally occurring lipid-soluble fatty acids with widespread distribution in mammalian tissues and diverse pharmacologic properties, can be involved in acute ocular inflammation. Prostaglandins can produce many of the signs of ocular inflammation, including vasodilatation, miosis, and increased vascular permeability.[5] In addition, topical administration of prostaglandins both elevates intraocular pressure and increases total outflow facility.[45] This suggests that an increase in aqueous humor production or a breakdown of the blood-aqueous barrier is responsible for the elevation of intraocular

290

pressure. The suggestion is supported by the finding that topical administration of arachidonic acid, a precursor of prostaglandin E_2, also increases intraocular pressure, total outflow facility, and aqueous humor protein.[81] Inhibitors of prostaglandin synthesis, such as aspirin or indomethacin, block the responses following topical arachidonic acid. This may be of particular clinical interest, since prostaglandin-like activity may be present in the aqueous humor of patients with acute anterior uveitis.[14] Prostaglandins also may be an etiologic factor in glaucomatocyclitic crises.[65] If prostaglandins are partly responsible for many of the clinical signs in acute anterior uveitis, then substances that antagonize either their synthesis or action may be of value in controlling these diseases.

Altered vascular permeability

The structural changes following ocular inflammatory disease may be permanent and could predispose the eye to subsequent recurrent inflammation. Altered vascular permeability may be present months after the cessation of active inflammation. The presence of aqueous protein in an apparently quiescent phase of chronic recurrent uveitis may be due to disruptions of the ciliary epithelium.[34] This in turn may alter the normal mechanisms for transporting prostaglandin and other substances from the eye.[6]

Structural changes

Uveitis, acute or chronic, can cause structural changes that lead to glaucoma. Clinical signs of acute iridocyclitis include perilimbal vascular injection, miosis, and photophobia. As stated, disruption of the blood-aqueous barrier results in cells and protein (flare) in the aqueous humor and anterior portion of the vitreous. Keratic precipitates are present. The inflammation causes more than mere trabecular damage. The presence of albumin and fibrin in aqueous humor can result in posterior or peripheral anterior synechiae.

Posterior synechiae

Adhesions of the iris to the lens occur earlier in the exudative types of iritis with a heavy aqueous flare, first by the formation of fibrinous adhesions and later by fibrovascular organization. The pupillary margin may be partially or completely involved. If the posterior synechiae are complete, they prevent aqueous humor from passing from the posterior to the anterior chamber through the pupil.

This causes increased pressure in the posterior chamber and a forward ballooning of the iris periphery (iris bombé). Anterior chamber depth is normal at the pupil, but elsewhere it is shallowed by the iris bombé. Forward movement of the peripheral iris can produce acute angle-closure glaucoma.

Peripheral anterior synechiae

Peripheral anterior synechiae, adhesions between the iris and the trabecular meshwork or cornea, can form secondary to the inflammatory process. Synechiae formation can be related to swelling of the iris periphery with the formation of adhesions, protein transudation and exudation in the angle (which pull the iris toward the cornea), or a bridge formation made by large-angle keratic precipitates. Synechiae resulting from iritis are not uniform in shape or in the height of their trabecular attachment. Peripheral anterior synechiae may be conical, cylindrical, or moundlike areas alternating with areas of completely open angle. The synechiae of intraocular inflammation differ from the synechiae of primary pupillary block, where iris segments are attached in a line parallel to Schwalbe's line. While the iridocorneal angle can be closed by peripheral anterior synechiae, it is often difficult to estimate the extent to which the decrease in outflow facility is due to synechiae or to inflammatory damage to the trabecular meshwork.

MANAGEMENT

Medical treatment of glaucoma secondary to active anterior uveitis is directed toward controlling the inflammation and preventing its consequences, as well as lowering the elevated intraocular pressure. Efforts are made to dilate the pupil and decrease the inflammatory reaction so that damage, scarring, and visual loss are minimized. In all inflammatory processes, one hopes that the damaged outflow mechanism will restore itself to normal. As long as the outflow channels are impaired, one should attempt to maintain the intraocular pressure within normal limits through antiglaucoma therapy. If medical therapy fails to control the elevated intraocular pressure, surgery may become necessary.

Pupillary dilation

Cycloplegic and sympathomimetic agents are used to break or prevent the formation of posterior synechiae and to prevent the development of a bound-down miotic pupil. They also reduce patient discomfort by decreasing spasms of the ciliary muscle and iris sphincter. Atropine 1% to 4%, homatropine 1% to 5%, and scopolamine 0.25% are effective cycloplegic agents. Phenylephrine 2.5% or 10% can be used to gain the added effect of sympathetic stimulation.

Corticosteroids

The introduction of corticosteroids revolutionized the management of intraocular inflammation. Almost all inflammatory reactions, regardless of cause, can be inhibited nonselectively by steroids. However, corticosteroids may not affect the underlying physiologic and biologic responses that caused the inflammation, and the eye often reverts to its original condition on their withdrawal.

The nonspecific antiinflammatory effect of corticosteroids on uveal inflammation has been ascribed to a decrease in capillary permeability,[15,59] to suppression of cellular exudates by interference with margination and "sticking" qualities of leukocytes,[15] and to an inhibition of the formation of granulation tissue.[58] Corticosteroids also exert a stabilizing effect on intracellular lysosomes associated with inflammatory responses.[101] This action may explain the inhibition of prostaglandin E release by antiinflammatory steroids.[18]

The antiinflammatory effect of corticosteroids on ocular structures can be obtained by topical, subconjunctival, or parenteral administration. Corticosteroids penetrate the cornea and sclera after topical administration. Penetration is increased in the inflamed eye. Experimental studies in rabbits suggest that phosphate derivatives may be less effective than acetate derivatives as topical antiinflammatory agents.[55] Most instances of anterior segment inflammation can be controlled with either topical dexamethasone 0.1% or prednisolone 1%. Tissue accumulation increases with the frequency of administration, and the drops should be instilled every 1 to 2 hours during the acute inflammatory process. When amelioration of the inflammation becomes evident, the time interval of administration may be lengthened. Frequently the inflammatory reaction can be controlled by a minimum dose of three to four drops daily.

Although corticosteroids have been shown to be effective in relieving inflammation, their administration can result in other ocular complications—particularly, increased intraocular pressure and cataract formation. These complications can occur regardless of whether the corticosteroid is administered topically or systemically. Approximately 20% to 30% of the population may show an elevation of intraocular pressure after the topical administration of corticosteroids.[4] Certain corticosteroids (such as medrysone) show less tendency to elevate intraocular pressure but may not be as effective in reducing inflammation.[82] Fluorometholone is an effective antiinflammatory agent, but it also causes significant elevations of intraocular pressure.[96] It may be difficult to determine whether an elevated intraocular pressure is caused by the original disease process or by topical corticosteroids. If the inflammation occurs only in one eye, the corticosteroid can be tested on the noninvolved eye.

If the inflammation does not respond adequately to topical steroids, either subconjunctival or systemic corticosteroid therapy may be required. Subconjunctival or sub-Tenon injection is effective in delivering high concentrations of steroids locally to the eye, resulting in a reduction of both systemic concentrations and potential systemic complications. The duration of the therapeutic effect may last for 1 to 6 weeks. Dexamethasone phosphate 4 mg (1 ml), prednisolone succinate 25 mg (1 ml), triamcinolone acetonide 4 mg (1 ml), and methylprednisolone acetate 20 mg (0.5 ml) are suitable steroid preparations. One should avoid using long-acting repository corticosteroids, since these may result in a delayed rise in intraocular pressure.[30] Systemic corticosteroids should be reserved for special situations when the other routes of administration have been ineffective. The physician should use the oral preparation with which he has the most experience. I prefer prednisone, starting at 80 to 100 mg daily. This is maintained until evidence of clinical remission occurs, at which time the daily dosage is decreased 5 mg every second or third day. The guiding principle for steroid therapy, either topical or systemic, is to use the minimum dose for the minimum time required to inhibit the inflammatory response.

The use of either systemic[71] or topical[3] corticosteroids for a prolonged period may induce posterior subcapsular cataracts. The systemic administration of corticosteroids may result in iatrogenic adrenal cortical insufficiency. Prolonged topical administration can cause considerable systemic absorption with resultant decreased plasma cortisol levels.[54] Titration of the corticosteroid is the most effective method of handling steroid complications while controlling the inflammation. However, corticosteroids themselves may induce anterior uveitis.[53] This is nongranulomatous and appears after termination of the steroid. If uveitis recurs on withdrawal of topical corticosteroids, the possibility of iatrogenic inflammation indistinguishable from that of the original ailment must be considered.

Immunosuppressive therapy

Unfortunately, corticosteroid side effects may preclude prolonged use. Also, steroid therapy may fail to control the inflammatory process and prevent progressive ocular damage. In this event, the physician may wish to consider immunosuppressive therapy. Immunologic mechanisms are involved in the pathogenesis of endogenous uveitis.[79] Immunosuppressive therapy has been employed with some success in a variety of eyes with chronic uveitis either intolerant or unresponsive to corticosteroids. Methotrexate[112] and combined low-dose prednisone with azathioprine or chlorambucil[2] result in a response rate of 60% to 70%. Careful hematologic monitoring is necessary.

Antiglaucoma therapy
Medical therapy

Treatment is directed first to either the cause of the inflammation or to the inflammation itself. Elevated intraocular pressure can be treated with topical epinephrine or timolol. Miotics are generally not recommended, since they may increase inflammation and lead to the formation of posterior synechiae. Systemic carbonic anhydrase inhibitors, with their effect of decreasing aqueous humor secretion, are very effective in treating glaucoma secondary to inflammatory disease with outflow obstruction.

Surgical therapy

Medical therapy may fail to control the secondary glaucoma, in which case surgery may become necessary. Iridectomy is the procedure of choice if pupillary block is a contributing factor. While iridectomy may not succeed in all such cases, it does not alter the prognosis if a subsequent filtering procedure becomes necessary. Iridectomy is a much safer and simpler procedure than filtration surgery, especially in inflamed eyes.

Filtration surgery is less successful in eyes with preexisting uveitis, where an increased postoperative inflammatory reaction may scar the filtering bleb. Filtration surgery is indicated when the intraocular pressure cannot be controlled medically at a level that prevents damage to the optic nerve or visual field. Standard filtration surgery (thermal sclerostomy or sclerectomy) has been reported to be more successful than filtering surgery under a scleral flap (trabeculectomy[33]), but I do not advocate it. Postoperative pupillary dilation and high-dose corticosteroids (topical and subconjunctival or systemic) are often necessary.

SPECIFIC INFLAMMATORY CONDITIONS

Anterior segment inflammation accounts for a large percentage of secondary glaucomas. Most conditions are nonspecific and have intervals of exacerbation and remission. Intraocular pressure may be acutely elevated, depending on the balance of trabecular impairment and ciliary body hyposecretion. In addition, pupillary block with obstruction of aqueous flow from the posterior to the anterior chamber may result in secondary acute angle-closure glaucoma. If the inflammatory process is chronic, it may result in damage to the trabecular meshwork and in secondary glaucoma. While most inflammatory conditions are purely ocular, some are associated with systemic disease.

Glaucoma in Fuchs' syndrome of heterochromic cyclitis

Fuchs' syndrome, a mild, chronic form of cyclitis associated with heterochromia iridis, often with cataracts and sometimes with glaucoma, was first recognized by Lawrence[57] in 1853 but was described by Fuchs[22] in 1906. The incidence is approximately 2% of all uveitis cases.[50] Fuchs' heterochromic cyclitis appears most frequently in the third and fourth decades of life. Men and women are equally affected.[19] The onset is insidious, and the clinical course is very long, mild, and chronic. Pain, irritation, photophobia, and redness of the affected eye are absent. The disease is thus usually present a long time before it is discovered. Some of the more observant patients may note the heterochromia, which develops gradually.

Signs

The fully developed syndrome presents with the following triad of signs: (1) heterochromia, (2) cyclitis, and (3) cataract.

HETEROCHROMIA. Heterochromia, which increases slowly over the years, is more noticeable when the irides are brown. Typically, the hypochromic eye is the affected eye. However, occasionally the involved eye may be darker (heterochromia inversa) because of iris stromal atrophy exposing the pigment epithelium. Stromal iris atrophy begins at the pupillary margin and spreads to the sphincter and iris periphery. This results in the characteristic moth-eaten appearance of the pupillary region and the lacunae-like holes of the iris by retroillumination. Atrophy leads to exposure of the iris radial vessels. In one third of the cases characteristic translucent grayish white nodules are present on the anterior surface of the iris, especially in the sphincter area. While most cases are unilateral, from 3.5%[20] to 13%[19] may be bilateral. It is almost always possible to recognize Fuchs' syndrome without considering the heterochromia if a careful ophthalmologic examination is made.

CYCLITIS. The one constant feature of this syndrome is very mild, chronic cyclitis. Aqueous flare and cells are always minimal. Posterior synechiae never occur except following intraocular surgery. Keratic precipitates, which are seen typically in the pupillary area and in the lower portion of the cornea, are a constant finding and are characteristically small or medium, round or star shaped, sharply circumscribed, never confluent, and white. Very fine filaments may be present between the precipitates. Of diagnostic value is the presence of anterior vitreous opacities, which appear biomicroscopically as white dots rather than as the brownish ones seen in other types of uveitis.[107]

CATARACT. This represents a frequent but late complication of Fuchs' syndrome. The cataract is a complicated type that starts in the posterior cortex beneath the capsule. It forms as a result of the long-standing cyclitis. This late development limits the value of a cataract as a diagnostic sign. Rapid progression can occur many years after the first cataract symptoms. In the hypermature stage, glaucomatous complications (phacolytic glaucoma, see Chapter 4) may be observed. Cataract surgery in patients with Fuchs' syndrome appears to be only slightly more complicated than routine surgery for senile cataracts. Elective removal of cataractous lenses in patients with this disease should not be delayed because of fear of a poor prognosis.[93]

Secondary glaucoma

The only serious late complication in Fuchs' syndrome is secondary glaucoma, with an incidence of 5% to 13% in unilateral cases and 25% to 33% in bilateral cases.[35] It usually resembles chronic open-angle glaucoma, with reduced outflow facility and normal episcleral venous pressure. The contralateral uninvolved eye may have abnormal tonometric or tonographic findings.[28]

Gonioscopic examination of the chamber angle may reveal the presence of multiple fine blood vessels, both radially and concentrically arranged, in the region of the trabecular meshwork. This may account for the apparently pathognomonic phenomenon in heterochromic cyclitis of a filiform hemorrhage in the angle following puncture of the anterior chamber. This usually occurs in the angle 180 degrees away from the site of puncture.[1]

In most instances, the glaucoma secondary to Fuchs' heterochromic cyclitis is a complication of the chronic inflammation. However, rubeosis iridis with secondary neovascular (hemorrhagic) glaucoma can occur in this disease.[60] While results following cataract removal are favorable, glaucoma may be a frequent postoperative complication.[28] It is difficult to assess the relation of glaucoma to cataract surgery, since glaucoma is frequently encountered as a late complication in the natural course of this disease.

Diagnosis

Like other syndromes, Fuchs' heterochromic cyclitis can be diagnosed when some of its characteristic manifestations are missing. Heterochromia is not a constant sign, and the disease can be identified in its absence. The character and course of the cyclitis identifies the disease (i.e., the quiet, white eye with mild iridocyclitis, minimal aqueous flare and cells, vitreous opacities, small white discrete keratic precipitates, and total absence of synechiae). Gonioscopic findings of vessels and the occurrence of an angle hemorrhage after anterior chamber puncture may be helpful in substantiating the diagnosis.

Fuchs' syndrome must be differentiated from the heterochromia secondary to uveitis of other causes in which there may be patchy iris stromal atrophy and posterior synechiae. None of the tests made in the usually exhaustive workup of a patient with uveitis are of any value in the diagnosis or management of heterochromic cyclitis. Therefore prompt recognition saves both the examiner and the patient much time and expense.

Glaucomatocyclitic crises must be considered in the differential diagnosis of Fuchs' syndrome. Three of nine patients in the original report by Posner and Schlossman[84] had definite heterochromia. Essential atrophy of the iris also must be considered in the differential diagnosis (see Chapter 6). However, other signs of eccentric pupil, ectropion of the pigment epithelium of the iris, and progressive peripheral anterior synechiae should eliminate any confusion with the secondary glaucoma in Fuchs' syndrome.

Etiology

The cause of heterochromic cyclitis is unknown. The association with status dysraphicus[78] or syringomyelia lends support to the theory of a degenerative or abiotrophic lesion. Pharmacologic studies have demonstrated a sympathetic denervation of the iris.[21,42] This sympathetic disturbance, whatever it may be, leads to changes in the blood vessels and atrophy of the iris stroma and chromatophores. Heterochromic cyclitis has been observed in families[42] and in identical twins.[66]

Pathology

Alterations of the iris are predominantly degenerative in character and include the following: decrease in the number of stromal melanocytes; degeneration of the iris pigment epithelium, especially the posterior layer; and thickening and hyalinization of the iris blood vessels with narrowing of their lumens.[25] Chronic, nongranulomatous iridocyclitis is present with active trabeculitis characterized by the presence of lymphocytes and plasma cells in the trabecular meshwork and an inflammatory membrane over the meshwork. Rubeosis of the iridocorneal angle is patchy and discontinuous.[80]

Management

Corticosteroids, whether administered topically or parenterally, are of no value in the treatment of heterochromic cyclitis. Indeed, long-term corticosteroid therapy may hasten cataract development and/or result in steroid-induced glaucoma. As stated, cataract surgery in patients with Fuchs' syndrome is only slightly more complicated than routine surgery for senile cataracts. The secondary glaucoma may be difficult to control medically. If medical therapy is ineffective in maintaining the intraocular pressure at a level that prevents optic nerve or visual field damage, then filtration surgery becomes necessary. Cases of Fuchs' syndrome with neovascular glaucoma are managed as outlined in Chapter 12.

Glaucomatocyclitic crises (Posner-Schlossman syndrome)

The syndrome of glaucomatocyclitic crises occupies a unique and important position among the many and heterogeneous types of glaucoma associated with uveitis. The syndrome was first fully described by Posner and Schlossman[84] in 1948. The condition typically occurs in individuals 20 to 50 years old and is seldom seen after the age of 60. The patient generally gives a history of recurrent attacks of unilateral blurred vision and haloes due to corneal edema. Symptoms are remarkably few and slight in relation to the height of the intraocular pressure. Some episodes may occur without symptoms. There seems to be an association of glaucomatocyclitic crises with primary open-angle glaucoma.

Signs

The features of this syndrome as described by Posner and Schlossman are listed below. However, a number of cases have been reported that deviate from this description.

Glaucomatocyclitic crises[84,85]

1. Unilateral involvement
2. Recurrent attacks of mild cyclitis
3. Findings of a slight decrease in vision, elevated intraocular pressure, open angles, and a few keratic precipitates; corneal edema, heterochromia, and a larger pupil on the affected side in some patients
4. Duration of crises from a few hours to a few weeks
5. Normal visual fields and optic discs
6. Between attacks all tests within normal limits, including intraocular pressure, outflow facility, and all provocative tests

UNILATERAL INVOLVEMENT. The process is usually unilateral with recurrent involvement of the same eye. Occasionally bilateral cases are seen, with both eyes involved at the same time or on different occasions.[44,62]

RECURRENT MILD CYCLITIS. A history of recurrent attacks of varying frequency is obtained.

Inflammatory signs are minimal, with occasional mild conjunctival injection. The signs of cyclitis do not precede glaucoma. Posterior synechiae are never found.

ATTACK. The most common presenting symptom is slight discomfort, but as a rule the patient does not complain of pain even at the height of the attack. Blurring of vision and haloes may occur if the intraocular pressure is high and corneal edema is present. The affected eye has a larger pupil during an attack. The most frequently observed initial intraocular pressures are between 40 and 60 mm Hg, and the iridocorneal angle is open. There is only a trace of aqueous flare and a slight increase in the number of aqueous cells. Clearing of the corneal edema with topical glycerin may be necessary to observe these anterior chamber findings. Keratic precipitates are generally noted within 3 days of the onset of the attack and begin to disappear soon after they are formed. They are small, discrete, well-defined, nonpigmented, flat, and round. There are seldom more than 25 precipitates, which tend to accumulate in the lower third of the cornea. Fresh precipitates may appear, however, with each exacerbation of the hypertension. Heterochromia, which was observed in three of the original nine cases studied by Posner and Schlossman,[84] is not characteristic for the syndrome. The attacks of hypertension last from a few hours to 1 month but very rarely persist for longer than 2 weeks.

AQUEOUS HUMOR DYNAMICS. Tonographic studies have shown a significant reduction in outflow facility during the attack.[23] The hypertension is also associated with a significant increase in the rate of aqueous humor formation.[95] The transfer coefficient of fluorescein in the anterior chamber by flow (volume of aqueous flowing into and out of the anterior chamber per unit time) and by diffusion (diffusional exchange between the anterior chamber and blood) are increased during attacks of glaucomatocyclitic crises.[68] During remission in these patients both coefficients return to normal.

RELATIONSHIP TO PRIMARY OPEN-ANGLE GLAUCOMA. Between attacks the affected eye has a normal intraocular pressure and outflow facility. Optic disc cupping or visual field loss does not occur during the course of the disease. However, there may be an association of glaucomatocyclitic crises with primary open-angle glaucoma. Patients with this syndrome have a higher than normal incidence of high-corticosteroid responsiveness to topical steroids similar to that of patients with primary

open-angle glaucoma.[44,86] There are a number of cases that deviate from the original clinical description. These patients show, between crises, an elevated intraocular pressure, decreased outflow facility, cupping of the optic nerve head, and visual field loss in the nonaffected as well as in the involved eye.[44,77,87] Careful follow-up of both eyes in patients with glaucomatocyclitic crises for evidence of primary open-angle glaucoma is important.

Diagnosis

The Posner-Schlossman syndrome represents a clinical entity that must be differentiated from other forms of glaucoma. Gonioscopy demonstrates an open iridocorneal angle in contrast to acute angle-closure glaucoma. In this syndrome the glaucoma is not a result or complication of the uveitis, but both manifestations are concomitant expressions of a single disease entity. Absent are signs of glaucoma secondary to uveitis, such as posterior synechiae, ciliary injection, small and irregular pupils, numerous aqueous cells and distinct aqueous flare, pigmented keratic precipitates, and peripheral anterior synechiae. Differentiation from heterochromic cyclitis is discussed earlier in the chapter.

Etiology

The mechanism responsible for the production of glaucomatocyclitic crises is obscure. A possible allergic factor has been entertained.[100] Recently prostaglandins, particularly prostaglandin E, have been found in high concentrations in aqueous humor during the attack and within normal limits during the remission.[65] In rabbit eyes prostaglandin E increases blood-aqueous humor barrier permeability and ultrafiltration in association with the elevation of intraocular pressure.[69] The increase in flow and diffusion coefficients for fluorescein in human eyes with glaucomatocyclitic crises is consistent with the observation of the response of animal eyes to prostaglandin E. The findings by angiography of iris congestion and fluorescein leakage at the pupillary border are also consistent with a prostaglandin-mediated response.[87] However, elevated prostaglandins, which in rabbits increase outflow facility, do not account for the reduced outflow facility in glaucomatocyclitic crises.

Management

A glaucomatocyclitic crisis is a self-limited glaucoma that usually subsides spontaneously regardless of treatment. Since the duration of the attack varies, it is difficult to provide well-matched control cases for drug effect studies. Topical corticosteroids may be effective in controlling the inflammatory process[100] but may elevate the intraocular pressure further. In the phase of high intraocular pressure, the use of systemic carbonic anhydrase inhibitors or topical therapy with epinephrine, timolol, or mild miotics usually reduces the intraocular pressure to normal.

Antiglaucoma therapy does not prevent recurrences and is not necessary between attacks. Prolonged treatment with corticosteroids should be avoided, since it may elicit a hypertensive ocular response in high-corticosteroid responders and complicate the condition.

Indomethacin, which inhibits the synthesis of prostaglandin E_2 from arachidonic acid, may be an effective treatment. Oral indomethacin 75 to 150 mg/day has been reported by Masuda et al.[65] to decrease intraocular pressure faster than the combination of acetazolamide and topical epinephrine and/or dexamethasone. These same authors have reported that a subconjunctival injection of polyphloretin phosphate, an inhibitor of prostaglandin E_2 effects, reduces intraocular pressure within a few hours. The effectiveness of prophylactic administration of prostaglandin synthesis inhibitors (indomethacin or aspirin) in preventing recurrent attacks is unknown. Glaucoma surgical procedures are not effective in preventing recurrences.[85]

Glaucoma associated with syphilis

Ocular involvement may result from congenital syphilis (infection of the fetus in utero) or from acquired adult disease. The association between secondary glaucoma and congenital syphilitic interstitial keratitis was first made by Hutchinson.[37] Glaucoma can occur with the early iritis or during the acute phase of interstitial keratitis and uveitis. After healing of the cornea, intraocular pressure elevation may not become a problem until years later.

Congenital syphilis

Congenital syphilis is caused by the transplacental transmission of the *Treponema pallidum* organism from the mother to the fetus. It usually occurs after the fourth gestational month and affects approximately 70% of affected infants born alive. Early congenital syphilis can present a variety of systemic signs and symptoms, including the following: maculopapular rash, mucopurulent discharge from the nose (snuffles), osteochrondritis and multiple fractures, meningitis, fever, anemia, hepatosplenomegaly with jaundice, nephritis, and pneumonitis. Ocular findings include acute and chronic iritis, interstitial keratitis, chorioretinitis ("salt and pepper retinopathy"), retinal periphlebitis, optic neuritis, and secondary cataracts. Pupillary abnormalities and optic atrophy may occur if neurosyphilis results. Acute iritis may be present at birth but more commonly begins when the infant is about 6 months of age.

The most characteristic ocular lesion of congenital syphilis is interstitial keratitis. This abnormality, together with peg teeth (Hutchinson's incisors, adult teeth) and labyrinthine deafness, form Hutchinson's triad. The keratitis, however, may be the only physical sign of the syphilitic condition.

Interstitial keratitis, which occurs in about 15% of cases, forms one of the late manifestations of congenital syphilis. It commonly appears between the sixth and twelfth years. While it may at first be unilateral, the condition becomes bilateral in at least 90% of patients. Its onset is heralded by lacrimation and photophobia. Corneal edema, infiltrates, and vascularization of the deep corneal layers are characteristic. Vessel formation may be so marked as to give the cornea a pink or "salmon patch" appearance. Anterior uveitis is almost invariable. The process may remain active from 1 week to several months. In healed lesions the vascular channels at the level of Descemet's membrane persist even though they may be devoid of circulating blood ("ghost vessels"). Local injury and nonspecific inflammation may cause a reopening of these vascular channels, leading to an apparent late relapse, which may in fact be only a nonspecific local vasomotor reaction.

Acquired syphilis

Acquired syphilis, with an incubation period of from 2 to 4 weeks, is divided into primary, secondary, and tertiary stages. The initial lesion is a chancre from which *T. pallidum* may be demonstrated on darkfield microscopic examination. During the secondary stage, 4 to 6 months after the appearance of the chancre, iridocyclitis may occur in association with the syphilitic skin rash. Meningitis with optic nerve and chiasm arachnoiditis can occur during the secondary stage, along with ocular findings of chorioretinitis followed by pigment proliferation and retrobulbar neuritis. The tertiary stage occurs 10 or more years after the chancre and is characterized by gumma formation. Central nervous system disease may develop as tabes dorsalis (degenerative involvement of the posterior columns) or general paresis (inflammatory central involvement with organic psychosis). Optic atrophy, Argyll Robertson pupils, and iridocyclitis are other ocular signs of tertiary syphilis.

Acquired syphilis may cause interstitial keratitis in approximately 3% of cases. Corneal disease can occur soon after the acquisition of the infection, but as a rule it is a late manifestation occurring, on the average, 10 years later. Interstitial keratitis in acquired syphilis resembles the congenital variety but is usually uniocular (6% of cases), frequently milder, and limited to a sector-shaped area of the cornea.

Diagnosis of syphilis

Diagnosis is based on the eye findings and other stigmata of congenital or acquired syphilis, together with positive serologic tests. Interstitial keratitis can occur as a complication of tuberculosis, leprosy, mumps, lymphogranuloma venereum, trypanosomiasis, onchocerciasis, and in association with Cogan's syndrome. The serum fluorescent treponemal antibody-absorption (FTA-ABS) test has become the definitive serologic test for syphilis, approaching 94% to 97% accuracy.[105] However, permanent false-positive FTA-ABS test results can occur in leprosy, Hashimoto's thyroiditis, and systemic lupus erythematosus. A false-positive result can also be seen in malaria, infectious mononucleosis, tuberculosis, and brucellosis; however, this result is transient, appearing only during the first 6 months of the disease.

Secondary glaucoma

ACTIVE UVEITIS. Secondary glaucoma may have multiple causes following systemic spirochetal infections. Iridocyclitis, with acutely elevated intraocular pressure, can occur in all stages and during the active phase of interstitial keratitis. In addition, anterior uveitis with secondary glaucoma can occur in late adult life in eyes that had interstitial keratitis in youth.[24] The relationship of this inflammatory type of glaucoma to the original keratitis is unknown.

LATE GLAUCOMA AFTER CONGENITAL SYPHILIS WITH INTERSTITIAL KERATITIS. The association of interstitial keratitis in young age with adult secondary glaucoma has been well documented. This glaucoma occurs in 15% to 20% of patients

years after the original inflammation has become inactive. The series by Tsukahara[104] indicates an average age of 16 years for the onset of interstitial syphilitic keratitis, with secondary glaucoma occurring an average of 27 years later. The clinical course suggests two main types of late glaucoma involvement: the predominantly deep-chamber open-angle type described by Knox[51] and the shallow-chamber angle-closure type reported by Sugar,[98] which occur with equal frequency.

OPEN-ANGLE TYPE. The onset is insidious, and the disease course resembles that of chronic simple glaucoma. Gonioscopy shows open angles. Evidence of the initial inflammatory condition may persist as old peripheral anterior synechaie and trabecular pigmentation. The open portions of the angle have a "dirty" appearance.[24] Similar gonioscopic findings are present with eyes with congenital syphilitic interstitial keratitis but without glaucoma. The degree of synechial closure may not accurately indicate the amount of outflow obstruction. One half of patients with open-angle glaucoma secondary to syphilis show involvement of both eyes. While the glaucoma damage may be progressive, there are no observations demonstrating an increase in the angle abnormalities with time.

These eyes show pathologic changes of congenital syphilis, such as interstitial keratitis and extensive atrophy of the choroid and retina. In addition to the peripheral anterior synechiae, there is extensive endothelialization and glass membrane formation in the anterior chamber overlying all angle structures and the iris.[51] These membranes cover the trabecular meshwork and extend along newly formed endothelium.[106]

In general, this type of glaucoma is reported to respond poorly to antiglaucoma medications, with control achieved in only 25% to 50% of cases.[24,104] Miotics are tolerated and used in combination with carbonic anhydrase inhibitors, epinephrine, or timolol. Filtration surgery is only successful in about 50% of cases. While surgery does not activate the old intraocular inflammation, these eyes are prone to more postoperative inflammation and external bleb scarring. Frequent topical and subconjunctival or parenteral corticosteroids are indicated.

ANGLE-CLOSURE TYPE. The angle-closure type of secondary glaucoma may have an acute onset with pain and high intraocular pressure, or it may present as chronic angle closure. The eyes characteristically have small anterior segments and shallow anterior chambers.[98] In addition to the angle closure, old inflammatory peripheral anterior synechiae and pigment residues are present in the angle. Interstitial keratitis in infancy may predispose these eyes to angle closure by resulting in abnormally small anterior segments[64] and vertically oval corneas.[31] Lichter and Shaffer[63] have described gonioscopic findings resembling cases of intraepithelial cysts of the iris and ciliary body, which may be an additional mode of angle closure in this disease.

Iridectomy is often successful in the angle-closure type of glaucoma. Approximately 60% to 70% of eyes are controlled following iridectomy and 80% to 90% of eyes with iridectomy and medical therapy.[24,104] The remaining eyes require filtration surgery. Prophylactic iridectomy is indicated in contralateral eyes with extremely narrow angles in which closure appears to be imminent.

Glaucoma in sarcoid uveitis

Sarcoidosis is a systemic noncaseating granulomatous disease of undetermined cause. Although the first description of sarcoidosis is attributed to Hutchinson,[38] its ocular features received little attention until 1936, when Herrfordt's syndrome of uveitis, salivary gland enlargement, and cranial nerve palsies was recognized as a sign of sarcoidosis.[9] Subsequently, sarcoidosis has been recognized as commonly having ocular involvement and as being a foremost cause of uveitis.

Systemic findings

Sarcoidosis is a multisystem disorder most commonly affecting young adults. The disease shows a number of immunologic changes, including depression of delayed-type hypersensitivity, hyperactive circulating antibody responses, and the Kveim skin test phenomenon.[41] The condition occurs more frequently in blacks than in whites. The most common systemic changes are diffuse fibrosis of the hili of the lungs and lymph nodes and cutaneous involvement, with soft, brown or red papules, nodules, and plaques. In addition there can be systemic involvement of the lung parenchyma (53%), liver (22%), spleen (13%), musculoskeletal system (7%), and central nervous system (9%).[70]

Ocular findings

Ocular manifestations are a prominent feature of this condition, occurring in 10% to 38% of patients with systemic sarcoidosis[40,70,92] and most commonly in blacks.

Approximately 20% of patients seek medical attention because of eye-related complaints, which are second only to pulmonary symptoms in frequency. Ocular abnormalities can be classified into three categories: (1) anterior segment disease, (2) posterior segment disease, and (3) orbital and other disease.

ANTERIOR SEGMENT DISEASE. Anterior segment structures are involved more frequently than other parts of the eye. Sarcoid anterior uveitis is a common and important ocular sign, occurring in 25% to 53% of patients.[40,70] The characteristic picture is nodular iritis that may be painless. Iris nodules are multiple small white superficial lesions in the crypts (Busacca nodules) and on the pupillary border (Koeppe nodules). Sarcoid nodules frequently involve the iris root and the iridocorneal angle.[67] In the acute stage, ocular inflammation can be unilateral. As the disease becomes chronic, bilateral involvement usually develops. Chronic granulomatous uveitis is exemplified by mutton fat keratic precipitates, iris nodules, and synechiae. Iris inflammatory changes often result in the formation of a pupillary membrane. Cataracts can be caused by chronic inflammation or treatment with corticosteroids. Conjunctival follicles or nodules and band keratopathy also occur.

POSTERIOR SEGMENT DISEASE. Involvement of the posterior segment occurs in approximately one fourth of patients with ocular sarcoidosis.[70] While retinopathy may be the sole ophthalmic expression of the ailment,[61] posterior segment disease usually accompanies anterior involvement. Predominant posterior manifestations are chorioretinitis and retinal periphlebitis. The chorioretinitis is clinically indistinguishable from that caused by other factors. Retinal periphlebitis, producing the ophthalmoscopic appearance of "candle wax drippings" in the more severe cases, is a hallmark of the disease.[26] Characteristic grayish white inferior vitreous opacities, occurring in chains like a "string of pearls," are frequently found.[56]

ORBITAL AND OTHER DISEASE. Lacrimal gland involvement in sarcoidosis is well established. Bilateral lacrimal enlargement may be the sole ophthalmic manifestation.[70] Orbital involvement is a rare cause of unilateral proptosis and problems with motility. Posterior segment sarcoidosis is accompanied by involvement of the central nervous system in 20% to 35% of cases.[26,70] This emphasizes the need for a thorough neurologic examination in patients with this form of ocular sarcoidosis. Optic nerve involvement is manifested by papilledema, papillitis, optic neuritis, and rarely by granulomas of the optic disc. When sarcoidosis affects the brain, the intracranial portion of the optic nerve may be involved by the inflammatory reaction.

Secondary glaucoma

Glaucoma is observed in approximately 11% of patients with ocular sarcoidosis at some time during the course of the disease. A higher incidence of secondary glaucoma, blindness, and subsequent enucleation occurs in blacks.[70] Mechanisms for impairment of aqueous humor outflow can include nodular infiltration of the trabeculum, peripheral anterior synechiae, or obstruction of the trabecular meshwork by particulate matter.[39] Secondary angle-closure glaucoma can result from dense posterior synechiae formation or occlusion of the pupil by a connective tissue pupillary membrane.

Diagnosis

Chest x-ray examination is the most important screening test and is abnormal in more than 90% of patients with ocular sarcoidosis.[70] A biopsy of accessible tissue, such as skin or lymph nodes, is essential for diagnosis. A conjunctival biopsy can confirm a histologic diagnosis if follicles are observed.[7] Because conjunctival biopsy is a safe and simple procedure, it has been advocated for the diagnosis of sarcoidosis even in the absence of clinically apparent conjunctival lesions. Positive conjunctival biopsy results are obtained in approximately one third of patients with histologically confirmed sarcoidosis, irrespective of the presence or absence of visible ocular lesions.[48]

Although the Kveim skin test is positive in 75% of patients with sarcoidosis, it may also be positive in other granulomatous conditions.[36] Also, although serum lysozyme is elevated in patients with sarcoidosis and active uveitis,[73,108] elevated serum lysozyme levels are not specific for sarcoidosis. They have also been correlated with disease activity in tuberculosis, uremia, Crohn's disease, megaloblastic anemia, myelomenocytic leukemia, rheumatoid arthritis, and osteoarthritis.[108]

Pathology

In sarcoidosis, one sees the typical nonnecrotic epithelioid tubercle. The tubercles are all the same size, although they may coalesce to form conglomerate masses that typically involve the iris and

ciliary body. The tubercles are surrounded by a small zone of inflammatory cells, mainly lymphocytes.

Management

Corticosteroids are usually effective in the treatment of systemic and ocular sarcoidosis. Patients with acute iritis, erythema nodosum, and hilar lymphadenopathy tend to have a benign, self-limiting course, whereas those individuals with chronic uveitis, skin plaques, pulmonary fibrosis, and bone cysts respond poorly to treatment with corticosteroids and almost invariably have a prolonged, complicated course.[40] Topical corticosteroids are effective in suppressing anterior segment inflammation, whereas periocular or systemic therapy is usually required for posterior involvement. Parenteral corticosteroids or other forms of immunosuppression are necessary for treating systemic sarcoidosis including central nervous system involvement. Steroid side effects can be frequent during therapy for this chronic condition.

Secondary glaucoma should be treated medically, with avoidance of the use of miotic therapy. Filtration surgery may become necessary in patients who are not medically controlled. Postoperative steroid therapy is necessary because of the chronically persistent inflammation of the iris and ciliary body. Iridectomy is the treatment of choice if the disease is complicated by secondary pupillary block glaucoma.

Glaucoma and anterior uveitis associated with arthritis

Anterior uveitis can be associated with various types of arthritis: ankylosing spondylitis, adult rheumatoid arthritis, and juvenile rheumatoid arthritis. The incidence of uveitis and associated complications as well as systemic manifestations differ for each of these conditions.

Ankylosing spondylitis (Marie-Strümpell disease)

Fifteen percent to 25% of patients with ankylosing spondylitis develop intermittent nongranulomatous anterior uveitis.[8] Cervical vertebrae involvement often makes it difficult for the patient to place his head at the slit lamp. However, the lumbosacral spine is involved as frequently as the cervical spine and easily escapes diagnosis. Recurrent attacks of uveitis may precede the onset of symptoms of ankylosing spondylitis, and the severity of the joint disease does not seem to be related to that of the eye disease. The HLA-B27 antigen, present in 5% of the white population, is found in 96% of patients with ankylosing spondylitis and in 58% of patients with uveitis.[8] Abnormal technetium bone scans of the sacroiliac joints have been reported in 60% of patients with the HLA-B27 antigen, acute nongranulomatous anterior uveitis, and normal lumbosacral spine x-ray films.[90] This suggests that acute anterior uveitis may represent a manifestation of spondylitic diathesis even in the complete absence of any suggestive symptomatic or radiologic joint change.

The uveitis is an acute nongranulomatous condition that responds to corticosteroid drops and pupillary dilation. Posterior synechiae, peripheral anterior synechiae, and trabecular damage can occur, leading to secondary glaucoma.

Adult rheumatoid arthritis

Adult rheumatoid arthritis, a chronic systemic disease of unknown cause, has an insidious onset in people between the ages of 25 and 50 and causes pain and swelling in one or more joints. Women are affected more commonly (75%). The disease may become chronic and involve all joints with contraction and deformity. Ocular manifestations are due to inflammatory and/or exudative alterations of connective tissue elements. About 5% of adults with rheumatoid arthritis develop iritis.[94]

Juvenile rheumatoid arthritis

The term juvenile rheumatoid arthritis covers a range of clinical syndromes. The spectrum can be divided into three major types based on the degree of articular and systemic involvement at the time of onset.[10]

ACUTE SYSTEMIC JUVENILE RHEUMATOID ARTHRITIS. This accounts for 20% of cases and occurs principally in young boys. The disease begins with a high fever, rash, anemia, lymphadenopathy, hepatosplenomegaly, and pericarditis. Most patients subsequently develop chronic polyarthritis. Still's original description[97] included this type of arthritis. Uveitis has not been reported in patients with this disease.

POLYARTICULAR-ONSET JUVENILE RHEUMATOID ARTHRITIS. This accounts for 50% of cases and occurs principally in girls. The polyarticular onset simultaneously involves five or more joints. There is a low incidence of systemic features, but the children appear ill. This variant has been called

adult-type–onset juvenile rheumatoid arthritis, but serum rheumatoid factor and subcutaneous nodules are rarely found. Uveitis occurs in a small percentage of cases.[91]

MONOARTICULAR-ONSET JUVENILE RHEUMATOID ARTHRITIS. This accounts for 30% of cases and is more common in girls than in boys (3:1 ratio). Characteristically, there is insidious swelling, pain, and stiffness in a large joint, most frequently the knee. Occasionally a small joint in the foot, hand, or elsewhere is affected. These children are apparently healthy, and their arthritis responds well to treatment. In most cases the disease remains monoarticular or pauciarticular, involving four or fewer joints. Antinuclear antibody and rheumatoid factor are absent. Systemic signs are rare. However, iridocyclitis is common, occurring in approximately 30% of cases.[91]

UVEITIS IN JUVENILE RHEUMATOID ARTHRITIS. In most children the iridocyclitis is a mild, insidious, chronic anterior segment inflammation that produces few symptoms. However, up to 45% of patients may have symptoms of severe pain, redness, and photophobia.[11,13] The iritis is nongranulomatous, with fine- or medium-keratic precipitates, cells, and flare, and in a few cases cells in the anterior vitreous. Posterior synechiae and pigment deposition on the anterior lens capsule are frequent. Arthritis precedes the uveitis in approximately 90% of cases, with the iridocyclitis developing 2 months to 12 years later. There is no parallel between the activity of the iridocyclitis and the joint disease. Whereas the arthritis tends to disappear in adult life, the iridocyclitis persists.[47] There can be extended periods of quiescence; however, these rarely last longer than 4 years. Eventually most patients have persistent aqueous flare, which probably indicates altered vascular permeability.

Chronic iridocyclitis can result in complications of band keratopathy (4% to 49%), posterior synechiae (38% to 61%), and rarely macular edema and papillitis.[13,43,47] Complicated cataracts are common, occurring in up to 50% of children. These cataracts can be related to chronic inflammation or to chronic corticosteroid therapy.

Secondary glaucoma

Glaucoma is a relatively common complication. The occurrence increases with the duration of the disease, approaching an incidence of 20%. Glaucoma may be secondary to posterior synechiae and iris bombé resulting in angle closure, to peripheral anterior synechiae, or to trabecular obstruction by particulate matter.

Management

ARTHRITIS. Systemic long-term corticosteroids are frequently necessary for treatment of the systemic manifestations. This therapy can be a causative factor in the development of posterior subcapsular cataracts. Both the dose and duration of systemic steroid therapy are important in the development of these cataracts. A high frequency of posterior subcapsular cataracts are observed in patients receiving more than 20 mg/day of prednisone (0.5 mg/kg/day). Cataracts do not occur in patients receiving corticosteroid therapy for less than 6 months. These cataracts may be reversible on withdrawal of the steroid.[72] This highlights the necessity of a team approach to meet the medical, orthopedic, and ophthalmologic needs of these patients.

UVEITIS. Approximately 50% of patients respond to topical corticosteroids and pupillary dilation. It is important to keep the pupil mobile to prevent the formation of posterior synechiae. In many eyes topical corticosteroids have no effect on anterior chamber cells and flare. Only about one third of the cases respond to treatment with systemic corticosteroids.[43] The results of immunosuppressive therapy (chlorambucil, cyclophosphamide, or azathioprine) have been disappointing.

CATARACTS. Surgical treatment of cataracts usually is discouraging.[13] However, more favorable results have been reported by Key and Kimura[47] with the use of periocular and often systemic corticosteroids both preoperatively and postoperatively to quell the surgical inflammatory response. These authors reported improved vision in 12 of 20 eyes subjected to extracapsular procedures.

GLAUCOMA. The possibility of a steroid-induced glaucoma should be kept in mind. Medical therapy avoids the use of miotics. Iridectomy is indicated if a pupillary block mechanism exists. There is no best method to achieve external filtration if it becomes necessary. A modified goniotomy technique has been described by Hass.[29] The incision is made at Schwalbe's line, and the knife is turned on edge to peel trabecular bands. This technique is reported to have been successful in 7 of 15 eyes for up to 2 years. However, these results are similar to goniotomy, thermosclerostomy, or trabeculectomy in this condition.[47]

Viral uveitis and secondary glaucoma

Various types of viral infections can cause uveitis and secondary glaucoma. The elevated intraocular pressure is related to the intraocular inflammation and can be secondary to pupillary block or to outflow damage as a result of peripheral anterior synechiae, trabecular inflammatory damage, or trabecular obstruction by inflammatory debris.

Herpesvirus

This group of viruses contains three members pathogenic for humans: (1) herpesvirus hominis, the virus of herpes simplex; (2) herpesvirus varicellae, which causes chickenpox and herpes zoster; and (3) herpesvirus simiae (b), which causes a subclinical infection in monkeys but a fatal central nervous system disease when transmitted to humans.

HERPES SIMPLEX. This endemic virus infection occurs in nonimmune individuals and usually results in a subclinical and self-limited disease. Type 1 virus causes herpetic infections of the eye, whereas type 2 virus is associated with genital infections. Up to 90% of adults have circulating antibodies to the type 1 virus and carry the virus in an inactive state. Secondary or recurrent ocular herpes simplex develops in patients with neutralizing antibodies and can result in conjunctivitis, keratitis (superficial or deep), uveitis (with or without keratitis), or trophic (postherpetic) keratitis.

Herpes simplex keratouveitis may be associated with an increased intraocular pressure. In a study by Falcon and Williams,[17] the associated herpetic ocular signs in 50 patients with secondary glaucoma included the following: disciform keratouveitis (44%), stromal keratouveitis (36%), disciform keratitis (10%), stromal keratitis (4%), scleral keratitis (2%), and metaherpetic ulcer (4%). These cases represented 28% of patients with herpes keratouveitis seen by Falcon and Williams. In this series, active corneal ulcers were not present at the time of raised intraocular pressure. Herpetic ocular hypertension is characterized by intermittent attacks with a mean duration of 8 weeks (range 1 to 124 weeks) of raised intraocular pressure. The frequency of ocular hypertensive attacks is greater in patients with irregular stromal keratitis than in patients with disciform keratitis.

Herpesvirus has been described as the causal agent in anterior uveitis.[49] Viral particles have been identified in the human iris,[109] and fluorescent antibody techniques provide a clinical method for establishing the diagnosis.[46,75] Elevated intraocular pressure is related to trabecular blockade or trabeculitis.[17,32,103] Angle closure is not implicated.[17]

The management of herpes simplex keratouveitis and glaucoma is directed initially toward halting or preventing activation of the viral disease. Two different antiviral drugs are currently available for treatment of herpetic keratitis: idoxuridine (IDU) and vidarabine (Ara-A). Neither of these drugs achieves therapeutic levels in the deep corneal stroma, anterior chamber, or iris. Preliminary research studies with trifluorothymidine demonstrate penetration through the cornea into the anterior chamber following topical application of 1% drops.[76,99] This may become the antiviral agent of choice for herpetic keratouveitis. Corticosteroids are effective in suppressing the associated intraocular inflammation. However, steroids can reactivate epithelial herpes simplex. Antiviral coverage with either IDU or Ara-A is given concurrently with topical corticosteroids to reduce reactivating epithelial herpes.[74] Supplementary hypotensive treatment with systemic carbonic anhydrase inhibitors and topical epinephrine or timolol may be required. While elevated intraocular pressure occurs before corticosteroid therapy, the possibility of corticosteroid-induced increases should be kept in mind.[102] The intraocular pressure usually returns to normal as the inflammation subsides. Approximately 12% of patients will develop a persistent secondary glaucoma requiring continued therapy after the uveitis has cleared. Filtration surgery may occasionally be required.[17]

HERPES ZOSTER. Herpes zoster ophthalmicus results from reinvasion or reactivation of the virus in the gasserian ganglion and the first (ophthalmic) branch of the trigeminal nerve. A vesicular rash on an erythematous base occurs along this division of the fifth nerve but does not cross the midline. Lancinating pain precedes the rash by 24 to 48 hours. The skin over the tip of the nose is supplied by the nasociliary branch of the fifth nerve, and lesions in this area frequently are followed by keratitis and uveitis. The iridocyclitis is associated with mutton fat keratic precipitates, posterior synechiae, and sector iris atrophy. Hypopyon may be present. Corneal sensation is lost and is never fully recovered.

Secondary glaucoma is stated to occur commonly in association with keratitis and uveitis from herpes zoster but perhaps not so frequently as herpes simplex.[12] Glaucoma is due to the intra-ocular inflammation and its consequences as previously described. The true incidence of glaucoma in herpes zoster ophthalmicus is not as well defined as in herpes simplex keratouveitis. However, as many as 25% of affected eyes may be found to have intraocular pressure elevation.[52]

Steroids are effective for the uveitic manifestation of herpes zoster. Topical steroids usually control the acute as well as the chronic form of uveitis. Occasionally subconjunctival or systemic corticosteroids are necessary. When maintaining patients with this disease on a regimen of long-term steroids, one must consider the possibility of steroid-induced glaucoma.

Rubella

The importance to the developing fetus of prenatal infection with rubella virus was first recognized by Gregg[27] in 1941. A large variety of congenital defects can occur in infants whose mothers contract the disease during the first trimester of pregnancy. The incidence of embryopathy varies and is more severe the earlier in pregnancy the disease occurs. Associated ocular disorders in decreasing rank of incidence include retinopathy, strabismus, cataracts, nystagmus, microphthalmus and microcornea, optic atrophy, corneal haze and leukomas, glaucoma, lid defects, and iris atrophy.[110] Besides ocular manifestations, other defects include congenital heart disease, deafness, mental retardation, and microcephaly.

The reported incidence of glaucoma in congenital rubella varies. Glaucoma seems to be associated with more advanced cases of the disease. A summary of retrospective studies up to 1969 reveals that of 730 reported cases of congenital rubella, 22 had glaucoma and 230 had cataracts.[110] Rubella keratitis, which results in corneal clouding, can present a problem in differential diagnosis with corneal edema of congenital glaucoma. Corneal haze, which is usually permanent, is deep, is diffuse or disciform, and resists attempts at clearing by removal of the epithelium. It can cause difficulty in measuring intraocular pressure. The MacKay-Marg tonometer may be the most accurate method.

Glaucoma can be transient or permanent. An inflammatory reaction is probably responsible for the transient condition. The iritis is nongranulomatous with diffuse and focal infiltration of the anterior uvea by lymphocytes, plasma cells, and histocytes.[113] The iritis may become chronic.[111]

This type of glaucoma is best managed medically with the combined use of corticosteroids and anti-glaucoma therapy. The permanent type of glaucoma is related to the developmental defects of the iridocorneal angle that occur in some rubella patients. Gonioscopically and pathologically the anterior chamber angle appears not unlike that of typical congenital glaucoma (see Chapter 5).

Mumps

Mumps is an acute contagious systemic disease characterized by painful enlargement of the salivary glands (most commonly the parotid gland) and, after puberty, by orchitis. Lymphocytic meningitis, pancreatitis, and involvement of other organs occur rarely. Ocular manifestations of mumps include dacryoadenitis, optic neuritis, keratitis, conjunctivitis, scleritis, and iritis.[89] Secondary glaucoma can occur in conjunction with the iritis.[88] There is one case reported of transient bilateral glaucoma occurring in a man during convalescence from mumps in which there were no signs of scleritis or iritis.[83] In this patient with open angles and reduced outflow facility, the glaucoma is reported to have responded to treatment with acetazolamide and topical corticosteroids.

REFERENCES

1. Amsler, M., and Verrey, F.: Hétérochromie de Fuchs et fragilité vasculaire, Ophthalmologica **111:**117, 1946.
2. Andrasch, R.H., Pirofsky, B., and Burns, R.P.: Immunosuppressive therapy for severe chronic uveitis, Arch. Ophthalmol. **96:**247, 1978.
3. Becker, B.: Cataracts and topical corticosteroids, Am. J. Ophthalmol. **58:**872, 1964.
4. Becker, B.: Intraocular pressure response to topical corticosteroids, Invest. Ophthalmol. **4:**198, 1965.
5. Beitch, B.R., and Eakins, K.E.: The effects of prostaglandins on the intraocular pressure of the rabbit, Br. J. Pharmacol. **37:**158, 1969.
6. Bito, L.Z.: The effects of experimental uveitis on anterior uveal prostaglandin transport and aqueous humor composition, Invest. Ophthalmol. **13:**959, 1974.
7. Bornstein, J.S., Frank, M.I., and Radner, D.B.: Conjunctival biopsy in the diagnosis of sarcoidosis, N. Engl. J. Med. **267:**60, 1962.
8. Brewerton, D.A., Caffrey, M., Hant, F.D., et al.: Ankylosing spondylitis and HL-A27, Lancet **1:**904, 1973.
9. Bruins Slot, W.J.: Ziekle van Besnier-Boeck en Febris uveoparotidea (Herrfordt), Ned Tijdschr. Geneeskd. **80:**2859, 1936.
10. Calabro, J.J., and Mareschano, J.M.: The early natural history of juvenile rheumatoid arthritis, Med. Clin. North Am. **52:**567, 1968.
11. Calabro, J.J., Parrino, G.R., Atchoo, P.D., et al.: Chronic iridocyclitis in juvenile rheumatoid arthritis, Arthritis Rheum. **13:**406, 1970,
12. Chandler, P.A., and Grant, W.M.: Glaucoma, Philadelphia, 1965, Lea & Febiger, p. 249.
13. Chylack, L.T., Bierfang, D.C., Bellows, H.R., and Stillman, J.S.: Ocular manifestations of juvenile rheumatoid arthritis, Am. J. Ophthalmol. **79:**1026, 1975.
14. Eakins, K.E., Whitelocke, R.A.F., Bennett, A., and Martenet, A.C.: Prostaglandin-like activity in ocular inflammation, Br. Med. J. **3:**452, 1972.
15. Ebert, R.H., and Barclay, W.R.: Changes in connective tissue reaction induced by cortisone, Ann. Intern. Med. **37:**506, 1952.
16. Epstein, D.L., Hashimoto, J.M., and Grant, W.M.: Serum obstruction of aqueous outflow in enucleated eyes, Am. J. Ophthalmol. **86:**101, 1978.
17. Falcon, M.G., and Williams, H.P.: Herpes simplex kerato-uveitis and glaucoma, Trans. Ophthalmol. Soc. U.K. **98:**101, 1978.
18. Floman, Y., Floman, N., and Zor, U.: Inhibition of prostaglandin E release by anti-inflammatory steroids, Prostaglandins **11:**591, 1976.
19. Franceschetti, A.: Heterochromic cyclitis: Fuchs' syndrome, Am. J. Ophthalmol. **39:**50, 1955.
20. Francois, J.: L'hétérochromie iriene de Fuchs, Ann. Ocul. **179:**559, 1946.
21. Francois, J.: Contribution à l'étude de l'hétérochromie de Fuchs et de ses troubles pupillaires (pathogénie sympathique), Ann. Ocul. **182:**585, 1949.
22. Fuchs, E.: Uber Komplikationen der Heterochromie, Z. Augenheilkd. **15:**191, 1906.
23. Grant, W.M.: Clinical measurements of aqueous outflow, Arch. Ophthalmol. **46:**113, 1951.
24. Grant, W.M.: Late glaucoma after interstitial keratitis, Am. J. Ophthalmol. **79:**87, 1975.
25. Goldberg, M.F., Erozan, Y.S., Duke, J.R., and Frost, J.K.: Cytopathologic and histopathologic aspects of Fuchs' heterochromic iridocyclitis, Arch. Ophthalmol. **74:**604, 1965.
26. Gould, H., and Kaufman, H.E.: Sarcoid of the fundus, Arch. Ophthalmol. **65:**453, 1961.
27. Gregg, N.McA.: Congenital cataract following German measles in the mother, Trans. Ophthalmol. Soc. Aust. **3:**35, 1941.
28. Hart, C.T., and Ward, D.M.: Intra-ocular pressure in Fuchs' heterochromic uveitis, Br. J. Ophthalmol. **52:**739, 1967.
29. Hass, J.S.: Surgical treatment of open-angle glaucoma. In Symposium on glaucoma: transactions of the New Orleans Academy of Ophthalmology, St. Louis, 1967, The C.V. Mosby Co.
30. Herschler, J.: Intractable intraocular hypertension induced by repository triamcinolone acetonide, Am. J. Ophthalmol. **74:**501, 1972.
31. Hoehne, H.: Ueber Keratitis parenchymatosa, Klin. Monatsbl. Augenheilkd. **105:**656, 1940.
32. Hogan, M.J., Kimura, S.J., and Thygeson, P.: Pathology of herpes simplex keratitis, Trans. Am. Ophthalmol. Soc. **61:**75, 1963.
33. Hoskins, H.D.: Secondary glaucomas. In Heilmann, K., and Richardson, K.T., editors: Glaucoma: concepts of a disease, Stuttgart, Germany, 1978, Georg Thieme, p. 377.

34. Howes, E.L., Jr., and Cruse, V.K.: The structural basis of altered vascular permeability following intraocular inflammation, Arch. Ophthalmol. **96:**1668, 1978.

35. Huber, A.: Glaucoma as a complication in heterochromia of Fuchs, Ophthalmologica **142:**66, 1961.

36. Hurley, T.H., Sullivan, J.R., and Hurley, J.V.: Reaction of Kveim test material in sarcoidosis and other diseases, Lancet **1:**494, 1975.

37. Hutchinson, J.: Diseases of the eye and ear consequent on inherited syphilis, London, 1863, Churchill, p. 170.

38. Hutchinson, J.: Anomalous disease of skin of fingers, etc. (papillary psoriasis?). In Illustrations of clinical surgery, vol. 1, London, 1878, Churchill, p. 42.

39. Iwata, K., Nanba, K., Sobue, K., and Abe, H.: Ocular sarcoidosis: evaluation of intraocular findings, Ann. N.Y. Acad. Sci. **278:**445, 1976.

40. James, D.G., Anderson, R., Langley, D., and Ainslie, D.: Ocular sarcoidosis, Br. J. Ophthalmol. **48:**461, 1964.

41. James, D.G., Neville, E., and Walker, A.: Immunology of sarcoidosis, Am. J. Med. **59:**388, 1975.

42. Jammes, J.L., and Nigam, M.P.: Pupillary autonomic functions in heterochromia iridis, Arch. Ophthalmol. **89:**291, 1973.

43. Kanski, J.J.: Anterior uveitis in juvenile rheumatoid arthritis, Arch. Ophthalmol. **95:**1794, 1977.

44. Kass, M.A., Becker, B., and Kolker, A.E.: Glaucomatocyclitic crisis and primary open-angle glaucoma, Am. J. Ophthalmol. **75:**668, 1973.

45. Kass, M.A., Podos, S.M., Moses, R.A., and Becker, B.: Prostaglandin E$_1$ and aqueous humor dynamics, Invest. Ophthalmol. **11:**1022, 1972.

46. Kaufman, H.E., Kanai, A., and Ellison, E.D.: Herpetic iritis: demonstration of virus in the anterior chamber by fluorescent antibody techniques and electron microscopy, Am. J. Ophthalmol. **71:**465, 1971.

47. Key, S.N. III, and Kimura, S.J.: Iridocyclitis associated with juvenile rheumatoid arthritis, Am. J. Ophthalmol. **80:**425, 1975.

48. Khan, F., Wessely, Z., Chazin, S.R., and Seriff, N.S.: Conjunctival biopsy in sarcoidosis: a simple, safe and specific diagnostic procedure, Ann. Ophthalmol. **9:**671, 1977.

49. Kimura, S.J.: Herpes simplex uveitis: a clinical and experimental study, Trans. Am. Ophthalmol. Soc. **60:**440, 1962.

50. Kimura, S.J., Hogan, M.J., and Thygeson, P.: Fuchs' syndrome of heterochromic cyclitis, AMA Arch. Ophthalmol. **54:**179, 1955.

51. Knox, D.L.: Glaucoma following syphilitic interstitial keratitis, Arch. Ophthalmol. **66:**44, 1961.

52. Kolker, A.E., and Hetherington, J., Jr.: Becker-Shaffer's diagnosis and therapy of the glaucomas, ed 4, St. Louis, 1976, The C.V. Mosby Co., p. 241.

53. Krupin, T., LeBlanc, R.P., Becker, B., et al.: Uveitis in association with topically administered corticosteroid, Am. J. Ophthalmol. **70:**883, 1970.

54. Krupin, T., Mandell, A.I., Podos, S.M., and Becker, B.: Topical corticosteroid therapy and pituitary-adrenal function, Arch. Ophthalmol. **94:**919, 1976.

55. Kupferman, A., and Leibowitz, H.M.: Anti-inflammatory effectiveness of topically administered corticosteroids in the cornea without epithelium, Invest. Ophthalmol. **14:**252, 1975.

56. Landers, P.H.: Vitreous lesion observed in Boeck's sarcoid, Am. J. Ophthalmol. **32:**1740, 1949.

57. Lawrence, W.: Treatise on diseases of the eye, ed. 3, Philadelphia, 1853, Isaac Hays.

58. Leopold, I.H.: Treatment of eye disorders with antiinflammatory steroids, Ann. N.Y. Acad. Sci. **82:**939, 1959.

59. Leopold, I.H., Purnell, J.E., Cannon, E.J., et al.: Local and systemic cortisone in ocular disease, Am. J. Ophthalmol. **34:**361, 1951.

60. Lerman, S., and Levy, C.: Heterochromic iritis and secondary neovascular glaucoma, Am. J. Ophthalmol. **57:**479, 1964.

61. Letocha, C.E., Shields, J.A., and Goldberg, R.E.: Retinal changes in sarcoidosis, Can. J. Ophthalmol. **10:**184, 1975.

62. Levatin, P.: Glaucomatocyclitic crises occurring in both eyes, Am. J. Ophthalmol. **41:**1056, 1956.

63. Lichter, P.R., and Shaffer, R.N.: Interstitial keratitis and glaucoma, Am. J. Ophthalmol. **68:**241, 1969.

64. Luyckx-Bacus, J., and Delmarcelle, Y.: Recherches biometriques sur des yeux présentant une microcornée ou une megalocornée, Bull. Soc. Belge Ophthalmol. **149:**433, 1968.

65. Masuda, K., Izawa, Y., and Mishima, S.: Prostaglandins and glaucomato-cyclitic crisis, Jpn. J. Ophthalmol. **19:**368, 1975.

66. Makley, T.A., Jr.: Heterochromic cyclitis in identical twins, Am. J. Ophthalmol. **41:**768, 1956.

67. Mizuno, K., and Watanabe, T.: Sarcoid granulomatous cyclitis, Am. J. Ophthalmol. **81:**82, 1974.

68. Nagataki, S., and Mishima, J.: Aqueous humor dynamics in glaucomato-cyclitic crisis, Invest. Ophthalmol. **15:**365, 1976.

69. Neufeld, A.H., and Sears, M.L.: Prostaglandin and eye, Prostaglandins **4:**157, 1973.

70. Obenauf, C.D., Shaw, H.E., Sydnor, C.F., and Klintworth, G.K.: Sarcoidosis and its ophthalmic manifestations, Am. J. Ophthalmol. **86:**648, 1978.

71. Oglesby, R.B., Black, R.L., von Sallmann, L., and Bunim, J.L.: Cataracts in patients with rheumatic diseases treated with corticosteroids, Arch. Ophthalmol. **66:**625, 1961.

72. Ohguchi, M., Ohno, S., Shiono, H., et al.: Posterior subcapsular cataracts in children on long-term corticosteroid therapy, Jpn. J. Ophthalmol. **19:**254, 1975.

73. Pascual, R.S., Gee, B.L., and Finch, S.C.: Serum lysozyme analysis and diagnosis and evaluation of sarcoidosis, N. Engl. J. Med. **289:**1074, 1973.

74. Patterson, A.: Management of ocular herpes simplex, Br. J. Ophthalmol. **51:**494, 1967.

75. Patterson, A., Sommerville, R.G., and Jones, B.R.: Symposium of kerato-uveitis, Trans. Ophthalmol. Soc. U.K. **88:**243, 1968.

76. Pavan-Langston, D., and Nelson, D.J.: Intraocular penetration of trifluridine, Am. J. Ophthalmol. **87:**814, 1979.

77. Perdviel, G., Raynaud, G., and Gayard, M.: Syndrome de Posner-Schlossman et glaucome, Bull. Soc. Ophthalmol. Fr. **62:**611, 1962.

78. Perkins, E.S.: Heterochromic uveitis, Trans. Ophthalmol. Soc. U.K. **81:**53, 1962.

79. Perkins, E.S.: Recent advances in the study of uveitis, Br. J. Ophthalmol. **58:**432, 1974.

80. Perry, H.D., Yanoff, M., and Scheie, H.B.: Rubeosis in Fuch's heterochromic iridocyclitis, Arch. Ophthalmol. **93:**337, 1975.

81. Podos, S.M., Becker, B., and Kass, M.A.: Prostaglandin synthesis, inhibition, and intraocular pressure, Invest. Ophthalmol. **12:**426, 1973.

82. Podos, S.M., Krupin, T., Asseff, C., and Becker, B.: Topically administered corticosteroid preparations: comparison of intraocular pressure effects, Arch. Ophthalmol. **86:**251, 1971.

83. Polland, W., and Thorburn, W.: Transient glaucoma as a manifestation of mumps: a case report, Acta Ophthalmol. **54:**779, 1976.

84. Posner, A., and Schlossman, A.: Syndrome of unilateral recurrent attacks of glaucoma with cyclitic symptoms, Arch. Ophthalmol. **39:**517, 1948.

85. Posner, A., and Schlossman, A.: Further observations on the syndrome of glaucomatocyclitic crises, Trans. Am. Acad. Ophthalmol. Otolaryngol. **57:**531, 1953.

86. Raitta, C., and Klemetti, A.: Steroidbelastung bei Posner-Schlossmanschem Syndrom, Albrecht Von Graefes Arch. Klin. Exp. Ophthalmol. **174:**66, 1967.

87. Raitta, C., and Vannas, A.: Glaucomatocyclitic crisis, Arch. Ophthalmol. **95:**608, 1977.

88. Riffenburgh, R.S.: Iritis and glaucoma associated with mumps, Arch. Ophthalmol. **51:**702, 1954.

89. Riffenburgh, R.S.: Ocular manifestations of mumps, Arch. Ophthalmol. **66:**739, 1961.

90. Russell, A.S., Lentle, B.C., Percy, J.C., and Jackson, F.I.: Scintigraphy of sacroiliac joints in acute anterior uveitis, Ann. Intern. Med. **85:**606, 1976.

91. Schaller, J., Kupfer, C., and Wedgewood, R.J.: Iridocyclitis in juvenile rheumatoid arthritis, Pediatrics **44:**92, 1969.

92. Siltzbach, L.E., James, D.G., Neville, E., et al.: Course and prognosis of sarcoidosis around the world, Am. J. Med. **57:**847, 1974.

93. Smith, R.E., and O'Connor, R.: Cataract extraction in Fuchs' syndrome, Arch. Ophthalmol. **91:**39, 1974.

94. Sorsby, A., and Gormaz, A.: Iritis in rheumatic affections, Br. Med. J. **1:**597, 1946.

95. Spivey, B.E., and Armaly, M.F.: Tonographic findings in glaucomatocyclitic crises, Am. J. Ophthalmol. **55:**47, 1963.

96. Stewart, R.H., and Kimbrough, R.L.: Intraocular pressure response to topically administered fluorometholone, Arch. Ophthalmol. **97:**2137, 1979.

97. Still, G.F.: On a form of chronic disease in children, Med. Chir. Trans. **80:**47, 1897.

98. Sugar, H.S.: Late glaucoma associated with inactive syphilitic interstitial keratitis, Am. J. Ophthalmol. **53:**602, 1962.

99. Sugar, J., Varnell, E., Centafanto, Y., and Kaufman, H.E.: Trifluorothymidine treatment of herpetic iritis in rabbits in intraocular penetration, Invest. Ophthalmol. **12:**532, 1973.

100. Theodore, F.H.: Observations of glaucomatocyclitic crises: Posner-Schlossman syndrome, Br. J. Ophthalmol. **36:**207, 1952.

101. Thomas, L.: The role of lysosomes in tissue injury. In Zeifach, B.W., Grant, L., and McCluskey, R.T., editors: The inflammatory process, New York, 1965, Academic Press, Inc., p. 449.

102. Thygeson, P.: Chronic herpetic kerato-uveitis, Trans. Am. Ophthalmol. Soc. **65:**211, 1967.

103. Townsend, W.M., and Kaufman, H.E.: Pathogenesis of glaucoma and endothelial changes in herpetic kerato-uveitis in rabbits, Am. J. Ophthalmol. **71:**904, 1971.

104. Tsukahara, S.: Secondary glaucoma due to inactive congenital syphilitic interstitial keratitis, Ophthalmologica **174:**188, 1977.

105. Tuffanelli, D.L., Wuepper, K.D., Bradford, L.L., and Wood, R.M.: Fluorescent treponemal-antibody absorption tests: studies of false-positive reactions to tests for syphilis, N. Engl. J. Med. **276:**258, 1967.

106. VanHorn, D.I., and Schultz, R.E.: Electronmicroscopy of syphilitic interstitial keratitis, Invest. Ophthalmol. **10:**469, 1971.

107. Vogt, A.: Lehrbuch und Atlas der Spaltlampenmikroskopie des levenden Auges, vol. 1, Berlin, 1930, Springer-Verlag, p. 1000.

108. Weinberg, R.S., and Tessler, H.H.: Serum lysozyme in sarcoid uveitis, Am. J. Ophthalmol. **82:**105, 1976.

109. Witmer, R., and Iwamoto, J.: Electron microscope observation of herpes-like particles in the iris, Arch. Ophthalmol. **79:**331, 1968.

110. Wolff, S.M.: The ocular manifestations of congenital rubella, Trans. Am. Ophthalmol. Soc. **70:**577, 1972.

111. Wolter, J.R., Insel, P.A., Willey, E.N., and Brittain, H.P.: Eye pathology following maternal rubella: a study of four children, J. Pediatr. Ophthalmol. **3**(2):29, 1966.

112. Wong, V.G., and Hersch, E.M.: Methotrexate in the therapy of cyclitis, Trans. Am. Acad. Ophthalmol. Otolaryngol. **69:**279, 1965.

113. Zimmerman, L.E., and Font, R.L.: Congenital malformations of the eye: some recent advances in the knowledge of the pathogenesis and histopathological characteristics, J.A.M.A. **196:**684, 1966.

Chapter 20

TRAUMA AND ELEVATED INTRAOCULAR PRESSURE

Jonathan Herschler and Michael Cobo

Trauma to the globe, both directly to the eye and indirectly to the orbit or head, is a frequent occurrence in everyday life. In blunt trauma, the severity of the injury to the ocular structures depends on several factors, including the size, weight, speed, and sharpness of the injuring object and its direction and point of impact. In addition, ocular injury may occur secondary to other forms of trauma such as chemical burns, therapeutic irradiation, and electrical injury. In this chapter situations in which trauma to the eye results in elevated intraocular pressure are considered. Knowledge of the mechanism of increased intraocular pressure is essential for proper choice of effective treatment.

BLUNT TRAUMA

Blunt trauma can be associated with anterior segment injuries, including hyphema, iris sphincter tear, iridodialysis, cyclodialysis, trabecular tear, inflammation, and zonular rupture with lens subluxation. A posttraumatic elevation in intraocular pressure may occur in association with these findings.

Hyphema

The most common presenting symptom after blunt trauma is reduction of visual acuity, and this in turn is usually due to a hyphema. If the intraocular pressure is measured shortly after injury accompanied by a hyphema, it may be elevated in comparison with the fellow eye; however, soon thereafter the intraocular pressure falls to a mildly subnormal level for approximately 5 days.[23] If a

pattern of intraocular pressure other than that described is seen, more than just a simple hyphema should be suspected. For example, if hypotony is severe or persistent, cyclodialysis, uveitis, or a missed global rupture should be strongly suspected.

The source of most bleeding is a tear into the face of the ciliary body between the longitudinal and circular fibers (Fig. 20-1). Small branches of the major arterial circle are torn and then bleed into the anterior chamber.[23] As the intraocular pressure rises in the globe, bleeding diminishes and a clot forms. Two to 4 days after the injury, clot lysis and retraction occur, and the maximal incidence of rebleeding of the injured vessels occurs at this time.[42] The rebleed is often more severe than the initial episode and can lead to the feared problem of total hyphema, also known as a ''blackball'' or ''eight-ball'' hyphema. Unlike the typical initial bleeding episode, total hyphema is usually associated with extreme pain, nausea, and other symptoms related to acute glaucoma.

The mechanism for the increase in intraocular pressure is mechanical obstruction of the trabecular meshwork by red blood cells and blood products (Fig. 20-2) and sometimes pupillary block from a clot.[17] Ghost cell glaucoma and hemolytic glaucoma are discussed in Chapter 21. The typical black appearance of the anterior chamber fluid is probably due to deoxygenated hemoglobin. Although many treatments have been suggested to lessen the incidence of rebleeding, none have yet been proved to alter the outcome significantly. At

307

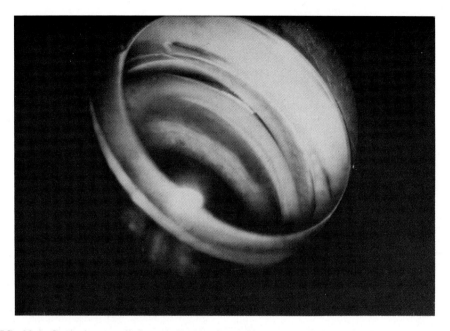

FIG. 20-1. Goniophotograph through Koeppe lens of human eye 2 days after blunt anterior segment trauma with mild hyphema. Large tear into face of ciliary body can be seen with raw, exposed longitudinal fibers remaining attached to scleral spur.

present, hospitalization with limitation of activity and a protective shield applied to the injured eye would appear prudent.[17] Preliminary reports suggest the use of ε-aminocaproic acid (a fibrinolysin inhibitor) to reduce the level of rebleeding.[10] The use of this agent is based on the belief that blocking lysis of the clot will reduce rebleeding; although this idea appears reasonable, similar logical arguments for the use of other agents in the past have not been substantiated by prolonged clinical trials.

Conservative treatment of elevated intraocular pressure with drugs that reduce aqueous formation and hyperosmotic agents frequently results in enough pressure lowering to allow for gradual resorption of the hyphema. Improvement is signaled by the appearance of a mixture of brighter blood and aqueous near the upper limbus. If no further rebleeding occurs, total resorption of the residual blood occurs within 7 to 10 days.[37]

The occurrence of a hyphema in a patient with the sickle cell disease or trait may be a special situation. Because of sludging and sickling, sickled red blood cells have been shown to have more difficulty in traversing the trabecular meshwork than do normal red blood cells.[29] In addition, the risk of vascular occlusion of the central retinal artery is greatly increased in patients with sickling.[18]

The optimal time and method of surgical intervention for medically unresponsive cases of total hyphema from blunt trauma is an often-debated subject, indicating no single best approach. Early intervention is to be avoided, since it is often accompanied by rebleeding; also, if intervention is delayed 3 to 5 days, a significant number of cases will resolve spontaneously. Severe, unremitting pain and early blood staining of the cornea are factors that, if present, argue for surgical intervention.

Experimental work by Sears[42] on clot retraction suggested optimum removal at 4 days. At this point the clot is freest of adherence to adjacent structures. However, it is clear that efforts at total removal of the clot are unnecessary for resolution of the glaucoma and expose the patient to an increased risk of rehemorrhage and loss of uveal tissue that may adhere to the clot.

Suggested surgical approaches include paracentesis,[31] irrigation with balanced salt solution or fibrinolytic agents,[35,36,40] or aspiration with an emulsification or vitrectomy type of instrument.[22,28] One of us (J.H.) favors draining the

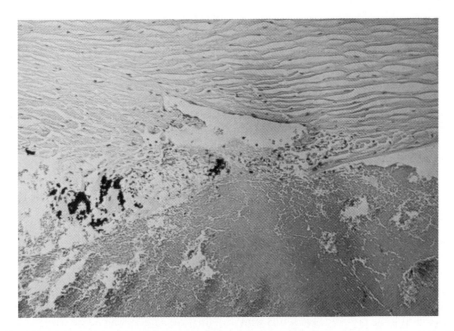

FIG. 20-2. Histologic section through trabecular meshwork and ciliary body of monkey eye following blunt anterior segment trauma. Note torn trabecular meshwork with large adherent blood clot blocking access of aqueous humor into that portion of Schlemm's canal.

anterior chamber through a trabeculectomy type of incision, since it allows a very controlled entrance and removal of debris with a minimum of instrumentation of the interior of the eye.

All techniques seem to yield favorable results in the hands of their proponents. The ultimate visual outcome is determined more frequently by retinal or optic nerve damage from the original injury than by problems related to the high-pressure episode.

Lens subluxation

Pupillary block can occur as a result of blunt trauma if there is subluxation of the lens. Rupture of a portion of the zonules may allow formed vitreous to herniate around the tilted lens equator, or the lens itself may become incarcerated in the pupil, thereby increasing the normal physiologic obstruction to aqueous flow through the pupil. This causes increased bulging of the peripheral iris and may lead to a full-blown angle-closure situation.

Miosis usually aggravates the problem. Dilation may allow vitreous to come through the pupil and fill the anterior chamber, and angle-closure attacks may be alleviated in this manner. Unfortunately, the eye may be at risk for repeated attacks of pupillary block and angle closure, depending on the relationship between the pupil, lens, and vitreous. Iridectomy (iridotomy) or lens extraction may be necessary in cases unresponsive to dilation. Treatment should be vigorous and timely so as to prevent synechiae formation in the angle.

If the lens becomes totally dislocated, it may fall into the vitreous cavity. This is usually not a problem unless the lens becomes hypermature and causes phacolytic glaucoma (see Chapter 9). However, it may fall forward into the anterior chamber and cause pupillary block and angle-closure glaucoma. This is an emergency due to early corneal decompensation from lens-endothelial touch. Additional details regarding the management of eyes with dislocation of the lens are provided in Chapter 10.

Forward movement of the lens-iris diaphragm

Angle closure due to forward displacement of the lens-iris diaphragm can occur after trauma.

Although not often recognized, it can be distinguished from pupillary block with lens subluxation by the shallowing of the central chamber and the lack of iridodonesis. The mechanism appears to be ciliary block, and although the exact cause has not been worked out, severe edema of the choroid, retina, and ciliary body secondary to the acute trauma could be the instigating factor. The condition is best treated with cycloplegics and corticosteroids and is self-limited in 3 to 5 days. Iridectomy is not helpful and should be avoided, since it may worsen the condition.

Inflammation

Inflammation from the trauma may cause compromise of the outflow structures due to obstruction by inflammatory cells, debris, or protein. At times the inflammatory cells can be difficult to distinguish from red blood cells. Inflammatory cells should be suspected if the pressure is elevated with only a moderate cellular count in the anterior chamber, since moderate quantities of fresh red blood cells do not elevate the intraocular pressure in eyes with normal outflow facility.

Treatment with topical corticosteroids helps to resolve the inflammation and decrease intraocular pressure. Chronic use of corticosteroids should be avoided, however, since individuals sensitive to these agents may show elevations of intraocular pressure within 2 weeks. If corticosteroids are employed, their possible adverse side effects must be borne in mind.

Occasionally, as the anterior chamber hemorrhage is resolving, the fresh red blood cells are gradually replaced with fine tan-colored cells. The intraocular pressure, which may have declined toward normal, may now start to rise. Rather than uveitis, a ghost cell problem (see Chapter 21) should be suspected. This is caused by degenerated red blood cell ghosts coming forward into the anterior chamber from a vitreous hemorrhage secondary to the original trauma.[9]

A rare cause of glaucoma several months after trauma is a retinal detachment related to traumatic retinal dialysis.[41] The resulting glaucoma shows inflammatory signs in the anterior segment and characteristically demonstrates major swings in intraocular pressure. Although rare, it is an important consideration in the diagnosis of mechanisms, since surgical reattachment cures this type of glaucoma (see Chapter 11).

Trabecular injury

The most common cause of elevated intraocular pressure in the early postinjury period is mechanical damage to the trabecular meshwork. Tears in the trabecular meshwork (Fig. 20-3) occur frequently after blunt trauma but are often overlooked.[3] One study reported evidence of trabecular injury in 13 of 17 patients with mild hyphemas examined gonioscopically within 48 hours of the injury.[19]

These trabecular tears themselves do not decrease outflow facility; however, the resultant scarring of the trabecular meshwork can lead to severe outflow obstruction (Fig. 20-4).

Increased intraocular pressure due to trabecular scarring does not respond well to medical therapy. However, if treated conservatively, this problem is usually self-limited—probably because of a recanalization of the damaged trabecular meshwork. Filtration surgery should be avoided if at all possible.

Tears in the ciliary body following trauma were first described in experimental animals in 1942.[23] However, the association of blunt ocular trauma and later-developing glaucoma was not noted clinically until 1945[12] and was not correlated pathologically until 1962.[44] The ciliary body tears noted histopathologically (and called angle recession) originally were thought to be evidence of past trauma but not the cause of the increased intraocular pressure.

Studies since these descriptions have tried to correlate the later-developing glaucoma with the extent of angle recession visible years after the initial injury.[7] They have concluded that glaucoma is more frequent in angle recession involving 270 degrees or more.[43] The only prospective studies available to date show an incidence of later-developing glaucoma after angle recession to be from 2% to 10%.[21,43]

The fresh tear into the ciliary body, which splits the longitudinal and circular fibers, begins to scar soon after injury.[19] The depth and extent of the visible cleft changes markedly in the first weeks and months following injury because of synechiae formation (Fig. 20-5). Some eyes show obliteration of the angle recess and sometimes even peripheral anterior synechiae (PAS) formation to the trabecular meshwork, which obscures the "angle recession."

Rather than looking solely for angle recession,

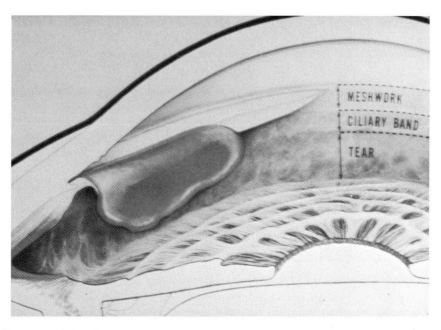

FIG. 20-3. Artist's conception of tear in trabecular meshwork following acute blunt anterior segment trauma. Note clot adherent to trabecular flap created by anterior segment trauma. Also note large tear into face of ciliary body with raw appearance of torn ciliary muscle.

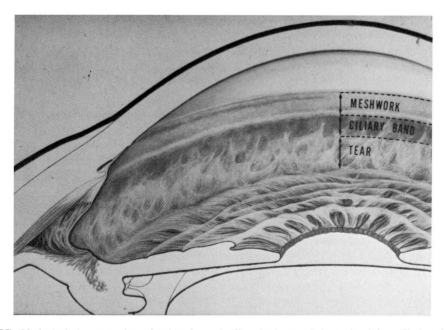

FIG. 20-4. Artist's conception of trabecular and ciliary body tear 9 days after injury. Trabecular tear is sealed, since trabecular flap has rotated back to its original position and scar tissue is forming. Note scar tissue formation in ciliary body tear with resultant narrowing of visible angle recession.

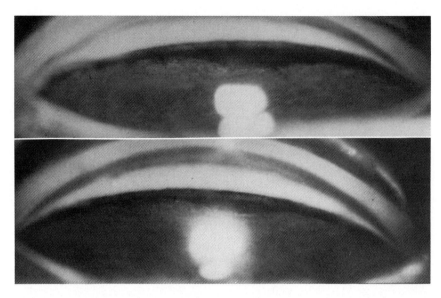

FIG. 20-5. Goniophotograph of monkey eye following blunt anterior segment trauma. Upper portion of figure is photographed 1 week following experimental blunt anterior segment injury with hyphema. Note both depth and horizontal extent of ciliary body tear. Lower portion of figure 5 shows same area pictured above 3 months following injury. Note narrowing of angle recession in areas beside deepest portion of ciliary body tear. This is caused by scar contraction. Peripheral anterior synechiae actually occlude portions of trabecular meshwork.

one can frequently recognize past trauma to the anterior segment by absent or torn iris processes, a localized depression or tear in the trabecular meshwork, and increased whitening and visibility of the scleral spur (Figs. 20-6 and 20-7).

Although asymmetric cupping and field loss are a common finding in simple open-angle glaucoma, asymmetry of pressure is not. When it is encountered, a secondary glaucoma (i.e., exfoliation syndrome) or an associated factor (i.e., trauma) should be considered. In our experience, careful gonioscopic examination of referred patients requiring surgery for chronic open-angle glaucoma shows that previous trauma is more frequently associated than was previously thought.

It is rare to find a truly unilateral glaucoma years after a blunt anterior segment injury. As mentioned earlier, decrease in outflow facility due to trauma probably occurs soon after the initial injury. The further loss in outflow facility is due to an underlying predisposition for the development of open-angle glaucoma. In a series of 18 patients suffering from glaucoma associated with previous trauma, an average 16.5 years elapsed between injury and discovery of increased intraocular pressure. Of interest was the finding that the fellow,

noninjured eye had an average intraocular pressure of 23.5 mm Hg, which is well above the statistical average.[19] An underlying predisposition for glaucoma in eyes with an intraocular pressure rise after trauma is further supported by the work of Armaly[1] indicating that the noninvolved eye of patients with traumatic glaucoma responded to steroid-provocative testing, as would the eye of a patient with primary open-angle glaucoma.

How does anterior segment trauma affect patients who already have established primary open-angle glaucoma? Initially, it may be more difficult to clear the anterior chamber of red blood cells with a resultant increase in intraocular pressure. However, if an extensive trabecular tear has occurred (in effect, a traumatic trabeculotomy), outflow facility may increase. Sometimes this increase in facility is only temporary, but occasionally a long-lasting improvement in intraocular pressure regulation may occur.

Cuticular membranes have been seen histopathologically in eyes enucleated for glaucoma due to trauma.[24] It is difficult to know if the membrane was the initial factor in decreasing the outflow, since eyes enucleated with traumatic glaucoma are usually blind and painful with long-standing glau-

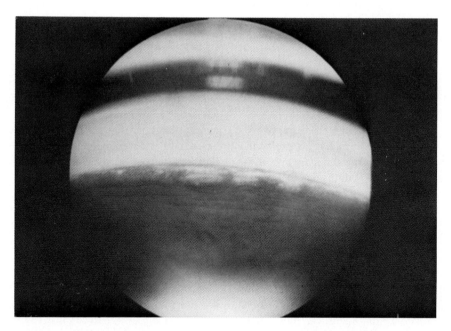

FIG. 20-6. Goniophotograph of human eye in patient with traumatic glaucoma 10 years after blunt anterior segment injury. Note area of torn iris processes with gray appearance of face of ciliary body. Also note whitening of trabecular meshwork and scleral spur in injured area.

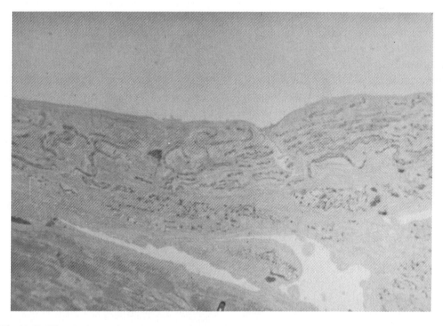

FIG. 20-7. Histologic section obtained at time of filtration surgery from area of filtration angle pictured in Fig. 20-6. Note collapse and scarring of adjacent trabecular sheets. Schlemm's canal is patent, but trabecular meshwork itself appears impermeable to aqueous humor flow.

coma. The pain is often due to bullous keratopathy and intraocular inflammation. It is known that many eyes with chronic inflammatory problems due to causes other than trauma will eventually develop cuticular membranes over the filtration meshwork.

PENETRATING INJURIES
Injury without a retained foreign body

The most significant glaucoma problem in a perforating injury to the globe is due to prolonged flattening of the chamber in an inflamed eye, leading to permanent PAS formation. The best treatment for this problem is prophylaxis. Adequate wound closure with fine permanent suture material lessens the incidence of glaucoma due to PAS formation.

Another cause for PAS formation is pupillary block. If the iris is not adequately dilated following injury and inflammation causes seclusion of the pupil, iris bombé with secondary angle closure will result. Prophylaxis is, again, the most effective way. to avoid this problem. However, if seclusion occurs, prompt surgical intervention (iridectomy or iridotomy) is imperative to avoid permanent angle closure by synechiae.

If the perforating object breaks the lens capsule, swelling of the lens may occur with a relative pupillary block resulting. This will also cause angle-closure glaucoma. The best treatment is aspiration of the swollen lens material.

As in blunt trauma, bleeding can occur from a perforating injury; thus total hyphema with glaucoma and ghost cell glaucoma can be seen in patients with perforating injuries.

Epithelial ingrowth (see Chapter 25), causing mechanical obstruction of the trabecular meshwork, is a rare complication of a perforating injury. It should be suspected as the cause of glaucoma if the eye remains chronically irritated after a perforating injury. A gray membrane may be seen on the posterior surface of the cornea.

Another rare cause for glaucoma seen after perforating trauma associated with a chronically inflamed eye is sympathetic ophthalmia. Usually the condition is bilateral, but one eye may be more affected than the other. This glaucoma, due to inflammatory obstruction of the trabecular meshwork, although rare, is never to be forgotten because of the potentially disastrous implications of the diagnosis. The recent advent of vitrectomy to rehabilitate severely traumatized eyes seems to be associated with a higher incidence of sympathetic ophthalmia than we have recognized in past years.[26]

Injury with a retained foreign body

A patient sustaining an intraocular foreign body may have early elevation in intraocular pressure either as a consequence of direct trauma to ocular structures or secondary to the effects of blunt trauma on the trabecular meshwork, as previously discussed. In addition, glaucoma may develop as a late sequela of a retained, often unsuspected, metallic foreign body.

A rupture of the lens capsule is present in about 50% of eyes injured by a metallic intraocular foreign body[33] and may result in a concurrent phacogenic glaucoma at the time of presentation. On occasion, this may be the presenting sign of an occult intraocular foreign body. The correct diagnosis may be suggested by a sealed corneal perforation site, a hole or transillumination defect in the iris, or direct visualization of the foreign body after pupillary dilation.[11] Appropriate x-ray studies, ultrasonography, and computerized axial tomography may confirm the clinical suspicion of an occult foreign body. However, it may not be possible to detect a minute foreign body in the anterior segment by these techniques in spite of strong clinical signs. In this situation an alternate approach is the use of a pediatric dental x-ray cassette, lodged lengthwise in the medial canthal region after the instillation of a topical anesthetic. On occasion, this may accurately localize an otherwise undetectable foreign body in the anterior segment. Such documentation is important, since appropriate therapy includes removal of the metallic foreign body to prevent the late complications of siderosis or chalcosis.

There are several mechanisms whereby intraocular foreign bodies may be responsible for the onset of late elevation in pressure. As in nonpenetrating injuries, the blunt trauma associated with the injury itself may damage the angle or trabecular meshwork. Flattening of the anterior chamber and concurrent inflammation may produce anterior synechiae.[39] Finally, it has been proposed that iron deposition in the trabecular meshwork of eyes with siderosis from a retained magnetic foreign body may directly explain the reduced aqueous outflow and secondary glaucoma.[14,15] This process, however, develops over months to years. In this era of vitreous surgery and increasingly sophisticated

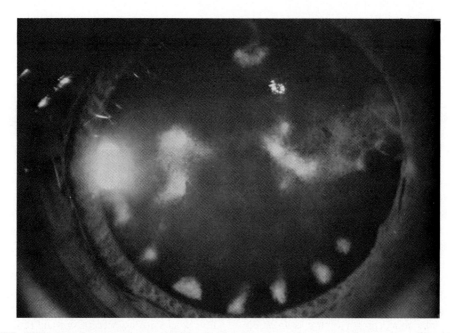

FIG. 20-8. Anterior segment photograph of siderotic cataract in construction worker with occult retained foreign body. Multiple small rust-colored spots are seen to lie subcapsularly, and non-pharmacologic mydriasis secondary to siderosis can be appreciated. Other features present but not demonstrated photographically include rusty staining of posterior corneal surface, heterochromia, and retained magnetic foreign body lodged in retina.

intraocular instrumentation, such complications are not common. Nevertheless, patients may have unsuspected intraocular foreign bodies and unilateral glaucoma.[30] Heterochromia, mydriasis, a rust-colored stain to the posterior corneal surface, and multiple rust-colored anterior subcapsular deposits (Fig. 20-8) are the classic clinical signs of siderosis and should lead the clinician to the appropriate diagnosis.

CHEMICAL INJURIES

Chemical burns of the eye carry a poor prognosis, in part because the early florid external manifestations of the injury may mask the internal damage from uncontrolled elevations in intraocular pressure. Recognition of the important role of elevated intraocular pressure necessitates its regular evaluation and treatment through all phases of the injury. The patient can only expect to reap the benefits of rehabilitative surgery if his physician is aware of the problems in early diagnosis and treatment of the secondary glaucoma associated with chemical ocular injuries.

The various pathogenic mechanisms potentially responsible for an elevation in intraocular pressure may come into play at different times after the injury, thus posing a constant threat to the visual potential of the chemically burned eye. To manage glaucoma secondary to a chemical injury, one must understand its pathogenesis, the difficulties in accurately measuring the intraocular pressure and documenting optic nerve damage, and, finally, the therapeutic modalities available. Glaucoma secondary to a chemical injury will be considered in the time frame of the three phases of the injury. The early phase (first hours to few days) is characterized by acute tissue destruction and the release of inflammatory mediators. It is followed by an intermediate phase (weeks to months) of repair, scarring, and ongoing inflammation. As inflammatory signs abate, the transition is made to a late phase characterized by extraocular and intraocular cicatrization and consequent functional disturbances.

Early damage

Structural damage to the anterior segment occurs within minutes after contact with the offending chemical and may be associated with an early rise in intraocular pressure. While early copious irrigation and removal of particulate matter is recommended, animal studies indicate that saponified alkaline chemicals are detected in the anterior chamber within seconds of the injury.[20,25] The severity of the injury is a function of the rapidity of ocular penetration, chemical concentration, and duration of exposure. Alkaline substances generally cause more profound damage through destruction of the lipid barriers of the anterior segment. Acids, on the other hand, coagulate the proteins of tissue with which they come in contact and generally result in a more superficial, corrosive injury.[16,25] However, if the eye is exposed to high concentrations of acid for more prolonged periods of time, deeper tissue destruction can occur, producing a clinical picture not unlike the more rapidly destructive alkali burn. The more severe injury, characteristically an alkali injury, results in ischemia of the anterior circulation, reflected in a whitened sclera and in death of the cellular elements of the anterior segment (Fig. 20-9).

Early elevations of intraocular pressure may result from scleral shrinkage secondary to the caustic injury, possibly coupled with the release of intraocular prostaglandins.[32] Conversely, in the most severely injured eyes, damage to the ciliary body may result in hypotony.[34]

Accurate documentation of the intraocular pressure may be difficult in this early period as a result of periorbital swelling and a thickened or irregular corneal surface. Conventional Schiøtz or applanation tonometry may be difficult in this setting, and the presence of corneal edema may result in underestimation of the intraocular pressure with these instruments. In the presence of corneal edema, measurements are more easily and accurately obtained with a MacKay-Marg or pneumatograph tonometer.[38] While tactile tension may allow one to discern extremes such as hypotony or profound elevation of intraocular pressure, it is highly subjective and inaccurate at intermediate pressure elevations and should not be relied on as the sole method of intraocular measurement.

Treatment of early elevation of intraocular pressure is limited to agents that decrease aqueous production, such as timolol and carbonic anhydrase inhibitors, and to epinephrine compounds. Miotics are contraindicated, since they augment the inflammatory response and may contribute to pupillary block if synechiae are formed between pupil and lens. If it is not possible to measure the intraocular pressure because of alterations of the anterior segment, prophylactic use of a carbonic anhydrase inhibitor may be reasonable until one can obtain accurate measurements.

Intermediate damage

During the intermediate or reparative phase, lid and conjunctival changes evolve while the cornea attempts to resurface in the face of potential stromal breakdown and concurrent endothelial damage. The trabecular meshwork may have been structurally damaged by the initial direct, toxic injury or from PAS formation as a result of inflammation and tissue necrosis. More inflamed eyes, in particular those with hypopyon formation, are prone to develop glaucoma in this phase.[8] Medical reduction of aqueous production remains the cornerstone of antiglaucoma therapy, coupled with antiinflammatory medications. However, topical corticosteroids may be contraindicated in the first few weeks in the face of corneal stromal lysis.[13] Empiric use of oral corticosteroids may reduce anterior chamber inflammation if one is not able to use topical corticosteroids because of stromal lysis.

Trabecular meshwork damage is the principal but not sole cause of elevation of intraocular pressure during the intermediate phase. The pupil, which frequently becomes unresponsive after a chemical injury, may become adherent to the lens, resulting in pupillary block glaucoma. This problem should be anticipated by the early use of mydriatics, with the effect on pupil size noted. If pupillary block develops nonetheless, intensive therapy with topical steroids and mydriatics should be undertaken. If this fails and if the media are sufficiently clear, laser iridectomy may be sufficient to break the pupillary block. As a last resort, one may be required to undertake a peripheral iridectomy.

Progressive cataract formation may occur and can contribute to increased intraocular pressure either on the basis of pupillary block from a swollen lens or from the release of lens material.[8] Medical therapy may allow surgery to be deferred. However, early lens extraction may be required; also, if possible, lens aspiration through a small wound is recommended.

Late damage

Once the anterior segment has stabilized relative to lid deformities and corneal resurfacing, it may become necessary to deal with more chronic

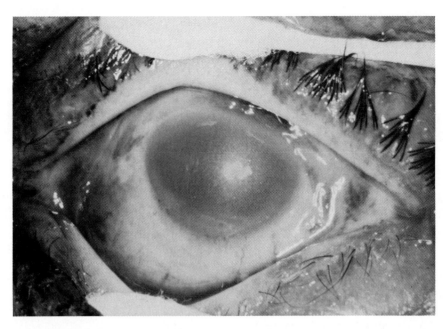

FIG. 20-9. External photograph of human eye 6 hours after chemical injury with potassium hydroxide. Whitening of inferior perilimbal sclera and conjunctiva can be seen, indicating ischemia. Cornea demonstrates typical beaten silver appearance seen after severe alkali chemical injury.

elevations of intraocular pressure. This is required not only to minimize optic nerve damage, but also to maximize the prognosis of a rehabilitative procedure such as a penetrating keratoplasty or keratoprosthesis.

If corneal surface irregularities exist, more correct readings of intraocular pressure are obtained with MacKay-Marg or pneumatograph tonometry. These instruments may be used with a (bandage) soft contact lens in situ without markedly altering accuracy. Scarred opaque media make following parameters such as visual fields and evaluation of the optic nerve head more difficult and less accurate. However, there are other, less precise parameters that may be helpful. If the injury is monocular, using the consensual response of the normal pupil may demonstrate an afferent defect, indicating significant optic nerve damage or coexisting retinal disease. A modified visual field, in which Goldmann perimetry (using larger peripheral isopters) is used to provide reproducible parameters that can be followed, may likewise be very helpful. If perimetry is not possible, confrontation fields with a bright light should discriminate between a residual temporal island or remaining central field. Ultrasound examination may detect advanced "beanpot" glaucomatous cupping, al-though a normal examination does not rule out advanced glaucomatous cupping.

In the chronic, noninflammatory phase of pressure elevation, miotics may be used to increase outflow through a damaged trabecular meshwork. Corticosteroids are less useful at this stage and may contribute to elevation of intraocular pressure.

Antiglaucoma surgery, which one would be hesitant to undertake in the acute or intermediate stages, may now be considered if the intraocular pressure is not adequately controlled medically. Since widespread conjunctival necrosis and subsequent scarring and symblepharon frequently occur, there is often no suitable site for a filtration operation. However, if damage is limited to the exposed interpalpebral fissure, there may be a reasonable site for filtration in an undamaged area. If not, the only alternative is cyclocryotherapy. However, because of ciliary body necrosis, aqueous production may already be reduced, and an elevated intraocular pressure may indicate concurrent damage of the trabecular meshwork. Consequently, cyclocryotherapy should be limited to treatment of no more than 90 to 180 degrees at one time. A freeze-thaw rather than a freeze-thaw-refreeze technique should be used. Cautious retreatment will lessen the likelihood of hypotony and phthisis.

RADIATION THERAPY

Radiation therapy for periocular and intracranial neoplasia may result in elevations of intraocular pressure from heterogeneous causes.[2] A secondary open-angle glaucoma, often associated with generalized conjunctival telangiectasis, can occur and may respond to conventional antiglaucoma treatment.[4] More intractable elevations in pressure may be due to rubeosis iridis or intraocular hemorrhage, presumably related to coexisting retinal radiation damage.[27] Generally this occurs in the presence of widespread ocular damage, and the prognosis for these eyes is understandably poor.

ELECTRICAL INJURY

While no conclusive data exist establishing glaucoma as a complication of electrical injury, abnormalities of the iris pigment due to accidental and therapeutic (cardioversion, electroconvulsive therapy) electrical trauma have been reported.[5,6] In these patients one may see mild to extensive loss of the iris pigment epithelium, which is best demonstrated by slit-lamp retroillumination. A concurrent dispersion of pigment onto the anterior lens capsule, anterior iris surface, and corneal endothelium is seen. While a transient elevation of intraocular pressure has been reported after cardioversion, and medically controllable elevations of intraocular pressure are noted in some patients who have had previous electroconvulsive therapy, a direct connection between electrical injury, dispersion of iris pigment, and glaucoma remains to be established.

REFERENCES

1. Armaly, M.F.: Steroids and glaucoma. In Symposium on glaucoma: transactions of the New Orleans Academy of Ophthalmology, St. Louis, 1967, The C.V. Mosby Co.
2. Barron, A., McDonald, J.E., and Hughes, W.F.: Long-term complications of beta radiation therapy in ophthalmology, Trans. Am. Ophthalmol. Soc. **68:**112, 1970.
3. Bechetoille, A.: Aspects gonioscopiques des lesions traumatiques de l'angle, Clin. Ophthalmol. **3:**17, 1971.
4. Bedford, M.A.: Corneal and conjunctival complications following radiotherapy, Proc. R. Soc. Med. **59:**529, 1966.
5. Berger, R.O.: Ocular complications of cardioversion, Ann. Ophthalmol. **10:**161, 1978.
6. Berger, R.O.: Ocular complications of electroconvulsive therapy, Ann. Ophthalmol. **10:**737, 1978.
7. Blanton, F.M.: Anterior chamber angle recession and secondary glaucoma: a study of the aftereffects of traumatic hyphemas, Arch. Ophthalmol. **72:**39, 1964.
8. Brown, S.I., Tragakis, M.P., and Pearce, D.B.: Treatment of the alkali burned cornea, Am. J. Ophthalmol. **74:**316, 1972.
9. Campbell, D.G., Simmons, R.J., and Grant, W.M.: Ghost cells as a cause of glaucoma, Am. J. Ophthalmol. **75:**205, 1973.
10. Crouch, E.R., and Frenkel, M.: Aminocaproic acid in the treatment of traumatic hyphema, Am. J. Ophthalmol. **81:**355, 1976.
11. Davidson, S.I.: Intraocular foreign bodies: clinical recognition, Int. Ophthalmol. Clin. **8**(1):171, 1968.
12. D'Ombrain, A.: Traumatic monocular chronic glaucoma, Trans. Ophthalmol. Soc. Aust. **5:**116, 1945.
13. Donshick, P.C., Berman, M.B., Dohlman, C.H., et al.: The effect of topical corticosteroids on ulceration in alkali-burned corneas, Arch. Ophthalmol. **96:**2117, 1970.
14. Duke-Elder, S.: System of ophthalmology, vol. 11, Diseases of the lens and vitreous; glaucoma and hypotony, St. Louis, 1969, The C.V. Mosby Co., p. 713.
15. Duke-Elder, S., and MacFaul, P.: Injuries, part 1, Mechanical injuries. Vol. 14 in Duke-Elder, S.: System of ophthalmology, St. Louis, 1972, The C.V. Mosby Co., p. 525.
16. Duke-Elder, S., and MacFaul, P.: Injuries, part 2, Nonmechanical injuries. Vol. 14 in Duke-Elder, S.: System of ophthalmology, St. Louis, 1972, The C.V. Mosby Co., p. 1011.
17. Edwards, W.C., and Layden, W.E.: Traumatic hyphema: a report of 184 consecutive cases, Am. J. Ophthalmol. **75:**110, 1973.
18. Goldberg, M.F.: The diagnosis and treatment of sickled erythrocytes in human hyphemas, Trans. Am. Ophthalmol. Soc. **76:**481, 1978.
19. Herschler, J.: Trabecular damage due to blunt anterior segment injury and its relationship to traumatic glaucoma, Trans. Am. Acad. Ophthalmol. Otolaryngol. **83:**239, 1977.
20. Hughes, W.F.: Alkali burns of the eye: I. Review of the literature and summary of the present knowledge, Arch. Ophthalmol. **35:**423, 1946.
21. Kaufman, J.H., and Tolpin, D.W.: Glaucoma after traumatic angle recession: a ten-year prospective study, Am. J. Ophthalmol. **78:**648, 1974.
22. Kelman, C.D., and Brooks, D.L.: Ultrasonic emulsification and aspiration of traumatic hyphema: a preliminary report, Am. J. Ophthalmol. **71:**1289, 1971.
23. Kilgore, G.L.: An experimental study of iridodialysis, Trans. Am. Ophthalmol. Soc. **40:**516, 1942.
24. Lauring, L.: Anterior chamber glass membranes, Am. J. Ophthalmol. **68:**308, 1969.
25. Lemp, M.A.: Cornea and sclera, Arch. Ophthalmol. **92:**158, 1974.
26. Lewis, M.L., Gass, J.D.M., and Spencer, W.H.: Sympathetic uveitis after trauma and vitrectomy, Arch. Ophthalmol. **96:**263, 1978.
27. Macfaul, P.A., and Bedford, M.A.: Ocular complications after therapeutic irradiation, Br. J. Ophthalmol. **54:**237, 1970.
28. McCuen, B.W., and Fung, W.E.: The role of vitrectomy instrumentation in the treatment of severe traumatic hyphema, Am. J. Ophthalmol. **88:**930, 1979.
29. Michelson, P.E., and Pfaffenbach, D.: Retinal arterial occlusion following ocular trauma in youths with sickle-trait hemoglobinopathy, Am. J. Ophthalmol. **74:**494, 1972.

30. Miles, D.R., and Boniuk, M.: Pathogenesis of unilateral glaucoma, Am. J. Ophthalmol. **62:**493, 1966.

31. Oksala, A.: Treatment of traumatic hyphema, Br. J. Ophthalmol. **51:**315, 1967.

32. Paterson, C.A., and Pfister, R.R.: Intraocular pressure changes after alkali burns, Arch. Ophthalmol. **91:**211, 1974.

33. Percival, S.P.B.: Late complications from posterior segment intraocular foreign bodies, Br. J. Ophthalmol. **56:** 462, 1972.

34. Pfister, R.R., Friend, J., and Dohlman, C.H.: The anterior segments of rabbits after alkali burns, Arch. Ophthalmol. **86:**189, 1971.

35. Polychronakos, D., and Razoglou, C.: Treatment of total hyphema with fibrinolysin, Ophthalmologica **154:**31, 1967.

36. Rakusin, W.: Urokinase in the management of traumatic hyphema, Br. J. Ophthalmol. **55:**826, 1971.

37. Read, J., and Goldberg, M.F.: Comparison of medical treatment of traumatic hyphema, Trans. Am. Acad. Ophthalmol. Otolaryngol. **78:**799, 1974.

38. Richter, R.C., Stark, W.J., Cowan, C., and Pollack, I.P.: Tonometry on eyes with abnormal corneas, Glaucoma **2:** 508, 1980.

39. Roper-Hall, M.J.: Intraocular foreign bodies: prognosis, Int. Ophthalmol. Clin. **8**(1):257, 1968.

40. Scheie, H.G., Ashley, B.J., and Burns, D.T.: Treatment of total hyphema with fibrinolysin, Arch. Ophthalmol. **69:**147, 1963.

41. Schwartz, A.: Chronic open-angle glaucoma secondary to rhegmatogenous retinal detachment, Am. J. Ophthalmol. **75:**205, 1973.

42. Sears, M.L.: Surgical management of black ball hyphema, Trans. Am. Ophthalmol. Otolaryngol. **74:**820, 1970.

43. Tonjun, A.M.: Intraocular pressure and facility of outflow late after ocular contusion, Acta Ophthalmol. **46:**886, 1968.

44. Wolff, S.M., and Zimmerman, L.E.: Chronic secondary glaucoma associated with retrodisplacement of iris root and deepening of the anterior chamber angle secondary to contusion, Am. J. Ophthalmol. **54:**547, 1962.

Chapter 21

GHOST CELL GLAUCOMA

David G. Campbell

Ophthalmologists have long known that blood and blood products in the form of a hyphema following trauma can raise the intraocular pressure. In 1963 Fenton and Zimmerman[9] reported that a form of glaucoma could be caused by degenerated blood products that originated in the vitreous and passed forward into the anterior chamber to obstruct the trabecular meshwork. Their light microscopic, histologic findings led them to believe that the glaucoma they were describing was due to red blood cell debris and macrophages, and noting the similarity to phacolytic glaucoma, they introduced the term hemolytic glaucoma. Follow-up reports seemed to confirm these findings.[1,8,10,12]

In 1975 Campbell and Grant[5] and in 1976 Campbell, Simmons, and Grant[16] described a secondary glaucoma associated with vitreous hemorrhage that they thought was caused primarily by degenerated red blood cells (ghost cells, erythrocyte ghosts). Their light and electron microscopic studies of anterior chamber aspirates showed little or no debris and few to no macrophages. They named this condition ghost cell glaucoma and defined it in the following manner: ghost cell glaucoma is a transient, secondary glaucoma resulting from obstruction of the trabecular meshwork by degenerated erythrocytes. The ghost cells develop within the vitreous cavity following several types of hemorrhage. They then enter the anterior chamber through a disruption in the anterior hyaloid face.

PATHOGENESIS
Red blood cell degeneration within the vitreous cavity

An understanding of ghost cell glaucoma requires knowledge of the fate of blood within the vitreous cavity following vitreous hemorrhage. Morphologic, colorimetric, and rheologic changes occur in the erythrocyte following its arrival in the vitreous cavity.[4] The normal erythrocytes degenerate from red, biconcave, pliable cells to tan or khaki-colored, spherical and hollow, less pliable ghost cells (Figs. 21-1 to 21-3). The conversion begins within days and is generally almost complete within 1 to 3 weeks. Once the ghost cells have formed, they do not degenerate further rapidly and can remain in this form within the vitreous cavity for many months. During the conversion to the ghost cell form, intracellular hemoglobin is lost, presumably through leaky membranes, into the extracellular vitreous space (Fig. 21-4). The hemoglobin that remains within the cell denatures and forms clumps called Heinz bodies, which adhere to the inner surface of the plasma membrane. The extracellular hemoglobin also becomes denatured and clumped, often forming small to large accumulations that tend to adhere to vitreous strands. The adherence to and the entrapment within vitreous strands (Fig. 21-5) prevents these extracellular clumps of hemoglobin from moving freely and from passing into the anterior chamber. In contrast, the red blood cell ghosts do not adhere to each other or to the vitreous strands and are free to move anteriorly. Erythrocyte ghosts are generally 4 to 7 μm in size, and the extracellular hemoglobin clumps are generally 2 to 20 μm in size. Studies of the vitreous show that macrophages are common and ingest both the extracellular clumps and the ghost cells (Fig. 21-6).

The anterior hyaloid face serves as a natural boundary for the products of vitreous hemorrhage. Laboratory studies show that neither fresh erythrocytes nor ghost cells are able to pass across the

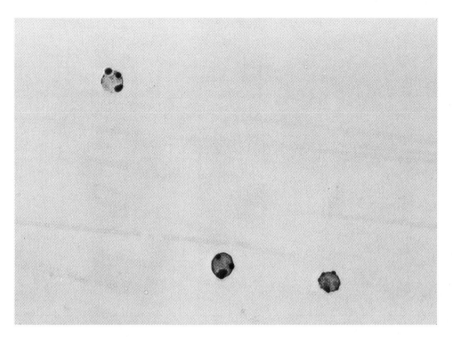

FIG. 21-1. Red blood cell ghosts, approximately 6 μm in size, as they appear viewed with phase-contrast microscopy. Dark Heinz bodies are at cell periphery.

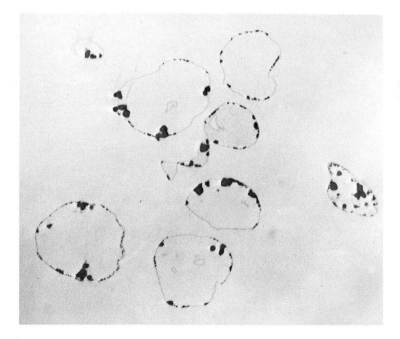

FIG. 21-2. Transmission electron micrograph of ghost cells withdrawn from anterior chamber of patient with traumatic ghost cell glaucoma.

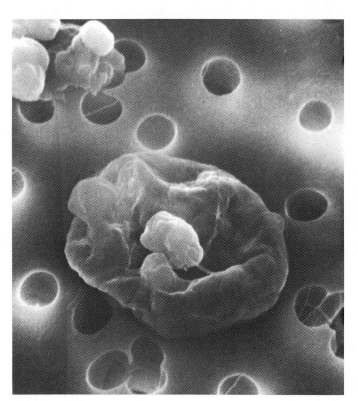

FIG. 21-3. Scanning electron micrograph of ghost cell collected on Nucleopore filter, showing protruding Heinz bodies. Specimen was taken from anterior chamber of patient with ghost cell glaucoma following cataract extraction.

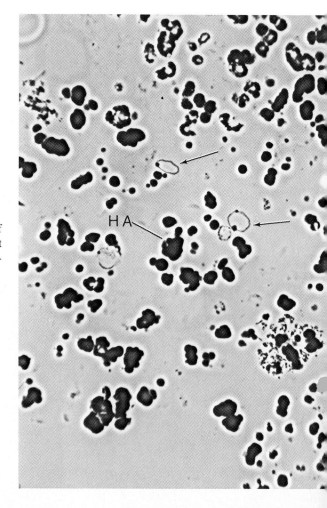

FIG. 21-4. Phase-contrast micrograph of vitreous hemorrhage specimen showing ghost cells *(arrows)*, much extracellular hemoglobin *(HA)*, and macrophage *(lower right)*.

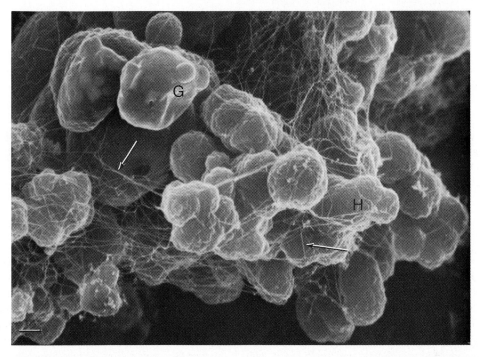

FIG. 21-5. Scanning electron micrograph of vitreous with hemorrhage showing free ghost cells *(G)*, enmeshed extracellular hemoglobin clumps *(H)*, and vitreous strands *(arrows)*.

FIG. 21-6. Macrophage removed from vitreous cavity of patient with vitreous hemorrhage. Cell has ingested both extracellular hemoglobin clump *(H)* and ghost cell *(G)*.

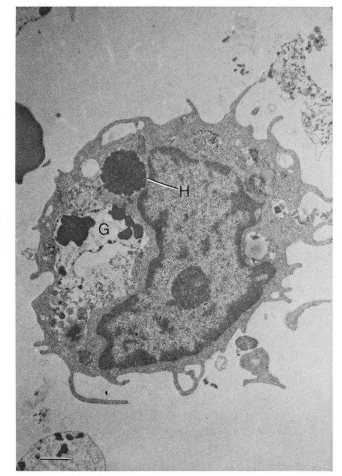

intact anterior hyaloid face. Clinical observations show further that if the anterior hyaloid face is intact following a vitreous hemorrhage, fresh or degenerated products of the hemorrhage are not seen in the anterior chamber. If, however, there has been a disruption of the anterior hyaloid face, caused by either trauma, surgery, or perhaps a rare spontaneous disruption, the cells pass forward in large numbers. Once in the anterior chamber, the ghost cells obstruct the trabecular meshwork and cause glaucoma.

Rheologic characteristics of the ghost cell

Ghost cells are less pliable than fresh red cells.[6] They cannot pass through a 5-μm Millipore filter and cannot pass through the human trabecular meshwork with ease, whereas fresh red blood cells do both. Ghost cells cause approximately three times more obstruction to outflow than an equal number of fresh erythrocytes. Histologic studies have shown that the ghosts tend to lodge in the outer and midportion of the trabecular meshwork, whereas fresh red blood cells pass to the inner meshwork and to Schlemm's canal with relative ease. Fixed ghost cells can be used to induce glaucoma in primates,[11] a finding that provides laboratory confirmation of previously reported clinical and laboratory observations.

CLINICAL FORMS

The clinical history of a patient with ghost cell glaucoma invariably includes a history of vitreous hemorrhage, usually due to trauma, surgery, or primary retinal disease such as diabetic retinopathy. The clinical history usually includes an event likely to have disrupted the anterior hyaloid face such as cataract extraction, vitrectomy, or trauma. A number of different clinical presentations of ghost cell glaucoma have been found; the majority of cases have followed vitrectomy, cataract extraction, or trauma.

Ghost cell glaucoma following vitrectomy

Following closed pars plana vitrectomy for vitreous hemorrhage, ghost cell glaucoma often occurs.[7] The surgical procedure generally disrupts the anterior hyaloid face, and ghost cells left behind at surgery pass into the anterior chamber and cause glaucoma within days to weeks following the procedure. The glaucoma generally lasts weeks to months. This glaucoma was relatively common when vitrectomy was first introduced, since in

some cases the initial procedure cleared away only a central corridor of hemorrhagic material, leaving much peripheral material, including ghost cells, behind. Later, as vitreous surgeons began removing more of the hemorrhagic content, the incidence of this entity following vitrectomy decreased considerably. This glaucoma occurred following vitrectomy with or without lensectomy but seemed slightly more common following lensectomy and the creation of a larger opening in the anterior hyaloid face.

Ghost cell glaucoma following cataract extraction: three presentations

The most common way that ghost cell glaucoma occurs following cataract extraction[4] involves the following sequence of events: A patient undergoes an uneventful intracapsular or extracapsular cataract extraction, which is followed by a large hyphema with extension into the vitreous within the first few days following the surgical procedure. Usually the anterior chamber hemorrhage clears at least partially, permitting a view of the vitreous hemorrhage. The elevation of intraocular pressure associated with the initial hemorrhage usually resolves within a week or two, but this is followed within 2 to 6 weeks postoperatively by an intraocular pressure elevation in association with the appearance of a multitude of tiny ghost cells in the anterior chamber. The pressure rise is due to obstruction of the trabecular meshwork by ghost cells that have reentered the anterior chamber. The original hyphema, which began in the anterior chamber, presumably extended back into the vitreous cavity through a disruption in the anterior hyaloid face created at the time of cataract removal. This same opening then allowed ghost cells to enter the anterior chamber at a later time.

The second presentation may occur following cataract extraction when a patient has a vitreous hemorrhage, usually from a retinal source existing before the cataract extraction. Large numbers of ghost cells existing within the vitreous cavity migrate into the anterior chamber immediately after the cataract extraction, which has disrupted the anterior hyaloid face, causing a marked elevation of intraocular pressure within days.

The third and least common presentation following cataract extraction occurs when a patient has a cataract extraction with disruption of the anterior hyaloid face and then develops a vitreous hemorrhage due to retinal disease at a later date. The red blood cells degenerate in the vitreous and then slowly pass forward into the anterior chamber. In this case the contents of the anterior chamber are mixed with fresher red blood cells as well.

Ghost cell glaucoma following trauma

Trauma to the eye, either blunt or penetrating, may result in the formation of a hyphema with hemorrhage into the vitreous cavity as well.[2] In some cases the hyphema clears, allowing a view of the vitreous cavity filled with blood. Ghost cells form in the vitreous cavity and begin to pass forward into the anterior chamber weeks to months following the original injury. Characteristically, the anterior chamber hyphema has cleared or almost cleared when the infusion of tan-colored ghost cells becomes apparent. The intraocular pressure, which may have been high after the hyphema, has spontaneously lowered, when the infusion of ghost cells causes it once more to rise.

Occasionally an eight-ball hyphema is complicated by ghost cell glaucoma in association with a vitreous hemorrhage.[3] A high pressure rise occurs in the immediate days following the injury, but this generally begins to ameliorate 1 to 2 weeks after the injury. The anterior chamber is typically still obscured by dark purple material when a second elevation of intraocular pressure occurs. Anterior chamber aspirate studies at this time have shown large numbers of ghost cells that presumably passed forward from the vitreous cavity, in addition to the contents of the eight-ball hyphema, consisting of fresher red blood cells, white blood cells, macrophages, and fibrin.

Rarely, ghost cell glaucoma has occurred without a known disruption of the anterior hyaloid face in association with a vitreous hemorrhage. In these rare cases a spontaneous disruption or dissolution of the anterior hyaloid face has been postulated.

CLINICAL FEATURES
Intraocular pressure

When a large number of erythrocyte ghosts exist within the anterior chamber, the patient may either be asymptomatic or complain of ocular pain due to high intraocular pressure. If large numbers of ghost cells have entered the chamber, the pressure rises quickly over a period of days to a level as high as 60 to 70 mm Hg. However, ghost cells do not always cause a pressure rise, especially if there is only a small number of them circulating in the anterior chamber.

Conjunctiva

The conjunctiva is generally white unless it has been inflamed by extreme elevation of intraocular pressure or previous surgery. The presence of ghost cells alone in the anterior chamber does not incite an inflammatory response, which explains the relatively quiet conjunctiva in the company of a markedly cellular anterior chamber.

Cornea

The cornea is typically normal but may be edematous with extreme elevation of intraocular pressure. If the cornea is edematous, topical glycerin is very useful in clearing it to allow examination of the contents of the anterior chamber, since the cells cannot be seen through an edematous cornea. The endothelium is either normal or has collections or layers of fine khaki-colored cells scattered on the surface. Keratic precipitates, characteristic of inflammation, do not form in association with ghost cells and when seen should lead the observer away from the diagnosis of ghost cell glaucoma toward an inflammatory cause.

Anterior chamber

The aqueous is typically filled with a multitude of tiny tan-colored cells, often circulating slowly. The characteristic red color of fresh erythrocytes is absent. The tan-colored cells may be mistaken for white blood cells, resulting in the misdiagnosis of uveitis or endophthalmitis. The cells are tiny, generally 4 to 6 μm in size, and may be overlooked unless high-power examination of the anterior chamber contents (generally $\times 25$ magnification) is used to examine the aqueous. If the cells exist in large quantities, a pseudohypopyon consisting of a layer of khaki-colored cells precipitated inferiorly is often mistaken for a true hypopyon. However, true hypopyons, which are collections of white blood cells, are white, and the khaki color of a layer of red blood cell ghosts is easily distinguished and pathognomonic for ghost cells. If fresher red blood cells exist, two or more different layers are often seen, with the lighter khaki-colored layer of ghosts appearing on top of a heavier, redder cell layer, imparting a candy-striped appearance.

Gonioscopy

Gonioscopic examination generally reveals either a normal-appearing open angle, an open angle covered by a fine layer of khaki-colored cells that have slightly to moderately discolored the trabecular meshwork, or a heavy layer filling the angle, generally inferiorly, with cells composing an early pseudohypopyon.

Vitreous

Examination of the vitreous cavity reveals the characteristic khaki color within, typical of degenerated hemorrhage. Often, many fine ghost cells, along with extracellular hemoglobin clumps frequently in sheets within the vitreous, can be seen. When the lens is absent, ghost cells can occasionally be seen streaming forward through a disruption in the anterior hyaloid face into the anterior chamber.

Anterior chamber aspiration studies

The diagnosis can often be confirmed by examination of an anterior chamber aspiration specimen, usually obtained in conjunction with a therapeutic irrigation of the anterior chamber.[4,6] The diagnosis is made most easily by immediate examination of an unstained drop of aqueous placed on a slide, covered by a slightly elevated cover slip, and examined with phase-contrast microscopy (Fig. 21-1). This generally reveals a multitude of ghost cells with characteristic Heinz bodies. Some specimens contain occasional macrophages. Noncellular debris is typically absent, but 1-μm Heinz bodies may occasionally be seen. Polymorphonuclear leukocytes and lymphocytes are not found. Large extracellular clumps of hemoglobin commonly found within the vitreous cavity are also not found within the aqueous specimens, presumably because they remain entrapped and attached to vitreous strands (Fig. 21-5). The diagnosis can also be made if the aspirate is filtered through a 1-μm Millipore filter and the surface is stained and examined by light microscopy. Characteristic ghost cells can be seen, but if, as is often the case, multitudes of cells are piled on each other, the cells appear to be amorphous debris. Scanning and transmission electron microscopic examination of the aspirates has confirmed the phase-contrast microscopic findings (Fig. 21-2 and 21-3).

Often, while collecting the aspirate, the surgeon may note that a volume greater than 0.2 cc, the volume of the anterior chamber, can be aspirated without causing collapse of the chamber. This indicates that free communication exists with the fluid within the vitreous and that this fluid is free to pass forward.

DIFFERENTIAL DIAGNOSIS

Ghost cell glaucoma must be differentiated from other glaucomas that occur in association with vitreous hemorrhage, including neovascular, hemosiderotic, inflammatory, and hemolytic glaucomas. Neovascular glaucoma, which is frequently associated with vitreous hemorrhage, can also be associated with extreme elevation of intraocular pressure. Neovascular glaucoma is differentiated from ghost cell glaucoma by the absence of ghost cells within the anterior chamber and the presence of neovascularization at the pupillary margin and in the angle.

Hemosiderosis causes a chronic open-angle glaucoma presumably due to iron deposition in and damage to the trabecular meshwork. This extremely rare glaucoma is more chronic, does not have ghost cells in the anterior chamber, and is characteristically associated with a slight discoloration of the meshwork. It occurs many years following the original injury, in contrast to ghost cell glaucoma, which occurs within weeks to months following the original injury.

Glaucoma secondary to uveitis has to be distinguished from ghost cell glaucoma. The tiny ghost cells may be misinterpreted as white blood cells, and the misdiagnoses of endophthalmitis and uveitis are not uncommon. The history of vitreous hemorrhage, disruption of the hyaloid face, a multitude of tiny khaki-colored cells, a relatively quite conjunctiva, and an absence of keratic precipitates, differentiates this condition from uveitis and endophthalmitis. The white hypopyon of uveitis or endophthalmitis is easily distinguished from the khaki-colored pseudohypopyon associated with ghost cell glaucoma.

In regard to hemolytic glaucoma, the major question has been whether a glaucoma, separate and distinguishable from the one described as being due to ghost cells, exists. I have not seen a patient with it or found an anterior chamber aspirate compatible with hemolytic glaucoma as originally described. It is possible that such a glaucoma exists, but if so, it is much rarer than ghost cell glaucoma. The diagnosis would be established by finding an anterior chamber tap specimen devoid of ghost cells but filled with macrophages and debris.

MANAGEMENT

The initial treatment of ghost cell glaucoma consists of standard medical therapy, including beta-adrenergic blocking agents, adrenergic agonists, parasympathomimetics, and carbonic anhydrase inhibitors. These may suffice to lower the pressure to a safe level until the supply of ghost cells within the vitreous cavity becomes exhausted and the glaucoma resolves.

Surgical intervention is often necessary because of persistently high and painful elevation of intraocular pressure despite maximum medical therapy. Thorough anterior chamber irrigation, repeated if necessary, is successful in most cases. Irrigation with 10 to 20 ml of fluid, directed toward the angle so that the fluid will circulate around it and help clear it of debris, is often effective. The initial paracentesis wound should be large enough to allow the aqueous and ghost cells to egress easily back around the needle. If this relatively simple and safe procedure is unsuccessful, vitrectomy to remove the contents of the vitreous cavity may be required. If anterior chamber washout lowers the intraocular pressure successfully but the pressure elevates again because of the further entrance of ghost cells from the vitreous, the procedure can be repeated.

Topical steroids have been tried but are ineffective, since this glaucoma is not inflammatory. If the patient is a steroid responder, long-term topical steroid use will cause further elevation of pressure. Steroids should be omitted or used in low doses only if concomitant inflammation is thought to exist.

PROGNOSIS

Ghost cell glaucoma is typically transient, although it may last many months. Eventually, the supply of erythrocyte ghosts in the vitreous cavity becomes exhausted and the cells stop passing forward into the anterior chamber. No permanent damage to the trabecular meshwork has been noted to date.

REFERENCES

1. Brucker, A.J., Michels, R.G., and Green, W.R.: Pars plana vitrectomy in the management of blood-induced glaucoma with vitreous hemorrhage, Ann. Ophthalmol. **10:**1427, 1978.
2. Campbell, D.G.: Ghost cell glaucoma following trauma, Ophthalmology **88:**1151, 1981.
3. Campbell, D.G., and Bellows, A.R.: Erythrocyte ghost cells in eight-ball hyphemas, read before the Association for Research in Vision and Ophthalmology, April 1977.
4. Campbell, D.G., and Essigmann, E.M.: Hemolytic ghost cell glaucoma, further studies, Arch. Ophthalmol. **97:** 2141, 1979.
5. Campbell, D.G., and Grant, W.M.: Alterations in red blood cells that prevent passage through the trabecular meshwork in human eyes, read before the Association for Research in Vision and Ophthalmology, April 1975.
6. Campbell, D.G., Simmons, R.J., and Grant, W.M.: Ghost cells as a cause of glaucoma, Am. J. Ophthalmol. **81:** 441, 1976.
7. Campbell, D.G., Simmons, R.J., Tolentino, F.I., and McMeel, J.W.: Glaucoma occurring after closed vitrectomy, Am. J. Ophthalmol. **83:**63, 1977.
8. Fenton, R.H., and Hunter, W.S.: Hemolytic glaucoma in CPC, Surv. Ophthalmol. **10:**355, 1965.
9. Fenton, R.H., and Zimmerman, L.E.: Hemolytic glaucoma, an unusual cause of acute open angle secondary glaucoma, Arch. Ophthalmol. **70:**236, 1963.
10. Phelps, C.D., and Watzke, R.C.: Hemolytic glaucoma, Am. J. Ophthalmol. **80:**690, 1975.
11. Quigley, H.A., and Addicks, E.M.: Chronic experimental glaucoma in primates, Invest. Ophthalmol. Vis. Sci. **19:** 126, 1980.
12. Wollensak, J.: Phakolytisches und hämolytisches Glaucom, Klin. Monatsbl. Augenheilkd. **168:**447, 1976.

GLAUCOMAS ASSOCIATED WITH OCULAR SURGERY

Chapter 22

MALIGNANT GLAUCOMA

Richard J. Simmons and John V. Thomas

Malignant glaucoma, first described by von Graefe[22] in 1869, is a rare but extremely serious form of glaucoma that has been responsible for the loss of one or frequently both eyes of many patients. It has been reported to occur in 2% to 4% of patients operated on for angle-closure glaucoma[10,22] and occurs regardless of the type of operation performed. The fact that it may occur in both phakic and aphakic eyes with potentially devastating consequences makes it an important form of glaucoma.

The following characteristics have played an important role in its unusual destructiveness: (1) difficulties in early recognition, (2) difficulties in early institution of optimal medical therapy for the involved eye, (3) difficulties in initiation of prompt prophylactic therapy for the fellow eye, and (4) difficulties in surgical management.

Knowledge of the unique characteristics of this form of glaucoma can help avoid many of these difficulties and ensure optimal success. Marked improvement in the management of malignant glaucoma has occurred over the past three decades and is largely due to the contributions of three men: Chandler, Grant, and Shaffer.

DEFINITION

The term malignant glaucoma is used here as von Graefe used it to identify a specific type of glaucoma that occurs in several settings, most commonly as a complication after surgery for angle-closure glaucoma. In the classic sense, malignant glaucoma is a certain type of postoperative shallowing or flattening of the anterior chamber with an accompanying rise in intraocular pressure.

It is referred to as ''malignant'' because of the difficulty with which it responds to conventional treatment. The name carries no implication of malignancy in the sense of neoplastic disease. Weiss and Shaffer[24] have suggested the term ciliary block glaucoma as a substitute for the term malignant glaucoma because it directs the attention of the clinician to the region of the ciliary body where, as is discussed below, some type of aqueous block appears to be present in this condition and because they find their term less alarming to the patient. However, thorough understanding of malignant glaucoma lies in the future, and many aspects of the presumed pathogenetic mechanism of malignant glaucoma remain unresolved or, as yet, unknown. In addition, it is a term widely understood by ophthalmologists. Therefore, at present we continue to retain the term malignant glaucoma.

PATHOPHYSIOLOGY

Although many details of the mechanism of malignant glaucoma are unknown, most investigators accept the hypothesis originally proposed by Shaffer.[18] According to this hypothesis, aqueous is diverted posteriorly into, behind, or beside the vitreous cavity (Figs. 22-1, 22-2, and 22-3). The specific mechanism that causes the posterior diversion of aqueous has not yet been identified. Some type of relative block to the anterior movement of aqueous near the junction of the ciliary processes, lens equator, and anterior vitreous face that causes aqueous to be diverted posteriorly is a possible mechanism that fits some of the clinical observations that have been made. Shaffer's hypothesis is supported by the success of Chandler's vitreous

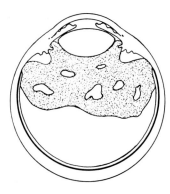

FIG. 22-1. Diagram of working hypothesis of fluid trapped in or behind vitreous body in phakic eye with malignant glaucoma.

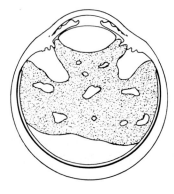

FIG. 22-2. Variation of same diagram as in Fig. 22-1, showing that fluid may, according to working hypothesis, occur at various sites in posterior segment.

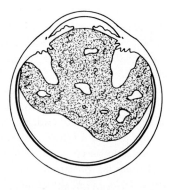

FIG. 22-3. Variation of same diagrams as in Figs. 22-1 and 22-2, in which eye is aphakic.

surgery (discussed on pp. 338-342), which is designed to remove aqueous trapped in the vitreous cavity and remedy the posterior diversion of aqueous by reestablishing the anterior flow of aqueous from the ciliary body to the anterior chamber.

Certain distinctive anatomic features have been regularly observed in the region of the ciliary processes, lens equator, and anterior vitreous face in eyes with malignant glaucoma. The tips of the ciliary processes may touch the lens when viewed through a peripheral iridectomy. The ciliary processes are frequently rotated anteriorly, their tips are sometimes flattened against the lens, and in one case, Grant observed some of the tips of the ciliary processes firmly adherent to the lens by synechiae after an attack of malignant glaucoma had subsided. The spaces between the ciliary processes, however, can be seen to be open, and through these spaces one can see the vitreous posteriorly. In phakic eyes with malignant glaucoma we, along with Chandler and Grant, have seen the anterior vitreous face to be abnormally forward behind the ciliary processes, and in aphakic eyes we have observed it touching and/or adherent to the ciliary processes.

Slit-lamp examination of the vitreous of certain eyes, both phakic and aphakic, with malignant glaucoma has revealed optically clear areas within the vitreous cavity, which have been interpreted as pockets of fluid. In a few cases in which the eye was unusually clear, a smooth vitreous face has been seen in the eye anterior to the middle of the vitreous cavity. We have interpreted this as the posterior hyaloid. The vitreous face in some eyes has been smooth and seemingly bowed forward, and an optically clear space has been present behind it.

Experimental perfusion studies in normal, enucleated human and calf eyes by Epstein et al.[6] have provided support for Grant's speculation that in malignant glaucoma there may be a decrease in the permeability of the vitreous body or of the anterior hyaloid membrane to the anterior flow of aqueous and that increased pressure in the space behind a posteriorly detached vitreous leads to a decrease in fluid movement through the vitreous gel. Epstein et al.[6] have also suggested that this resistance to the forward flow of aqueous could be further increased by apposition of the peripheral anterior hyaloid to the ciliary body and the peripheral lens, since there would be a decrease in available hyaloid surface area for fluid flow.

Fatt[7] measured the hydraulic flow conductivity of vitreous in vitro and noted that with increased pressure on the vitreous gel, the vitreous became dehydrated and fluid conductivity through the dehydrated vitreous decreased.

With the above experimental data in mind, Quigley[14] has postulated that one possible explanation for the occurrence of malignant glaucoma may be the following sequence of events: (1) an initiating event occurs to increase the posterior force applied to the vitreous gel (for example, increased fluid pressure in the cavity posterior to the detached vitreous); (2) fluid flows through the vitreous toward the anterior chamber at an increased rate, but some compaction (in effect, dehydration) of the gel occurs; (3) because of the dehydration, the fluid conductivity of the vitreous gel decreases, and with continued higher pressure posteriorly, the gel undergoes a further decrease in conductivity, setting up a vicious cycle; and (4) the compressed vitreous gel is moved forward physically by the posterior-to-anterior pressure difference, leading to shallowing of the anterior chamber.

According to this explanation, osmotic agents are effective in malignant glaucoma, since they decrease the fluid content of the vitreous cavity, thereby lowering pressure behind the vitreous. The decrease in pressure would produce a decrease in the compaction or dehydration of the vitreous, thereby allowing improved fluid conductivity and possibly restoring normal tissue relationships and intraocular pressure. Surgical disruption of the vitreous gel structure would prevent the recurrence of the cycle, since there would be no intact vitreous gel to act as a diaphragm across the entire globe. An important detail that remains unexplained by the above proposed hypothetical sequence of events is how the initial increased pressure behind the vitreous body occurs.

Although much basic information on the mechanism of malignant glaucoma awaits firm documentation, much practical progress has been made in the recognition, medical management, and surgical therapy of this once hopeless condition.

Attention to the phenomena associated with malignant glaucoma has led a number of ophthalmologists to the recognition of forms of glaucoma identical to, very similar to, or related to classic malignant glaucoma. While classic malignant glaucoma was first and is still most commonly seen after surgery on phakic eyes with primary angle-closure glaucoma, it was realized years ago that the condition could persist after lens extraction on eyes afflicted with malignant glaucoma. In recent years conditions similar to classic malignant glaucoma have been identified after cataract extraction alone on eyes without preexisting glaucoma, in eyes operated on for open-angle glaucoma, in eyes receiving miotic therapy,[16] in eyes being treated with miotics after surgery for open-angle glaucoma,[11] in eyes with spasm and swelling of the ciliary body,[13] in cases where inflammation and trauma have been prominent predecessors,[9] and in eyes without previous surgery or miotic therapy.[9,17]

Whether these conditions should be classified as forms of malignant glaucoma or as conditions that have similarity to classic malignant glaucoma will be definitively answered only as new knowledge becomes available.

DEVELOPMENT OF MALIGNANT GLAUCOMA

The chance of malignant glaucoma after surgery for angle-closure glaucoma is greatest in eyes where some of the angle is closed at the time of operation. In our experience, if the angle is open or has been opened by medical therapy at the time of operation, malignant glaucoma usually does not occur; however, when some of the angle remains closed, the danger of development of malignant glaucoma after surgery is still present. Its development as a consequence of surgery seems to have little relationship to the type of procedure performed, since it occurs after iridectomy, cyclodialysis, and filtering surgery of the conventional type with a full-thickness sclerostomy as well as with a scleral flap, such as trabeculectomy.

The level of tension at the time of surgery for angle-closure glaucoma is not a reliable indicator of the possible occurrence of malignant glaucoma. Although frequently elevated at the time of surgery, the tension may in some cases be normal or low. In some eyes the tension has become normal because of a low rate of aqueous formation, which may be a spontaneous reaction to a previous acute attack of angle-closure glaucoma, or it may be due to the use of carbonic anhydrase inhibitors, topical drops that reduce aqueous production, or hyperosmotic solutions, either oral or intravenous.

Malignant glaucoma may be detected during

surgery or at any time following surgery. Some cases have been known to develop months after the initial operation. These later cases generally are thought to result from the discontinuance of mydriatic-cycloplegic drops. Once the medication is stopped, the anterior chamber shallows or flattens and tension rises. In other instances the development of malignant glaucoma is noticed when a regimen of miotic drops is begun long after surgery.

DIFFERENTIAL DIAGNOSIS

Before the diagnosis of malignant glaucoma is accepted in any eye with elevated or normal tension and a flat or shallow anterior chamber, several entities in the differential diagnosis should be considered.

The three most important entities that may be confused with malignant glaucoma are choroidal separation, pupillary block, and suprachoroidal hemorrhage. Accuracy in diagnosis may depend on consideration of a combination of (1) the characteristics of each condition, (2) the response of the eye to medical therapy, and (3) the use of a surgical confirmation procedure that will allow the most precise and certain differentiation possible at surgery through the performance of several specific steps before vitreous surgery for the malignant glaucoma itself.

Choroidal separation

Choroidal separation is common after filtering surgery and is usually found in a hypotonous eye. On direct and indirect ophthalmoscopy, elevations of the choroid in the peripheral fundus are usually visible, although in some cases the choroidal separation is shallow or low and cannot be easily discerned. At surgery one may distinguish choroidal separation from malignant glaucoma by the presence of a characteristic straw-colored fluid of variable viscosity in the suprachoroidal space. In malignant glaucoma, such suprachoroidal fluid is almost never present, and when fluid is present in the suprachoroidal space, the diagnosis is almost always choroidal separation.

In the combined experience of Chandler and Grant,[5] only one case of malignant glaucoma showed any fluid in the suprachoroidal space, and in this case the quantity of fluid was very small. When a shallow anterior chamber with hypotony and choroidal separation persist, it should be treated by drainage of the suprachoroidal fluid from one or more sclerotomies and reformation of the anterior chamber through a paracentesis incision with saline.

Pupillary block

Pupillary block is more difficult to distinguish from malignant glaucoma than is choroidal sepa-

TABLE 22-1
Differential diagnosis

	Malignant glaucoma	Choroidal separation	Pupillary block	Suprachoroidal hemorrhage
Anterior chamber	Flat or shallow	Flat or shallow	Flat or shallow	Flat or shallow
Intraocular pressure	Normal or elevated	Subnormal	Normal or elevated	Normal or elevated
Fundus appearance	No choroidal elevation	Large, smooth, light brown choroidal elevations	Normal	Dark brown or dark red choroidal elevations
Suprachoroidal fluid	Absent	Straw-colored fluid present	Absent	Light red or dark red blood present
Relief by drainage of suprachoroidal fluid	No	Yes	No	Yes
Relief by iridectomy	No	No	Yes	No
Patent iridectomy present	Yes	Yes	No	Yes
Onset	At surgery or first 5 days postoperatively (but sometimes weeks to months postoperatively)	First 5 days postoperatively, occasionally later	Early or late postoperatively	At surgery or first 5 days postoperatively (rarely later)

ration because it characteristically occurs as a flat or shallow anterior chamber with normal or elevated pressure. It is essential to rule out this diagnosis before accepting the diagnosis of malignant glaucoma. Pupillary block is more common than malignant glaucoma. If there is no patent iridectomy in the iris, it is impossible with currently available means to reliably distinguish between pupillary block and malignant glaucoma. Pupillary block is relieved by a patent iridectomy, and malignant glaucoma is not; therefore, the coloboma in the iris should be inspected carefully for its presence and patency. If there is any doubt about the presence of a patent iridectomy, another should be performed.

While usually a patent iridectomy is intended at the time of glaucoma surgery, in some instances a functional, patent communication between the posterior and anterior chamber through the iris is not in fact present. In a few instances the attempt at iridectomy during surgery results only in a hole in the anterior stroma of the iris, and the posterior pigment epithelium is left intact. Should this be the case, careful inspection by slit-lamp biomicroscopy and by gonioscopy will usually reveal the presence of the posterior pigment epithelium in the iridectomy. When this is the case, blockage will persist until disruption of the posterior pigment epithelium is accomplished rather neatly and cleanly by a knife puncture or even more simply by laser iridectomy. In some cases the surgical wound is too far posterior for the creation of a patent iridectomy, and uveal tissue from the ciliary body is inadvertently excised at the time of intended iridectomy. This may result in hemorrhage into the anterior or posterior chambers or vitreous cavity and the absence of a patent coloboma in the peripheral iris. This can be avoided by carefully identifying anatomic landmarks before surgery to be sure that the intended incision into the anterior chamber is not posterior to the scleral spur. In other cases a correctly performed iridectomy may be nonpatent if the iris becomes incarcerated in the wound. In addition, the iridectomy may be obstructed by intraocular tissue such as Descemet's membrane, anterior hyaloid surface, or ciliary processes, and this may result in its lack of patency. In all of these instances, the lack of patency of the intended iridectomy can usually be identified by careful biomicroscopy with the slit lamp and by gonioscopy.

If pupillary block is present, the anterior chamber will readily deepen after iridectomy is performed. This deepening is usually associated with the sudden escape of aqueous humor through the iridectomy and the surgical wound. This dramatic deepening confirms the diagnosis of pupillary block.

The suggestion has been made by some that vitrectomy be used for the relief of pupillary block in aphakia, but this therapy appears to us to be unnecessary and excessive for cases of simple pupillary block, since iridectomy relieves the block in nearly all such cases.

Suprachoroidal hemorrhage

Hemorrhage into the suprachoroidal space, like malignant glaucoma, may be characterized by a flat or shallow anterior chamber in the presence of a normal or elevated pressure. Hemorrhage into the suprachoroidal space can occur at the time of surgery, or it may occur in the early hours or days after surgery. It is sometimes associated with pain, but at other times it is not. In addition, eyes with suprachoroidal hemorrhage may have the sudden onset of a flat anterior chamber on the first, second, or third postoperative day and are usually quite injected. Ophthalmoscopy or ultrasonography may reveal the presence of single or multiple elevations of the choroid in the periphery of the fundus. The choroidal elevations secondary to hemorrhage may be similar in size and distribution to those in simple choroidal separation. Ophthalmoscopically, however, they are frequently dark reddish brown in color as opposed to the lighter brown color of ordinary choroidal separations. The presence of these features should make one suspect suprachoroidal hemorrhage.

Suprachoroidal hemorrhage and choroidal separation can sometimes be differentiated by ultrasonography. However, this is usually unnecessary, since the treatment will be the same as outlined below, regardless of the results of ultrasonography.

If suprachoroidal hemorrhage is present, sclerotomy into the suprachoroidal space reveals liquified or partially liquified blood, which is usually dark red or black. Occasionally the fluid obtained is a mixture of clear straw-colored fluid and reddish to black liquefied blood. All the fluid obtained from the suprachoroidal space should be drained from two sclerotomies and the anterior chamber formed with saline as outlined on p. 339.

In a few very rare cases intrachoroidal hemorrhage occurs without major penetration of the hemorrhage into the suprachoroidal space itself. In such cases all clinical features are identical to those associated with suprachoroidal hemorrhage except that little or no free blood is found in the suprachoroidal space, and drainage of the blood is not possible. Spontaneous absorption will occur slowly.

Table 22-1 summarizes the differential features of the clinical entities mentioned above.

MANAGEMENT
Medical therapy

When one suspects malignant glaucoma and is faced with a patient with a shallow or flat anterior chamber and normal or elevated pressure, one should employ the medical regimen for malignant glaucoma.

Miotic therapy was used for many years with uniformly unsuccessful results in malignant glaucoma, and this experience suggested to Chandler and Grant that miotics might in fact precipitate or aggravate malignant glaucoma. With the advent of acetazolamide in the 1950s, carbonic anhydrase inhibitors were tried in combination with miotics, but this combination was also disappointingly ineffective in the relief of malignant glaucoma.

The first major success in medical therapy for malignant glaucoma came with the report by Chandler and Grant[4] in 1962 of the successful relief of this condition with mydriatic-cycloplegic drops. Mydriatic-cycloplegic treatment is beneficial in malignant glaucoma presumably because it tightens the zonules, tending to pull the lens back into the plane of the ciliary body against the force of the vitreous, which tends to push it forward. In cases of aphakic malignant glaucoma, mydriatic-cycloplegic drops are of little benefit. However, it is reasonable to use them for their effect on relaxation of the ciliary body muscle.

The initial treatment consisted of 4% atropine and 10% phenylephrine drops, each four or five times a day.[4] This treatment was uniformly successful in the first eight cases in which it was tried and has been effective in many other cases since that time. In our series, it soon became apparent that continuation of cycloplegia permanently or for an indefinite period of time was important. Generally, when atropine was continued, the anterior chamber retained normal depth and the tension was lowered. However, on discontinuation of atropine, the chamber became shallow or flat and

tension rose. In most cases, but not all, this process was reversed by reestablishing the use of atropine.

Our experience with these cases has emphasized the importance of continuing atropine or scopolamine indefinitely, since one cannot be certain that a recurrence of malignant glaucoma can be relieved by resumption of the drops. We now believe that in cases successfully treated with medical therapy, 1% atropine drops should be continued indefinitely once a day or every other day to prevent recurrence of malignant glaucoma.

We have also found that if mydriatic-cycloplegic drops alone do not relieve the malignant glaucoma, the addition of a carbonic anhydrase inhibitor such as acetazolamide or methazolamide will relieve the condition in some patients. The addition of hyperosmotic agents to the regimen has been found to relieve an additional number. More recently we have added timolol to our regimen in the expectation that it will decrease aqueous production, lower the pressure, and help relieve the malignant glaucoma.

From this experience we believe that the optimal regimen of medical therapy for malignant glaucoma consists of the concurrent use of mydriatic-cycloplegic drops, timolol, carbonic anhydrase inhibitors, and hyperosmotic solutions in full dosage from the very beginning of treatment. Our preferred initial dosages consist of atropine 1%, 1 drop four times daily, phenylephrine 10% 1 drop four times daily, timolol ½% 1 drop two times daily, acetazolamide 250 mg by mouth four times daily, and hyperosmotic solutions in maximal dosage. Undiluted 50% oral glycerol (1 ml per pound of body weight) should be given cold for palatability and consumed over a period of no more than 5 minutes. Mannitol 20%, 2 g (10 ml) per kilogram may be administered intravenously over a 45-minute period. The patient is not given any oral food or fluids for 2 hours before and after the administration of the hyperosmotic agent to ensure that its osmotic effect is not altered. The hyperosmotic agents are given every 12 hours.

The dose of any of the above medications should be reduced if the patient is intolerant to it. Where no contraindications exist, the entire regimen is surprisingly well tolerated by the average patient for a period of 4 to 5 days. In some patients who complain of nausea with the administration of oral glycerol, the use of antiemetics 1 hour before administration can reduce this unpleasant side effect.

This regimen should be continued until the anterior chamber forms and the pressure improves, or until this regimen has been tried for 4 to 5 days.

If the condition is relieved, the regimen is gradually tapered and discontinued over several days. Hyperosmotic agents are discontinued first, and then carbonic anhydrase inhibitors are tapered and discontinued. Mydriatic (phenylephrine) drops are stopped, but the cycloplegic (atropine) drops are continued indefinitely. If the anterior chamber does not deepen and tension does not improve with the medical treatment outlined above, one must not consider the treatment a failure until it has been tried for 4 or 5 days. We have seen cases in which the condition was relieved only after 2 or 3 days of treatment and one case in which the condition was relieved only after 5 days of treatment. With the use of this optimal medical regimen for 4 to 5 days, about 50% of cases of malignant glaucoma are relieved.

If medical therapy is unsuccessful, and if the ocular media are clear and the iridectomy visible, it may be reasonable to use the argon laser to shrink the ciliary processes. Recently Herschler[8] reported success with this technique in five of six cases of malignant glaucoma unresponsive to medical therapy.

If the ciliary processes are visible through the peripheral iridectomy without the aid of a gonioscopy lens, the laser beam may be applied directly through the cornea. Before the ciliary processes are treated with the laser beam, topical glycerin may be required to clear corneal edema. The power used varies from 300 mW to 1000 mW. The duration of treatment is 0.1 second, and the spot size varies from 100 to 200 μm. In the cases reported that were successfully treated, shrinkage of two to four ciliary processes was produced by the laser. Immediately after laser treatment, slight deepening of the anterior chamber occurred, and medical therapy was continued. Full restoration of the depth of the anterior chamber, however, occurred after 3 to 5 days of continued medical therapy.

Herschler[8] has suggested that the efficacy of laser shrinkage of the ciliary processes in treating malignant glaucoma may be due to relief of relative ciliolenticular block to the anterior flow of aqueous humor. However, these observations do not provide clear evidence delineating any specific mechanism, since, as we have stated,[20] many unanswered questions remain. For example, does laser therapy contract the adjacent hyaloid membrane, which is in apposition to the ciliary processes? Does the heat of the laser on the ciliary processes rupture the hyaloid membrane itself? Does it alter the permeability of the adjacent vitreous? Does it rupture adhesions of the hyaloid to the ciliary processes? Does it act by lysis of the lens zonules in this region? Does the laser procedure followed by 2 to 3 days of medical therapy merely allow time for continued medical therapy to have effect? In regard to this last possibility, we have seen cases that have responded to medical therapy only on the fifth day of the therapy. In the cases reported by Herschler, medical therapy was given for a few days both before and after laser therapy. This leaves the distinct possibility that medical therapy itself was responsible for relief of the malignant glaucoma. However, in spite of these hypothetical issues regarding the mechanism of malignant glaucoma, laser therapy to the ciliary processes involves little risk in such cases, and we believe it should be tried in eyes in which medical therapy has failed and in which the ciliary processes are visible in the coloboma.

If medical and laser therapy fail to relieve the condition, we recommend the use of a sequence of surgical steps that we call the "surgical confirmation procedure." This procedure will eliminate with certainty at surgery the other diagnostic possibilities in the differential diagnosis of malignant glaucoma (i.e., choroidal separation, pupillary block, and suprachoroidal hemorrhage) and allow the immediate performance of surgery for malignant glaucoma in cases where the diagnosis is confirmed. If, however, one of the other diagnostic possibilities is present, it can be treated surgically at that time and the procedure terminated.

Surgical therapy

Many surgical procedures have been employed for malignant glaucoma since its description in 1869. A simple posterior sclerotomy 8 to 10 mm from the limbus was recommended in 1877 by Weber,[23] who employed this procedure successfully in one case in which he applied pressure on the cornea for 2 minutes after making the posterior sclerotomy, presumably with the loss of vitreous through the wound site. This procedure was repeated by other surgeons but proved unreliable.

Lens extraction was first recommended by Pagenstecher[12] (1877) and first used by Rheindorf[15] (1887), possibly after a decade of cautious contemplation. Many eyes have been saved from malignant glaucoma by lens extraction. In 1951 Chandler[2] reported a series of cases of malignant glaucoma in which he employed lens extraction. In those cases where vitreous was lost anteriorly, the malignant glaucoma was relieved. However, where vitreous was not lost anteriorly, the malignant glaucoma usually continued.

In 1954 Shaffer[18] called attention to the importance of the role of the vitreous in phakic and aphakic eyes affected by malignant glaucoma. In such cases he noted that when lens extraction was performed without vitreous loss, the malignant course persisted, but it would respond to a subsequent deep incision into the vitreous. This incision presumably disrupted the anterior and posterior hyaloid membranes. Because this incision into the vitreous relieved the malignant glaucoma, he postulated that aqueous was trapped in or behind the detached vitreous body in both phakic and aphakic eyes.

Based on his own experience and the experience of Shaffer, Chandler[3] devised a new surgical technique in 1964 involving puncture and aspiration of the vitreous body without removal of the lens. Since the primary disorder appeared to be one involving the relationship of aqueous humor and the vitreous, removal of the lens seemed superfluous. He postulated that extraction of the lens itself did not relieve the malignant glaucoma but that the disturbance of the vitreous associated with vitreous loss at the time of cataract extraction for malignant glaucoma produced the beneficial effect. He reported six cases in which a needle was passed into the vitreous around the lens and vitreous and/or fluid aspirated. He postulated that the needle puncture would pierce the anterior hyaloid and the posterior hyaloid where it was displaced anteriorly and that the vitreous body would be decompressed by aspiration of fluid and/or vitreous. This procedure was successful in relieving malignant glaucoma, but because of a high incidence of postoperative cataract formation, he abandoned the procedure. However, Balakrishnan and Abraham[1] successfully employed this operation in a series of cases without complication.

In an effort to avoid damage to the lens and yet retain the beneficial effect of his 1964 operation, in 1965 Chandler devised and first used the procedure currently recommended for malignant glaucoma. In 1968 Chandler et al.[5] reported the uniform success of this procedure in a series of cases

where medical therapy had failed to relieve malignant glaucoma. Chandler's procedure for malignant glaucoma includes as its initial steps the sequence of surgical diagnostic maneuvers referred to above as the surgical confirmation procedure. These initial steps help differentiate with certainty at the time of surgery malignant glaucoma from the other entities to be considered in its differential diagnosis. Since the initial report of success with this procedure, the operation has been used in many eyes. The combined experience of Chandler, Grant, and ourselves includes over 70 patients in whom some form of malignant glaucoma has played a role in one or both eyes. In over 30 of these eyes, Chandler's procedure has been used. In the vast majority of cases it has been successful in relieving the malignant glaucoma without complication, but we have learned that the operation must be performed precisely according to the recommended protocol and that steps must not be altered or eliminated if its characteristics of safety and efficacy are to be preserved.

The following is Chandler's procedure for malignant glaucoma—the current surgical procedure of choice for this disorder.

Confirmation of communication between the posterior and anterior chamber

Before the patient enters the operating room, the anterior segment of the eye is studied carefully by slit-lamp biomicroscopy and by gonioscopy for the presence or absence of a patent coloboma, since it is imperative that there be communication between the posterior and anterior chambers. If any question exists about the patency of a peripheral coloboma in the iris, an additional iridectomy is performed. A laser iridectomy may be attempted initially. If that is unsuccessful, a surgical peripheral iridectomy should be done in order to rule out pupillary block, since there is no reliable way currently known to distinguish between pupillary block and malignant glaucoma in the absence of a patent coloboma.

At the time of iridectomy, if pupillary block is present, aqueous will be released from the posterior chamber and the anterior chamber will deepen in response to the iridectomy. The wound can then be closed and the procedure terminated. The diagnosis of pupillary block is confirmed and its treatment accomplished simultaneously. If the anterior chamber remains flat, the surgeon must proceed with the other surgical steps described below.

Sclerotomy to confirm the absence of suprachoroidal fluid or blood

A beveled incision is made in the peripheral cornea with a Wheeler knife or a similar instrument to allow access to the anterior chamber for later injection of fluid and air. The incision is kept in the periphery of the cornea and can be made roughly parallel to the limbus. No suture is required to close this beveled incision at the end of the procedure, since if the bevel follows a path through the cornea, the wound so made will be self-sealing as the anterior chamber is formed. This incision should be tested to be sure that easy access with a syringe can be obtained. Later, access to the anterior chamber through this wound will be more difficult, when the eye is hypotonous.

At the sites chosen for sclerotomies, conjunctiva and Tenon's capsule should be incised with a radial incision (a radial incision is least traumatic and most convenient). Usually a site away from the area of previous ocular surgery is chosen (i.e., both lower quadrants are most commonly used when a filtering procedure or iridectomy has been previously performed above). A radial incision through the sclera to the suprachoroidal space, about 3 mm in length with its center a carefully measured distance of 3.5 mm behind the external limbus, is then made in both quadrants (Figs. 22-4 and 22-5). The incision should not be more posteriorly placed for reasons to be pointed out later.

When sclerotomies are made in a case of malignant glaucoma, no fluid will be present in the suprachoroidal space. However, if straw-colored fluid is encountered in the suprachoroidal space, the diagnosis is choroidal separation, and the fluid should be drained completely from the suprachoroidal space through both sclerotomies. The anterior chamber is deepened through the previously placed beveled incision in the cornea with saline and in some cases air. The diagnosis of choroidal separation is confirmed, and the case is terminated after closure of the conjunctival incision. The sclerotomy wounds themselves are left open without suturing in the hope that any future reaccumulation of fluid in the suprachoroidal space will be encouraged to drain spontaneously from the eye through the freshly formed sclerotomy wound.

If suprachoroidal hemorrhage is present, blood or a mixture of old blood and suprachorodial fluid will be found in the suprachoroidal space. This old blood should then be drained from the supra-

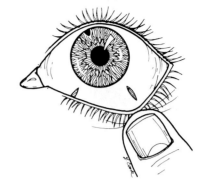

FIG. 22-4. Sclerotomy incisions. Note their relationship to limbus, as well as their circumferential positions.

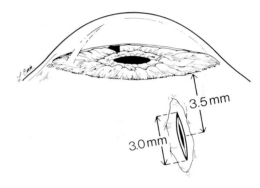

FIG. 22-5. Size of sclerotomy incision and its distance from limbus.

chorodial space, the anterior chamber reformed with saline, and the conjunctival incision closed. As with choroidal separation, the sclerotomy wounds should not be sutured. The diagnosis of suprachoroidal hemorrhage is thus confirmed, and the operation is terminated.

If no fluid flows from the sclerotomies, a smooth spatula such as a standard cyclodialysis spatula should be passed circumferentially through the lips of the sclerotomy into the suprachoroidal space parallel to the limbus. Occasionally fluid or blood can be present in the suprachoroidal space but is loculated and does not flow freely from the sclerotomy until this maneuver with a cyclodialysis spatula is performed. If iridectomy has been done and yet the anterior chamber remains shallow or flat, and if sclerotomies into the suprachoroidal space have been made and fluid or blood are not found, the diagnosis of malignant glaucoma is established.

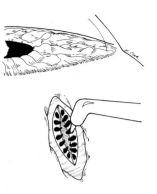

FIG. 22-6. Placement of diathermy to inner edges of scleral wound to cauterize inner scleral layers, as well as vessels in adjacent choroid. Diathermy should not be directly applied to choroid, since it may cause and stimulate bleeding.

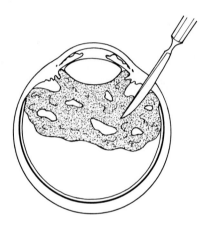

FIG. 22-7. Wheeler knife is used to pierce uvea and enter vitreous cavity. Knife is kept away from lens by aiming it toward optic nerve head.

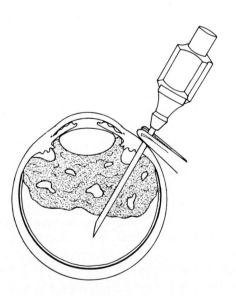

FIG. 22-8. Eighteen-gauge needle is inserted 12 mm into eye. Hemostat guard to control depth of needle is shown.

Using the sclerotomies made for tapping of the suprachorodial space, one should then carry out deep vitreous surgery for malignant glaucoma with the assurance that it is necessary and that other diagnostic possibilities have been eliminated with surgery.

The operation of choice is Chandler's deep vitreous surgery for malignant glaucoma as described below. This can be performed by using the paracentesis entry into the anterior chamber and the sclerotomies made for the suprachoroidal drainage, without making additional incisions into the globe.

Vitreous surgery for malignant glaucoma

The vitreous surgery is performed through one of the sclerotomies previously made. The site most frequently chosen is the lower temporal sclerotomy because it is convenient and has been successfully used in most of our cases. At one of the sclerotomy wounds, a ring of surface diathermy is placed around the inner layers of the scleral wound using a strong RF diathermy current with a conical electrode and sufficient power to produce brown discoloration of the sclera and slight coagulation of the vessels in the underlying choroid (Fig. 22-6). This diathermy is used to try to avoid bleeding from the uvea when the uvea is later pierced. When this has been correctly performed, bleeding of the uvea has not been a problem. Next, a Wheeler knife is plunged into the vitreous cavity to a depth of about 10 mm through the ciliary body (Fig. 22-7), the knife being aimed toward the optic nerve to avoid contact with the lens. The wound in the uvea is enlarged slightly anteriorly and posteriorly to a length, in a radial direction, of about 3 mm with its center 3.5 mm behind the external limbus.

An 18-gauge needle is next used, and a hemostat is placed around its shaft a measured distance of 12 mm behind its tip in order to prevent excessively deep penetration into the globe. The needle is then passed through the scleral-uveal wound into the vitreous cavity toward the optic nerve (Fig. 22-8). When the needle is fully inserted to the measured depth of 12 mm, its tip is moved back and forth about 4 mm in an arc of about 4 mm to allow slight separation of the vitreous membranes in its path; a syringe such as a 5-cc Luer-Lok syringe is then attached to the base of the needle by the assistant. The surgeon carefully controls the position of the needle within the eye with both hands and is not free to attach the syringe to the needle. After the syringe is attached to the needle by the assistant, the surgeon continues to maintain the position of the needle with one hand and with the other hand aspirates 1 to 1½ ml; if necessary, the assistant may aspirate while the surgeon holds the needle in place with both hands. The fluid thus obtained may be waterlike fluid, fluid vitreous, or vitreous (Fig. 22-9).

Before the needle is withdrawn from the eye, ¼ ml of aspirated fluid is reinjected into the eye in order to clear the tip of the needle of any vitreous strands engaged within its lumen. The needle is then carefully withdrawn from the eye exactly along its path of entry. The eye at this point will be markedly hypotonous, with folds in the cornea and sclera. A small amount of saline is then injected into the anterior chamber through the previously placed beveled incision in order to partially restore the shape and configuration of the globe. It is important, however, at this time that the eye not be filled out completely with saline, because in some cases saline will flow back into and behind the vitreous cavity and recreate the original malignant glaucoma. The quantity of saline injected should be just enough to partially restore the globe. A very large air bubble is then placed in the anterior chamber to fill the anterior chamber completely and force the iris and lens posteriorly (Figs. 22-10 and 22-11). The air bubble should be large enough to deepen the chamber to a depth greater than that usually encountered in the normal myopic eye. After injection of the air, the eye should still be hypotonous, since it is important not to fill out the eye completely to normal contour and tensions. A sterile Schiøtz tonometer can be placed on the eye at the end of the procedure, or a muscle hook can be used to test the pressure in the eye. If there is measurable pressure within the eye, too much saline has been injected.

The procedure is the same in aphakic eyes except that the wound of entry into the vitreous can be made at the limbus through a newly formed iridectomy or an existing iridectomy, since there is no lens to be injured by the anterior placement of the vitreous puncture. In such an aphakic eye, the needle is passed into the eye for a distance of 15 mm instead of 12 mm, since the wound of entry is at the limbus rather than 3.5 mm behind the limbus.

The scleral wounds are each closed with a single interrupted suture, and the conjunctival wounds are then closed with simple running or interrupted sutures.

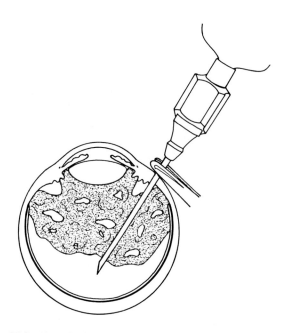

FIG. 22-9. Syringe is attached to 18-gauge needle, and 1.0 to 1.5 ml of vitreous is aspirated.

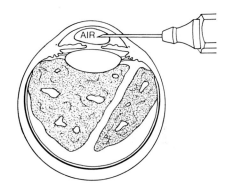

FIG. 22-10. Air bubble is placed in anterior chamber to deepen it.

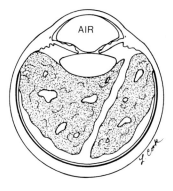

FIG. 22-11. Size of air bubble should be large enough to deepen chamber to depth greater than usually encountered in normal myopic eye.

Postoperative care

Atropine is instilled at the end of the operation and is continued postoperatively for weeks or months. We do not know with certainty whether cycloplegics can later be discontinued in all cases after this procedure has been performed, but it has been our experience that after the eye has been stable for several weeks following surgery, the cycloplegics can be tapered and stopped with careful observation of the anterior chamber. Should reshallowing of the anterior chamber occur, of course, one would immediately restart cycloplegics, but in our experience this has not been necessary in patients relieved of malignant glaucoma by this procedure. In addition, our experience has shown that miotics, including phospholine iodide, can be used after the eye has stabilized from this surgical procedure without recurrence of malignant glaucoma. Topical steroids to suppress inflammation can be of value, since they not only improve comfort postoperatively, but also may encourage significant beneficial filtration from the sclerotomy sites.

Results of therapy

Since 1965, when it was first introduced, Chandler's procedure has been used numerous times by us and by our colleagues. The operation is predictable and reliable as long as exacting attention is given to details. Complications or lack of efficacy of the procedure can almost always be traced to a lack of diligent attention to the details of the procedure. For example, if diathermy is not applied around the wound, hemorrhage into the suprachoroidal space and vitreous may occur. If the air bubble used at the end of the procedure is too small to force the lens, iris, and vitreous posteriorly, the procedure may not be successful. If the initial incision in the sclera is too far posterior, the procedure may become less effective or ineffective because the anterior vitreous is not affected adequately. The anterior placement of the wound for vitreous puncture in this procedure may be essential, since it is calculated to be anterior to the anterior portion of the vitreous base, thereby allowing disruption of the anterior hyaloid membrane as the instrument is placed into the vitreous cavity. Therefore the site of this wound should be measured carefully. If the scleral incision is too anterior (i.e., if it is centered less than 3 mm from the limbus), injury to the lens with cataract formation may result.

At surgery, or postoperatively in some cases, the anterior chamber will appear to have flattened, but careful inspection will show that the air bubble instilled during surgery has slipped behind the iris. This is in no way an indication that the malignant glaucoma has recurred. Manipulation of the patient's head or eye or prolonged dilation of the pupil will often shift the air bubble back into the anterior chamber. Otherwise, it will gradually reabsorb, and the anterior chamber will gradually reform.

A few small transient punctate fundus hemorrhages have been encountered in a few cases on careful postoperative examination by indirect ophthalmoscopy, but these have not resulted in any permanent damage.

Transient postoperative choroidal separation has occurred in about a third of our cases. It is important to distinguish choroidal separation after the procedure from recurrence of malignant glaucoma. If choroidal separation follows this procedure, the eye is soft; and although the anterior chamber is shallow or flat, suprachoroidal elevation in the peripheral fundus is present, and the condition will gradually clear spontaneously with improvement in the anterior chamber depth.

In several cases malignant glaucoma has not responded to the first performance of Chandler's procedure, but we have merely resumed medical therapy for 2 to 3 days and then repeated the procedure. Following the second operation, these eyes have responded with relief of the malignant glaucoma.

In three cases, when we were attempting aspiration through a disposable 18-gauge needle, no fluid or vitreous entered the needle and syringe. When this occurred, we merely withdrew the needle from the vitreous and attempted to instill as much air as possible into the flat anterior chamber. We then resumed atropine therapy and the full medical regimen for malignant glaucoma, and in each of these three cases the eye responded to medical therapy whereas it had not before the procedure. In one of these cases we were able to resume miotic therapy some months after the procedure was performed.

Chandler's procedure for malignant glaucoma in our hands has been considerably simpler, safer, and more effective than lens extraction in an eye with malignant glaucoma. In many of these cases the lens was clear before surgery, and by our avoiding lens extraction, a phakic eye with a clear lens resulted following relief of the malignant glaucoma. Even in cases where a cataract suitable for removal is present in the eye at the time of malignant glaucoma, we believe it is safer to carry out Chandler's procedure to relieve the malignant glaucoma and then some months later, when the eye is stabilized, remove the cataract as a separate surgical procedure. We have some years later removed cataracts that had been present before surgery and have found a normal response of these eyes to lens extraction.

This procedure has been surprisingly complication free as well as effective in our hands when carried out precisely as described. It is probably important, however, that the details of the procedure as outlined on pp. 338-342 be followed precisely, for it is not known with certainty how far one can depart from the protocol and still retain the efficacy and safety of the procedure.

At the time that this procedure was devised, the sophisticated instruments for vitrectomy were not available; since their advent, many colleagues have mentioned to us the thought that vitrectomy, rather than Chandler's procedure, might be the treatment of choice for malignant glaucoma. Our belief in this regard at the present time is that vitrectomy is not necessary in order to relieve malignant glaucoma and can be more traumatic to the external ocular tissues, existing filtration blebs, and so on. In our hands, the recommended procedure has been atraumatic and has avoided substantial conjunctival surgery, thereby sparing these delicate tissues to allow successful filtration surgery such as trabeculectomy when indicated. It must be remembered that often these eyes have hazy anterior segments and that visualization for vitrectomy in the usual manner is frequently impossible. We have so far had no case in which the malignant glaucoma could not be relieved by a combination of medical therapy followed when necessary by Chandler's procedure, with repeated surgery in a few cases and postoperative cycloplegic therapy in all cases. Should a case be encountered in which a trial of medical therapy and Chandler's procedure fails, we recommend that one repeat the medical therapy for an additional 3 days and then repeat Chandler's procedure. If, after these two trials of medical therapy and two trials of Chandler's procedure, the malignant glaucoma still does not respond, the use of vitrectomy,

lens extraction, or cyclocryotherapy (in aphakic eyes) should be strongly considered.

THE FELLOW EYE

All precautions must be taken to protect the fellow eye, since a patient who has malignant glaucoma in one eye is likely to develop the same condition in the other eye. To provide a greater margin of safety, it is reasonable to attempt to create a laser iridectomy in the fellow eye before surgical intervention. Two iridectomy sites can be created. If one is unsuccessful in creating a laser iridectomy, surgical prophylactic peripheral iridectomy is imperative. Miotics may precipitate angle-closure and malignant glaucoma in a predisposed eye. Therefore "prophylactic" miotic drops, used in the belief that they will protect the fellow eye are contraindicated. This practice is unwise in ordinary primary angle-closure glaucoma and is particularly dangerous and proscribed in malignant glaucoma.

We have never known malignant glaucoma to occur in the fellow eye when iridectomy was performed with an entirely open angle and normal ocular tension. If glaucoma is allowed to develop in the fellow eye, the treatment becomes much more difficult and the results far more uncertain. To prepare for iridectomy in the fellow eye, if some of the angle is already closed and the tension is rising, all possible medical therapy to open the angle and lower the tension should be used. Medical measures to be used in such a circumstance include maximum doses of carbonic anhydrase inhibitors, hyperosmotic agents, and timolol. Miotics should not be used. If the angle can be opened and the tension normalized with these medical measures, a peripheral iridectomy can be performed without the expectation of postoperative malignant glaucoma.

If glaucoma is present in the fellow eye and the angle does not open on medical treatment, one can anticipate malignant glaucoma after surgery whether or not tension has been brought to normal. In such cases an iridectomy is done, atropine is instilled at the conclusion of the operation, and the full optimal medical regimen for malignant glaucoma outlined on pp. 336-337 is begun at the end of surgery. This regimen of mydriatic-cycloplegic drops, carbonic anhydrase inhibitors, and hyperosmotics is continued in the hope of aborting the expected malignant course. If one is successful in aborting the malignant course, the intensive medical regimen is tapered as outlined on pp. 336-337. If malignant glaucoma occurs and persists in spite of the full medical regimen for 4 to 5 days, one must resort to laser or surgical therapy.

It is most important that the best opportunity for effective treatment of the fellow eye be seized promptly and that the opportunity not be lost because of preoccupation with the involved eye or procrastination. Since prophylactic surgery on a fellow eye is ideally performed when the angle is open and tension is normal, one should not allow conditions to become less favorable before performing the surgery. Even if some closure of the angle and an elevated intraocular pressure are already present in the fellow eye, the immediate employment of medical measures to open the angle followed by prompt iridectomy gives the best chance for avoiding the full development of malignant glaucoma. For these reasons, prompt attention to the fellow eye should be employed immediately after institution of the optimal medical regimen for the eye with malignant glaucoma.

When an eye is badly involved with malignant glaucoma, there is a tendency in all of us, because the first eye is in such severe difficulty, to wait and do nothing to the second eye until we are sure of the outcome of the first, for fear of encountering unavoidable risk. This tendency must be strongly resisted, since it leads to the absolutely erroneous course of inaction; instead, the opposite course of prompt therapy for the fellow eye is the most conservative, prudent, and risk free. The greater risk lies in inaction toward the fellow eye. The absence, for one reason or another, of prompt appropriate therapy for the fellow eye has resulted in bilateral blindness in many patients.

REFERENCES

1. Balakrishnan, E., and Abraham, J.E.: Chandler's operation for malignant glaucoma, Arch. Ophthalmol. **82:**723, 1969.
2. Chandler, P.A.: Malignant glaucoma, Am. J. Ophthalmol. **34:**993, 1951.
3. Chandler, P.A.: A new operation for malignant glaucoma: a preliminary report, Trans. Am. Ophthalmol. **62:**408, 1964.
4. Chandler, P.A., and Grant, W.M.: Mydriatic-cycloplegic treatment in malignant glaucoma, Arch. Ophthalmol. **68:**353, 1962.
5. Chandler, P.A., Simmons, R.J., and Grant, W.M.: Malignant glaucoma: medical and surgical treatment, Am. J. Ophthalmol. **66:**496, 1968.
6. Epstein, D.L., Hashimoto, J.M., Anderson, P.J., and Grant, W.M.: Experimental perfusions through the anterior and vitreous chambers with possible relationships to malignant glaucoma, Am. J. Ophthalmol. **88:**1078, 1979.
7. Fatt, I.: Hydraulic flow conductivity of the vitreous gel, Invest. Ophthalmol. Vis. Sci. **16:**565, 1977.
8. Herschler, J.: Laser shrinkage of the ciliary processes— a treatment for malignant (ciliary block) glaucoma, Ophthalmology **87:**1155, 1980.
9. Levene, R.: A new concept of malignant glaucoma, Arch. Ophthalmol. **87:**497, 1972.
10. Mehner, A.: Beitrag zu den Komplikationen bie Glaucomoperationen Speziell bie der Iridectomie, Klin. Monatsbl. Augenheilkd. **70:**491, 1923.
11. Merrit, J.C.: Malignant glaucoma induced by miotics postoperatively in open-angle glaucoma, Arch. Ophthalmol. **95:**1988, 1977.
12. Pagenstecher, H.: Ueber Glaukoms, Arch. Ophthalmol. **10:**7, 1877.
13. Phelps, C.D.: Angle-closure glaucoma secondary to ciliary body swelling, Arch. Ophthalmol. **92:**287, 1974.
14. Quigley, H.A.: Malignant glaucoma and fluid flow rate (letter to the editor), Am. J. Ophthalmol. **89:**879, 1980.
15. Rheindorf, O.: Ueber Glaukom, Klin. Monatsbl. Augenheilkd. **25:**148, 1887.
16. Rieser, J.C., and Schwartz, B.: Miotic induced malignant glaucoma, Arch. Ophthalmol. **87:**706, 1972.
17. Schwartz, A.L., and Anderson, D.R.: "Malignant glaucoma" in an eye with no antecedent operation or miotics, Arch. Ophthalmol. **93:**379, 1975.
18. Shaffer, R.N.: Role of vitreous detachment in aphakic and malignant glaucoma, Trans. Am. Acad. Ophthalmol. Otolaryngol. **58:**217, 1954.
19. Simmons, R.J.: Malignant glaucoma, Br. J. Ophthalmol. **56:**263, 1972.
20. Simmons, R.J.: Discussion of Herschler, J.: Laser shrinkage of the ciliary processes—a treatment for malignant (ciliary block) glaucoma, Ophthalmology **87:**1158, 1980.
21. Simmons, R.J., and Dallow, R.L.: Primary angle closure glaucoma. In Duane, T.D., Clinical ophthalmology, vol. 3, New York, 1976, Harper & Row, Publishers, Inc.
22. von Graefe, A.: Beitrage zur Pathologie und Therapie des Glaucoms, Arch. Ophthalmol. **15:**108, 1869.
23. Weber, A.: Die Ursache des Glaukoms, Arch. Ophthalmol. **23:**1, 1877.
24. Weiss, D.I., and Shaffer, R.N.: Ciliary block (malignant) glaucoma, Trans. Am. Acad. Ophthalmol. Otolaryngol. **76:**450, 1972.

Chapter 23

SECONDARY GLAUCOMA IN APHAKIA

Morris M. Podolsky and Robert Ritch

Various complications of cataract extraction, postoperative inflammation, and preexisting propensities of the aphakic eye may lead to temporary or permanent elevations of intraocular pressure after cataract extraction. Although this phenomenon is commonly called "aphakic glaucoma," this rubric is misleading, since it implies that aphakia itself is the cause of the elevated intraocular pressure. In actuality, a variety of mechanisms link aphakia and glaucoma. It can be stated categorically that aphakia itself does not cause elevated intraocular pressure, and we concur with Chandler and Grant[12] in calling for abandonment of the term aphakic glaucoma in favor of a more precise description of the mechanism of intraocular pressure elevation in the aphakic eye. The types of glaucoma emphasized in this chapter are those that would not be present in an eye if it were not aphakic.

As is the case with the primary glaucomas, the mechanisms of secondary elevation of intraocular pressure in aphakic eyes can be broadly divided into open- and closed-angle categories. Glaucomas associated with aphakia may develop immediately after cataract extraction or weeks to months later (see outline below). Their onset may be acute or insidious. It is also possible for both open-angle and angle-closure mechanisms to be involved in the same eye. Careful examination is therefore imperative so that the optimal method of treatment may be instituted.

Causes of glaucoma in aphakia

A. Open-angle glaucoma
  1. Early onset
    a. Preexisting open-angle glaucoma
    b. Early postoperative pressure rise
    c. Alpha-chymotrypsin–induced glaucoma
    d. Hyphema
  2. Intermediate onset
    a. Vitreous filling anterior chamber
    b. Hyphema
    c. Inflammation
    d. Lens particle glaucoma
    e. Steroid-induced glaucoma
    f. Ghost cell glaucoma
  3. Late onset
    a. Primary open-angle glaucoma
    b. Ghost cell glaucoma
    c. Epithelial ingrowth
    d. Fibrous proliferation
B. Angle-closure glaucoma
  1. Early onset
    a. Preexisting peripheral anterior synechiae
    b. Air block
    c. Pupillary block
    d. Vitreociliary block (malignant glaucoma)
  2. Intermediate and late onset
    a. Pupillary block
    b. Neovascular glaucoma

OPEN-ANGLE GLAUCOMA ASSOCIATED WITH APHAKIA
Preexisting open-angle glaucoma

Primary open-angle glaucoma may either preexist or coincidentally present at the time of cataract extraction. One must take care to rule out the various secondary causes before making this diagnosis, which is essentially one of exclusion.

Careful preoperative evaluation, including tonometry and gonioscopy, as well as tonography and perimetry when applicable, should be performed. This determination is important for preoperative preparation, intraoperative care, and evaluation of any postoperative rise in intraocular pressure. Precautions may be taken to minimize those factors that increase the likelihood of a secondary glaucoma in the postoperative period.

The effect of cataract extraction on intraocular pressure has been a controversial subject. In the immediate postoperative period there is often a self-limited episode of elevated pressure (see below). In regard to long-term effects, some studies have suggested that intraocular pressure may be reduced for a period of a few weeks to several months.[33,37,62,68] In one study, intraocular pressure was found to be reduced for up to 6 years postoperatively in patients in whom the pressure had been controlled preoperatively with mild miotics.[70] Bigger and Becker[7] thought that cataract extraction commonly improved intraocular pressure control, presumably on the basis of decreased aqueous production. They recommended cataract extraction alone for most glaucoma patients no matter what the state of the intraocular pressure control preoperatively.

Other studies, however, have indicated that cataract extraction per se does not lower the intraocular pressure.[30,46] Indeed, Galin et al.[29,30] concluded that if intraocular pressure was lower postoperatively, inadvertent filtration had probably occurred. It appears that the hypotensive effect formerly observed after cataract extraction was due to inadvertent filtration, which is less common with the watertight closure of the cataract incision now commonly obtained with fine, nonabsorbable sutures.[30,43,55]

The presence of aphakia does have an indirect influence on intraocular pressure control. Cholinesterase inhibitors, such as echothiophate, which are relatively contraindicated in the phakic eye, may be used in the aphakic eye. Epinephrine may be tried in patients in whom it could not be used preoperatively because of narrow angles. However, aphakia is also a relative contraindication to the use of epinephrine, and one must be alert to the development of epinephrine-induced cystoid macular edema.

Cataract extraction may have an adverse effect on functioning filtering blebs. Overall experience suggests a 50% loss or reduction of functioning blebs. A variety of techniques for cataract extraction in the presence of a bleb have been suggested, including incision through the bleb, corneal incision anterior to the bleb, and incision in an area away from the bleb (e.g., inferiorly or inferotemporally).[23,78] Whatever the technique, postoperative hypotony may lead to collapse of the bleb, and concomitant inflammation may lead to sealing of the walls of the bleb to the underlying episclera. In addition, vitreous may herniate into the filtration site, occluding it. Our preference is to remove the cataract from below so as to avoid surgery in the immediate region of the bleb.

Transient postoperative rise in intraocular pressure

A transient rise in intraocular pressure occurs after uncomplicated intracapsular cataract extraction.[79,81,82] Rich et al.[81] demonstrated elevated intraocular pressure in every one of 20 eyes within several hours after surgery. Alpha-chymotrypsin was not used in any of these eyes, whereas acetylcholine was injected after lens removal in all cases. The intraocular pressure rose to 26 to 50 mm Hg at a mean of 6.8 hours after surgery. Pain and corneal edema were present at the time of the rise but may not necessarily have been caused by it.

A number of etiologic factors have been suggested. First, watertight closure of the corneoscleral wound is a sine qua non. Exact reapproximation of the incisional margins with multiple fine nonabsorbable sutures under the high magnification available with the operating microscope precludes the "safety valve" of aqueous leakage allowed by earlier techniques of wound closure.

Second, "plasmoid aqueous" formed in the first hours after surgery may contribute to the intraocular pressure elevation by obstructing the trabecular meshwork.[30] Prostaglandins may also play a role. Aspirin and indomethacin have been found to blunt the postoperative pressure rise,[80] although this has been disputed.[30]

Third, there is a deformational effect on the aqueous outflow structures in the region of the corneoscleral incision because of edema.[50,51] A white ridge resembling an inverted snowbank can be seen to protrude into the anterior chamber with the internal lips of the wound at the crest of the ridge (Fig. 23-1). This ridge usually recedes within 2 weeks. The edema of the inner lips of the incision may be unrelated to the sutures closing the incision, since no ridge developed when a corneoscleral incision in an enucleated eye was closed with sutures. Campbell and Grant[10] have suggested that tight corneoscleral sutures themselves may deform the outflow structures enough to raise

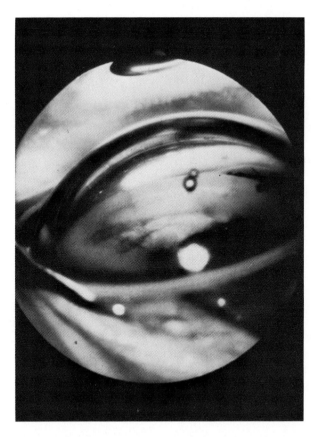

FIG. 23-1. ''White ridge'' after cataract extraction. In this gonioscopic view ridge is present at right of photograph and represents edema of inner lips of cataract incision. Suture is visible as dark mass in angle recess visible through trabecular meshwork. (Courtesy Ralph E. Kirsch, M.D.)

the intraocular pressure. In eyes in which cataract extraction through a corneal incision has been made, theoretically precluding an effect on the outflow structures by the incision or the closing sutures, elevated intraocular pressure may[79] or may not[84] follow.

The patient who experiences a significant rise in intraocular pressure immediately after cataract extraction will have ocular pain. Postoperative pain, therefore, may not necessarily be due to operative trauma or postoperative inflammatory reaction, but to the height of the pressure rise. The cornea may be edematous. The angle is open on gonioscopy, but a ridge of edema may be noted in the area of the corneoscleral incision.

One may wish to avoid watertight closure in a patient with extensive visual field loss from glaucoma, since even a transient postoperative rise in pressure may obliterate the remaining field.[53] The surgeon should measure the intraocular pressure a few hours after cataract extraction and also insti-

tute prophylactic treatment to blunt the rise. Patients with severe postoperative pain should not be given routine injections of narcotics but should be examined at the slit lamp. The use of alpha-chymotrypsin should also be approached cautiously in these patients.

A transient postoperative rise in intraocular pressure is the most likely diagnosis when the pressure is elevated several hours after surgery and should be suspected when the angle is open and the anterior chamber is unremarkable. The diagnosis is most certain in retrospect, when the pressure returns to normal the following day. As a practical matter, the rise in pressure will remain undetected if the pressure is not measured several hours after surgery. In most patients it is inconsequential, but it may cause further damage in a patient with a compromised visual field. The incidence of wound complications, such as iris prolapse and wound leak, may be increased.[48]

Since this pressure rise usually resolves spontaneously within 36 hours, in the absence of pre-existing glaucomatous damage no treatment is necessary unless the level of pressure is high enough to threaten the integrity of the incision or cause the patient pain. In addition to aspirin or indomethacin, timolol may be useful.[35a] If necessary, carbonic anhydrase inhibitors and hyperosmotic agents can also be used.

Alpha-chymotrypsin–induced glaucoma (zonulytic glaucoma)

Alpha-chymotrypsin is commonly used for zonulysis during intracapsular cataract extraction. Pressure elevations of 20 to 30 mm Hg have been observed in up to 72% of patients in whom it has been used.* The rise in intraocular pressure usually occurs from 2 to 5 days after cataract extraction.

The mechanism by which alpha-chymotrypsin causes a rise in pressure remains controversial. Obstruction of the trabecular meshwork with zonular fragments has been postulated. Anderson[2] found by scanning electron microscopy a flufflike material in the meshwork of owl monkeys treated with intraocular alpha-chymotrypsin, Worthen[102] injected enucleated human eyes with alpha-chymotrypsin and demonstrated a similar material in the trabecular meshwork.

Other mechanisms proposed for zonulytic glaucoma include direct toxic effects on the meshwork and ciliary body, damage to the meshwork from contaminants in the enzyme preparation, alpha-chymotrypsin–induced inflammation, and mechanical damage to the meshwork from instillation of the enzyme. Damage to the meshwork and ciliary body after injection of alpha-chymotrypsin into the anterior chamber has been demonstrated experimentally.[24,60] Other studies have failed to corroborate these findings.[36,61] Kirsch[47] found no change in the incidence of zonulytic glaucoma after running the preparation through a Millipore filter before intraocular instillation. He also observed no change in aqueous flare when zonulytic glaucoma occurred, and topical steroids had no ameliorating effect on the intraocular pressure rise.[48] Mechanical damage from the instillation of alpha-chymotrypsin is unlikely, since instillation of the diluent alone does not result in elevated intraocular pressure.[47] Normal amounts of anti-alpha-chymotrypsin have been demonstrated in the aqueous of responders to alpha-chymotryp-

sin,[28] and Kirsch[48] ruled out hypersensitivity to the enzyme by demonstrating negative skin tests.

Investigations of the effect of alpha-chymotrypsin in patients with preexisting glaucoma have shown either no increase in the incidence of zonulytic glaucoma[31] or only a slightly increased incidence.[47] No long-term effects on aqueous humor dynamics have been demonstrated in eyes that have had zonulytic glaucoma.[45]

Prevention is the most effective treatment. Judicious use of alpha-chymotrypsin only when indicated by the patient's age or the state of maturity of the cataract should be encouraged. Attention to the use of minimum volumes and the use of a 1:10,000 solution instead of a 1:5000 solution will decrease the incidence of pressure elevation.[49]

Irrigation of the anterior chamber before lens extraction may remove zonular fragments. Irrigation does not diminish the incidence of zonulytic glaucoma by removing the enzyme itself, since anti-alpha-chymotrypsin activity in the anterior chamber inactivates the enzyme within minutes after instillation.

When zonulytic glaucoma develops, temporizing measures are indicated, since it is self-limited, usually abating within 48 to 72 hours. Medical therapy with timolol and/or carbonic anhydrase inhibitors usually suffices. Extreme caution should be used in patients with severe glaucomatous damage.

Several investigators have studied the use of prophylactic treatment to blunt the intraocular pressure rise expected after the use of alpha-chymotrypsin. In one study, intraocular acetylcholine did not prevent zonulytic glaucoma.[28] Preoperative acetazolamide or mannitol and postoperative acetazolamide, pilocarpine, or topical steroid also failed to prevent it.[8] Acetazolamide given after the onset of the intraocular pressure rise failed to shorten the duration of the glaucoma in comparison with that of untreated eyes.[5] However, Packer et al.[69a] found prophylactic treatment with timolol and acetazolamide to blunt the rise in intraocular pressure due to the use of alpha-chymotrypsin.

Vitreous in the anterior chamber

Free vitreous in the anterior chamber may rarely be associated with open-angle glaucoma.[34,89] Vitreous in the anterior chamber usually results from spontaneous rupture of the anterior hyaloid face. Intraoperative loss of vitreous may also lead to free vitreous in the anterior chamber when an ante-

---

*References 41, 47, 49, 58, 65.

rior vitrectomy is not performed. Vitreous often is present in the anterior chamber without causing glaucoma, and this diagnosis is difficult to prove.

This form of secondary glaucoma most commonly begins in the first few weeks after cataract surgery but may not appear until months postoperatively. The mechanism appears to be direct obstruction of the trabecular meshwork by vitreous. Grant[34] introduced vitreous into the anterior chamber of enucleated eyes and produced a significant outflow obstruction attributed to vitreous in the trabecular meshwork.

When vitreous in the anterior chamber results from intraoperative loss of vitreous, coincident intraocular inflammation may exacerbate the intraocular pressure elevation. In addition, vitreous loss leads to elevated intraocular pressure by predisposing the eye to pupillary block and peripheral anterior synechiae (PAS) formation.[64,89] The glaucoma may thus be complicated by more than one mechanism.

On slit-lamp examination, the anterior chamber is filled with vitreous. The angle is open, and vitreous appears to extend into the meshwork, but this is difficult to confirm by direct visualization.

The usual agents for control of open-angle glaucoma in the aphakic eye may be used. Mydriatics, by allowing withdrawal of the vitreous from the anterior chamber, may also be effective,[43,89] as may hyperosmotic agents. Miotics, by causing the iris to draw the vitreous away from the meshwork, may occasionally be efficacious, but their effect is often unpredictable. When recondensation of the vitreous face occurs, the vitreous will spontaneously retract from the angle with subsequent resolution of the glaucoma. If the glaucoma is not controlled medically, anterior vitrectomy is indicated.

Hyphema

A hyphema most commonly occurs in the first week after surgery. The source of the hemorrhage is usually the site of the iridectomy or, less commonly, the cataract incision. A hyphema may also occur spontaneously or in association with minor trauma or heavy physical exercise many months after surgery.[72,90,94] The source of the late hyphema is fine neovascularization of the interior aspect of the cataract incision. Fine lacy new vessels may be visible on gonioscopy at the site of the cataract incision. If the hyphema is chronic and intermittent, these may occasionally bleed if

light pressure is applied with a goniolens, a maneuver with which one must be cautious.

Most postoperative hyphemas are limited in extent. These small hyphemas are asymptomatic beyond blurring of vision and are not associated with elevations in intraocular pressure. More extensive hyphemas, however, may cause the intraocular pressure to rise, and the patient may experience severe pain. Gonioscopy, when possible, typically reveals an open angle. A cellular response of variable severity may occur in response to the blood in the anterior chamber, and the mechanism of the pressure rise is believed to be due to obstruction of the trabecular meshwork by hemosiderin-laden macrophages. If the hyphema is extensive, there may be direct obstruction of the meshwork by clotted blood. In addition, chronic intermittent hyphemas may lead to secondary angle closure from PAS formation in the inferior angle where the blood settles. If a hyphema occurs in a patient with a broken anterior hyaloid face, the vitreous may fill with blood. This may cause delayed restoration of vision, as well as ghost cell glaucoma.

The hyphema and the associated secondary glaucoma are usually self-limited. Treatment is therefore aimed at tiding the patient over the acute episode. Medical treatment is preferred, timolol and carbonic anhydrase inhibitors being the agents of first choice. Pilocarpine should probably not be used, since this exacerbates the postoperative inflammation. Hyperosmotic agents may be used to blunt an acute rise in intraocular pressure. Since clearance of the hyphema may be dependent on a sufficient rate of aqueous flow, medical therapy should be reserved for patients in whom the pressure level threatens corneal blood staining, the integrity of the wound, or visual field loss.

Surgical intervention should be reserved for those patients in whom medical therapy fails to control the pressure. Evacuation of the hyphema by irrigation and aspiration with a vitrectomy instrument may be attempted with less risk than in the phakic patient. In patients with a hyphema secondary to wound neovascularization, photocoagulation of the offending vessels with the argon laser has been evaluated with variable results.[72,96]

Uveitis

Intraocular inflammation causes elevation of intraocular pressure in the aphakic eye by the same mechanisms as those found in phakic eyes. These include obstruction of the meshwork by inflammatory cells and fibrinous aqueous, peripheral anterior synechiae, and pupillary block. The intraocular inflammation may be part of the postoperative course or may represent an exacerbation of preexisting uveitis. Inflammation usually must be severe in order to result in a significant elevation of intraocular pressure. Sometimes a diagnosis must remain presumptive. A detailed discussion of glaucoma secondary to uveitis is given in Chapter 19.

Steroid-induced open-angle glaucoma

Numerous studies have demonstrated that topical corticosteroid treatment causes an elevation of intraocular pressure in susceptible patients. Those with primary open-angle glaucoma are characteristically prone to such elevations. This topic is discussed fully in Chapter 17.

Topical steroids are commonly used in the postoperative period after cataract extraction, and patients who are high (gg) responders may secondarily develop an elevated intraocular pressure. In some cases postoperative effects of corticosteroids on aqueous outflow may be masked by concomitant secretory hypotony and not be revealed until aqueous production has restored itself or may not be evident at all if decreased aqueous production continues until after the steroids have been discontinued.

It is conceivable that increased absorption of topical steroids by an inflamed eye may make the eye more susceptible to their hypertensive effects. Partial blockage of the trabecular meshwork due to inflammation may result in a higher pressure elevation than would otherwise ordinarily be seen. Cycloplegics, which may induce pressure elevations in glaucomatous patients, may also be an aggravating factor. Steroid-induced alterations in the trabecular meshwork may be masked by secretory hypotony due to inflammation and become manifest only when the inflammation has cleared. These phenomena need further investigation.

Ocular examination does not reveal anything that would otherwise not be present in the eye. Precautionary measures require judicious use of steroids in the postoperative period. If the intraocular pressure is elevated because of the use of steroids, their discontinuation should result in a lowering of the pressure. The degree of inflammation and the use of cycloplegics should be kept in mind when one is confronted with this situation. The use of steroids that have a lesser effect than dexamethasone on intraocular pressure, such as fluorometholone, should be considered. If neces-

sary, concomitant use of antiglaucoma agents, especially inhibitors of aqueous secretion, may be employed.

Lens particle glaucoma

A secondary glaucoma may develop after either planned or unplanned extracapsular cataract extraction due to lens cortex remnants in the anterior chamber. Not all eyes with retained cortical material after cataract extraction, however, will demonstrate a rise in intraocular pressure. A variety of mechanisms may account for this rise, including obstruction of the meshwork with free lens particles, obstruction with macrophages swollen with lens material, and plugging of the meshwork in inflammatory debris. Angle-closure glaucoma may result from the development of a pupillary membrane, causing pupillary block, or from PAS formation. See Chapter 9 for a detailed discussion of the mechanism of lens particle glaucoma.

The patient has an anterior chamber filled with retained cortical material. In general, there is also a marked inflammatory response in the anterior chamber, and prominent white keratic precipitates are present on the corneal endothelium and vitreous face.

Medical therapy is usually sufficient to control the intraocular pressure. In addition to the usual ocular hypotensive agents, topical steroids should be employed when an inflammatory component is prominent. Eventually the glaucoma resolves as the retained cortical material is removed by the inflammatory process.

When medical therapy fails to control the glaucoma, surgical removal of the retained cortical material is indicated. Currently available infusion-suction cutting instruments are excellent for this purpose.

Ghost cell glaucoma

Ghost cell glaucoma is due to physical blockage of the outflow channels of the trabecular meshwork by the plasma membranes of degenerated erythrocytes (erythrocyte ghosts). These result from bleeding into the vitreous, either from a vitreous hemorrhage or from an anterior chamber hemorrhage that gains access to the vitreous. Blood in the vitreous may be present before the cataract extraction or may occur at the time of surgery or long afterward. The onset of ghost cell glaucoma depends on the presence of defects in the anterior hyaloid face, which allow the ghost cells to gain access to the anterior chamber. Such breaks may occur during the cataract extraction or post-operatively. This topic is discussed fully in Chapter 21.

Epithelial ingrowth and fibrous proliferation

The onset of glaucoma in the late postoperative period should alert the examiner to rule out fibrous proliferation and epithelial ingrowth. These fearsome late complications of cataract extraction are discussed in Chapter 25.

Pseudophakia

Glaucoma in the presence of an intraocular lens may occur at any time and may or may not be related to the lens. Primary open-angle glaucoma is a relative contraindication to intraocular lens implantation. Preexisting glaucoma may be affected by the presence of an intraocular lens, depending on its type and position within the eye. Also, glaucoma may result from the presence of the lens itself. This topic is covered in Chapter 24.

ANGLE-CLOSURE GLAUCOMA ASSOCIATED WITH APHAKIA
Preexisting angle-closure glaucoma

Cataract extraction serves as definitive therapy for eyes with angle-closure glaucoma that have not previously undergone surgery. Such eyes might be those that have had an attack of angle closure but have not undergone iridectomy for one or another reason, eyes with narrow angles that develop closure as the cataract swells, fellow eyes that might have been treated with miotics, eyes with chronic angle closure, and eyes with narrow angles that may be predisposed to angle closure. Peripheral anterior synechiae and secondary damage to the trabecular meshwork are not altered by the surgery. Residual glaucoma is managed as open-angle glaucoma.

An eye with previous angle closure that has had normal intraocular pressure may also develop secondary open-angle glaucoma after cataract extraction. If there has been irreversible damage to the meshwork as a result of the angle-closure component, the resulting secondary glaucoma may be proportionately worsened. The degree to which this occurs depends on the preoperative status of the meshwork.

Careful preoperative evaluation of the patient should reveal any previously undiscovered element of angle closure. Gonioscopy and tonography are essential in assessing the risk of postoperative exacerbation of elevated pressure. Prevention of further compromise of trabecular function is paramount and is accomplished by intensive control of postoperative inflammation and precautionary measures to avoid a postoperative flat anterior chamber and subsequent extension of peripheral anterior synechiae. Surgical intervention for a postoperative flat anterior chamber should be considered earlier in a patient with significant preoperative peripheral anterior synechiae.

Pupillary block

Pupillary block may be defined as the failure of aqueous to pass from the posterior to the anterior chamber because of blockage of the pupil and iridectomy. The block may be functional, as when air is involved, but is usually accompanied by the formation of adhesions between the hyaloid face and the iris. These adhesions may be strong or weak.

Aphakic pupillary block was described in 1865 by Bowman[9] and was discussed by Knapp[52] in 1895. Hudson[40] (1911) described vitreopupillary block. Significant observations on the pathophysiology and treatment of pupillary block were made by Chandler[11] and Sugar.[91,92]

Pupillary block is the single most common cause of angle closure after cataract extraction.[26] Its incidence has been reported as being between 1% and 7%,[85] depending on the type of closure of the cataract incision, when the intraocular pressure was measured postoperatively, and the length of follow-up. It is most common in the immediate postoperative period but may occur at any time. Cotlier[20] found 76% of cases to occur within 2 weeks of surgery.

A number of conditions may predispose an eye to aphakic pupillary block (see below). A wound leak is probably the most frequent cause of early pupillary block, since it permits the anterior hyaloid to adhere to the posterior iris. A flat anterior chamber with hypotony and choroidal detachment is often followed by pupillary block. Conversely, pupillary block may cause a wound leak and flat anterior chamber, especially when the intraocular pressure is elevated soon after surgery.

Causes of pupillary block
1. Wound leak
2. Postoperative inflammation
3. Pupillary occlusion
4. Posterior vitreous detachment
5. Air

6. Incomplete iridectomy
7. Iris prolapse
8. Iridectomy too anterior
9. Lens remnants

Air in the anterior and/or posterior chambers may cause pupillary block within 24 to 48 hours of surgery.* Intumescent retained lens material may obstruct the iridectomy and induce greater inflammation, leading to adhesions.[42] Pupillary occlusion by a dense membrane may occur from such causes as marked inflammation or a hyphema. Postoperative inflammation is a frequent cause of later pupillary block. The anterior hyaloid may adhere to the iris at the pupillary border or may adhere to much of the posterior iris surface.

Chances of pupillary block are enhanced when the iridectomy is incomplete (Fig. 23-2), too anterior, or included in an iris prolapse (Fig. 23-3). A basal iridectomy is protected from the vitreous face by the ciliary processes. Pupillary block is most likely to occur if the iridectomy does not extend to within 1 mm of the iris root.[93] Even a sector iridectomy does not ensure against pupillary block if it is not truly basal (Fig. 23-4).

A posterior vitreous detachment may be associated with pooling of aqueous behind the vitreous, which forces the vitreous more anteriorly, making pupillary block a more likely development.

Pupillary block by air

Air often enters the anterior chamber as the lens is extracted, or it is placed into the anterior chamber at the end of the procedure. An eye in which the vitreous volume has been decreased by massage and hyperosmotics may be soft at the end of the procedure, even with a large air bubble. However, when the vitreous volume reconstitutes itself, the aqueous can pass out of the trabecular meshwork but the air cannot; it becomes confined to a relatively smaller volume. Since it is not compressible, the intraocular pressure may rise. A bubble filling the anterior chamber will block the flow of aqueous through the pupil, much as does a lens in the anterior chamber (Fig. 23-5). In this case aqueous behind the iris causes peripheral bombé and angle closure. If some or all of the air is in the posterior chamber, the air itself may cause

the iris to flatten against the trabecular meshwork (Fig. 23-6). If the bubble is large, air may be present in both the anterior and posterior chambers. In this situation the air in the anterior chamber maintains central chamber depth while that in the posterior chamber, in concert with the aqueous, acts to produce angle closure by distributing behind the peripheral iris.

In the former case the clinical appearance may be misleading, since the anterior chamber depth is maintained centrally, and it may not be immediately apparent that the cause of elevation of intraocular pressure is blockage of the trabecular meshwork. Slit-lamp examination and gonioscopy, however, will reveal peripheral iris bombé and closure of the angle.

Intensive mydriasis may relieve the pupillary block until the air has been resorbed. Air in the posterior chamber may be released into the anterior chamber. If this is insufficient, the air may be removed, with the patient under topical anesthesia, by paracentesis with a 30-gauge needle. When the air is in the posterior chamber, it may sometimes be massaged into the anterior chamber if the bubble is small enough. Otherwise, paracentesis combined with gentle massage should suffice. If too much air is drawn off, the anterior chamber may be reconstituted with balanced salt solution if necessary.

Pupillary block by vitreous

When the pupil and iridectomy are obstructed by vitreous, the anterior vitreous face is almost invariably intact. A formed anterior hyaloid acts as a relatively impermeable barrier to the forward flow of aqueous. A broken vitreous face is only rarely associated with pupillary block.[71] Eyes with preexisting uveitis or iris neovascularization are especially susceptible to pupillary block from posterior synechiae due to more severe postoperative inflammation.

Pupillary block may be diagnosed at various stages in its progression. The patient may experience a decrease in vision and pain in the involved eye or may be asymptomatic. The common clinical picture is a shallow or flat anterior chamber with an elevated intraocular pressure and a middilated, nonreactive pupil. However, the classic presentation is by no means the rule, and it is important to be able to recognize the various earlier stages in order to minimize consequences to the eye.

---

*References 4, 44, 86, 88, 103.

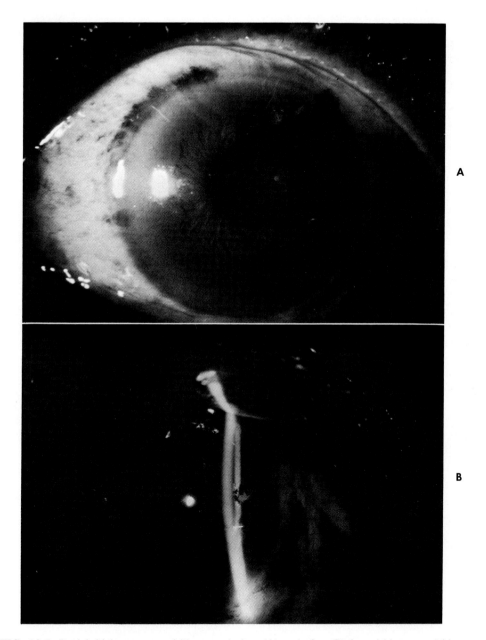

FIG. 23-2. Partial-thickness sector iridectomy before **(A)** and after **(B)** laser iridectomy. Iridectomy was easily performed with only six spots of 100-μm spot size, 0.1 second's duration, and 300 mW power. (From Ritch, R., and Podos, S.M.: Perspect. Ophthalmol. **4**:129, 1980.)

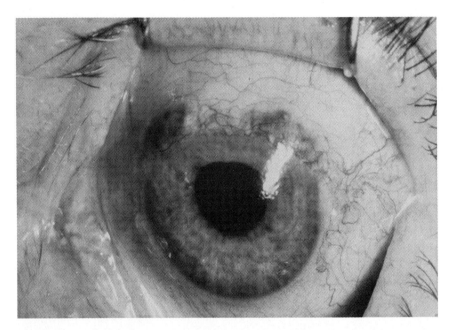

FIG. 23-3. Two peripheral iridectomies (10 o'clock and 2 o'clock position) incarcerated in wound with resultant pupillary block glaucoma. (Courtesy Max Forbes, M.D.)

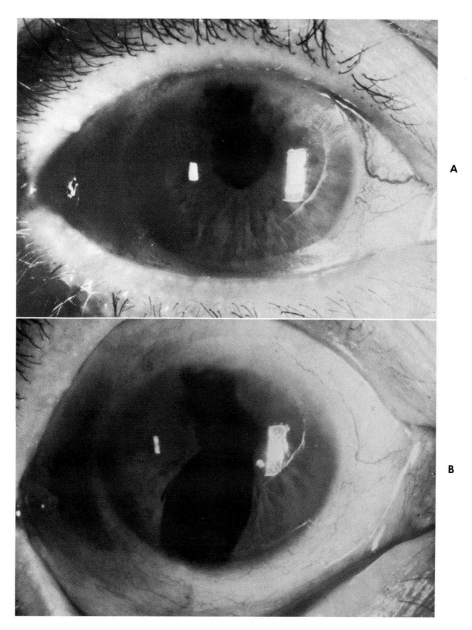

FIG. 23-4. Even sector iridectomy does not necessarily guarantee that pupillary block will not occur, as in this patient before **(A)** and after **(B)** second sector iridectomy relieved block. (Courtesy Max Forbes, M.D.)

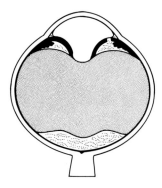

FIG. 23-5. Artist's conception of air bubble in anterior chamber causing pupillary block. Posterior aspect of bubble occludes both pupil and iridectomy.

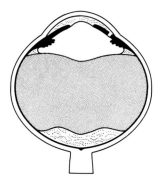

FIG. 23-6. Pupillary block secondary to air in posterior chamber.

• • •

The intraocular pressure is most likely to be high if no wound leak is present. If a wound leak is present, or if there is marked secretory hypotony, the intraocular pressure may be low. It may be normal if the block is early, or if a small fistula exists.

The anterior chamber may be flat, shallow, or deep. When the chamber is shallow or flat, pupillary block glaucoma must be distinguished from a postoperative flat anterior chamber due to a wound leak. A wound leak is suggested by the presence of a filtering bleb, a positive Seidel test, or visualization of a wound gape on gonioscopy. However, the Seidel test will be negative in some instances when there is insufficient aqueous to create a visible rivulet in the fluorescein-stained tear film.

A deep chamber is most likely to be found early in the sequence of pupillary block, and the examiner is easily misled at this time. If the trabecular meshwork is blocked by angle closure, restricted ability of aqueous to exit from the anterior chamber may result in temporary maintenance of the chamber. However, it will more or less rapidly shallow and flatten as aqueous exits by uveoscleral outflow or a wound leak even if the meshwork is completely blocked. If broad adhesions between the hyaloid face and posterior iris are present in some areas but not in others, the depth of the chamber may be irregular. Chandler and Grant[12] believe that this latter appearance is pathognomonic for pupillary block.

The cornea may be clear or edematous, or it may exhibit folds in Descemet's membrane, depending on the intraocular pressure and the state of corneal compensation. The pupil and iridectomy may be occluded with vitreous, inflammatory membranes, or retained lens remnants (Fig. 23-7), although occasionally the pupillary margin may not appear to be sealed over its entire circumference. In such situations posterior synechiae to the vitreous occur from the posterior surface of the iris rather than from the pupillary margin. The vitreous face is characteristically intact, and posterior synechiae or a pupillary membrane may be visible.

On gonioscopy, the angle is usually closed, but it may be open if the block is diagnosed early enough. The choroid may be intact or detached. If the anterior chamber is shallow or flat with separation of the choroid or ciliary body, the intraocular pressure is usually low.

If the diagnosis is in doubt, an intravenous injection of fluorescein can be given.[75] Fluorescein will appear in the anterior chamber of a normal aphakic eye in about 20 seconds, whereas in pupillary block, it may be absent entirely or slowly trickle in.

It is often difficult to decide whether the flat chamber or pupillary block came first when both are present. If the intraocular pressure is high, one must think of pupillary block or vitreociliary block, whereas if the pressure is low, one should think of a wound leak. However, a secondary wound leak may lead to a low pressure, and a prolonged flat chamber predisposes the eye to pupillary block.

The incidence of a flat chamber due to a wound leak after cataract extraction has been greatly reduced with the advent of tight wound closure and nonabsorbable sutures. The wound leak may result from faulty closure, premature dissolution of absorbable sutures, pressure on the globe, Valsalva's maneuver, or an elevated intraocular pressure postoperatively. Cotlier[19] found the incidence to be

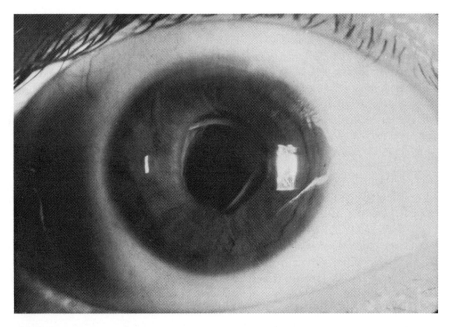

FIG. 23-7. Lens remnants after congenital cataract extraction. No iridectomy was performed. Patient developed pupillary block several years after surgery. (Courtesy Max Forbes, M.D.)

higher in patients with preexisting glaucoma. A chain of events may ensue whereby transient pupillary block leads to an elevated intraocular pressure, which causes a wound leak. Loss of the chamber due to a wound leak predisposes the eye to further pupillary block, which may remain after the chamber is spontaneously or surgically reformed, and which may initiate the cycle again. The intraocular pressure in an eye caught in this cycle may be within normal limits or even low because of the "escape valve" of the inciting wound leak.

Choroidal detachments may also cause shallowing of the chamber, initiating the chain of events cited above. In some instances, the low intraocular pressure due to a wound leak allows transudation of fluid into the suprachoroidal space by reversing the pressure gradient between the intravascular pressure within the choroidal vessels and the intraocular pressure. The detachment may develop at the time of surgery by the same mechanism. The choroidal detachment then produces forward pressure on the iris, causing shallowing of the anterior chamber.[14,19] Production of aqueous is diminished because of ciliary detachment, further shallowing the chamber, and may initiate the sequence leading to pupillary block.[15]

Prophylactic measures should be taken to guard against pupillary block. These include making sure that the iridectomy is basal and/or making more

than one iridectomy. Wound closure should be adequate, and not too much air should be allowed to remain in the anterior chamber. Postoperative inflammation should be vigorously treated, as should wound leaks. Tonometry should be performed routinely postoperatively, as should gonioscopy as soon as is feasible, particularly if the intraocular pressure is elevated.

Medical therapy is the first line of treatment. Intensive mydriasis will often break the block if adhesions between the anterior hyaloid and posterior iris are not too extensive.* Mydriasis may have only a temporary effect, since iridovitreal adhesions can still form, and topical steroids should be used to reduce inflammation. Movement of the pupil by alternating mydriatics and miotics may be more effective than mydriatics alone in preventing adhesions. Miotics alone may be effective in breaking a pupillary block if the pupil is moderately dilated to begin with, or if the iridectomy is functionally blocked or caught up in an iris prolapse. Because short-acting mydriatics are easier to reverse than long-acting ones, we prefer to use the former in the early postoperative period routinely.

Hyperosmotic agents may dehydrate the vitreous sufficiently to retract the anterior hyaloid and break adhesions. If the chamber is flat, hyperos-

*References 11, 13, 15, 77, 91, 99.

motics may convert it to a shallow one, permitting pupillary movement or allowing one to treat with the laser.

If this treatment is insufficient, a regimen of topical 0.25% echothiophate followed by subconjunctival injection of 0.2 ml of 5% pralidoxime (Protopam), a potent replenisher of cholinesterase, has been suggested.[43] This can be extremely irritating to the eye, and our experience with it is limited.

Gentle stroking of the cornea with the lubricated tip of a glass rod midway between the pupillary margin and limbus with the patient under topical anesthesia may suffice to break adhesions at the pupillary margin and is a reasonably safe procedure.[93]

If a wound leak is a factor, pressure patching the eye may aid in breaking the cycle of the wound leak and pupillary block. The use of strong miotics and patching to deepen a shallow or flat chamber has often been reported to be successful.* Surgical repair of the wound leak should be performed if this is unsuccessful.

If medical treatment is unsuccessful, we prefer to attempt to break the pupillary block with the laser before proceeding to surgery. If the block is present because of a partial-thickness iridectomy, a few spots of 50- or 100-μm spot size, 0.1 or 0.2 second's duration, and 300 to 400 mW power will succeed in penetrating the pigment epithelium. Laser procedures should never be performed in the presence of a flat chamber, since the first burn will result in corneal endothelial opacification. Hyperosmotics and pressure patching for an hour will often allow a shallow chamber to form. Even a shallow chamber may be deep enough to permit laser treatment if it is performed carefully. Whenever the chamber is shallow, the corneal endothelium is more predisposed to burns. These may often be prevented by keeping the power low and spacing the burns a few seconds apart rather than "machine-gunning" them. This allows heat to dissipate from the treated site and, although more burns and a longer treatment session are necessary, the increased success is well worth it.

Laser pupilloplasty,[96] photomydriasis[17,71] and laser iridectomy[3,74,82,87] have been advocated for breaking pupillary block. Pupilloplasty consists of placing a few low-power stretch burns on the sphincter to peak the pupil and may be useful if the

synechiae are only at the pupillary margin and easy to break. Photomydriasis requires a larger number of burns and may increase inflammation without breaking the block. If photomydriasis is attempted but success early in the procedure is not achieved, one should not persist.

Our own preference is to attempt to break the block by peaking the pupil and, if this is unsuccessful, to go directly to creating a new iridectomy with the laser. The major advantage of the laser over a surgical iridectomy is that it does not involve reopening an already-inflamed eye. The technique is basically that used for creating a laser iridectomy in a phakic eye,[82] with a few additional considerations.

The site chosen for the iridectomy should be opposite the site of the previous iridectomy. If only point adhesions are present at the pupillary margin (Fig. 23-8), then penetration of the iris at any point should result in release of aqueous and breakage of the block. However, broad adhesions, as mentioned, may also be present. Examination of Fig. 23-9 will show that penetration of the iris over an area of such adhesions will open a path only to the anterior hyaloid face, and the block will remain. Such adhesions are more likely to be present in the region of the previous iridectomy, which is already blocked, and are less likely to occur 180 degrees away. Adhesions may be scattered about also, and it is possible that a laser iridectomy at one site will be unsuccessful, whereas one a short distance away might be successful. If the first iridectomy is unsuccessful in releasing trapped aqueous but was not difficult to perform, we prefer to attempt a second one 90 degrees away before considering surgical intervention. The cornea must be reasonably clear to perform laser treatment.

Laser iridectomy can be quite difficult to perform when the pupil is middilated or wider, since the iris stroma is correspondingly thicker. An attempt should be made to bring down the pupil with miotics. Stretch burns of 500-μm spot size, 0.5 second's duration, and 150 mW power, placed on either side of the selected site, may succeed in thinning the stroma at the selected site. It is also possible that the "humping" effect on either side of the burns may assist in breaking adhesions to the hyaloid.

If two laser iridectomies do not succeed in breaking the block, surgical iridectomy is indicated. Since it has already been shown that large

---

*References 15, 18, 32, 56, 76.

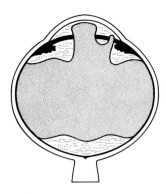

FIG. 23-8. Pupillary block secondary to vitreous occlusion of pupil and iridectomy. Point adhesions are present between anterior hyaloid face and iris at pupillary margin.

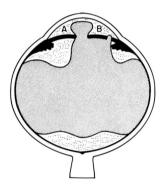

FIG. 23-9. Pupillary block with broad adhesions between anterior hyaloid face and iris in one area and point adhesions in another. Laser iridectomy will be unsuccessful when performed over these adhesions **(B),** but successful when performed over the region of sequestered aqueous **(A).**

pockets of aqueous are not present, we prefer a sector iridectomy in order to have the greatest chance of finding smaller pockets. Surgical iridectomy has long been used in the treatment of pupillary block.* If this is unsuccessful, incision of the anterior hyaloid face† or a partial anterior vitrectomy[21] may be performed to allow aqueous trapped behind the vitreous to reach the anterior chamber. Infusion-suction cutters can also be used to remove membranes occluding the pupil.[42]

Transfixion of the iris has been advocated as a simple method of alleviating pupillary block, but we find it superfluous when following the above

*References 11, 15, 20, 26, 92.
†References 1, 22, 89, 92, 95.

protocol, and it may lead to problems with the vitreous. A retroiridial sweep with a spatula to break adhesions has also been reported to be successful.[39]

Vitreociliary block (malignant glaucoma)

If iridectomy is unsuccessful in relieving the suspected pupillary block, a diagnosis of vitreociliary block (aphakic malignant glaucoma) must be entertained. This is fully discussed in Chapter 22. Briefly, forward movement of the ciliary body, aggravated by posterior vitreous detachment, results in blockage of the posterior chamber and pupil by vitreous. Aqueous is misdirected posteriorly and pools either retrovitreally, intravitreally, or both. This leads to a further increase in forward pressure by the vitreous, and a cycle is created. Mydriatic-cycloplegic treatment, successful in treating malignant glaucoma in the phakic patient,[16] is of no use in the aphakic patient. Surgical treatment is necessary once the diagnosis has been established.

Flat anterior chamber with peripheral anterior synechiae

Peripheral anterior synechiae are seen most often in aphakic eyes when a flat chamber from any cause has complicated the postoperative period. The incidence of PAS formation is related to the length of time that the chamber remains flat. Exacerbating factors include the degree of intraocular inflammation, vitreous loss, and iris prolapse.[38]

There is no fixed length of time during which the anterior chamber must remain flat before peripheral anterior synechiae will form. It may be as short as 2 to 3 days in some patients and as long as 2 weeks in others. Cotlier[19] found that secondary glaucoma did not develop if the anterior chamber was flat for less than 6 days but did develop in 13.5% of his patients when the chamber was flat for longer than 5 days. Kronfeld[56] found an incidence of glaucoma of 53% if the chamber was absent for 9 or more days.

Peripheral anterior synechiae can also be seen as a result of cataract extraction in eyes in which no flat chamber has supervened. Adherence of the peripheral iris to the cataract incision due to incorporation of the iris into the closing sutures or due to partial prolapse of the iris is a contributing factor.

In some eyes the elevation of intraocular pressure is lower than one would expect from the apparent extent of the PAS formation.[15] In these eyes the peripheral iris is adherent to the peripheral cornea anterior to the meshwork and does not occlude the meshwork itself. Although broad peripheral anterior synechiae may be present on gonioscopy, the angle itself is not closed, and the intraocular pressure may remain normal, since aqueous has access to the meshwork in the tunnel behind the iris adhesion. Chandler and Simmons[15] believe that bridging peripheral anterior synechiae are especially likely when choroidal detachment accompanies a flat chamber.

Attempts to free the meshwork from the synechiae by dissecting the peripheral iris have been largely regarded as unproductive. The impairment of aqueous outflow seems to result not only from actual occlusion of the meshwork but also from intrinsic damage to it. Medical therapy is the first line of treatment for this form of glaucoma, but surgical treatment may be required in severe cases.

Neovascular glaucoma

As in phakic eyes, iris neovascularization leads to elevated intraocular pressure by direct occlusion of the meshwork and by closure of the angle by peripheral anterior synechiae, which result from contraction of the neovascular membrane. In aphakic eyes, pupillary block due to iridovitreal synechiae with new vessels is an additional mechanism.

The angle may be open or closed. The central anterior chamber usually remains deep. In those eyes with pupillary block, classic signs such as adherence of the pupil and margins of the iridectomy to the vitreous face, marked iris bombé, and appositional and/or synechial closure of the angle may be observed.

Treatment of neovascular glaucoma in the aphakic eye is similar to that discussed for the phakic eye in Chapter 12.

CONGENITAL CATARACT AND GLAUCOMA

Glaucoma following surgical treatment of congenital cataract is common.[25,73] François[25] reported a 5% incidence whether discission or linear extraction was employed. Data is scanty for the more modern techniques using infusion-suction cutters. Mechanisms for the glaucoma include:

1. Swelling of lens remnants
2. Uveitis
3. Seclusion or occlusion of the pupil
4. Delayed reformation of the anterior chamber
5. Peripheral anterior synechiae
6. Pupillary block
7. Epithelial ingrowth
8. Recurrent hyphema

Chandler has emphasized that pupillary block frequently leads to a secondary glaucoma after surgery for congenital cataract, since iridectomy is often not performed. Even if an iridectomy is created, postoperative inflammation often causes it to become occluded.

Kurz and Einaugler[57] reported one case of recurrent hyphemas and secondary glaucoma in a patient who had undergone a needling operation for congenital cataract 37 years previously. The recurrent hyphemas arose from fibrovascular connective tissue that had invaded the lenticular remnants from the iris.

DIFFERENTIAL DIAGNOSIS

The differential diagnosis is based on a consideration of the patient's ophthalmic history, ocular examination, the temporal relationship of the intraocular pressure rise to surgery, and postoperative examination of the anterior chamber and angle.

In many patients with glaucoma, the diagnosis of elevated intraocular pressure in the early postoperative period can be made on the basis of the patient's complaint of pain and the gross appearance of the corneal edema. Gonioscopy should also be performed when elevated intraocular pressure develops, since the determination as to whether the angle is open or closed establishes the glaucoma in one of two broad categories, the approach to which may be quite different. The presence of inflammation, hyphema, lens remnants, or vitreous in the anterior chamber will guide the examiner toward the correct management.

The interval between cataract extraction and the rise in intraocular pressure is helpful in elucidating the cause of the pressure rise when the diagnosis is in doubt (Table 23-1).

MANAGEMENT
Medical therapy

The treatment of specific entities is discussed above and in the appropriate chapters. In this final section we wish to provide a few generalizations.

In the immediate postoperative period, an open-angle glaucoma of any cause need be treated only if the intraocular pressure is high enough to cause pain or corneal edema, to threaten the integrity

TABLE 23-1

Temporal relationship of glaucoma after cataract extraction

Open-angle glaucoma	
Transient postoperative intraocular pressure	Several hours
Alpha-chymotrypsin–induced	24 to 48 hours
Hyphema	2 to 7 days
Uveitis	Days to weeks
Lens particle glaucoma	Days to weeks
Steroid-induced glaucoma	Weeks
Vitreous in anterior chamber	Weeks to months
Ghost cell glaucoma	Weeks to months
Epithelial ingrowth or fibrous proliferation	Months
Primary open-angle glaucoma	Anytime
Angle-closure glaucoma	
Flat anterior chamber	1 day to 2 weeks
Pupillary block	Days to weeks; occasionally late onset
Vitreociliary block	Days to weeks
Neovascular glaucoma	Anytime

of the incision, or to compromise the vasculature of the optic nerve and retina. If a patient has damage from preexisting glaucoma, however, it becomes much more imperative to lower the intraocular pressure to prevent further damage.

The agents of choice for treatment of elevated intraocular pressure in the early postoperative period are those that decrease aqueous production. Timolol and carbonic anhydrase inhibitors may be supplemented by hyperosmotics on a temporary basis. Oral glycerin or isosorbide, or parenteral mannitol can be helpful in blunting spikes of pressure or when rapid diminution of pressure is indicated. These will successfully tide most patients over the acute episode.

Epinephrine may also be considered on a short-term basis when other agents are contraindicated for systemic reasons. The risk of cystoid macular edema makes epinephrine relatively unsuitable for long-term treatment of glaucoma in aphakic patients.* The maculopathy is dose related and develops weeks to months after the initiation of treatment. The incidence is approximately 20% to 30% of patients treated and varies with the concentration of epinephrine used.[54] Fortunately, with

*References 54, 63, 67, 69, 97.

rare exception, this entity is reversible after discontinuation of the drug.[63]

When inflammation is judged to contribute to an elevation of intraocular pressure, intensive steroid treatment is indicated. Although studies are inconclusive regarding the effects of steroids on routine postoperative inflammation, they should certainly be used when inflammation is severe. Caution needs to be exercised with regard to prolonged or intensive use after the inflammation has cleared, since some patients may develop a secondary steroid-induced elevation of pressure.

Miotics do not have a place in the treatment of early-onset open-angle glaucoma, since these tend to exacerbate intraocular inflammation. Nevertheless, the use of echothiophate to control open-angle glaucoma in the early postoperative period has been advocated.[32]

In intermediate- and late-onset glaucoma, when the eye has quieted from postoperative inflammation, cholinergic agents, when indicated, can be used effectively. Strong cholinergics, such as echothiophate, no longer contraindicated on the basis of cataractogenesis, become useful and may have a more potent effect than in the phakic eye.[35] Because the incidence of retinal detachment is higher in the aphakic eye, a thorough peripheral retinal examination should be performed before miotic therapy is initiated.

Surgical therapy

Only rarely are open-angle glaucomas in the early postoperative period not self-limited or readily controlled with medical therapy. In cases where surgery does become necessary, a simple anterior chamber paracentesis may suffice to lower pressure for a long-enough period to allow the process to ameliorate. This is also a useful procedure in air block, whereas a hyphema or ghost cell glaucoma may be treated by anterior chamber washout.

Most patients with glaucoma associated with aphakia who come to surgery in the late postoperative period have either primary open-angle glaucoma or chronic angle-closure glaucoma that cannot be controlled medically. A number of procedures have been suggested for the treatment of these entities.

Trabeculectomy

The success rate of trabeculectomy for glaucoma in aphakia has often been reported to be approximately 50%. The major cause for failure has been scarring of the conjunctiva due to previous intraocular surgery. Other factors include vitreous plugging of the filtration site, increased postoperative inflammation leading to sealing of the bleb, and technical difficulties encountered in performing the surgery.

It is our impression that trabeculectomy performed in the aphakic eye has nearly the same success rate as that performed in the phakic eye if certain precautions are taken. The technical aspects of the procedure are essentially the same as in phakic eyes. Preoperative preparation with hyperosmotic agents may aid in keeping the vitreous away from the operative site. Our preference is to operate from below to avoid a previously scarred conjunctiva, unless a corneal incision was used for the cataract extraction. Either a limbus-based or a fornix-based flap may be used. When the latter is the case, we prefer to suture it back to the cornea with several 11-0 nylon sutures. The patient's head should be tilted back to prevent the vitreous face from coming too close to the trabeculectomy site, where it might be inadvertently cut when the iridectomy is made.

If there is any question of the vitreous face not being intact, it is useful to perform an anterior vitrectomy with an infusion-suction cutter through the filtration site after a broad-based iridectomy has been made. Certainly, if vitreous presents at the time of creation of the iridectomy, an anterior vitrectomy should be performed. If cataract extraction has been extracapsular, a vitrectomy is not necessary unless vitreous is lost during the trabeculectomy procedure. Inflammation should be vigorously controlled with periocular steroids at the time of surgery and with both topical and systemic steroids postoperatively. Gentle massage to keep the filtration site open and the bleb expanded should be used when the intraocular pressure rises above 15 mm Hg postoperatively.

Cyclocryotherapy

Cyclocryotherapy has been primarily advocated for eyes with uncontrolled glaucoma that have undergone unsuccessful attempts at surgery and for eyes with neovascular glaucoma. Its effects are unpredictable, and the procedure is associated with a high incidence of complications. These include cataract formation in the phakic patient and phthisis, anterior segment necrosis, intraocular hemorrhage, and macular edema, particularly in patients with neovascular glaucoma. Many variations of the technique, differing in the temperature and placement of the probe, duration and number of applications, and circumferential extent of treatment, have been reported.

Bellows and Grant[6] have recently recommended cyclocryotherapy as the primary procedure for glaucoma in the nonneovascular aphakic eye. Crucial considerations regarding the procedure are placement of the anterior edge of the probe tip 2.5 mm from the limbus to ensure freezing over the pars plicata, a single-freeze technique rather than a freeze-thaw-refreeze technique, and initial treatment of an area over 180 degrees rather than 360 degrees to avoid overtreatment. The entire 360-degree circumference should never be treated, even with repeated treatments if the first is unsuccessful. Bellows and Grant have hypothesized that the effectiveness of the procedure might be due to the decreased blood supply to the ciliary body in elderly patients, particularly after cataract extraction, and that after zonular rupture the ciliary processes might retract to a location more readily frozen than that found in the phakic patient.

Although our first choice of surgical procedure is trabeculectomy, cyclocryotherapy, when performed carefully, provides a reasonable backup in uncomplicated aphakic patients when the former fails.

Cyclodialysis

Cyclodialysis has been advocated as the surgical procedure of choice for glaucoma associated with aphakia.[27,92] It has gradually been declining in popularity over the last few years, since its results are highly unpredictable and often temporary. Prolonged hypotony, leading to ciliary detachment, macular edema, and papilledema, is a common complication. Frequently the cyclodialysis cleft seals, resulting in an elevation of intraocular pressure. The procedure may have a place in the management of aphakic eyes with peripheral anterior synechiae in which trabeculectomy has failed.

Argon laser photocoagulation of ciliary processes

Successful reduction of intraocular pressure by photocoagulation of the ciliary processes has been reported.[59,66] Because the ciliary epithelium may be capable of regeneration, and because extensive photocoagulation is necessary to achieve a measurable reduction in aqueous production, a longer follow-up is necessary before this procedure can be generally recommended.

Laser trabeculoplasty

Argon laser treatment of the trabecular meshwork has now been shown to produce excellent results in primary open-angle glaucoma in phakic patients with reported follow-ups of as long as 4 years.[100,101] The rationale of this procedure is predicated on the hypothesis that senile collapse of the trabecular meshwork leads to blockage of aqueous outflow and a resultant elevation of intraocular pressure. Reversal of trabecular collapse should then increase the facility of aqueous outflow and reduce intraocular pressure. The hypothesized mechanism of action of laser treatment is based on the presumption that heat absorption by the corneoscleral meshwork leads to scarring of the internal portion of the trabecular meshwork. This in turn causes shrinkage of the corneoscleral meshwork, physically pulling open the juxtacanalicular meshwork and Schlemm's canal. There is some histologic evidence for this hypothesis.[100] In one study, outflow facility increased by 50% in 13 eyes in which tonography was performed before and after the procedure.[99]

The procedure does not work as well in aphakic patients but still has a success rate of approximately 50%,[101] and side effects are minimal when it is properly performed. The results in the small numbers of pseudophakic patients treated to date appear to be at least as good as those in aphakic patients and perhaps better.[100a] This may be related to the degree of tension transmitted to the trabecular meshwork through the iris root by the weight of the lens. It will be interesting eventually to compare the results of the procedure in patients with iris plane lenses with those in patients with posterior chamber lenses, in whom a significant portion of the zonular system remains intact.

With regard to the secondary glaucomas, laser treatment works well in the treatment of exfoliation syndrome and pigmentary glaucoma. It does not appear to be successful in the treatment of glaucoma secondary to uveitis, even when the angle is open and not visibly affected by inflammatory precipitates. Wise (personal communication, 1981) has reported success in two patients with angle recession, but two patients of ours have not been controlled. The degree of scarring of the meshwork may be the determining factor. Laser treatment has not yet been sufficiently evaluated in other forms of secondary open-angle glaucoma. At the time of this writing, we advocate laser trabeculoplasty as the initial procedure in the aphakic patient with primary open-angle glaucoma, exfoliation syndrome, and pigmentary glaucoma in whom surgery is considered necessary. However, it is not successful in those cases in which vitreous fills the anterior chamber.[101] In general, if the meshwork is "collapsed," there is a reasonable chance of success, whereas if the meshwork is physically obstructed, such as by scarring, inflammation, or endothelialization, the procedure would not be expected to be successful.

Patients undergoing laser trabeculoplasty have not been routinely pretreated with aspirin as they are before laser iridectomy but are routinely posttreated with topical steroids for 1 week.

The patient is given a topical anesthetic, and an antireflective gonioscopy lens is used. The laser is set initially at a 50-μm spot size, 0.1 second's duration, and 1000 mμ power. One should aim for the pigmented portion of the trabecular meshwork, attempting to hit on its anterior aspect toward Schwalbe's line rather than the posterior aspect, since burns on the scleral spur and ciliary face result in postoperative uveitis and PAS formation.

The desired result is blanching and small-bubble formation on the pigmented portion of the meshwork. If large bubbles are obtained, the power should be turned down. If there is no effect, it should be turned up. Our range has been between 700 and 1200 mW. Although a total of 100 spots over 360 degrees of the meshwork was originally recommended,[101] we have also obtained good results with 50 spots and usually place somewhere between 50 and 80 spots on the theory that more can be added later if necessary. Success is better in older patients and in those with more pigment on the trabecular meshwork.

Patients should be continued on a regimen of antiglaucoma medication after the procedure rather than having it tapered rapidly, since it may take up to 3 weeks for the pressure to stabilize. Some patients have an immediate drop, whereas others may have a transient rise in pressure immediately after the procedure, presumably because of edema of the meshwork and further lowering of the outflow facility. For this reason, patients should be kept in the office for an hour or two after the procedure so that their intraocular pressures can be measured and appropriate treatment instituted if the pressure rises.

REFERENCES

1. Allen, J.C.: Surgical treatment of pupillary block, Ann. Ophthalmol. **9:**661, 1977.
2. Anderson, D.R.: Experimental alpha-chymotrypsin glaucoma studied by scanning electron microscopy, Am. J. Ophthalmol. **71:**470, 1971.
3. Anderson, D.R., Forster, R.K., and Lewis, M.L.: Laser iridotomy for aphakic pupillary block, Arch. Ophthalmol. **93:**343, 1975.
4. Barkan, O.: Glaucoma induced by air blockade, Am. J. Ophthalmol. **34:**567, 1951.
5. Beidner, B., Rothkoff, L., and Blumenthal, M.: The effect of acetazolamide on early increased intraocular pressure after cataract extraction, Am. J. Ophthalmol. **83:**565, 1977.
6. Bellows, A.R., and Grant, W.M.: Cyclocryotherapy of chronic open-angle glaucoma in aphakic eyes, Am. J. Ophthalmol. **83:**615, 1978.
7. Bigger, J.F., and Becker, B.: Cataracts and primary open-angle glaucoma: the effect of uncomplicated cataract extraction on glaucoma control, Trans. Am. Acad. Ophthalmol. Otolaryngol. **75:**260, 1971.
8. Bloomfield, S.: Failure to prevent enzyme glaucoma, Am. J. Ophthalmol. **65:**405, 1968.
9. Bowman, W.: On extraction of cataract by a traction-instrument with iridectomy with remarks on capsular obstructions and their treatment, Ophthalmic Hosp. Rec. (London) **4:**332, 1863-1865.
10. Campbell, D.G., and Grant, W.M.: Trabecular deformation and reduction of outflow facility due to cataract and penetrating keratoplasty sutures, Invest. Ophthalmol. Supp. **16:**126, 1977.
11. Chandler, P.A.: Glaucoma from pupillary block in aphakia, Arch. Ophthalmol. **67:**44, 1962.
12. Chandler, P.A., and Grant, W.M.: Glaucoma, ed. 2, Philadelphia, 1979, Lea & Febiger, pp. 224-235.
13. Chandler, P.A., and Johnson, C.C.: A neglected cause of secondary glaucoma in eyes in which the lens is absent or subluxated, Arch. Ophthalmol. **37:**740, 1947.
14. Chandler, P.A., and Maumenee, A.E.: A major cause of hypotony, Am. J. Ophthalmol. **52:**609, 1961.
15. Chandler, P.A., and Simmons, R.J.: Gonioscopy during surgery for aphakic eyes with pupillary block, Am. J. Ophthalmol. **74:**571, 1972.
16. Chandler, P.A., Simmons, R.J., and Grant, W.M.: Malignant glaucoma: medical and surgical treatment, Am. J. Ophthalmol. **66:**495, 1968.
17. Cleasby, G.W.: Photocoagulation coreoplasty, Arch. Ophthalmol. **83:**145, 1970.
18. Cotlier, E.: Aphakic flat anterior chamber. II. Effect of spontaneous reformation and medical therapy, Arch. Ophthalmol. **87:**124, 1972.
19. Cotlier, E.: Aphakic flat anterior chamber. III. Effect of inflation of the anterior chamber and drainage of choroidal detachments, Arch. Ophthalmol. **88:**16, 1972.
20. Cotlier, E.: Aphakic flat anterior chamber. IV. Treatment of pupillary block by iridectomy, Arch. Ophthalmol. **88:**22, 1972.
21. Cotlier, E.: Anterior vitriotomy for aphakic flat anterior chamber, Br. J. Ophthalmol. **56:**347, 1972.
22. Cotlier, E., and Herman, S.: Aphakic flat anterior chamber: treatment by anterior vitriotomy, Arch. Ophthalmol. **86:**507, 1971.
23. Étienne, R.: Conduite à tenir en presence de l'association glaucome et cataracte, Ann. Ocul. **196:**1154, 1963.
24. Fanta, H., and Herold, I.: Spätfolgen nach enzymatischer Zonulolyse in histologischen Schnitt, Klin. Monatsbl. Augenheilkd. **142:**1011, 1963.
25. François, J.: Glaucoma and uveitis after congenital cataract surgery, Ann. Ophthalmol. **3:**131, 1971.
26. François, J.: Aphakic glaucoma, Ann. Ophthalmol. **6:**429, 1974.
27. Galin, M.A.: Surgical technique of cyclodialysis and lens extraction, Ann. Ophthalmol. **7:**1257.
28. Galin, M.A., Barasch, K.R., and Harris, L.S.: Enzymatic zonulysis and intraocular pressure, Am. J. Ophthalmol. **61:**690, 1966.
29. Galin, M.A., Hung, P.T., and Obstbaum, S.A.: Cataract extraction in glaucoma, Am. J. Ophthalmol. **87:**124, 1979.
30. Galin, M.A., Lin, L.L., and Obstbaum, S.A.: Cataract extraction and intraocular pressure, Trans. Ophthalmol. Soc. U.K. **98:**124, 1978.
31. Gombos, G.M., and Oliver, M.: Cataract extraction with enzymatic zonulolysis in glaucomatous eyes, Am. J. Ophthalmol. **64:**69, 1967.
32. Gorin, G.: Echothiophate iodide for glaucoma or flat anterior chamber following cataract extraction, Am. J. Ophthalmol. **67:**392, 1969.
33. Gormaz, A.: Ocular tension after cataract surgery, Am. J. Ophthalmol. **53:**832, 1962.
34. Grant, W.M.: Open-angle glaucoma with vitreous filling the anterior chamber following cataract extraction, Trans. Am. Ophthalmol. Soc. **61:**96, 1963.
35. Guyton, J.S.: Choice of operation for primary glaucoma combined with cataract extraction, Arch. Ophthalmol. **33:**265, 1945.
35a. Haimann, M.H., and Phelps, C.D.: Prophylactic timolol for the prevention of high intraocular pressure after cataract extraction, Ophthalmology **88:**233, 1981.
36. Hervouet, F.: Nouvelles précisions histologiques sur l'action de l'alpha chymotrypsine sur les tissues oculaires, An. Inst. Barraquer **3:**194, 1962.
37. Hilding, A.C.: Reduced ocular tension after cataract surgery, Arch. Ophthalmol. **53:**686, 1955.
38. Hitchings, R.A.: Aphakic glaucoma: prophylaxis and management, Trans. Ophthalmol. Soc. U.K. **98:**118, 1978.
39. Hitchings, R.A.: Acute aphakic pupil block glaucoma: an alternative surgical approach, Br. J. Ophthalmol. **63:**31, 1979.
40. Hudson, A.C.: Injury to the vitreous body as a factor in the production of secondary glaucoma, R. London Ophthalmic Hosp. Rep. **18:**203, 1911.
41. Iglesios, F.G.: La zonulolisis enzimatica de Barraquer, An. Inst. Barraquer **1:**3, 1960.

42. Jacklin, H.N.: Excision of pupillary membrane after cataract extraction with the vitreous infusion suction cutter, Am. J. Ophthalmol. **79:**1050, 1975.

43. Jaffe, N.S.: Cataract surgery and its complications, ed. 3, St. Louis, 1981, The C.V. Mosby Co.

44. Jaffe, N.S., and Light, D.S.: The danger of air pupillary block glaucoma in cataract surgery with osmotic hypotonia, Arch. Ophthalmol. **76:**633, 1966.

45. Jocson, V.L.: Tonography and gonioscopy before and after cataract extraction with alpha-chymotrypsin, Am. J. Ophthalmol. **60:**318, 1965.

46. Kaufman, I.H.: Intraocular pressure after lens extraction, Am. J. Ophthalmol. **59:**722, 1965.

47. Kirsch, R.E.: Glaucoma following cataract extraction associated with use of alpha chymotrypsin, Arch. Ophthalmol. **72:**612, 1964.

48. Kirsch, R.E.: Further studies on glaucoma following cataract extraction associated with the use of alpha chymotrypsin, Trans. Am. Acad. Ophthalmol. Otolaryngol. **69:** 1011, 1965.

49. Kirsch, R.E.: Dose relationship of alpha-chymotrypsin in production of glaucoma after cataract extraction, Arch. Ophthalmol. **75:**774, 1966.

50. Kirsch, R.E., Levine, O., and Singer, J.A.: The ridge at the internal edge of the cataract incision, Arch. Ophthalmol. **94:**2098, 1976.

51. Kirsch, R.E., Levine, O., and Singer, J.A.: Further studies on the ridge at the internal edge of the cataract incision, Trans. Am. Acad. Ophthalmol. Otolaryngol. **83:** OP-224, 1977.

52. Knapp. H.: Ueber Glaucom nach Discission des Nachstarrs und seine Heilung, Arch. Augenhielkd. **30:**1, 1895.

53. Kolker, A.E.: Visual prognosis in advanced glaucoma: a comparison of medical and surgical therapy for retention of vision in 101 eyes with advanced glaucoma, Trans. Am. Ophthalmol. Soc. **75:**539, 1977.

54. Kolker, A.E., and Becker, B.: Epinephrine maculopathy, Arch. Ophthalmol. **79:**552, 1968.

55. Kornzweig, A.C., and Schneider, J.: Cataract extraction in glaucoma cases, Ann. Ophthalmol. **6:**959, 1974.

56. Kronfeld, P.C.: Delayed restoration of the anterior chamber, Am. J. Ophthalmol. **38:**483, 1954.

57. Kurz, G.H., and Einaugler, R.B.: Intralenticular hemorrhage following discussion of congenital cataract, Am. J. Ophthalmol. **66:**1163, 1968.

58. Lantz, J.M., and Quigley, J.H.: Intraocular pressure after cataract extraction: effects of alpha-chymotrypsin, Can. J. Ophthalmol. **8:**339, 1973.

59. Lee, P.F.: Argon laser photocoagulation of the ciliary processes in cases of aphakic glaucoma, Arch. Ophthalmol. **97:**2135, 1979.

60. Lessell, S., and Kuwabara, T.: Experimental alpha-chymotrypsin glaucoma, Arch. Ophthalmol. **81:**853, 1969.

61. Leydhecker, W.: Histologische Untersuchung am Trabekelsystem nach kurzfristiger Einwiklung von alphachymotrypsin, Klin. Monatsbl. Augenheilkd. **142:**554, 1963.

62. Linn, J.G.: Cataract extraction in management of glaucoma, Trans. Am. Acad. Ophthalmol. Otolaryngol. **75:** 273, 1971.

63. Mackool, R.J., Muldoon, T., Fortier, A., and Nelson, D.: Epinephrine-induced cystoid macular edema in aphakic eyes, Arch. Ophthalmol. **95:**791, 1977.

64. Mamo, J.G.: Late effects of vitreous loss, Ann. Ophthalmol. **6:**935, 1974.

65. Manezo, J.L., Marco, M., and Mascarell, E.V.: Enzymatic ocular hypertension: a statistical study, J. Fr. Ophthalmol. **1:**289, 1978.

66. Merritt, J.C.: Transpupillary photocoagulation of the ciliary processes, Ann. Ophthalmol. **8:**325, 1976.

67. Michels, R.G., and Maumenee, A.E.: Cystoid macular edema associated with topically applied epinephrine in aphakic eyes, Am. J. Ophthalmol. **80:**379, 1975.

68. Miller, J.R., and Morin, J.D.: Intraocular pressure after cataract extraction, Am. J. Ophthalmol. **66:**523, 1968.

69. Obstbaum, S.A., Galin, M.A., and Poole, T.A.: Topical epinephrine and cystoid macular edema, Ann. Ophthalmol. **8:**455, 1976.

69a. Packer, A.J., Fraioli, A.J., and Epstein, D.L.: The effect of timolol and acetazolamide on transient intraocular pressure elevation following cataract extraction with alpha-chymotrypsin, Ophthalmology **88:**239, 1981.

70. Palimeris, G., Chimonidou, E., Magouritsas, N., and Velissaropoulos, P.: Cataract extraction in chronic simple glaucoma, Ophthalmic Surg. **5:**62, 1974.

71. Patti, J.C., and Cinotti, A.A.: Iris photocoagulation therapy of aphakic pupillary block, Arch. Ophthalmol. **93:**347, 1975.

72. Petrelli, E.A., and Wiznia, R.A.: Argon laser photocoagulation of inner wound vascularization after cataract extraction, Am. J. Ophthalmol. **84:**58, 1977.

73. Phelps, C.D., and Arafat, N.I.: Open-angle glaucoma following surgery for congenital cataracts, Arch. Ophthalmol. **95:**1985, 1977.

74. Pollack, I.P.: Use of argon laser energy to produce iridotomies, Trans. Am. Ophthalmol. Soc. **77:**674, 1979.

75. Ray, R.R., and Binkhorst, R.D.: The diagnosis of pupillary block by intravenous injection of fluorescein, Am. J. Ophthalmol. **61:**481, 1966.

76. Reese, A.B.: Herniation of the anterior hyaloid membrane following uncomplicated intracapsular cataract extraction, Trans. Am. Ophthalmol. Soc. **46:**73, 1948.

77. Reese, A.B.: Herniation of the anterior hyaloid membrane following uncomplicated intracapsular cataract extraction, Am. J. Ophthalmol. **32:**933, 1949.

78. Regan, E.F., and Day, R.M.: Cataract extraction after filtering procedures, Trans. Am. Ophthalmol. Soc. **68:** 96, 1970.

79. Rich, W.J.: Further studies on early postoperative ocular hypertension following cataract extraction, Trans. Ophthalmol. Soc. U.K. **89:**639, 1969.

80. Rich, W.J.: Prevention of postoperative ocular hypertension by prostaglandin inhibitors, Trans. Ophthalmol. Soc. U.K. **97:**268, 1977.

81. Rich, W.J., Radtke, N.D., and Cohan, B.E.: Early ocular hypertension after cataract extraction, Br. J. Ophthalmol. **58:**725, 1974.

82. Ritch, R., and Podos, S.M.: Argon laser treatment of angle-closure glaucoma, Perspect. Ophthalmol. **4:**129, 1980.

83. Roberts, W.: An unusual form of glaucoma in aphakics, Trans. Am. Acad. Ophthalmol. Otolaryngol. **69:**1024, 1965.

84. Rothkoff, L., Beidner, B., and Blumenthal, M.: The effect of corneal section on early increased intraocular pressure after cataract extraction, Am. J. Ophthalmol. **85:**337, 1978.

85. Scheie, H.G., and Ewing, M.Q.: Aphakic glaucoma, Trans. Ophthalmol. Soc. U.K. **98:**111, 1978.

86. Scheie, H.G., and Frazier, W.: Ocular hypertension induced by air in the anterior chamber, Arch. Ophthalmol. **44:**691, 1950.

87. Schwartz, L.W., Rodriguez, M.M., Spaeth, G.L., et al.: Argon laser iridotomy in the treatment of patients with primary angle-closure or pupillary block glaucoma: a clinicopathologic study, Trans. Am. Acad. Ophthalmol. Otolaryngol. **85:**294, 1978.

88. Selinger, E.: Ocular hypertension induced by air in the anterior chamber after cataract extraction, Am. J. Ophthalmol. **20:**827, 1937.

89. Simmons, R.J.: The vitreous in glaucoma, Trans. Ophthalmol. Soc. U.K. **95:**422, 1975.

90. Speakman, J.S.: Recurrent hyphema after surgery, Can. J. Ophthalmol. **10:**299, 1975.

91. Sugar, H.S.: Pupil block in aphakic eyes, Am. J. Ophthalmol. **46:**831, 1958.

92. Sugar, H.S.: Pupillary block and pupil-block glaucoma following cataract extraction, Am. J. Ophthalmol. **61:** 435, 1966.

93. Swan, K.C.: Relationship of basal iridectomy to shallow chamber following cataract extraction, Arch. Ophthalmol. **69:**191, 1963.

94. Swan, K.C.: Hyphema due to wound vascularization after cataract extraction, Arch. Ophthalmol. **89:**87, 1973.

95. Theodore, F.H.: Complications after cataract extraction, Boston, 1965, Little, Brown & Co., p. 289.

96. Theodossiadis, G., Kouris-Borgkati, E., and Velissaropoulos, P.: Clinical and pathologic-anatomical results following the application of a mobile argon-laser beam in aphakic pupillary block glaucoma, Klin. Monatsbl. Augenheilkd. **175:**180, 1979.

97. Thomas, J.V., Gragoudas, E.S., Blair, N.P., and Lapus, J.V.: Correlation of epinephrine use and macular edema in aphakic glaucomatous eyes, Arch. Ophthalmol. **96:** 625, 1978.

98. Wiesel, J., and Swan, K.C.: Mydriatic therapy of shallow chamber after cataract extraction, Arch. Ophthalmol. **58:**126, 1957.

99. Wilensky, J.T., and Jampol, L.M.: Laser therapy for open angle glaucoma, Ophthalmology **88:**213, 1981.

100. Wise, J.B.: Long-term control of adult open angle glaucoma by argon laser treatment, Ophthalmology **88:**197, 1981.

100a. Wise, J.B.: Personal communication, 1981.

101. Wise, J.B., and Witter, S.L.: Argon laser therapy for open-angle glaucoma, Arch. Ophthalmol. **97:**319, 1979.

102. Worthen, D.M.: Scanning electron microscopy after alpha-chymotrypsin perfusion in man, Am. J. Ophthalmol. **73:**637, 1972.

103. Wyman, G.J.: Glaucoma induced by air injections into the anterior chamber, Am. J. Ophthalmol. **37:**424, 1954.

Chapter 24

GLAUCOMA AND INTRAOCULAR LENS IMPLANTATION

William E. Layden

Ridley reported the first intraocular lens (IOL) implantation in 1949.[18] Following its inception, the technique was pursued principally in Europe. Initial complication rates were high, but with technical evolution there has been a significant reduction in operative and postoperative problems. During the past decade lens implantation has become an increasingly popular procedure in the United States.

Developmentally there has been considerable variation in lens design, technique of implantation, and anatomic location of intended implantation site within the eye.[18] Originally lenses were placed in the posterior chamber. This was followed by a proliferation of surgical procedures and lens designs that have in common the placement of the implant at or about the pupil with fixation to the iris by several means. This type of IOL implantation has been widely employed in the United States and accounts for the bulk of available data on complication rates. Other techniques that have evolved include IOL placement in the anterior chamber with angle support, and, more recently, a return to posterior chamber placement with support by the ciliary body and/or posterior lens capsule. Posterior chamber insertion is associated with extracapsular lens removal, whereas iris fixation is performed with either intracapsular or extracapsular cataract extraction.

Glaucoma is a recognized complication following IOL implantation as it has been with the traditional extracapsular and intracapsular methods of cataract removal where visual correction is accomplished by spectacle or contact lens. There are several distinct considerations regarding the analysis of glaucoma associated with lens implantation. These include (1) lens placement in eyes with preexisting glaucoma, (2) implantation in eyes without preexisting glaucoma but with secondary glaucoma resulting postoperatively, and (3) how the latter compares with cataract extraction without lens implantation.

LENS IMPLANTATION WITH PREEXISTING GLAUCOMA

Assessment of the effect of IOL placement in eyes with preoperative glaucoma is somewhat difficult because of the uncertain effects of cataract extraction without pseudophakia on the postoperative pressure in normal and glaucomatous eyes.[3,13,24] The degree and duration of the possible pressure-lowering tendency in cataract extraction is quite variable. The amount of medication needed postoperatively to control preexisting glaucoma is a factor commonly used to analyze the relationship of surgery to later pressure problems. Other parameters to be studied are the same as those defining any form of glaucoma, such as progression of field loss, optic nerve head changes, chamber angle and corneal alterations, and visual acuity loss.

A number of studies that provide information on pseudophakia and glaucoma are now available. The majority of these indicate that the incidence of postoperative glaucoma in the pseudophakic patient with preexisting glaucoma is the same or

TABLE 24-1
Pseudophakia and glaucoma: preexisting glaucoma

Author	Eyes	Precontrol	Postcontrol
Smith and Anderson[37]	24	23/24*; 1/24	14/24*; 8/24 (2 lost)
Clayman et al[7]	48	36/48*; 12/48	18/48* 30/48
Taylor et al.[39]	43	(O) 31/32*; 1/32	24/32*; 8/32
		(N) 6/11*; 5/11	4/11*; 7/11
Drews[10]	22	(O) 14 ⎫ 5/16†; 11/16	14/16; 2/16* (1 lost)
		(N) 7 ⎬ 5/16*; 11/16†	"50% complication rate"
		(S) 1 ⎭	
Alpar[1,2]	27	(L) 27/27	9/27 bleb failure (7/27*)
	32	(NL) 32/32	11/32 bleb failure (9/32*)

*Medical therapy required.
†Number of eyes adequately followed.
O, Open-angle glaucoma; *N,* narrow-angle glaucoma; *S,* secondary glaucoma; *L,* implantation; *NL,* no implantation.

less than before surgery.* In these studies postoperative control of the glaucoma often required less medication (Table 24-1). Therefore IOL implantation in certain carefully selected glaucoma patients may be reasonable. The results of four-loop implants in open-angle glaucoma patients compared with those in a control group were similar in regard to preoperative and postoperative intraocular pressure values.[37] In a series of patients who had miosis and open-angle glaucoma, other than the mechanical difficulty of implantation of iris plane lenses associated with miosis, there were no significant problems in controlling the intraocular pressure postoperatively.[7] Other series have confirmed this finding.[9,26,28] In contrast, there is some suggestion that lens implantation in patients with chronic open-angle glaucoma is not worth the attendant risk.[15] Most series, however, show no significant difference in the preoperative and postoperative control of intraocular pressure, although it is important to note that all patients studied had controlled open-angle glaucoma before IOL implantation, usually with minimal antiglaucoma therapy.

One report, in which angle-closure glaucoma occurred preoperatively, indicated that control was easier postoperatively and that the pseudophakia did not affect these eyes adversely.[39] However, the effect of lens implantation on angle-closure glaucoma patients is less certain because of the

small number of cases reported. Lens implantation in treated acute angle-closure glaucoma patients should be approached with caution.

Even though the postoperative control of open-angle glaucoma and possibly angle-closure glaucoma may not be adversely affected in the majority of cases, there are some important considerations regarding surgical selection and postoperative management. Miotic agents, if employed following lens implantation, may produce synechiae and membranes around the implant, rendering fundus examination difficult. Drugs that dilate the pupil to facilitate visualization of the optic nerve head may cause lens dislocation. In addition to some of these postoperative medical quandaries, there are potential surgical difficulties. The iris of the medically treated glaucoma patient may be rigid because of long-standing miosis. Iris surgery may be required, resulting in the risk of excessive manipulation and corneal endothelial damage. In such instances some surgeons have performed radial iridotomies, employing iris repair with fine sutures for a pupil-supported lens.[7,10] Such surgery requires considerable experience.

Eyes that have required multiple antiglaucoma medications preoperatively and that have significant visual field and optic nerve damage may be at a greater risk with IOL implantation. Studies of such eyes are not available, but I believe that patients with severe, advanced glaucoma should not be considered for pseudophakos. A major reason for avoiding implantation in such patients is the

*References 1, 2, 7, 10, 37, 39.

possibility of further compromise of the trabecular meshwork as the result of lens placement, leading to increased intraocular pressure. Peripheral anterior synechiae (PAS) and new vessel formation in 30% of patients with anterior chamber lens implants have been reported.[23,29] The significance of this effect on long-term glaucoma control is unknown. Another reason for avoiding implantation in such patients is the surgical difficulty encountered in patients with advanced glaucoma requiring filtering surgery. Flat anterior chambers and corneal compromise may result.[19,27] Implantation in children with glaucoma is believed to be contraindicated at this time.[17]

Alpar[1] compared 15 previously filtered eyes in glaucoma patients who underwent IOL implantation with 25 previously filtered eyes in patients who underwent routine cataract extraction without IOL implantation. The study employed four different types of lenses, including iris-supported and anterior chamber lenses. Bleb failure occurred in 40% of patients receiving IOL implants and in an equal number of patients not receiving implants. The specific ease of pressure control postoperatively in 27 eyes with filtering blebs and subsequent lens implants was also studied by Alpar.[2] In these eyes nine (33%) had failure of blebs, and, of these, seven required postoperative glaucoma medication (26%). By comparison, in the same study of 32 eyes with filtering blebs and cataract extraction alone, nine (28%) required postoperative therapy. Only one eye had superior pseudophakia–corneal touch with localized edema.

Clinical picture and pathophysiology
Visual acuity

The visual acuity of eyes with preexisting glaucoma undergoing lens implantation has been reported. In one study, 89% of patients achieved a visual acuity of 6/6 to 6/12.[7] Only two eyes (4.2%) had a visual acuity of 6/60 or less. Pupillary membranes, macular degeneration, and corneal edema were cited as causes of decreased vision. In another series, 20 of 32 eyes with chronic open-angle glaucoma and IOL implants had a vision of 6/12 or better.[39] Visual acuities of 6/18 or less were due to macular degeneration or varying degrees of glaucomatous optic atrophy and field loss. It appeared that the postoperative vision was consistent with the status of the posterior segment and not a consequence of the surgical pro-

cedure. In this same report, 9 of 11 eyes with chronic angle-closure glaucoma and lens implants demonstrated a postoperative vision of 6/12 or better.[39] In another series, approximately half of 16 glaucoma patients had a postoperative vision of 6/12 or better, and in three instances visual function was worse following the procedure.[10]

It appears that in the majority of cases, visual acuity is not affected adversely by lens implantation in eyes with preexisting glaucoma if the status of the cornea, optic nerve head, visual field, and retina is judiciously correlated preoperatively.

Cornea, iris and pupil

Postoperative corneal edema has occurred in some patients with preexisting glaucoma and lens implantation (Fig. 24-1). This is more likely to occur where pressure elevations are in the range of 35 to 45 mm Hg or higher. The edema may result from corneal endothelial compromise due to either implantation surgery, glaucoma that is difficult to control, or a combination of both factors. As already noted, iris surgery, consisting of a sector iridotomy and suturing of the iris wound before or after lens implantation, may be necessary to facilitate pseudophakos placement. In regard to surgical technique, the pupil should allow secure fixation but still be large enough to permit atraumatic lens insertion.[7] When faced with the extremely miotic pupil that does not dilate, the surgeon may elect to perform iris surgery to permit cataract extraction and then place a 9-0 or 10-0 polypropylene suture, which can be tied to reform the pupil for lens implantation, in the margin of the iridotomy.[10] It is important to assess the degree of pupillary dilation preoperatively, and miotics should be discontinued several days before IOL surgery.

Anterior chamber angle

The anterior chamber angle does not appear to be affected adversely unless the mechanics of IOL implantation have been unduly complicated. There may not be a significant amount of PAS formation as compared with that of routine cataract extraction without lens implantation. Notwithstanding, the anterior chamber angle should be inspected meticulously in patients with preoperative glaucoma for the presence of peripheral anterior synechiae, which should be an indicator for caution in determining whether or not a lens should be inserted. Implant surgeons should perform careful gonioscopy on all possible candidates, particularly when employing anterior chamber lenses.[33] Contact with anterior synechiae should be avoided because superior peripheral synechiae, aggravated by IOL implantation, have been followed by late superior displacement of lenses and corneal edema.

Mechanism of glaucoma

Aggravation of preexisting glaucoma may be caused by inflammation, pigment release as a result of IOL implantation, PAS formation, pseudophakodonesis leading to prominent neovascularization (Fig. 24-2), iritis, and, questionably, biodegradation of the lens material.

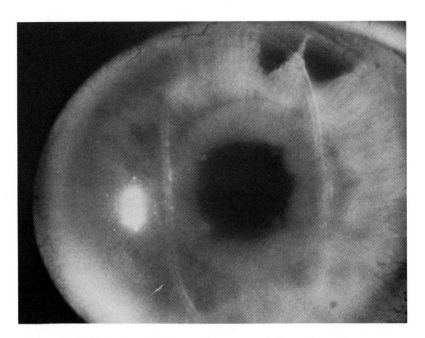

FIG. 24-1. Corneal edema with pressure of 40 to 45 mm Hg.

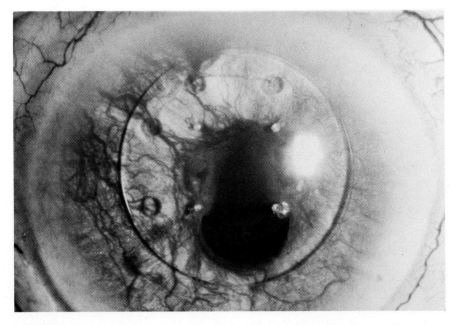

FIG. 24-2. Marked pseudophakodonesis with chronic iritis and subsequent neovascularization only in anterior segment.

LENS IMPLANTATION CAUSING SECONDARY GLAUCOMA

The FDA study comparing implant procedures with cataract controls without implants (core study) was presented to the American Academy of Ophthalmology by Worthen et al.[42] in 1979. The data in Table 24-2 indicate that iris-supported lenses and posterior chamber lenses are similar to the control rate in the occurrence of secondary glaucoma, hyphema, and uveitis. Anterior chamber lenses, however, appear to have almost twice the incidence of secondary glaucoma, as well as higher rates of hyphema and uveitis. This has been partly attributed to lens manufacture techniques

and to the association of the uveitis-glaucoma-hyphema (UGH) syndrome[11,20] (Fig. 24-3). Pupillary block (Fig. 24-4) in the FDA study was highest with this type of lens (0.6%). Pupillary block, as reported by a variety of authors (Table 24-3), has ranged from 0.2% to 6.94%. Iris-supported lenses can also produce pupillary block. The Kelman anterior chamber lens has not been found to produce pupillary block glaucoma.[6] My experience parallels that of the FDA study in that anterior chamber lenses of the Choyce design have been more often implicated in secondary pupillary block glaucoma. Data on the Choyce style of anterior chamber lens have failed to reveal sufficient in-

TABLE 24-2
Pseudophakia and glaucoma: core study—FDA

Control	Lens type			
	AC	IF	ICF	PC
3132	6650	14,360	5722	1182
Pupillary block (%) 0.4	0.6	0.3	0.3	0.0
Secondary glaucoma (%) 3.6	6.3	3.9	2.1	3.5
Hyphema (%) 2.4	5.0	3.3	2.7	0.9
Uveitis (%) 1.7	2.3	1.7	1.3	0.8
Macular edema (%) 3.2	4.9	3.0	2.2	4.3

From Worthen, D.M., Boucher, J.A., Buxton, J.N., et al.: Ophthalmology **87:**267, 1980.
AC, Anterior chamber; *IF,* iris fixation; *ICF,* iridocapsular fixation; *PC,* posterior chamber.

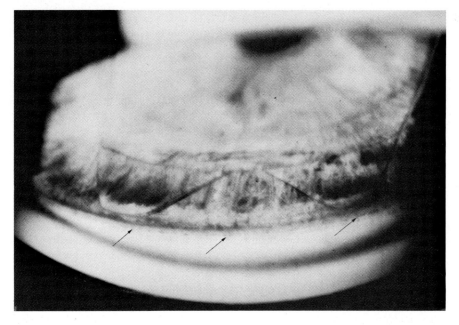

FIG. 24-3. UGH syndrome with neovascularization along feet of implant and meshwork *(arrows).*

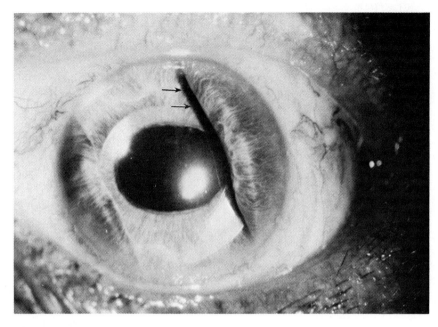

FIG. 24-4. Iris bombé secondary to pupillary block *(arrows).*

TABLE 24-3
Pseudophakia and glaucoma: pupillary block

Author	Eyes with glaucoma (lens type)	Pupillary block
Smith and Anderson[37]	26/606 iris	1/26 (1%)
Kraff et al.[22]	5/613 iris	5/5 (8%)
Werner and Kaback[41]	4/106 iris	4/4 (3.8%)
Binkhorst[4]	—iris	(0.2%)
Nordlohne[26]	—iris	(6.94%)
Phyodorov et al.[31]	3000 (L) iris	(1.8%)
	2000 (NL) iris	(0.9%)
Pearce and Ghost[30]	4/537 iris	(0.7%)
François[12]	(Review of aphakic glaucoma)	(1% to 7%)
Dagasan[8]	Extracapsular	(0.7%)
	Intracapsular	(1.5%)

L, Implantation; *NL,* no implantation.

dexes of pupillary block glaucoma. Pupillary block may result from wound leaks[14] (Fig. 24-5), improper placement of iridotomies, or a forward shift of the iris-lens diaphragm, which may follow a retinal detachment procedure.

The overall association of pseudophakia and secondary glaucoma has been studied by a number of authors. This information is summarized in Table 24-4. The incidence of secondary glaucoma following IOL implantation as a result of various mechanisms ranges from 0 to 4.3%. In comparison, François[12] has described the many causes of glaucoma in aphakia in eyes without implants, which in his study ranged from 0.7% to 7%. Dagasan[8] differentiated between extracapsular and intracapsular extractions without IOL implantation and found an incidence of 0.7% and 1.5%, respectively. It appears that most styles of lenses have been implicated in postoperative secondary glaucoma. Further studies are needed on the newer posterior chamber lenses.

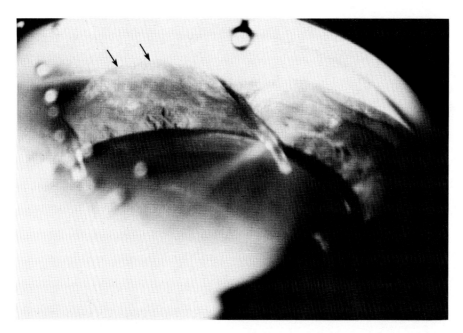

FIG. 24-5. Suspected wound leak in eye with shallow anterior chamber initially with iris incarcerated into surgical wound *(arrows)*.

TABLE 24-4
Pseudophakia and glaucoma: secondary glaucoma

Author	Eyes (lens type)	Incidence (%)
Smith and Anderson[37]	26/606 iris	4.3
Phyodorov et al.[31]	6/2700 iris	0.3
Binkhorst[4]	6/500 iris	1.2
Tennant[40]	0/160 anterior chamber	0
Kern[21]	6/200 iris	3
Taylor et al.[38]	0/100 iris	0
Drews[10]	21/300 iris	0.7
Praeger[32]	8/300 iris	0.3
Shepard[34]	5/500 iris	1
François[12]	(Review of aphakic glaucoma)	0.7 to 7 (range)

Clinical picture and pathophysiology

Visual acuity

In a series of patients with pseudophakia and pupillary block, three fourths of the patients had a visual acuity of 6/15 or greater.[41] Most reports of secondary glaucoma and pseudophakia do not contain final visual acuities. More reports are needed to gauge the effect of the induced glaucoma on vision.

In my experience, visual acuity can be severely compromised when lenses are inserted in eyes with severe preexisting secondary glaucoma and compromised corneal endothelium and corneal edema. Secondary glaucoma is a relative contraindication to lens implantation.[27] Unless the underlying secondary glaucoma is well controlled, further deterioration might occur in an already-damaged optic nerve. The visual acuity again depends on the posterior pole factors; consequently, the lens is not the sole criteria for safety or success of the IOL implant technique.

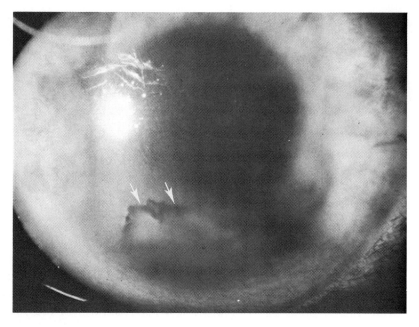

FIG. 24-6. Anterior chamber lens with hyphema that cleared medically *(arrows)*. Pressure was controlled medically.

Cornea, iris and pupil

The cornea can be severely compromised by either a secondary glaucoma or the presence of blood in the anterior chamber (Fig. 24-6). Pre-existing endothelial compromise may be a significant factor in IOL placement and secondary glaucoma.

The iris can be prominently involved in glaucoma after IOL implantation (Fig. 24-7), especially in those cases where either iris-supported or anterior chamber lenses are associated with pupillary block. A posterior chamber lens could cause pupillary block because of inflammatory response involving iris and lens material, which become adherent to the lens. In my experience, causes of glaucoma secondary to IOL implantation include obstruction of the pupil by inflammation, hemorrhage, and vitreous, as well as lens material in those cases of prior extracapsular lens extraction.

Anterior chamber angle

After lens implantation the anterior chamber angle may be compromised severely. In patients with anterior chamber lenses and pupillary block glaucoma, permanent residual PAS formation may lead to secondary glaucoma (Fig. 24-8). In patients with anterior chamber lenses, the presence of a small wound leak may explain the complica-

tions of a flat anterior chamber in sectors of the angle other than where the feet of the lens implant are situated. Bleeding or severe inflammation may result in sufficient debris in the anterior angle to cause a permanent secondary glaucoma.

The most common cause of secondary glaucoma has been some form of pupillary block. This appears to be more common with the anterior chamber lenses; however, it may be seen with iris fixation lenses and possibly with posterior chamber lenses. The mechanical presence of a lens in a pupil may create synechiae to the lens, resulting in a pupillary membrane and obstruction of flow of aqueous from posterior to anterior chamber. Inadequate iridectomies or iridotomies or coverage of these openings by feet of the lenses can contribute to the problem.

Other causes of secondary glaucoma include vitreous and lens material obstructing the trabecular meshwork. Secondary glaucoma may also result from epithelialization of the anterior chamber. In an early report, 4 of 10 eyes enucleated for intractable postoperative glaucoma showed epithelialization of the anterior chamber.[5] These eyes contained anterior chamber acrylic implants.

Many of the same factors that cause aggravation of preexisting glaucoma can also contribute to the deterioration of secondary postoperative pressure problems. The relationship of postopera-

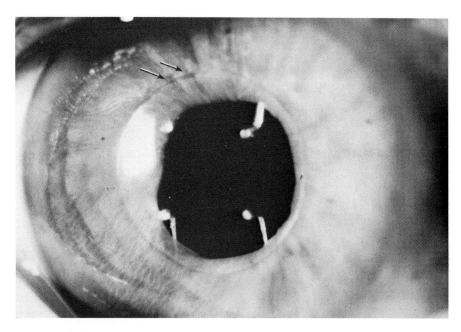

FIG. 24-7. Chronic iritis thought to be due to iris erosion with a metal loop lens *(arrows)*.

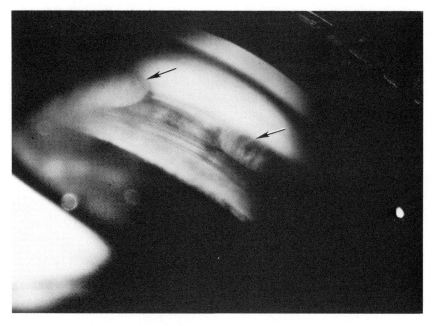

FIG. 24-8. Prominent bowing forward of iris around anterior chamber lens with subsequent residual synechiae *(arrows)*.

tive steroid medication to intraocular pressure should also be taken into consideration. On the one hand, steroids are known to be a cause of intraocular pressure elevation and should be suspected when the cause is uncertain. Conversely, topical steroids may be helpful in the control of pressure elevation when uveitis is playing a role.

Diagnosis

Slit-lamp examination

Slit-lamp examination is essential in evaluating the status of the anterior segment postoperatively and should be performed in an orderly and meticulous manner. Corneal edema and corneal endothelial compromise should be noted, as well as the presence of any inflammatory precipitates or pigment debris. It is essential to survey the surface of the iris and pupil in regard to the type and position of the implanted lens in order to detect early iris bombé with pupillary block (Fig. 24-9). One should also search for the presence of lens material around the pupil and vitreous in the anterior chamber.

Gonioscopy

Gonioscopy is fundamental to the evaluation of complications of lens implantation. Neovascularization of the angle, trabecular debris, pigment, and PAS formation may all be recognized. Gonioscopy may aid in determining whether a peripheral iridotomy is obstructed by a portion of the implant. The presence of a large amount of pigmentation in the meshwork would point suspicion toward the pigment dispersion syndrome and/or exfoliation. Gonioscopic examination of the uninvolved or unoperated eye is often helpful for comparison.

Optic nerve head evaluation

Optic nerve head evaluation is often difficult in eyes with either preexisting or secondary glaucoma after lens implantation. Inflammation, blood in the anterior segment, or vitreous debris may prevent adequate visualization of the optic nerve head. In eyes with clear anterior and posterior segments, extreme miosis or synechiae of the iris to the implant may prevent adequate fundus visualization. I use a contact lens and slit-lamp direct view of the optic nerve head whenever possible in these situations. Use of a direct ophthalmoscope with a Koeppe lens is another valuable technique that permits visualization of the optic nerve head through compromised pupillary openings. When the pupil can be dilated easily (and without fear of lens implant subluxation), visualization of the optic nerve head is readily accomplished through the usual methods, such as with Hruby lens.

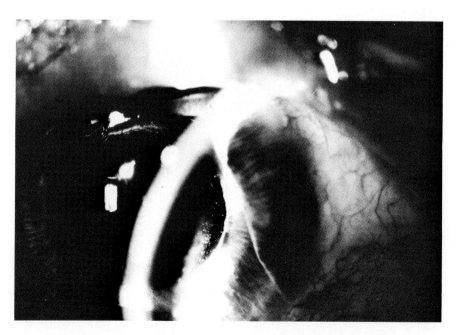

FIG. 24-9. Slit-lamp view of pupillary block.

Differential diagnosis

Recognition of hidden disorders usually presents no difficulty. The elevation of intraocular pressure is the common denominator, and the examiner should consider the various mechanisms that are known to cause glaucoma after cataract extraction with or without lens implantation. Adequate records and preoperative examinations should be helpful in distinguishing preexisting from secondary glaucoma. Again, examination of the uninvolved eye is valuable for comparison and for case analysis.

MANAGEMENT
Medical therapy

Cholinergic agents may occasionally be helpful in the control of postoperative glaucoma if the pressure elevation is not severe. However, in eyes with inflammation and synechiae, cholinergic agents are usually contraindicated, since they may aggravate the inflammatory response and increase both peripheral anterior and posterior synechiae formation. In addition miosis may increase posterior synechiae, causing pupillary block to occur more readily. Visualization of the optic nerve head and/or retina is compromised. Retinal separation is an additional hazard. In view of these problems, cholinergic agents are seldom the primary mode of medical management postoperatively in implanted eyes.

The adrenergic agents are generally preferred as the initial treatment. Beta-adrenergic blocking agents and adrenergic agonists are used. The adrenergic agents appear to help control the pressure elevation without aggravating underlying iritis and vitreous inflammation. Less pain is experienced by patients. The concomitant use of cycloplegics can be employed. Two dangers with epinephrine are the occurrence of aphakic maculopathy and the possible dislocation of some iris-supported lenses. The increasing use of anterior chamber and posterior chamber lenses as well as iris suture lenses may obviate the latter complication.

Topical steroids are used to control postoperative glaucoma caused by uveitis. The double-edged effect of steroids on intraocular pressure must be reiterated. There is a pressure-elevating effect in susceptible eyes, and the clinician must use good judgment and probably employ the minimum amount of medication necessary to control the problem. Cycloplegics and mydriatics are specifically indicated in those cases of postoperative

glaucoma caused by pupillary block. Release of the pupillary block with deepening of the anterior chamber is frequently achieved medically. Cycloplegics are also useful to combat the irritation and pain associated with inflammatory glaucoma.

The carbonic anhydrase inhibitors are a valuable adjunct in the treatment of many transient glaucoma problems and may be quite helpful with certain cases of pupillary block before surgical intervention. These agents are often useful in the long-term control of postoperative glaucoma with IOL implantation because of the numerous problems and sometimes limited effect of topical drugs.

Surgical therapy

One report has described the fate of eyes in which IOL removal was necessary.[35] In this report, visual acuity improved in 46% of patients after the lens was removed. The most common cause for lens removal was iritis and corneal decompensation. Twelve percent of patients had glaucoma requiring lens removal.

My own experience with eyes that have required removal of an implant due to uncontrolled glaucoma has not been satisfactory. Vitreous loss, deformation of the iris, further PAS formation, and corneal decompensation can all be expected in such eyes (Fig. 24-10). Anterior chamber lenses are easier to remove than other types. Iris-supported lenses and iridocapsular lenses are difficult to remove without further complications. Posterior chamber lenses must, of necessity, have severance of their haptics before they can be dislodged. However, control of the glaucoma may be easier after removal.

In those eyes in which pupillary block is recognized early, laser or surgical iridectomy can be useful to prevent further synechiae formation (Fig. 24-11).

In pseudophakic eyes, as in other forms of glaucoma, filtration procedures can be considered for the control of pressure elevation that resists all medical therapy. With the advent of the newer guarded sclerotomies such as trabeculectomy, continued surgical formation of the chamber can be accomplished, guarding against lens implant–corneal endothelial touch. Before the eye is entered, paracentesis with anterior chamber air or Healon insertion may also aid in the prevention of iris-supported or iridocapsule lenses from touching the corneal endothelium (Fig. 24-12). Anterior chamber air injection before trabeculectomy should

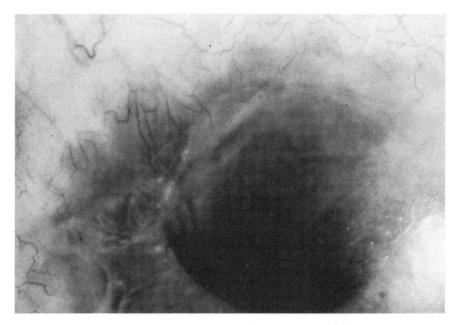

FIG. 24-10. Severe corneal damage from pseudophakos removal.

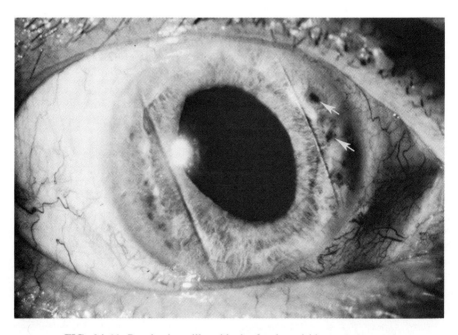

FIG. 24-11. Resolved pupillary block after laser iridectomy *(arrows)*.

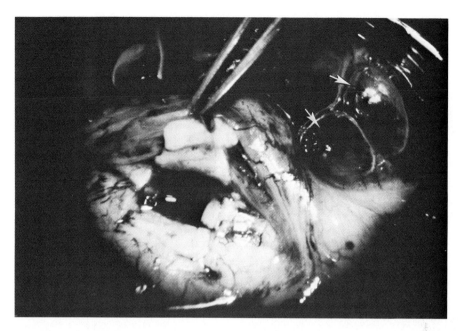

FIG. 24-12. Surgeon's view of trabeculectomy opening with air *(arrows)* retained in anterior chamber in pseudophakic eye.

also be considered in patients with anterior chamber lenses. While it is true that this lens is mechanically unable to come forward, the air blocks iris "escape" around the lens. Retention sutures, wires, and "skewer" immobilization of lenses have been described.[36] Posterior chamber lenses are a newer modality and have not yet been associated with the occurrence of glaucoma. It is not certain whether these or other techniques would be required should glaucoma develop. Other types of filtration procedures should be avoided because of the danger of collapse of the anterior chamber and endothelium–pseudophakos contact.

Cyclodialysis with simultaneous IOL implantation has been reported by Montgomery and Gills.[25] However, these authors state that the procedure necessitates an extreme amount of technical skill and should not be performed by the "ordinary surgeon." Cyclodialysis with lens implantation may be complicated by hyphema, closure of the cleft, or ocular hypotony. Cyclocryotherapy has been recommended by some.[16] Cyclocryotherapy is a destructive procedure, causing anterior chamber and vitreous inflammation. It may be used as a last resort in selected eyes. More experience is needed before a clear rationale and definitive surgical technique can be recommended with confidence for the control of refractory glaucoma in a pseudophakic eye.

REFERENCES

1. Alpar, J.J.: Cataract extraction and lens implantation in eyes with pre-existing filtering blebs, J. Am. Intraocul. Implant Soc. **5:**33, 1979.
2. Alpar, J.J.: Person communication, 1980.
3. Bigger, J.F., and Becker, B.: Cataracts and primary open angle glaucoma: the effect of uncomplicated cataract extraction on glaucoma control, Trans. Am. Acad. Ophthalmol. Otolaryngol. **75:**260, 1971.
4. Binkhorst, C.D.: Five hundred planned extracapsular extractions with irido-capsular and iris-clip lens implantation in senile cataract, Ophthalmic Surg. **8:**37, 1977.
5. Bresnick, G.H.: Eyes containing anterior chamber acrylic implants, Arch. Ophthalmol. **82:**726, 1969.
6. Buxton, J.N., Barer, C.F., Jaffe, M.S., and Manopoli, F.A.: Clinical evaluation of the Kelman anterior chamber intraocular lens, J. Am. Intraocul. Implant Soc. **4:**216, 1978.
7. Clayman, H.M., Jaffe, N.S., Light, D.S., and Eichenbaum, D.B.: Lens implantation, miosis and glaucoma, Am. J. Ophthalmol. **87:**121, 1979.
8. Dagasan, V.: Aphakic glaucoma, Ankara Univ. Tip. Fak. Goz. Klin. Yill. **18:**135, 1966.
9. Dallas, N.L.: Five year trial of the Binkhorst iris-clip lens in aphakia, Trans. Ophthalmol. Soc. U.K. **90:**725, 1970.
10. Drews, R.C.: Personal communication from transactions of the St. Vincent's Hospital meeting, 1977.
11. Ellington, F.T.: Complications with the Choyce Mark VIII anterior chamber lens implant, J. Am. Intraocul. Implant Soc. **3:**199, 1977.
12. François, J.: Aphakic glaucoma, Ann. Ophthalmol. **6:**429, 1974.
13. Galin, M.A., Lin, L.L.K., and Obstbaum, S.A.: Cataract

extraction and intraocular pressure, Trans. Ophthalmol. Soc. U.K. **98:**124, 1978.

14. Giovinco, J.: Personal communication, 1980.
15. Herschler, J.: Glaucoma and the intraocular lens, Ann. Ophthalmol. **11:**1058, 1979.
16. Herschler, J.: Personal communication, 1979.
17. Hiles, D.A.: Implant surgery in children, Int. Ophthalmol. Clin. **19**(3):95, 1979.
18. Jaffe, N.S.: The changing scene of intraocular implant lens surgery, Am. J. Ophthalmol. **88:**819, 1979.
19. Junge, J.: Combined intraocular lens implantation and trabeculectomy, J. Am. Intraocul. Implant. Soc. **3:**105, 1977.
20. Keates, R.H., and Ehrlich, R.R.: "Lenses of chance": complications of anterior chamber implants, Ophthalmology **85:**408, 1978.
21. Kern, R.: Iridocapsular lenses versus iris-clip lenses: comparison of the results and complications of 100 of each, Ophthalmic. Surg. **8:**82, 1977.
22. Kraff, M.C., Sanders, D.R., and Liebermann, H.L.: The Medallion suture lens: management of complications, Ophthalmology **86:**643, 1979.
23. Kraff, M.C., and Sanders, D.R., and Liebermann, H.L.: 300 primary anterior chamber lens implantations: gonioscopic findings and specular microscopy, J. Am. Intraocul. Implant Soc. **5:**207, 1979.
24. Miller, J.R., and Morin, J.D.: Intraocular pressure after cataract extraction, Am. J. Ophthalmol. **66:**523, 1968.
25. Montgomery, D., and Gills, J.P.: Extracapsular cataract extraction lens implantation and cyclodialysis, Ophthalmic. Surg. **11:**343, 1980.
26. Nordlohne, M.D.: The intraocular implant lens development and results with special reference to the Binkhorst lens, Doc. Ophthalmol. **38:**1, 1974.
27. Obstbaum, S.A., and Galin, M.A.: Glaucoma, cataract surgery and the intraocular lens, Int. Ophthalmol. Clin. **19**(3):139, 1979.
28. Pearce, J.L.: Long term results of the Binkhorst iris-clip lens in senile cataracts, Br. J. Ophthalmol. **56:**319, 1972.
29. Pearce, J.L.: Long term results of the Choyce anterior chamber lens implants Mark V, VII, and VIII, Br. J. Ophthalmol. **59:**99, 1975.

30. Pearce, J.L., and Ghost, T.: Surgical and postoperative problems with Binkhorst 2 and 4 loop lenses, Trans. Ophthalmol. Soc. U.K. **97:**84, 1977.
31. Phyodorov, S.N., Yegorov, E.V., and Feldman, B.G.: Analysis of 3000 operations on implantation of intraocular pupillary lens after removal of senile, congenital and complicated cataracts (Phyodorov-Zacharov lens), J. Continu. Ed. Ophthalmol., June 1979, p. 36.
32. Praeger, D.L.: Extracapsular cataract extraction with simultaneous implantation of 300 Copeland iris plane lenses: five year follow-up, a retrospective study, Ophthalmic, Surg. **10:**59, 1979.
33. Rousey, J.J.: Peripheral anterior synechiae and intraocular lenses, Am. Intraocul. Implant Soc. J. **5:**307, 1979.
34. Shepard, D.D.: Intraocular lens implantation—analysis of 500 consecutive cases, Ophthalmic. Surg. **8:**57, 1977.
35. Shepard, D.D.: The fate of eyes from which intraocular lenses have been removed, Ophthalmic. Surg. **10:**58, 1979.
36. Simcoe, C.W.: Retaining devices for protection of corneal endothelium, J. Am. Intraocul. Implant Soc. **5:**234, 1979.
37. Smith, J.A., and Anderson, D. R.: Effect of the intraocular lens on intraocular pressure, Arch. Ophthalmol. **94:**1291, 1976.
38. Taylor, D.M., Dalburg, L.A., Consentino, R.T., and Howard, R.O.: Intraocular lenses: one hundred consecutive cases of intracapsular cataract extraction with Copeland iris plane lens implantation, Ophthalmic. Surg. **6:**13, 1975.
39. Taylor, D.M., and Stein, A.L.: Long term follow-up of 43 intraocular lenses in eyes with primary glaucoma, J. Am. Intraocular Implant Soc. **5:**313, 1979.
40. Tennant, J.L.: Results of primary and secondary implants using Choyce Mark VIII lenses, Ophthalmic. Surg. **8:**54, 1977.
41. Werner, D., and Kaback, M.: Pseudophakic pupillary block glaucoma, Br. J. Ophthalmol. **61:**329, 1977.
42. Worthen, D.M., Boucher, J.A., Buxton, J.N., et al.: Interim FDA report on intraocular lenses, Ophthalmology **87:**267, 1980.

Chapter 25

EPITHELIAL INGROWTH AND FIBROUS PROLIFERATION

Walter J. Stark and William E. Bruner

Epithelial ingrowth and fibrous proliferation are two complications that can follow anterior segment surgery or penetrating injuries to the globe. Both complications are rather rare, but they can lead to secondary glaucoma. Epithelial ingrowth often leads to loss of the eye if it is not diagnosed and treated early, whereas fibrous proliferation is usually a less serious complication and is not as likely to cause severe glaucoma or loss of the eye. However, fibrous proliferation may occur after an injury to the eye that is severe enough in itself to result in loss of the eye. The term epithelial downgrowth is synonymous with epithelial ingrowth, which is now the preferred term.

HISTORICAL BACKGROUND

Rothmund[51] (1872) postulated that anterior chamber cysts resulted from implantation of epithelium into the anterior chamber during trauma. This was confirmed histopathologically in 1891.[16] Perera[46] (1937) established a classification of epithelial involvement of the eye in which he divided the problem into three types: (1) "pearl" tumors of the iris, (2) epithelial posttraumatic cysts, and (3) epithelialization of the anterior chamber. Since then, a number of case reports have appeared in the literature on the diagnosis and treatment of the disease. Recent advances have included the use of photocoagulation[14,41,45] in the diagnosis and treatment of epithelial invasion and also the use of cryotherapy and vitrectomy instrumentation in its treatment.[8,57]

Fibrous ingrowth, or proliferation, which includes retrocorneal fibrous membrane and stromal ingrowth, was not really recognized until 1914, when Henderson[31] first discussed its pathogenesis. He differentiated between the healing processes of limbal and corneal incisions and found that prolapse of the lens capsule or iris into a limbal wound allowed the growth of subconjunctival fibrous tissue into the anterior chamber. Several authors later reported the incidence of fibrous ingrowth after intraocular surgery to be 25% to 30% in eyes enucleated after surgery.[5,20,71] There are two basic types of fibrous proliferation in the anterior segment.[69] One is that seen after severe penetrating ocular trauma or faulty wound closure at the time of surgery. The other is the retrocorneal membrane caused by endothelial metaplasia.[36] Epiretinal and posterior vitreal fibrous proliferation are not discussed here in detail.

PATHOPHYSIOLOGY
Epithelial invasion
Pearl tumors

Pearl tumors of the iris may result from traumatic implantation of a piece of skin or hair follicle into the anterior chamber.[43] These lesions are extremely rare and clinically appear as solid, pearly white tumors on the iris surface and are not connected with any entrance wound. They are slow growing and usually quite benign, although they may be accompanied by an inflammatory reaction. Histologically the tumors are encapsulated, consisting of layers of epithelium. There is usually a central core of amorphous necrotic tissue or of keratinized cells arranged in concentric layers. The course of pearl tumors is benign and generally not

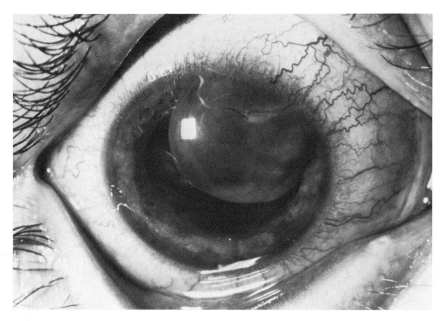

FIG. 25-1. Large epithelial cyst in patient following penetrating injury.

associated with secondary glaucoma or loss of an eye. No treatment is necessary.

Epithelial cysts

Epithelial cysts and true epithelial ingrowth need to be differentiated because of their vastly different clinical courses, treatments, and prognoses. However, the pathophysiologies of the two are probably very similar. Epithelial cysts appear as translucent or gray cysts in the anterior chamber, and they may connect with an area of previous perforation of the globe (Fig. 25-1). They are usually readily diagnosed. The rate of growth of these cysts is highly variable, some showing virtually no growth and others becoming large enough to cause secondary glaucoma.

Numerous attempts have been made to reproduce epithelial cysts experimentally in animals.* Those few experiments that were successful required the implantation of full-thickness conjunctiva, an in-turned conjunctival flap, or a large gaping wound with iris prolapse.[50] Free implants of pure conjunctival or corneal epithelium almost always were reabsorbed.

Mechanical factors rather than a difference in cell type seem to determine whether an epithelial cyst occurs or, instead, a sheet of ingrowth develops.[13,30] These factors are still not fully under-

stood, but Harbin and Maumenee[30] reported on six cases in which typical epithelial cysts of the anterior chamber were unintentionally converted into epithelial downgrowth by attempted surgical removal. This study showed that the epithelial cells in epithelial cysts are capable of producing typical epithelial ingrowth if the cyst wall is opened and the cyst is not completely removed from the eye.

Histopathologically epithelial cysts are thin walled and lined with epithelium, and they contain a yellowish or serous fluid (Fig. 25-2). They can vary in size from less than 1 mm in diameter to larger cysts filling almost all of the anterior chamber.

Epithelial ingrowth

The reported incidence of histologically proved epithelial ingrowth after cataract extraction varies from 0.09% to 0.11%.[4,63] In eyes enucleated for complications after cataract extraction, epithelial ingrowth has been reported in from 8% to 26% of cases.*

The exact pathogenesis of epithelial ingrowth is unknown, but probably it requires the presence of a wound leak,[33] and a patent fistula has been found to be present in one third to one half of cases at the time of diagnosis (Fig. 25-3).[57] An eye with

---

*References 15, 17, 20, 21, 29, 50.

*References 2, 4, 20, 22, 46, 63.

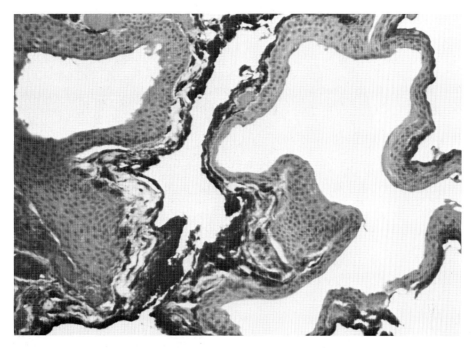

FIG. 25-2. Histologic section of epithelial cyst seen in Fig. 25-1, showing epithelium lining cyst.

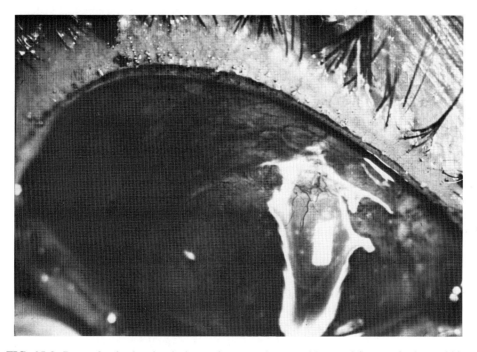

FIG. 25-3. Patent fistula showing leakage of aqueous humor with use of fluorescein dye and blue light. (From Stark, W.J., Michels, R.G., Maumenee, A.E., and Cupples, H. Published with permission from the American Journal of Ophthalmology **85:**772-780. Copyright by the Ophthalmic Publishing Co.)

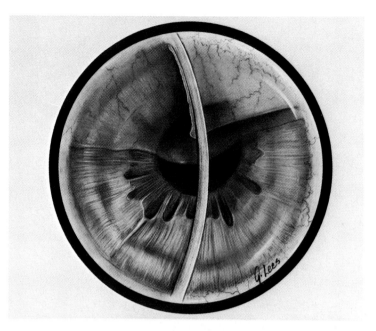

FIG. 25-4. Epithelial ingrowth involving posterior surface of cornea, superior iris, and vitreous face. (From Stark, W.J., Michels, R.G., Maumenee, A.E., and Cupples, H. Published with permission from the American Journal of Ophthalmology **85:**772-780, 1978. Copyright by the Ophthalmic Publishing Co.)

epithelial ingrowth may have undergone penetrating trauma or a complicated postoperative course, such as a flat anterior chamber, hyphema, iris or vitreous incarceration, hypotony, and/or iritis; however, epithelial ingrowth can also occur after uneventful intraocular surgery.

Ferry[24] demonstrated that instruments bearing fragments of epithelium may also play a role in causing epithelial ingrowth. Islands of epithelial cells have been found growing on the iris after uncomplicated cataract extraction.[28] Epithelial ingrowth has also been seen in association with intraocular cellulose sponge material left in the eye after cataract surgery[18] and with suture tracts.[3] The type of conjunctival flap used (limbal or fornix based) has not been shown to be a factor in the development of epithelial ingrowth.[4,42] Epithelial ingrowth has been reported most commonly to develop after a penetrating injury or cataract surgery; however, it has also been documented after penetrating keratoplasty[58] and glaucoma surgery.[22]

Histologic examination of eyes with epithelial ingrowth shows stratified squamous epithelial cells, in a layer of one, two, or three cells in thickness, extending onto the back of the cornea, replacing the endothelium. At the advancing edge, this ingrowth may be five or more cells in thickness, accounting for the apparent increase in thickness of the membrane as seen clinically on slit-lamp examination (Fig. 25-4). Often the epithelial ingrowth is far more extensive on the iris surface than on the cornea[13] (Fig. 25-5). Peripheral anterior synechiae are often present because of trauma and chronic inflammation. Portions of the trabecular meshwork are usually lined by epithelium, causing blockage of aqueous outflow and occasionally glaucoma (Fig. 25-6). Occasionally epithelium may extend posteriorly over the ciliary processes and pars plana.[34,58] A fistulous tract, present in up to 50% of cases, is also lined by stratified squamous epithelium,[12,57] and in these cases hypotony may be present.

There have not been any satisfactory experimental reproductions of epithelial ingrowth in animals. In monkeys Regan[50] produced two cases that were histologically similar to, but not clinically like, the disease as seen in humans.

Electron microscopic studies show the invading cells in epithelial ingrowth to be ultrastructurally very similar to normal conjunctival epithelium. Frequent hemidesmosomes and a well-developed basal lamina are seen along the base of the epithelial ingrowth.[34] Similar ultrastructural studies of epithelial ingrowth following keratoplasty have not been reported.

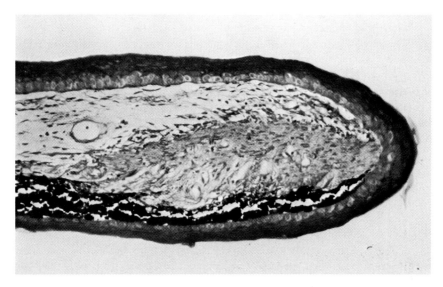

FIG. 25-5. Extensive epithelial ingrowth on iris surface. (Courtesy William R. Green, M.D., Eye Pathology Lab, The Wilmer Institute.)

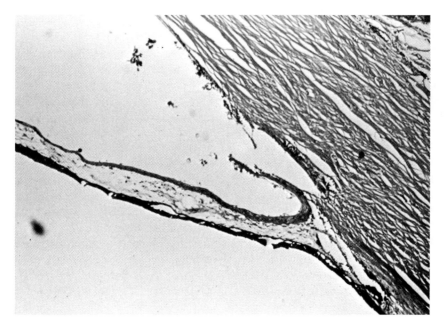

FIG. 25-6. Epithelium growing on anterior iris and into angle. (Courtesy William R. Green, M.D., Eye Pathology Lab, The Wilmer Institute.)

Fibrous proliferation or metaplasia

There are two types of fibrous ingrowth. One is the ingrowth of stromal fibrous tissue through a faulty wound closure or after trauma.* The other type is the retrocorneal membrane that sometimes occurs after chemical burns,[39] herpes keratitis,[65] cryotherapy to the cornea,[44] graft failure,[37,48] or pars plana vitrectomy[36] and in the vitreous touch syndrome.[56]

The incidence of fibrous ingrowth or metaplasia is difficult to assess clinically, but histopathologic studies have reported it as frequently being present in eyes enucleated after anterior segment surgery. Allen[2] reported stromal ingrowth in 30% of eyes enucleated after cataract extraction, and Dunnington[20] observed it in 33% of eyes enucleated after cataract extraction. Bettman[5] found that 25% of eyes enucleated after various kinds of intraocular surgery and 32% of those enucleated after cataract surgery contained fibrous ingrowth. In the same study, epithelial invasion was found in only 1% of the eyes.

Fibrous ingrowth is sometimes associated with poor wound closure and incarceration of lens capsule, iris, or vitreous in the wound. Clinically fibrous ingrowth can be confused with epithelial ingrowth but is generally less progressive and less destructive.

The source of the fibroblasts in fibrous ingrowth is still disputed. The three possible sources are subepithelial connective tissue,[61] corneal or limbal stroma,[53] and metaplastic endothelium.[44] When Descemet's membrane is intact, the fibroblasts probably arise from metaplastic endothelium. In surgical cases Brown and Kitano[7] found that destruction of endothelium was critical in allowing fibrous ingrowth to occur. Swan[61] reported four clinical causes of fibrous ingrowth after cataract extraction: (1) poor wound apposition, (2) uveitis, (3) recurrent hemorrhage, and (4) tissue incarceration. He gave evidence supporting subepithelial connective tissue as the source of fibrous ingrowth.

Experimentally fibrous ingrowth was produced in rabbits by Sherrard and Rycroft,[52] who found that the ingrowth initially consisted of fibroblasts; later, however, as the membranes "matured," they resembled corneal stroma. The factors important in promoting the fibrous ingrowth were said to be (1) healthy corneal stroma capable of producing excess collagenous material, (2) a perforation in Descemet's membrane large enough to allow material into the anterior chamber, and (3) damage to the corneal endothelium around the area of the wound.

Histopathologically the two types of fibrous ingrowth can be distinguished. Eyes with true fibrous ingrowth associated with faulty wound closure or a penetrating injury show an area of defect in Descemet's membrane, with fibrous tissue growing along the back of the cornea, posterior to the endothelium (Fig. 25-7). The membranes are often vascularized and can extend into the angle, over the iris, and into the vitreous cavity (Fig. 25-8 and 25-9). The fibrous membrane may in some cases attach to the retina and cause a traction detachment. Peripheral anterior synechiae are often present.[27] These fibrous membranes consist of collagen fibrils, with an irregular arrangement relative to each other, and fibroblasts that are indistinguishable from corneal stromal fibroblasts. Frequently the space between the back of the cornea and the membrane is lined with endothelial cells.[52] Experimental perforating injuries of the globe have been used to demonstrate the development of intraocular fibrous proliferation in the posterior segment.[64] The vitreous can act as a scaffold for fibrous extension throughout the globe (Fig. 25-10).

In those cases of retrocorneal membrane unassociated with a penetrating injury or faulty wound closure, the pathologic findings are somewhat different. Michels et al.[44] found that after rabbit corneas were frozen, a retrocorneal fibrous membrane formed between Descemet's membrane and a layer of regenerated endothelium. In their study, electron microscopy showed that the fibroblasts within the fibrous membrane had many ultrastructural similarities to endothelial cells, including the formation of junctional complexes between adjacent cells and the deposition of a basement membrane material similar to Descemet's membrane. They found no breaks in Descemet's membrane and no evidence that stromal fibroblasts were involved in the membrane formation; therefore they theorized that metaplastic endothelial cells were responsible for the cellular and extracellular components of the membrane. Other studies in which no perforation or break in Descemet's membrane was present also support the endothelial metaplasia theory as an explanation for these kinds of fibrous proliferations.*

---

*References 2, 5, 20, 27, 52, 53.

*References 36, 37, 44, 54, 56, 65.

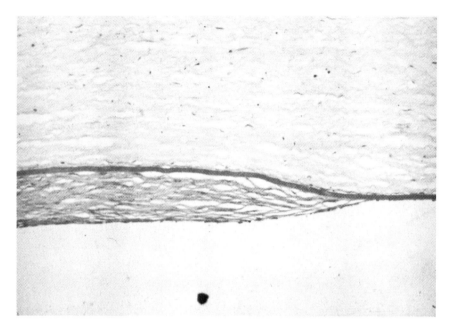

FIG. 25-7. Retrocorneal fibrous membrane on posterior surface of cornea. (Courtesy William R. Green, M.D., Eye Pathology Lab, The Wilmer Institute.)

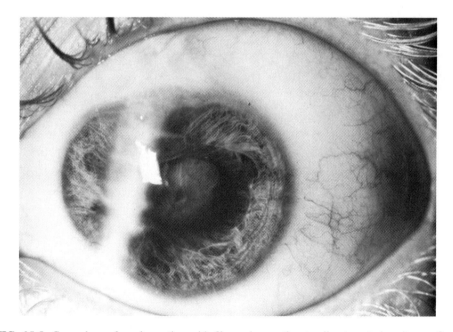

FIG. 25-8. Corneal scar from laceration with fibrous ingrowth extending to anterior vitreous face.

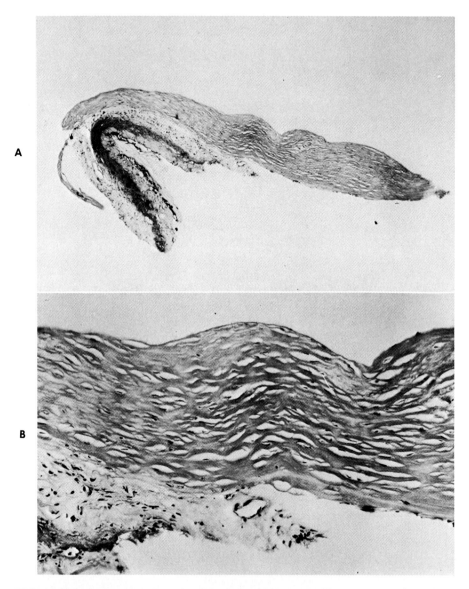

FIG. 25-9. Low (**A**) and medium (**B**) power view of fibrous ingrowth attached to iris tissue. (Courtesy William R. Green, M.D., Eye Pathology Lab, The Wilmer Institute.)

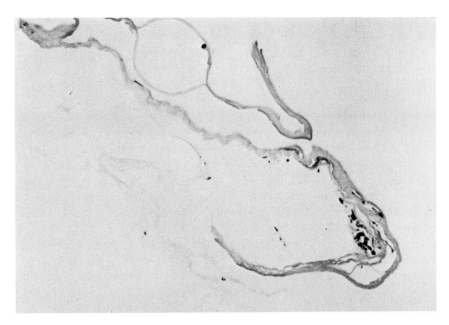

FIG. 25-10. Fibrous ingrowth extending onto vitreous surface. (Courtesy William R. Green, M.D., Eye Pathology Lab, The Wilmer Institute.)

MECHANISM OF GLAUCOMA
Epithelial cysts and ingrowth

Glaucoma rarely occurs as a result of epithelial cysts. The cysts may occasionally enlarge and block the angle or cause iridocyclitis and a secondary elevation of pressure. Attempted surgical removal of a cyst can promote its conversion to proliferation and lead to secondary glaucoma.[30]

Glaucoma frequently complicates epithelial ingrowth unless a fistula is present. Bernardino et al.[4] found glaucoma in 12 of 24 cases of epithelial ingrowth. The cause of the glaucoma was (1) epithelium lining the trabecular meshwork, (2) dense anterior synechiae closing the angle, (3) a pupillary block mechanism,[11] and/or (4) blockage of the angle by ''desquamating epithelium in the form of particulate matter,'' as described by Terry et al.[62] In one third to one fourth of cases, epithelial ingrowth may present with hypotony or normal pressure and a fistulous tract into the anterior chamber.[9,12,57] If the fistula closes or is closed during treatment, glaucoma may subsequently develop. Untreated, the natural course of the disease is usually that of uncontrolled glaucoma if a fistula is not present, massive epithelial invasion of the eye, inflammation, and loss of the eye. When a fistula is present in an untreated eye, the fistula may later

close from intraocular inflammation, leading to uncontrolled glaucoma.

Fibrous proliferation or metaplasia

The true incidence of glaucoma in eyes with fibrous ingrowth or metaplasia is difficult to determine, but it seems to be high in those eyes that have ultimately needed enucleation.[33] The glaucoma is usually caused by angle changes from the surgery or injury that led to the fibrous ingrowth, but glaucoma can also result from invasion of the angle structures by fibrous tissue and from angle closure by progressive peripheral anterior synechiae (PAS) formation. Friedman and Henkind[27] reported on two cases of stromal ingrowth following cataract extraction. In both cases the eye had secondary glaucoma and required enucleation. On histopathologic study, the eye in one case showed closure of the angle by PAS formation, and the eye in the other case showed extensive fibrous tissue in the angle, as well as peripheral anterior synechiae occluding the angle.

Glaucoma is less likely to be associated with the retrocorneal fibrous membrane that may occur after ocular insult or injury that causes no break in Descemet's membrane. However, any eye that has undergone sufficient trauma may, of course, develop secondary glaucoma from angle recession, PAS formation, or other causes.

DIAGNOSIS
Epithelial cysts and ingrowth

The diagnosis of epithelial cysts is made on a clinical basis and is rarely difficult, because the cyst is usually visible in the anterior chamber with the slit lamp (Fig. 25-11). The cyst is translucent and may be partially filled with epithelial debris, which is sometimes layered (Fig. 25-12). If secondary, the cyst is usually attached to an incision or perforation site.

The typical patient with epithelial ingrowth has had ocular trauma or surgery and may complain of prolonged tearing, pain, and photophobia after anterior segment surgery or trauma. One early warning sign of possible epithelial ingrowth is a persistently soft eye after surgery with a fistula present. One may also see iris drawn up toward the wound. When the ingrowth is more advanced, the proliferating epithelial cells usually appear as a thin gray translucent or transparent membrane on the back of the cornea, with a scalloped, thickened leading edge (Fig. 25-13). The cornea is often clear over the ingrowth, but occasionally the stroma becomes vascularized and cloudy, and a

drop of glycerin is useful in clearing the cornea to observe the line of ingrowth. A fistula is present with the Seidel test in about 30% to 50% of cases.[57] When testing for a fistula, one should use 2% fluorescein with slight external pressure on the eye (Fig. 25-3).

Iris involvement may be difficult to detect by slit-lamp examination. Flattening of the iris surface, a translucent membrane, and graying of the anterior vitreous are suggestive of iris involvement. In all cases of suspected epithelial ingrowth, the iris should be tested with laser burns to detect the presence of intraocular epithelium and to delineate the extent of involvement (Fig. 25-14). This was first demonstrated by Maumenee,[41] who advocated the use of the photocoagulator to determine where epithelium was growing on the iris. With xenon photocoagulation or argon laser application, the epithelium on the iris turns white, whereas normal iris turns light brown. With the argon laser, a spot size of 200 or 500 μm is used with a power setting just high enough to cause a burn on normal iris. This technique is used to demarcate normal iris from involved iris.

Other diagnostic aids of value when the diagnosis is uncertain on clinical grounds include scraping the back of the involved cornea with a curette through a small peripheral corneal incision and submitting the tissue for cytopathologic examina-

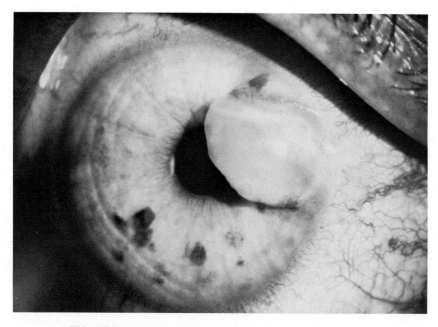

FIG. 25-11. Moderate-sized epithelial cyst in anterior chamber.

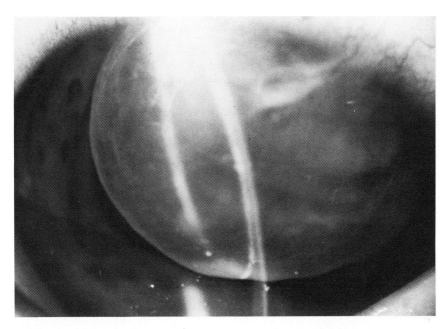

FIG. 25-12. Large epithelial cyst showing layering of whitish keratin debris at inferior portion of cyst.

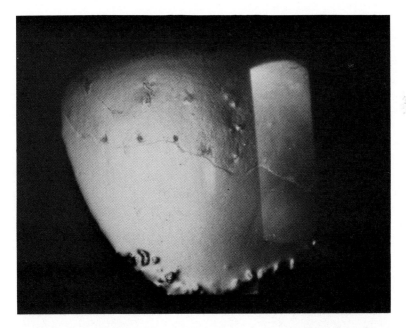

FIG. 25-13. Appearance of epithelial ingrowth advancing down posterior surface of cornea. (Leading edge is scalloped and thickened. (From Stark, W.J., Michels, R.G., Maumenee, A.E., and Cupples, H. Published with permission from the American Journal of Opthalmology **85:**772-780, 1978. Copyright by the Ophthalmic Publishing Co.)

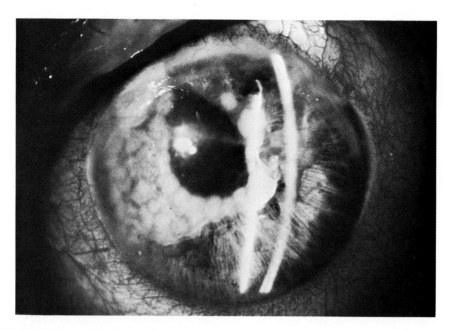

FIG. 25-14. Argon laser burns placed on anterior iris surface to delineate extent of epithelial involvement. Laser causes epithelium to turn white, whereas noninvolved iris turns brown. (From Stark, W.J., Michels, R.G., Maumenee, A.E., and Cupples, H. Published with permission from the American Journal of Ophthalmology **85:**772-780, 1978. Copyright by the Ophthalmic Publishing Co.)

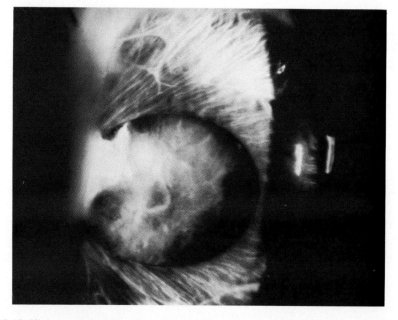

FIG. 25-15. Higher power of Fig. 25-8, showing fibrous ingrowth extending over anterior vitreous face.

tion.[10] The tissue must be fixed on a slide quickly and then sent for hematoxylin-eosin staining. Paracentesis of the anterior chamber with cytopathologic examination of anterior chamber cells may also be helpful. Specular microscopy can be used as a noninvasive method but requires a clear cornea and is often not diagnostic.[55]

Fibrous proliferation or metaplasia

The clinical presentation of fibrous proliferation, or ingrowth, can be extremely variable—depending on its cause, location, and severity.[61] When it extends onto the iris and vitreous, it can easily be recognized (Fig. 25-15). However, when it presents as a sheet on the back of the cornea, it may be hard to differentiate from epithelial ingrowth. The irregular fibroblastic membrane tends to have a "characteristic interlacing network of fine gray fibers having the appearance of woven cloth."[61] Bullous keratopathy may be present, making the diagnosis more difficult. A careful ocular history and examination are essential, but there are no specific tests that are useful, other than those mentioned for epithelial ingrowth.

Differential diagnosis

The differential diagnosis of epithelial cysts includes neuroepithelial cysts of the pigment epithelium of the iris, parasitic cysts, and congenital iris cysts, which may be lined by epithelium.[43] The differential diagnosis of both stromal and epithelial ingrowth includes detachment of Descemet's membrane, inflammatory glassy membranes, vitreocorneal adhesions, and excessively shelved corneal incisions. None of these entities except inflammatory membranes involve the iris, so differentiation is usually not difficult. Endothelium and Descemet's membrane can proliferate after trauma and can cover the anterior chamber angle and iris.[69] Such "descemetization" is rare after surgery, but it may be difficult to distinguish from epithelial and fibrous ingrowth.

MANAGEMENT
Epithelial cysts

Epithelial cysts of the anterior chamber often remain small for many years, and cysts should be observed initially for signs of growth (Fig. 25-16). The cysts are best left untreated unless they enlarge and block the pupillary space, decreasing vision, or unless they cause uncontrolled glaucoma or iritis.[8]

In the past, a number of treatment modalities were tried, including x-ray therapy, chemical cautery, electrolysis, and diathermy.[32,35,68,70] These methods have generally been abandoned for the

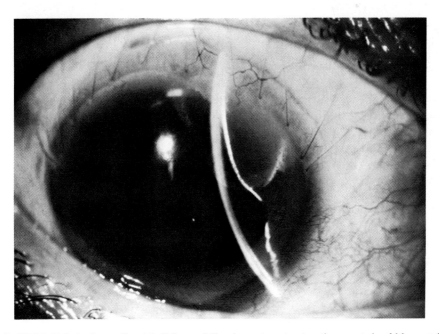

FIG. 25-16. Relatively small epithelial cyst following cataract extraction; cyst should be watched initially for signs of growth or other complications.

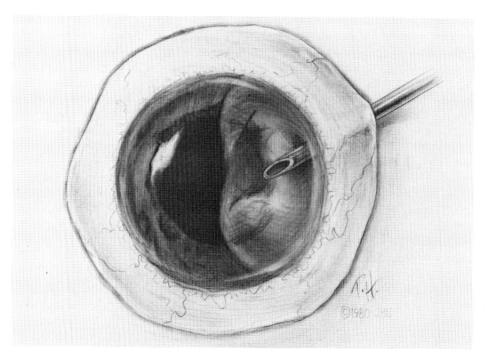

FIG. 25-17. Cyst is aspirated through limbal approach. (From Bruner, W.E., Stark, W.J., Michels, R.G., and Maumenee, A.E.: Ophthalmic Surg. **12:**279, 1981. © 1980, The Johns Hopkins University.)

current treatment options, which are photocoagulation,[14,45] aspiration with cryodestruction, and surgical excision.[8,32,43,59]

Cleasby[14] described four cases successfully treated with the xenon photocoagulator. He applied six to eight burns to the cyst and then repeated the treatment in 1 month. One cyst required a third treatment. All four cysts collapsed with this method. Okun and Mandell[45] described the treatment of three eyes with cysts, also with the xenon photocoagulator. With multiple treatments they were able to collapse the cysts in all cases, but the cysts were not entirely eliminated. None of the above-mentioned authors noted serious complications.

Our preferred surgical approach to epithelial cysts involves either a closed-eye or an open-eye technique,[8] depending on the status of the lens. In the closed-eye technique, which is useful in aphakic patients, the cyst is aspirated through a limbal approach (Fig. 25-17). A partial vitrectomy is then performed (Fig. 25-18). Air is injected into the anterior chamber to tamponade the collapsed cyst and to act as insulation for cryodestruction of the cyst. The cryoprobe is then used to freeze the cyst through the cornea or in the angle (Fig. 25-19). Fig. 25-20 illustrates an eye treated by this technique.

In phakic eyes when preservation of the lens

is desired, and in certain aphakic cases, an open-eye technique is used. The cyst contents are aspirated as in the closed-eye technique (Fig. 25-21). Through a second Ziegler puncture the anterior chamber is filled with air (Fig. 25-22), and the cyst is dissected bluntly from its attachments to the cornea, angle, and iris (Fig. 25-23). Often the iris adhesions cannot be broken, but it is important to pull the cyst away from the angle so as not to cut into the cyst when entering the eye. The eye is opened (Fig. 25-24), and the entire cyst is removed, along with adherent iris if necessary (Fig. 25-25). After the cyst is removed, a small piece of tissue is excised from both edges of the remaining iris and sent separately for pathologic examination to be sure that the margins are free of epithelium. The wound is closed tightly with multiple interrupted sutures (Fig. 25-26). The anterior chamber is formed with air, which acts as an insulator and helps protect the lens from the freeze. Cryotherapy can then be applied through the cornea or limbus if areas of possible cyst remnants are suspected. Fig. 25-27 illustrates an eye that was treated in this manner.

One of the most serious complications of cyst removal is its conversion to a sheetlike epithelial ingrowth.[8,30] Other complications include corneal edema, hypotony, and retinal detachment.

Text continued on p. 400.

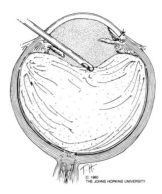

FIG. 25-18. Partial vitrectomy is performed. (From Bruner, W.E., Stark, W.J., Michels, R.G., and Maumenee, A.E.: Ophthalmic Surg. **12:**279, 1981.)

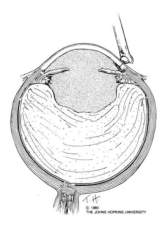

FIG. 25-19. With air in anterior chamber, cryoprobe is used to freeze cyst through cornea or limbus. (From Bruner, W.E., Stark, W.J., Michels, R.G., and Maumenee, A.E.: Ophthalmic Surg. **12:**279, 1981.)

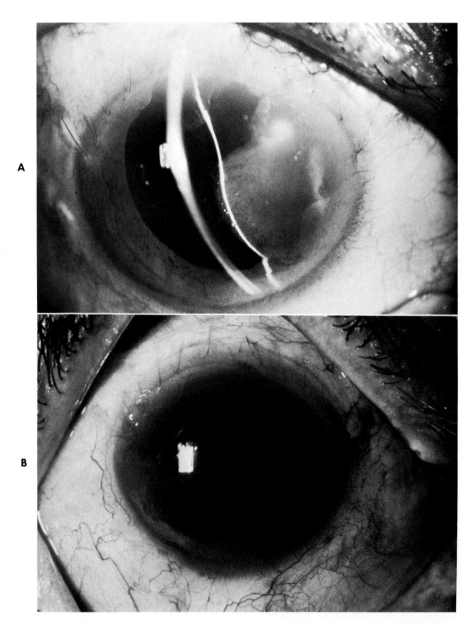

FIG. 25-20. A, Preoperative appearance of cyst. **B,** Eye 2 years after closed-eye technique with no evidence of recurrence and with corrected visual acuity of 20/20. (From Bruner, W.E., Stark, W.J., Michels, R.G., and Maumenee, A.E.: Ophthalmic Surg. **12:**279, 1981.)

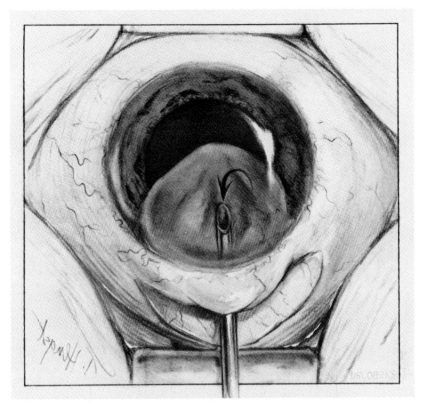

FIG. 25-21. Cyst contents are aspirated. (From Bruner, W.E., Stark, W.J., Michels, R.G., and Maumenee, A.E.: Ophthalmic Surg. **12**:279, 1981. © 1980, The Johns Hopkins University.)

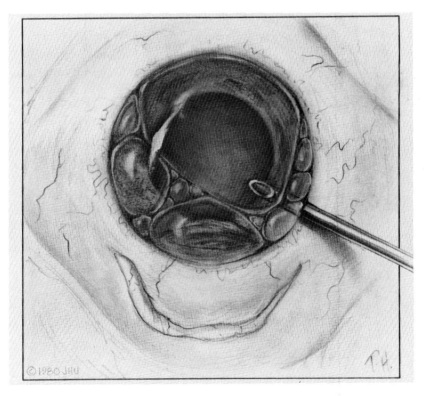

FIG. 25-22. Anterior chamber is filled with air through second Ziegler puncture. (From Bruner, W.E., Stark, W.J., Michels, R.G., and Maumenee, A.E.: Ophthalmic Surg. **12**:279, 1981. © 1980, The Johns Hopkins University.)

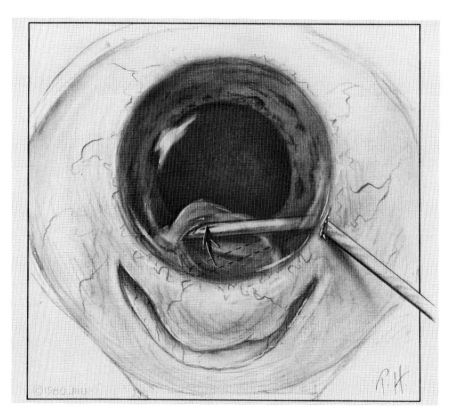

FIG. 25-23. Cyst is dissected bluntly from its attachments to cornea, angle, and iris if possible. (From Bruner, W.E., Stark, W.J., Michels, R.G., and Maumenee, A.E.: Ophthalmic Surg. **12:** 279, 1981. © 1980, The Johns Hopkins University.)

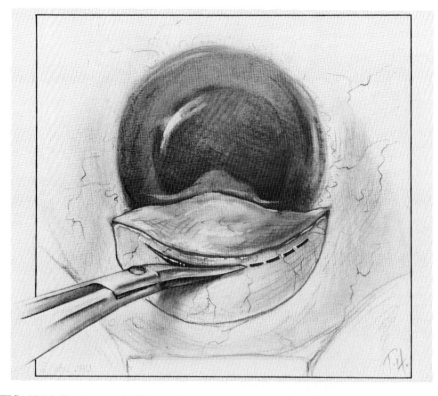

FIG. 25-24. Eye is opened with razor blade and scissors, with care taken not to cut into cyst. (From Bruner, W.E., Stark, W.J., Michels, R.G., and Maumenee, A.E.: Ophthalmic Surg. **12:**279, 1981. © 1980, The Johns Hopkins University.)

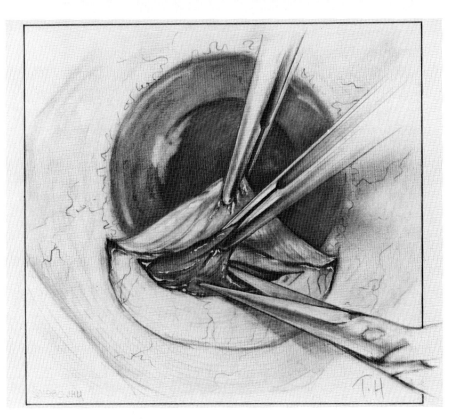

FIG. 25-25. Cyst is then removed from anterior chamber and adherent iris is also excised if necessary. (From Bruner, W.E., Stark, W.J., Michels, R.G., and Maumenee, A.E.: Ophthalmic Surg. **12:**279, 1981. © 1980, The Johns Hopkins University.)

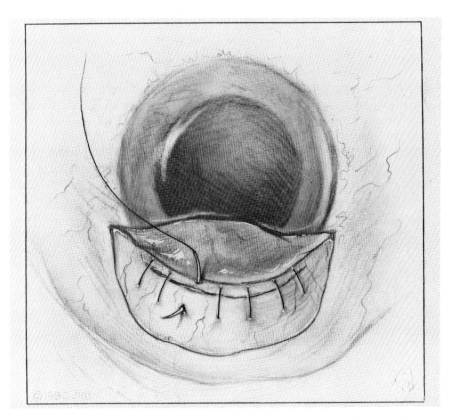

FIG. 25-26. Wound is closed tightly with multiple interrupted 10-0 monofilament nylon sutures. (From Bruner, W.E., Stark, W.J., Michels, R.G., and Maumenee, A.E.: Ophthalmic Surg. **12:** 279, 1981. © 1980, The Johns Hopkins University.)

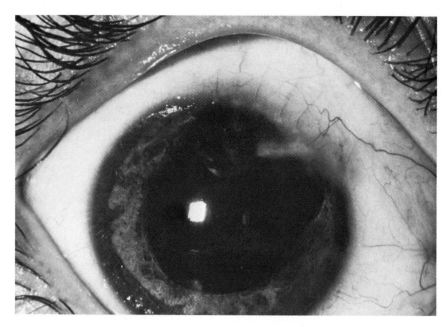

FIG. 25-27. Postoperative appearance of patient in Fig. 25-1, 6 months after surgery. Patient has corrected visual acuity of 20/25. (From Bruner, W.E., Stark, W.J., Michels, R.G., and Maumenee, A.E.: Ophthalmic Surg. **12:**279, 1981.)

Epithelial ingrowth

The treatment of epithelial ingrowth has included irradiation* and various surgical methods.† Irradiation is probably ineffective and is no longer used. Surgical treatments have been modified and revised at various times. Maumenee et al.[42] reported a series of 40 cases of "epithelial downgrowth" treated by diagnostic photocoagulation of the areas of the iris surface, excision of the involved iris, and destruction of the epithelium on the back of the cornea by chemical cauterization or cryotherapy. Treatment was considered successful in 27% of the cases, and the patients had a postoperative visual acuity of 20/50 or better, absence of recurrence of ingrowth, and control of intraocular pressure. Brown[6] modified this technique by exposing and excising the affected chamber angle tissues en bloc. He reported on three cases. One patient had a postoperative visual acuity of 20/80; the second patient's visual acuity was 20/400; the third patient's visual acuity was not reported. In all three cases there was no evidence of recurrence.

Following the surgery all three patients developed glaucoma, which was controlled medically. Friedman[26] described treating three patients with a

radical surgical method involving en bloc excision of involved cornea, sclera, iris, ciliary body, and vitreous, as well as the use of a freehand corneoscleral graft for reconstruction. The patients' postoperative visual acuities were 20/50, 20/60, and 20/100. None of these patients had recurrence of the epithelial ingrowth.

Stark et al.[57] reported on 10 patients treated with a modification of Maumenee's technique. Preoperatively the iris was treated with argon laser photocoagulation to define the extent of the epithelial ingrowth involvement (Fig. 25-12). Fluorescein dye was used topically to identify any fistulas, and any fistulas found were closed with sutures or a scleral flap (Fig. 25-3). With the use of a vitrectomy instrument, the area of involved iris and vitreous was removed (Fig. 25-28). The anterior eye was then filled with sterile air, which acted as a thermal insulator to enhance cryotherapy, which was then applied in a transcorneal and transscleral fashion to destroy any epithelium remaining on the back of the cornea, in the angle, or on the ciliary body (Fig. 25-29). The epithelial sheet on the back of the cornea appeared white on the first day after surgery and began to slough by the second day (Fig. 25-30). The sheet usually disappeared by the fifth day.

Postoperatively visual acuity improved in 8 of 10 cases, and four eyes achieved a final visual

---

*References 19, 25, 47, 49, 66, 67.
†References 23, 38, 40, 42, 60.

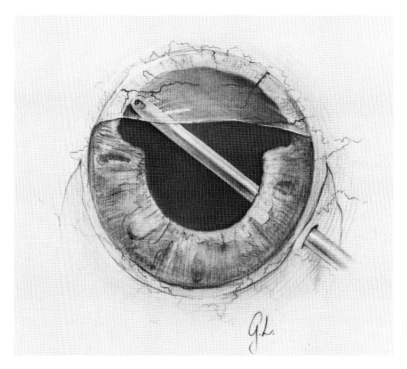

FIG. 25-28. With vitrectomy instrumentation, area of iris and vitreous involved by epithelial ingrowth is excised. Peripheral iris is not excised.

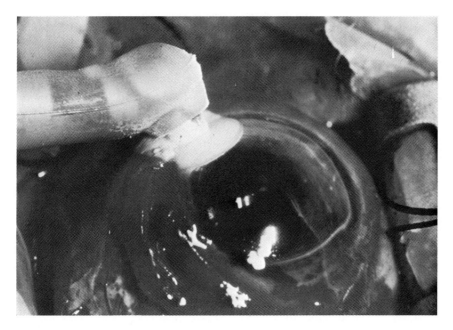

FIG. 25-29. After anterior eye is filled with air to act as insulator, cryotherapy is applied in a transcorneal and transscleral fashion to destroy epithelium on back of cornea, in angle, or on ciliary body. (From Stark, W.J., Michels, R.G., Maumenee, A.E., and Cupples, H. Published with permission from the American Journal of Ophthalmology **85:**772-780. Copyright by the Ophthalmic Publishing Co.)

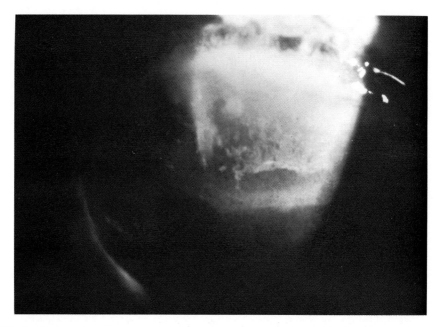

FIG. 25-30. One day after cryotherapy, epithelium on posterior surface of cornea turns white and starts to slough. (From Stark, W.J., Michels, R.G., Maumenee, A.E., and Cupples, H. Published with permission from the American Journal of Ophthalmology **85:**772-780. Copyright by the Ophthalmic Publishing Co.)

acuity of 6/12 (20/40) or better. Intraocular pressure was less than 21 mm Hg in all cases, and only two eyes required topical antiglaucoma medications. There were no intraoperative or early postoperative complications reported, with longest follow-up of 33 months (Fig. 25-31). Decompensation of the central cornea occurred in four eyes, which subsequently required penetrating keratoplasty. With longer follow-up, only one of eight patients retained vision of 20/40. Three have 20/200 or better vision. Long-term problems causing reduced vision included cloudy cornea (two eyes), optic atrophy (one eye), macular membrane (one eye), cystoid macular edema (two eyes), and phthisis bulbi (one eye).

The most important prognostic factor to successful management of epithelial ingrowth appears to be early diagnosis and treatment.[57] If the diagnosis can be made when only a small area of the anterior segment is involved, more conservative methods, such as cryotherapy alone, can be successful. If the disease is far advanced (e.g., with total iris and angle involvement), it may be preferable to avoid extensive surgery if the fellow eye has good visual acuity. The pressure in extensively involved eyes can often be controlled by cyclocryotherapy if medical therapy is not adequate.

If the involved eye is the patient's only eye, then surgical therapy is usually recommended as soon as possible.

Fibrous proliferation or metaplasia

There is, as yet, no satisfactory treatment for fibrous proliferation, or ingrowth. Specific factors that might lead to fibrous ingrowth should be kept in mind during surgery. Preventive measures include careful suture placement, good wound closure, and care to avoid injuring the endothelium. Topical steroid therapy has generally been ineffective in treatment, and surgical excision of fibroblastic membranes has not been universally successful. Therefore the best treatment is prevention.[61]

Secondary glaucoma may be treated by cyclocryotherapy if medical therapy alone fails to control the pressure. If the fibrous ingrowth reaches the posterior chamber and causes retinal detachment by traction, it can be excised with the use of vitrectomy instrumentation. In rabbits transvitreal fibrous proliferation produced by experimental perforation of the posterior segment has been successfully treated by early vitrectomy.[1] Generally radical surgery is not advised for fibrous proliferation, and glaucoma should be managed medically if possible or surgically if necessary.

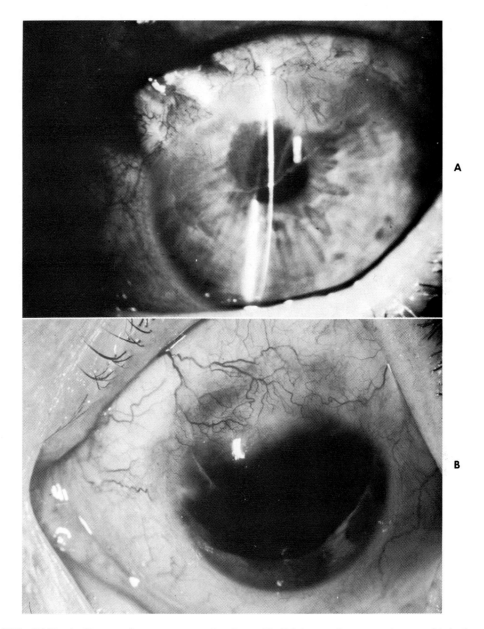

FIG. 25-31. A, Preoperative appearance showing epithelial ingrowth on superior one third of posterior cornea. **B,** Appearance 2 years after surgery, with clear central cornea and opaque vascularized cornea in area of previous epithelial ingrowth. Vision is limited because of cystoid macular edema. (From Stark, W.J., Michels, R.G., Maumenee, A.E., and Cupples, H. Published with permission from the American Journal of Ophthalmology **85:**772-780. Copyright by the Ophthalmic Publishing Co.)

REFERENCES

1. Abrams, G.W., Topping, T.M., and Machemer, R.: Vitrectomy for injury: the effect of intraocular proliferation following perforation of the posterior segment of the rabbit eye, Arch. Ophthalmol. **97:**743, 1979.
2. Allen, J.C.: Epithelial and stromal ingrowths, Am. J. Ophthalmol. **65:**179, 1968.
3. Allen, J.C., and Duehr, P.A.: Sutures and epithelial downgrowth, Am. J. Ophthalmol. **66:**293, 1968.
4. Bernardino, V.B., Kim, J.C., and Smith, T.R.: Epithelialization of the anterior chamber after cataract extraction, Arch. Ophthalmol. **82:**742, 1969.
5. Bettman, J.W.: Pathology of complications of intraocular surgery, Am. J. Ophthalmol. **68:**1037, 1969.
6. Brown, S.I.: Treatment of advanced epithelial downgrowth, Trans. Am. Acad. Ophthalmol. Otolaryngol. **77:**618, 1973.
7. Brown, S.I., and Kitano, S.: Pathogenesis of the retrocorneal membrane, Arch. Ophthalmol. **75:**518, 1966.
8. Bruner, W.E., Stark, W.J., Michels, R.G., and Maumenee, A.E.: Management of epithelial cysts of the anterior chamber, Ophthalmic Surg. **12:**279, 1981.
9. Calhoun, F.P.: The clinical recognition and treatment of epithelialization of the anterior chamber following cataract extraction, Trans. Am. Ophthalmol. Soc. **47:**498, 1949.
10. Calhoun, F.P.: An aid to the clinical diagnosis of epithelial downgrowth into the anterior chamber following cataract extraction, Am. J. Ophthalmol. **61:**1055, 1966.
11. Chandler, P.A., and Grant, W.M.: Lectures on glaucoma, Philadelphia, 1965, Lea & Febiger.
12. Chee, P.H.Y.: Epithelial downgrowth, Arch. Ophthalmol. **78:**492, 1967.
13. Christensen, L.: Epithelization of the anterior chamber, Trans. Am. Ophthalmol. Soc. **58:**284, 1960.
14. Cleasby, G.W.: Photocoagulation of iris-ciliary body epithelial cysts, Trans. Am. Acad. Ophthalmol. Otolaryngol. **75:**638, 1971.
15. Cogan, D.G.: Experimental implants of conjunctiva into the anterior chamber, Am. J. Ophthalmol. **39:**165, 1955.
16. Collins, E.T., and Cross, F.R.: Two cases of epithelial implantation cyst in the anterior chamber after extraction of cataract, Trans. Ophthalmol. Soc. U.K. **12:**175, 1892.
17. Corrado, M.: Glaucoma secondario a penetrazione e proliferazione de epitelio in c.a. in occhio operato di cataratta, Ann. Ottal. **59:**706, 1931.
18. Dixon, W.S., and Speakman, J.S.: Epithelial downgrowth following cataract surgery, Arch. Ophthalmol. **84:**303, 1970.
19. Dollfus, M.A., and Vail, D.: Roentgen therapy of epithelial invasion of the anterior chamber, Trans. Am. Ophthalmol. Soc. **64:**50, 1966.
20. Dunnington, J.H.: Healing of incisions for cataract extraction, Am. J. Ophthalmol. **34:**36, 1951.
21. Dunnington, J.H., and Regan, E.F.: The effect of sutures and of thrombin upon ocular wound healing, Trans. Am. Acad. Ophthalmol. Otolaryngol. **55:**761, 1951.
22. Eldrup-Jørgensen, P.: Epithelialization of the anterior chamber, Acta Ophthalmol. **47:**328, 1969.
23. Fazakas, S.: Epitheliosis of the anterior chamber following cataract operation, Orv. Hetil. **76:**776, 1932.
24. Ferry, A.P.: The possible role of epithelium-bearing surgical instruments in pathogenesis of epithelialization of the anterior chamber, Ann. Ophthalmol. **3:**1089, 1971.
25. Fleming, K.O.: Epithelial downgrowth, Can. Med. Assoc. J. **74:**209, 1956.
26. Friedman, A.H.: Radical anterior segment surgery for epithelial invasion of the anterior chamber: report of three cases, Trans. Am. Acad. Ophthalmol. Otolaryngol. **83:**216, 1977.
27. Friedman, A.H., and Henkind, P.: Corneal stromal overgrowth after cataract extraction, Br. J. Ophthalmol. **54:**528, 1970.
28. Friedman, A.H., Takerka, H.B., and Henkind, P.: Epithelial implantation membrane on the iris surface following cataract extraction with report of two cases, Am. J. Ophthalmol. **71:**482, 1971.
29. Gundersen, T.: Results of autotransplantation of cornea into the anterior chamber: their significance regarding corneal nutrition, Trans. Am. Ophthalmol. Soc. **36:**207, 1938.
30. Harbin, T.S., and Maumenee, A.E.: Epithelial downgrowth after surgery for epithelial cyst, Am. J. Ophthalmol. **78:**1, 1974.
31. Henderson, T.: Discussion of Collins, E.T.: Discussion on postoperative complications of cataract extraction, II, Trans. Ophthalmol. Soc. U.K. **34:**18, 1914.
32. Hogan, M.J., and Goodman, E.K.: Surgical treatment of epithelial cysts of the anterior chamber, Arch. Ophthalmol. **64:**286, 1960.
33. Jaffe, N.S.: Cataract surgery and its complications, ed. 3, St. Louis, 1981, The C.V. Mosby Co.
34. Jensen, P., Minckler, D.S., and Chandler, J.W.: Epithelial ingrowth, Arch. Ophthalmol. **95:**837, 1977.
35. Kennedy, P.J.: Treatment of cysts of the iris with electrolysis, Arch. Ophthalmol. **55:**527, 1956.
36. Kenyon, K.R., Stark, W.J., and Stone, D.L.: Corneal endothelial degeneration and fibrous proliferation after pars plana vitrectomy, Am. J. Ophthalmol. **81:**486, 1976.
37. Kurz, G.H., and D'Amico, R.A.: Histopathology of corneal graft failures, Am. J. Ophthalmol. **66:**184, 1968.
38. Long, J.C., and Tyner, G.S.: Three cases of epithelial invasion of the anterior chamber treated surgically, Arch. Ophthalmol. **58:**396, 1957.
39. Matsuda, H., and Smelser, G.K.: Endothelial cells in alkali-burned corneas: ultrastructural alterations, Arch. Ophthalmol. **89:**402, 1973.
40. Maumenee, A.E.: Symposium: Postoperative cataract complications; epithelial invasion of the anterior chamber, retinal detachment, corneal edema, anterior chamber hemorrhages, changes in the macula, Trans. Am. Acad. Ophthalmol. Otolaryngol. **61:**51, 1957.
41. Maumenee, A.E.: Treatment of epithelial downgrowth and intraocular fistula following cataract extraction, Trans. Am. Ophthalmol. Soc. **62:**153, 1964.
42. Maumenee, A.E., Paton, D., Morse, P.H., and Butner, R.: Review of 40 histologically proven cases of epithelial downgrowth following cataract extraction and suggested surgical management, Am. J. Ophthalmol. **69:**598, 1970.
43. Maumenee, A.E., and Shannon, C.R.: Epithelial invasion of the anterior chamber, Am. J. Ophthalmol. **41:**929, 1956.
44. Michels, R.G., Kenyon, K.R., and Maumenee, A.E.: Retrocorneal fibrous membrane, Invest. Ophthalmol. **11:**822, 1972.
45. Okun, E., and Mandell, A.: Photocoagulation as a treatment of epithelial implantation cysts following cataract

surgery, Trans. Am. Ophthalmol. Soc. **72:**170, 1974.

46. Perera, C.A.: Epithelium in the anterior chamber of the eye after operation and injury, Trans. Am. Acad. Ophthalmol. Otolaryngol. **42:**142, 1937.

47. Pincus, M.H.: Epithelial invasion of anterior chamber following cataract extraction: effect of radiation therapy, Arch. Ophthalmol. **43:**509, 1950.

48. Polack, F.M.: Scanning electron microscopy of corneal graft rejection: epithelial rejection, endothelial rejection, and formation of posterior graft membranes, Invest. Ophthalmol. **11:**1, 1972.

49. Reese, A.B.: The treatment of complications of ocular surgery (round-table conference), Am. J. Ophthalmol. **35:**715, 1952.

50. Regan, E.F.: Epithelial invasion of the anterior chamber, Arch. Ophthalmol. **60:**907, 1958.

51. Rothmund, A.: Ueber Cysten der Regenbogenhaut, Klin. Monatsbl. Augenheilkd. **10:**189, 1872.

52. Sherrard, E.S., and Rycroft, P.V.: Retrocorneal membranes. I. Their origin and structure, Br. J. Ophthalmol. **51:**379, 1967.

53. Sherrard, E.S., and Rycroft, P.V.: Retrocorneal membranes. II. Factors influencing their growth, Br. J. Ophthalmol. **51:**387, 1967.

54. Silbert, A.M., and Baum, J.L.: Origin of the retrocorneal membrane in the rabbit, Arch. Ophthalmol. **97:**1141, 1979.

55. Smith, R.E., and Parrett, C.: Specular microscopy of epithelial downgrowth, Arch. Ophthalmol. **96:**1222, 1978.

56. Snip, R.C., Kenyon, K.R., and Green, W.R.: Retrocorneal fibrous membrane in the vitreous touch syndrome, Am. J. Ophthalmol. **79:**233, 1975.

57. Stark, W.J., Michels, R.G., Maumenee, A.E., and Cupples, H.: Surgical management of epithelial ingrowth, Am. J. Ophthalmol. **85:**772, 1978.

58. Sugar, A., Mayer, R.F., and Hood, I.: Epithelial downgrowth following penetrating keratoplasty in the aphake, Arch. Ophthalmol. **95:**464, 1977.

59. Sugar, H.S.: Further experience with posterior lamellar resection of the cornea for epithelial implantation cyst, Am. J. Ophthalmol. **64:**291, 1967.

60. Sullivan, G.L.: Treatment of epithelialization of the anterior chamber following cataract extraction, Trans. Ophthalmol. Soc. U.K. **89:**445, 1973.

61. Swan, K.C.: Fibroblastic ingrowth following cataract extraction, Arch. Ophthalmol. **89:**445, 1973.

62. Terry, T.L., Chisholm, J.F., and Schonberg, A.L.: Studies on surface-epithelium invasion of the anterior segment of the eye, Am. J. Ophthalmol. **22:**1083, 1939.

63. Theobald, G.D., and Haas, J.S.: Epithelial invasion of the anterior chamber following cataract extraction, Trans. Am. Acad. Ophthalmol. Otolaryngol. **52:**470, 1948.

64. Topping, T.M., Abrams, G.W., and Machemer, R.: Experimental double-perforating injury of the posterior segment in rabbit eyes: the natural history of intraocular proliferation, Arch. Ophthalmol. **97:**735, 1979.

65. Townsend, W.M., and Kaufman, H.E.: Pathogenesis of glaucoma and endothelial changes in herpetic keratouveitis in rabbits, Am. J. Ophthalmol. **71:**904, 1971.

66. Vail, D.: Epithelial downgrowth into the anterior chamber following cataract extraction arrested by radium treatment, Trans. Am. Ophthalmol. Soc. **33:**306, 1935.

67. Vail, D.: Epithelial downgrowth into the anterior chamber following cataract extraction: arrest by radium treatment, Arch. Ophthalmol. **15:**270, 1936.

68. Vail, D.: Treatment of cysts of the iris with diathermy coagulation, Trans. Am. Ophthalmol. Soc. **51:**522, 1953.

69. Waring, G.O., Laibson, P.R., and Rodrigues, M.: Clinical and pathological alterations of Descemet's membrane: with emphasis on endothelial metaplasia, Surv. Ophthalmol. **18:**325, 1974.

70. Wilson, W.: Iris cyst treated by electrolysis, Br. J. Ophthalmol. **48:**45, 1964.

71. Wood, D.J.: An unusual result following traumatic iridocyclitis, Br. J. Ophthalmol. **16:**546, 1932.

Chapter 26

GLAUCOMA FOLLOWING PENETRATING KERATOPLASTY

Alan Sugar

Elevated intraocular pressure can be a significant problem following penetrating keratoplasty. While the success of keratoplasty has improved greatly because of technical advances over the past several decades, improved technology has also led to increased recognition of glaucoma. The recent improvements, especially in aphakic graft success,[13] have also led to increased recognition of glaucoma in primarily aphakic grafted eyes.[8] In the decade since the problem was first emphasized, our understanding of the cause, treatment, and prevention has greatly increased.

For the purposes of this discussion, glaucoma is defined as elevated intraocular pressure, with or without optic nerve head damage and visual field loss. While structural and functional changes undoubtedly occur frequently, they are not well documented in most studies, partly because of the complex optical problems of patients with corneal grafts.

INCIDENCE

It is difficult to determine the true incidence of glaucoma following keratoplasty in reports made before the introduction of electronic tonometry (MacKay-Marg) for graft patients.[8] Stallard,[33] based on experiences from an early era of transplantation, advised against grafts larger than 7 mm in diameter because of the high probability of glaucoma related to synechiae to the graft. Mortada's[16] findings support this: 3 of 30 patients with grafts with diameters of 5.0 to 5.5 mm but 7 of 20 patients with grafts with diameters of 6.5 to 7.5 mm

developed glaucoma. Although most grafts now are 7.5 mm or larger in diameter, current wound closure techniques have made such synechiae a less frequent problem. Thomas and Purnell[36] noted a 5% incidence of glaucoma in 100 patients with penetrating grafts performed from 1957 to 1962. Raab and Fine[31] reported an 11.6% incidence, with most cases occurring with interstitial keratitis. These authors examined primarily phakic eyes and stressed the need to control synechiae if glaucoma was to be prevented.

Irvine and Kaufman,[8] using the MacKay-Marg tonometer, documented a remarkably high incidence of elevated intraocular pressure in the early postkeratoplasty period. The average maximum intraocular pressure in the first week was 24 mm Hg in phakic eyes, 40 mm Hg in aphakic eyes, and 50 mm Hg in eyes undergoing combined cataract extraction and keratoplasty. They found no evidence of angle closure in the majority of their patients. Wood et al.[43] and Olson and Kaufman[22] found that while pressures tended to decrease in the weeks following surgery, a significant number of aphakic patients developed long-standing glaucoma. Patients having glaucoma preoperatively had only a slightly higher chance of having postoperative glaucoma. Of those patients having a pressure greater than 35 mm Hg in the first week, 76% still required glaucoma therapy at 6 months and 19% required cyclocryotherapy. The patients having the best prognosis with respect to glaucoma after aphakic grafts were those without preoperative glaucoma who had an initial postoperative pressure of 28 mm Hg or less, although 20% of these still required treatment for glaucoma at 6 months.[22] Polack,[30] in a long-term study of aphakic grafts, noted pressure elevation in 60% of early postoperative eyes and in 42% at 6 months. Thoft et al.[35] found glaucoma in 10% or less of keratoplasty patients without preexisting intraocular pressure problems. This low incidence may relate to differences in surgical technique, which are discussed below.

The significance of postoperative intraocular pressure elevation is not limited to glaucomatous damage per se. Glaucoma in the keratoplasty patient can have a devastating effect on graft clarity. Heydenreich,[7] in 112 grafts performed from 1957 to 1965, achieved 60% graft clarity in patients without glaucoma but only 11% clarity in those with postoperative glaucoma. Fine[5] found glaucoma to be the single factor most responsible for failure of aphakic grafts. Polack[29] and Paton[27] also stressed the reduced prognosis for graft clarity in the presence of an elevated intraocular pressure. At least one reason for this effect may be direct damage to the corneal endothelium caused by either acute or chronic intraocular pressure elevation. Svedbergh[34] showed endothelial cell loss in monkeys with artificially elevated intraocular pressures. Endothelial loss has also been demonstrated in humans with chronic glaucoma by clinical specular microscopy.[32,38] Glaucoma does not appear to alter the incidence of immunologic graft rejection.[4]

It is interesting that in the initial few weeks following keratoplasty, elevated intraocular pressure, at least before endothelial destruction, does not cause corneal thickening. The corneal stroma is actually thinned by the compressing effect of increased intraocular pressure.[21] This finding is consistent with our current understanding of the forces controlling corneal stromal hydration. Epithelial edema, however, may be a sign of glaucoma, even when the stroma is thin.[44]

ETIOLOGY

The cause of glaucoma following keratoplasty can be variable (see outline). In phakic eyes it may be related to any of the forms of postsurgical glaucoma discussed in the previous chapters of this book. These include pupillary block, lens-induced glaucoma, uveitis, anterior synechiae, hemorrhage, and steroid-induced glaucoma.[11] Preexisting primary open-angle glaucoma may be detected postoperatively or exacerbated by steroid therapy. In addition, many corneal diseases that may require keratoplasty can be associated with glaucoma. These include anterior segment anomalies, herpetic keratitis, and trauma.

Etiology of postkeratoplasty glaucoma
A. Phakic grafts
   1. Preexisting glaucoma
      a. Primary glaucoma
      b. Glaucoma related to corneal disease (Fuchs', interstitial keratitis, iridocorneal endothelial syndrome, herpes, etc.)
   2. Postsurgical glaucoma
      a. Pupillary block
      b. Iritis
      c. Hemorrhage
      d. Synechiae
      e. Lens-induced glaucoma
      f. Steroid-induced glaucoma
      g. Prostaglandin-related glaucoma
B. Aphakic grafts
   1. As above
   2. Trabecular collapse
   3. Secondary angle-closure glaucoma

It has been shown that an aspirin-inhibitable protein rise occurs in the aqueous humor of patients undergoing anterior segment surgery.[46] This suggests that prostaglandin release may be a factor in the early intraocular pressure rise following keratoplasty. In a double-blind study, however, aspirin failed to prevent this intraocular pressure rise in aphakic graft patients.[45]

The factors causing glaucoma in aphakic grafts include those discussed above and in Chapter 23. The finding of Irvine and Kaufman[8] that intraocular pressure rises more often after aphakic than after phakic grafts, however, suggests some unique situation in the aphakic eye undergoing keratoplasty. Zimmerman et al.[47] postulated that the interruption of Descemet's membrane by a keratoplasty incision caused a lack of anterior support for the trabecular meshwork. They hypothesized that the loss of zonular tension due to lens removal could alter the posterior trabecular support in the aphakic eye. The combination of these two factors would lead to trabecular "collapse" and decreased aqueous outflow. To test this hypothesis, outflow facility was measured in eye bank eyes with a constant pressure perfusion system after phakic or aphakic keratoplasty. Suturing was performed either with conventional deep stromal placement or with through-and-through sutures including Descemet's membrane. In phakic eyes the outflow facility was unaltered by either technique. In aphakic eyes, however, through-and-through suturing failed to alter facility of outflow, whereas conventional suturing decreased facility significantly. To test this effect clinically in aphakic grafts, 10 patients received through-and-through sutures and 15 received conventional sutures. Those with through-and-through sutures had significantly lower pressures for the first ·5 postoperative days; only one had a detectable wound leak.[50]

An alternative approach to the prevention of posterior wound gaping and trabecular collapse is to use a donor button for keratoplasty that is larger than the recipient bed. This also tends to deepen the iridocorneal angle. Olson and Kaufman[20] developed a mathematical model to predict the effect of various factors on angle distortion by keratoplasty. From their formula they determined that the following factors would increase anterior trabecular support or decrease angle narrowing: (1) larger host corneal diameter; (2) looser or shorter suture bites, decreasing tissue compression at the wound; (3) smaller trephine sizes; (4) thinner peripheral host cornea; and (5) larger-donor-than-recipient button size.[25,26]

Surgical variables proposed to relate to glaucoma following aphakic keratoplasty[18,20,25]

1. Corneal diameter (recipient)
2. Size of recipient bed
3. Thickness of recipient bed
4. Size of donor button relative to host bed
5. Suture bite length
6. Suture tightness

The concept of a larger-donor-than-recipient button size was tested in the same in vitro system used to test through-and-through sutures. With the use of conventional suturing, 8.0-mm buttons in 7.5-mm recipient beds of aphakic eye bank eyes did not lower the outflow facility,[48] whereas same-size buttons did.[47] When this concept was then applied to human grafts,[49] with the use of 8.0-mm buttons in 7.5-mm recipient beds, the average intraocular pressure for the first 6 days postoperatively was 18.3 mm Hg in aphakic eyes and 21.2 mm Hg in eyes with combined cataract extraction and keratoplasty. When 7.5-mm donor buttons were used in 7.5-mm beds, the corresponding pressures were 26.6 and 34.4 mm Hg, respectively. A larger donor button appeared to be of no advantage in aphakic grafts, which did not have marked pressure elevation. Applying this same

technique to 8.0-mm recipient beds with the use of 8.5-mm donor grafts only partially prevented intraocular pressure elevation. Same-size aphakic and combined 8.0-mm grafts had an average pressure of 44.6 mm Hg, whereas 0.5-mm-larger grafts in 8.0-mm beds had an average pressure of 34.2 mm Hg.

This discrepancy in the effect of a larger-donor-than-recipient graft at a greater diameter is consistent with Olson and Kaufman's calculations.[20] The predicted donor size for an 8.0-mm recipient bed to prevent angle flattening to less than 15 degrees for an average corneal diameter is 8.2, 8.6, or 9.0 if wound compression is 0.2, 0.3, or 0.4 mm, respectively.[18] Thus the tighter the sutures, the larger the relative donor size must be. The calculation of appropriate donor diameter for clinical use is made more complex by many variables, including the intraocular pressure, plunger height, and blade sharpness, which alter the true button size cut by a given trephine.[19] The use of oversized grafts does not significantly affect postoperative refractive error, and it decreases the incidence of wound leak and synechiae contributing to prevention of long-term angle damage.[6,24] Some surgeons have noted little difference in intraocular pressure between same-size and larger-donor-than-recipient button groups, but their low glaucoma incidence in both groups may reflect differences in other factors, such as suture tightness.[15] Perl et al.[28] retrospectively compared 25 same-size with 95 oversized aphakic grafts. Pressure greater than 30 mm Hg occurred in 56% of the same-size and in 31% of the oversized graft eyes in the early postoperative period.

While Irvine and Kaufman[8] did not find angle closure to be a problem in their initial study, they were examining primarily the short-term situation. Angle compression and trabecular collapse are probably short-term effects in most cases. Thoft et al.[33] and Lass and Pavan-Langston[11] found synechial angle closure to be the basis for long-term glaucoma requiring late therapy. All of their patients without preexisting glaucoma had from 30 to 270 degrees of synechial angle closure. They believed that intensive topical steroid therapy was responsible for their low incidence of approximately 10% chronic glaucoma by decreasing synechiae formation.

DIAGNOSIS

There are special problems in detecting intraocular pressure elevation in patients with corneal disease either with or without keratoplasty. Goldmann applanation tonometry is difficult or inaccurate when the corneal surface is irregular or edematous, and Schiøtz tonometry requires a regular corneal curvature within the normal range. Buxton et al.[2] compared Schiøtz and Goldmann tonometry in grafted eyes and found readings to be comparable and reliable. Their patients, however, all had clear grafts and were not in the early postoperative period, and none had glaucoma. Kaufman et al.[10] compared pressure measurements in eyes with irregular or scarred corneas taken with Schiøtz, Goldmann, and MacKay-Marg tonometers with pressure measurements obtained by direct cannulation of the anterior chamber. Only the MacKay-Marg readings were accurate, confirming a similar study in rabbits.[41] The same technique was used in two patients following keratoplasty, again showing MacKay-Marg tonometry to be accurate over a wide range of pressures.[42] The pneumatic applanation tonometer has also given accurate results in patients with corneal disease and is preferred by some surgeons.[13] There has been some question of its accuracy, however, in several carefully controlled laboratory situations.[17] Some groups have found none of the tonometers consistently useful and feel forced to rely on tactile tension in many cases.[35]

MANAGEMENT
Medical therapy

Therapy for glaucoma following penetrating keratoplasty should follow a logical stepwise progression, as does therapy for other glaucomas. It is complicated, however, by the tendency of the glaucoma to be severe when it occurs, though not quite the "all or none" situation that some have described,[26] and by the difficulty of using disc or field changes as the chief guides to treatment and possibly thereby risking graft damage. If a specific treatable cause of glaucoma, such as pupillary block, is present, it may be treated in the same manner as in other situations, but this is unusual. Steroid-induced glaucoma may be difficult to distinguish, and the use of steroids may be necessary despite the glaucoma.

The most widely used agents for medical therapy in these patients have been the oral carbonic anhydrase inhibitors. However, their ability to lower pressure in the initial postoperative period was not impressive in the study of Wood et al.[43] and negligible in that of Olson et al.[23] Many elderly patients develop lethargy, weakness, and anorexia that they do not mention or relate to these agents until they note improvement after discontinuation of the drug. Since most aphakic graft patients are elderly and often infirm, they should be specifically questioned about possible signs of drug toxicity. The next step has usually been to add miotics, beginning with 2% pilocarpine and progressing as necessary to higher concentrations, and then to cholinesterase inhibitors. These are usually well tolerated in aphakic eyes and do not appear clinically to increase anterior chamber activity or synechiae formation. Epinephrine may be of some value. Oral hyperosmotic agents may be helpful for temporary control of severe pressure elevation, but they are impractical for prolonged use.[43]

When added to carbonic anhydrase inhibitors in the acute postoperative phase of glaucoma, timolol had no more effect than a placebo alone.[23] In the chronic phase, however, it may be of great benefit. Lass and Pavan-Langston[11] studied 13 aphakic graft patients with a mean intraocular pressure of 39.6 mm Hg at 22 months following keratoplasty. Timolol was added to the previous oral and topical therapy, and the mean intraocular pressure fell to 25.8 mm Hg after the first week. Four patients required cyclocryotherapy, but all 13 would have required it if timolol had not been added. The mean pressure fell from 38 to 16 mm Hg in the controlled eyes by the end of the 30-week study. When timolol is used in postkeratoplasty eyes, especially those with epithelial vulnerability, care should be taken to watch for possible epithelial toxicity.[14,37] I have observed a patient with postkeratoplasty glaucoma who, with the use of 0.5% timolol, repeatedly developed punctate keratopathy, which cleared when the concentration was reduced to 0.25%.

Surgical therapy

Surgical therapy is indicated when disc and field changes occur, the graft appears to be threatened by elevated pressure, or marked pressure elevation persists despite medical therapy. As in most glaucoma surgery, individualized decisions are required. Cyclodialysis was considered an appropriate procedure in the past and was used by Kandori et al.[9] prophylactically at the time of keratoplasty. Casey and Gibbs[3] performed 100 cyclodialyses for postkeratoplasty glaucoma, especially in aphakia, but only 22 were successful. Filtering procedures may be likely to fail in these aphakic eyes with secondary glaucoma. It has been suggested, moreover, that any intraocular surgery in a patient with a clear graft has a 30% risk of causing graft failure.[12]

Cyclocryotherapy has become the most widely used procedure for medically uncontrollable post-keratoplasty glaucoma.[1,13,35] It may also be used preoperatively in patients with uncontrolled glaucoma, since prior filtering procedures may fail postoperatively.[40] In the initial report of West et al.,[40] nine eyes were treated preoperatively. After grafting, seven remained controlled, one required repeated cryotherapy, and one became phthisic. Fourteen eyes were treated postoperatively, requiring a total of 23 treatments, and 12 were controlled, whereas two became phthisic. Most eyes received 360-degree single-freeze treatment, and those having repeated freeze-thaw-refreeze treatment were more likely to become phthisic. Binder et al.[1] treated a series of 36 patients, all of whom had precryotherapy pressures of greater than 40 mm Hg with 28 having intraocular pressures greater than 50 mm Hg. Twelve applications at $-50°$ to $-60°$ C for 60 seconds were made for 360 degrees. Thirty eyes were controlled by one treatment, five by two, and one by three, and 82% of the grafts remained clear. Fourteen percent developed complications including phthisis bulbi (one), vitreous hemorrhage (two), transplant failure (two), and macular edema (one). Thoft et al.[35] used 180-degree cyclocryotherapy in 15 eyes. Nine were controlled by one procedure, and six by multiple treatments. One eye became phthisic, and three developed visual loss following uveitis. Despite these complications, most groups recommend cyclocryotherapy as the primary surgical procedure for control of secondary glaucoma following keratoplasty.[1,13,35]

It appears from the above discussion that the problem of glaucoma following penetrating keratoplasty should lessen with the application of recent advances. Each surgeon should be able to apply the principles outlined by Olson and Kaufman[20] to alter the graft size or suturing technique if necessary. Appropriate use of steroids may decrease long-term problems.[35] When these preventive measures fail, careful use of medical therapy and, when necesssry, cyclocryotherapy should salvage vision in many eyes that would previously have been lost.

REFERENCES

1. Binder, P.S., Abel, R., and Kaufman, H.E.: Cyclocryotherapy for glaucoma after penetrating keratoplasty, Am. J. Ophthalmol. **79:**489, 1975.
2. Buxton, J.N., Riechers, R.J., and Aaron, S.D.: Corneal grafts and their effect upon the applanation Schiotz disparity, Arch. Ophthalmol. **86:**28, 1971.
3. Casey, T.A., and Gibbs, D.: Complications in corneal grafting, Trans. Ophthalmol. Soc. U.K. **92:**517, 1972.
4. Cherry, P.M., Pashby, R.C., Tadros, M.L., et al.: An analysis of corneal transplantation. I. Graft clarity, Ann. Ophthalmol. **11:**461, 1979.
5. Fine, M.: Problems of keratoplasty in aphakic eyes. In Symposium on the cornea: transactions of the New Orleans Academy of Ophthalmology, St. Louis, 1972, The C.V. Mosby Co., p. 144.
6. Foulks, G.N., Perry, H.D., and Dohlman, C.H.: Oversize corneal donor grafts in penetrating keratoplasty, Ophthalmology **86:**490, 1979.
7. Heydenreich, A.: Hornhautregeneration und Augendruck, Klin. Monatsbl. Augenheilkd. **145:**500, 1966.
8. Irvine, A.R., and Kaufman, H.E.: Intraocular pressure following penetrating keratoplasty, Am. J. Ophthalmol. **68:** 835, 1969.
9. Kandori, F., Kurimoto, S., Fukunaga, K., et al.: Preventive procedure to postoperative secondary glaucoma on penetrating keratoplasty, Acta Soc. Ophthalmol. Jpn. **71:** 1189, 1967.
10. Kaufman, H.E., Wind, C.A., and Waltman, S.R.: Validity of MacKay-Marg electronic applanation tonometer in patients with scarred irregular corneas, Am. J. Ophthalmol. **69:**1003, 1970.
11. Lass, J.H., and Pavan-Langston, D.: Timolol therapy in secondary angle-closure glaucoma post penetrating keratoplasty, Ophthalmology **86:**51, 1979.
12. Lemp, M.A., Pfister, R.R., and Dohlman, C.H.: The effect of intraocular surgery on clear corneal grafts, Am. J. Ophthalmol. **70:**719, 1970.
13. Maumenee, A.E.: Recent advances in corneal transplantation, Trans. Ophthalmol. Soc. U.K. **96:**462, 1976.
14. McMahon, C.D., Shaffer, R.N., Hoskins, H.D., et al.: Adverse effects experienced by patients taking timolol, Am. J. Ophthalmol. **88:**736, 1979.
15. Minaai, L., and Doughman, D.J.: Penetrating keratoplasty: the effect of donor buttons being larger than recipient beds on intraocular pressure and refraction, unpublished manuscript.
16. Mortada, A.: Results of partial penetrating keratoplasty related to the size of the graft, Br. J. Ophthalmol. **54:** 66, 1970.
17. Moses, R.A., and Grodzki, W.J.: The pneumatonograph, a laboratory study, Arch. Ophthalmol. **97:**547, 1979.
18. Olson, R.J.: Aphakic keratoplasty, determining donor size to avoid elevated intraocular pressure, Arch. Ophthalmol. **96:**2274, 1979.
19. Olson, R.J.: Variation in corneal graft size related to trephine technique, Arch. Ophthalmol. **97:**1323, 1979.
20. Olson, R.J., and Kaufman, H.E.: A mathematical description of causative factors and prevention of elevated intra-

ocular pressure after keratoplasty, Invest. Ophthalmol. Vis. Sci. **16:**1085, 1977.

21. Olson, R.J., and Kaufman, H.E.: Intraocular pressure and corneal thickness after penetrating keratoplasty, Am. J. Ophthalmol. **86:**97, 1978.

22. Olson, R.J., and Kaufman, H.E.: Prognostic factors of intraocular pressure after aphakic keratoplasty, Am. J. Ophthalmol. **86:**510, 1978.

23. Olson, R.J., Kaufman, H.E., and Zimmerman, T.J.: Effects of timolol and Daranide on elevated intraocular pressure after aphakic keratoplasty, Ann. Ophthalmol. **11:** 1833, 1979.

24. Olson, R.J., Mattingly, T.P., Waltman, S.R., et al.: Refractive variation and donor tissue size in aphakic keratoplasty, Arch. Ophthalmol. **97:**1480, 1979.

25. Olson, R.J., Zimmerman, T.J., and Kaufman, H.E.: Elevated intraocular pressure after aphakic keratoplasty: iatrogenic disease and prevention, Ann. Ophthalmol. **10:**931, 1978.

26. Olson, R.J., Zimmerman, T.J., and Kaufman, H.E.: Intraocular pressure and aphakic keratoplasty. In Kaufman, H.E., and Zimmerman, T.J., editors: Current concepts in ophthalmology, vol. 6, St. Louis, 1979, The C.V. Mosby Co., p. 97

27. Paton, D.: The prognosis of penetrating keratoplasty, Ophthalmic Surg. **7:**36, 1976.

28. Perl, T., Charlton, K.H., and Binder, P.S.: Disparate diameter grafting; astigmatism, intraocular pressure, and visual acuity, Ophthalmology **88:**774, 1981.

29. Polack, F.M.: Corneal transplantation, New York, 1977, Grune & Stratton, Inc., p. 165.

30. Polack, F.M.: Keratoplasty in aphakic eyes with corneal edema, Ophthalmic Surg. **11:**701, 1980.

31. Raab, M.F., and Fine, M.: Penetrating keratoplasty in interstitial keratitis, Am. J. Ophthalmol. **67:**907, 1969.

32. Setala, K., and Vannas, A.: Endothelial cells in the glaucomato-cyclitic crisis, Adv. Ophthalmol. **36:**218, 1978.

33. Stallard, H.B.: Eye surgery, ed. 5, Baltimore, 1973, The Williams & Wilkins Co., p. 404.

34. Svedbergh, B.: Effects of artificial intraocular pressure elevation on the corneal endothelium in the vervet monkey, Acta Ophthalmol. **53:**839, 1975.

35. Thoft, R.A., Gordon, J.M., and Dohlman, C.H.: Glaucoma following keratoplasty, Trans. Am. Acad. Ophthalmol. Otolaryngol. **78:**352, 1974.

36. Thomas, C.I., Purnell, E.W.: Prevention and management of early and late complications of keratoplasty, Am. J. Ophthalmol. **60:**385, 1965.

37. Van Buskirk, E.M.: Corneal anesthesia after timolol maleate therapy, Am. J. Ophthalmol. **88:**739, 1979.

38. Vannas, A., Setala, K., and Ruusuvaara, P.: Endothelial cells in capsular glaucoma, Acta Ophthalmol. **55:**951, 1978.

39. West, C.E., Capella, J.A., and Kaufman, H.E.: Measurement of intraocular pressure with a pneumatic applanation tonometer, Am. J. Ophthalmol. **74:**505, 1972.

40. West, C.E., Wood, T.O., and Kaufman, H.E.: Cyclocryotherapy for glaucoma pre- or postpenetrating keratoplasty, Am. J. Ophthalmol. **76:**485, 1973.

41. Wind, C.A., and Irvine, A.R.: Electronic applanation tonometry in corneal edema and keratoplasty, Invest. Ophthalmol. **8:**620, 1969.

42. Wind, C.A., and Kaufman, H.E.: Validity of MacKay-Marg applanation tonometry following penetrating keratoplasty in man, Am J. Ophthalmol. **72:**117, 1971.

43. Wood, T.O., West, C., and Kaufman, H.E.: Control of intraocular pressure in penetrating keratoplasty, Am. J. Ophthalmol. **74:**724, 1972.

44. Ytteborg, J., and Dohlman, C.H.: Corneal edema and intraocular pressure. II. Clinical results, Arch. Ophthalmol. **74:**477, 1965.

45. Zimmerman, T.J., Binder, P.S., and Abel, R., et al.: Aspirin and the intraocular pressure rise following aphakic keratoplasty: a negative report, Ann. Ophthalmol. **8:** 611, 1976.

46. Zimmerman, T.J., Gravenstein, N., Sugar, A., et al.: Aspirin stabilization of the blood-aqueous barrier in the human eye, Am. J. Ophthalmol. **79:**817, 1975.

47. Zimmerman, T.J., Krupin, T., Grodzki, W., et al.: The effect of suture depth on outflow facility in penetrating keratoplasty, Arch. Ophthalmol. **96:**505, 1978.

48. Zimmerman, T.J., Krupin, T., Grodzki, W., et al.: Size of donor corneal button and outflow facility in aphakic eyes, Ann. Ophthalmol. **11:**809, 1979.

49. Zimmerman, T.J., Olson, R., Waltman, S., et al.: Transplant size and elevated intraocular pressure post keratoplasty, Arch Ophthalmol. **96:**2231, 1978.

50. Zimmerman, T.J., Waltman, S.R., Sachs, U., et al.: Intraocular pressure after aphakic penetrating keratoplasty "through-and-through" suturing, Ophthalmic Surg. **10:** 49, 1979.

INDEX

A

Aborigine, Australian, incidence of exfoliation syndrome in, 99-100

Acetazolamide
  angle closure treated with, 152
  effects of, on eye, 250
  episcleritis treated with, 272
  Fuchs' endothelioepithelial dystrophy treated with, 82
  hyphema-induced glaucoma treated with, 234
  malignant glaucoma treated with, 336
  venous pressure and, 211

Acetophenazine maleate, effects of, on eye, 247

Acetylcholine, glaucoma treated with, 346

Acetylsalicylic acid, effects of, on eye, 250, 254-255

Acid, eye injury from, 316

Acne rosacea, glaucoma associated with, 236

Acromegaly, glaucoma associated with, 222, 223

ACTH; *see* Adrenocorticotropic hormone

Acuity, visual, following lens implant, 369, 373

Adenoma
  adrenal, Cushing's syndrome and, 223
  pituitary, 222-223

Adenoma sebaceum, tuberous sclerosis indicated by, 45

Adrenal hyperplasia, 223

Adrenalectomy, Cushing's syndrome treated with, 223

Adrenergic agonist drugs
  aniridia treated with, 26
  exfoliation syndrome glaucoma treated with, 118
  ghost cell glaucoma treated with, 327
  glaucoma following lens implant treated with, 377

Adrenocorticotropic hormone
  Cushing's syndrome and, 223
  intraocular pressure in patients treated with, 258

AF; *see* Angiogenesis factor

Akineton; *see* Biperiden hydrochloride

Aldactone; *see* Spironolactone

Alkaline substance, eye injury from, 316

Alpha-chymotrypsin
  effects of, on eye, 254
  use of, in phacolytic glaucoma surgery, 126

Alport's syndrome, 134, 137

Amblyopia, Stickler's syndrome indicated by, 159

ε-aminocaproic acid, 308

Amitril; *see* Amitriptyline

Amitriptyline, effects of, on eye, 248

Ammonia, corneal burn from, 287

Amphetamine drugs, effects of, on eye, 249

Amyl nitrate, effects of, on eye, 251

Amyloidosis, primary familial, 234-235

Anesthetic drugs, effects of, on eye, 253

Angiogenesis factor, neovascularization and, 175, 179-181

Angioma, facial, 37

Angiomatosis retinae, 44-45

Angle
  abnormality in, 18, 24-26, 86
  closure of
    choroidal enlargement as cause of, 37
    ectropion uveae and, 171
    pupillary block as cause of, 154
    synechial, 164, 171-172
    trauma as cause of, 145
  developmental anomalies of, 51
  effect of iridocorneal endothelial syndrome on, 70, 76
  effect of neurofibromatosis on, 36
  effect of Peters' anomaly on, 21
  embryonal tissue in, 34
  faulty development of, 53
  formation of, 12
  involvement of, in exfoliation syndrome, 103-105
  malformations of, 39
  narrowing of, 131, 132
  neovascular formation in, 162, 164, 166

Aniridia
  ectopia lentis and, 134
  glaucoma and, 5, 24-27
  management of, 26-27
  Rieger's syndrome compared with, 18

Ankylosing spondylitis, 300-301

Antazoline phosphate, effects of, on eye, 249

Anterior chamber
  changes in, following scleral buckling operation, 154
  effects of ghost cell glaucoma on, 325, 326
  effects of lens implant on, 369-370, 374-376
  effects of retrolental fibroplasia on, 60
  epithelialization of, 374
  flare in, due to phacolytic glaucoma, 122
  flat
    following lens implantation, 369
    with peripheral anterior synechiae, 359-360
  intraocular lens implant in, 367